D1479538

Commonsense Approach to

CORONARY CARE

A Program

FIFTH EDITION

Commonsense Approach To
CORONARY CARE
A Program

MARIELLE ORTIZ VINSANT, R.N., M.S.

Instructor, Department of Nursing Education
Baptist Hospital
Miami, Florida

MARTHA I. SPENCE, R.N., M.N., C.C.R.N.

Clinical Nurse Specialist
University of Alabama Hospitals
Coronary Care Unit
Birmingham, Alabama

FIFTH EDITION

with 591 illustrations

The C. V. Mosby Company

ST. LOUIS · BALTIMORE · PHILADELPHIA · TORONTO   1989

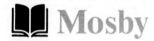

Editor: Don Ladig
Assistant Editor: Audrey Rhoades
Project Manager: Carlotta Seely
Production Editor: Cynthia A. Miller
Book and Cover Design: Rey Umali

FIFTH EDITION

Copyright © 1989 by The C.V. Mosby Company

All rights reserved. No part of this publication may be reproduced, stored in a retrieval system, or transmitted, in any form or by any means, electronic, mechanical, photocopying, recording, or otherwise, without prior written permission from the publisher.

Previous editions copyrighted 1972, 1975, 1981, 1985

Printed in the United States of America

The C.V. Mosby Company
11830 Westline Industrial Drive, St. Louis, Missouri 63146

Library of Congress Cataloging-in-Publication Data

Vinsant, Marielle Ortiz.
  Commonsense approach to coronary care.

Includes bibliographies and index.
  1. Coronary heart disease—Nursing. I. Spence,
Martha I. II. Title. [DNLM: 1. Coronary Disease—
nurses' instruction. 2. Coronary Disease—programmed
instruction. WG 18 V788c]
RC685.C6V56 1988   616.1′23′0024613   88-31507
ISBN 0-8016-5324-X

C/D/D 9 8 7 6 5 4 3

To
Louis Lemberg, M.D.
Agustin Castellanos, Jr., M.D.
Azucena G. Arcebal, M.D.
Gloria Steffens, R.N., M.S.
who gave us the autonomy and inspiration to grow

I would like to dedicate my efforts
on this fifth edition to the
memory of my late father
Harold S. Inglis
—M.I.S.

Foreword

This book is a good example of a premise that arose twenty-two centuries ago, namely, that teaching is an art rather than a science. Unfortunately, this principle is often neglected in our technified age. To achieve their purpose the authors of this book have addressed human beings as individuals, not anonymous persons. Readers must be well aware of these aims if they are to obtain full benefit from the material presented. They must also recognize that it is dangerous and antididactic to apply the goals and methods of science to all aspects of learning. Gilbert Highet has repeatedly emphasized that a strictly scientific relationship (either verbal or written) between teacher and pupil is inadequate and undesirable. Naturally, some coherence is required in all presentations, but this requisite does not remove the emotional ingredient.

The "system" used in this book arose after hundreds of live encounters in the form of spontaneous (or conventional) lectures, dialogues, and discussions. Hence it was based on a person-to-person relation in which readers must act as inquisitive pupils, true interlocutors who can find themselves— whether believing or doubting—persistently *thinking* about the various approaches to coronary care, which they would not have looked at in exactly the same fashion. Unless readers work themselves into the proper mental framework, it is possible that this approach might appear too complex, highly dogmatic, or, for some, extraordinarily simple. But in any case, the stimulation created in the minds of readers is even more important than the factual information. Whereas not every scientific statement can be proven, the desire to learn can be experienced by all.

Agustin Castellanos, Jr., M.D.

Preface

We first became aware of the need for a new approach to coronary care training while teaching nurses in a course sponsored by the Florida Regional Medical Program and the Florida Heart Association. Initially we used a traditional, fragmented approach, but this method met with only moderate success. It did not provide the nurse with a basis for realistically and systematically solving patient problems. Subsequently, we developed our own methods for simplification, organization, and practical presentation of the subject matter. When this approach met with success, we wondered if others might also find it meaningful. It has been gratifying to find, through comments made on previous editions, that this approach has been found valid by many of our readers.

Our approach is based on a thorough knowledge of normal anatomy and physiology. Utilizing knowledge of anatomy and physiology, the student is able to deduce the clinical consequences of pathological changes. For example, knowledge of the anatomy of the coronary artery system enables the practitioner to anticipate the type of complications that will be associated with coronary artery occlusion. Knowledge of the role of electrolytes in cardiovascular tissue enables the practitioner to better understand newer diagnostic tests as well as the effects and side effects of recent advancements in drug therapy. Information in this area has been updated in this edition to reflect current knowledge and modes of therapy.

It is our aim to simulate as closely as possible our classroom situation. We believe that students' interest increases as they are encouraged to participate. By participating, students are also given a means of evaluating their understanding of the topics discussed. We chose the programmed format for this book because we felt that it would be the best to fulfill these aims. Information is presented in a comprehensive, correlated form. We believe that memorization is a crutch, not an effective learning tool. Therefore readers are encouraged to use their reasoning powers to a maximum and keep memorization to a minimum.

This text is constructed so that each unit is built on the preceding one, and the student is cautioned not to read isolated segments of the book. Cross references, reviews, and repetition are provided to maintain the continuity of the units. Readers who do not understand the answer given should refer to the previous unit discussing that topic. Also, an index has been provided with this edition.

This book is directed to both beginner and advanced practitioner. No previous knowledge of cardiology is necessary, although we believe that those who have some experience will also find this book useful. Because recent advances in coronary care have expanded the scope and comprehensiveness of this field of nursing, a more in-depth knowledge of physiology is required. If beginners find some of this material complex, we strongly urge that they pace themselves to facilitate comprehension of basic concepts. The text remains structured so that the more complex areas may be omitted without loss of continuity.

Our primary focus, as with previous editions is still the patient with acute myocardial infarction in the coronary care unit. However, in this edition with the addition of a new unit, we have expanded the scope beyond coronary artery disease to other problems primarily seen with patients in coronary care units and/or related areas. The type of patients admitted to these areas has expanded in more recent years to include many more with these diagnoses as well as coronary artery disease since their physiologic problems are similar. These diagnoses include malignant ventricular arrhythmias with a focus on torsades de pointes, pre-excitation syndrome (W-P-W, etc.), cardiomyopathy, and mitral prolapse. Information provided throughout the text on related coronary artery syndromes and functional disorders, such as angina, arrhythmias, and congestive heart failure, and their therapy will continue to be valuable in any setting dealing with the patient with heart disease.

This fifth edition contains several revisions. A section on SvO2 monitoring has been added to Unit 3, oxygenation. This information is a natural extension and completion to our previously existing unit on oxygenation which has always emphasized the clinical significance of the O2 saturation. This addition also expands the practical aspects of our text and supports our basic premise of integrating clinical concepts with sound physiologic principles. The sections of Unit 9, mechanical complications in coronary artery disease: heart failure and shock, on hemodynamic monitoring and IABP have been updated and expanded to include more practical information from the authors' own clinical experiences. However, the information on hemodynamic monitor-

ing is still intended as an introduction/overview of this information with a focus on myocardial infarction. The authors recommend that this be supplemented by one of the many excellent complete texts available on the subject as indicated on the bibliography. Unit 10, pharmacologic intervention, has been heavily updated to include new anti-arrhythmic, beta-blocking, inotropic, and thrombolytic drugs. The discussion of countershock in Unit 11 has been expanded to include the use of the automatic implantable cardioverter/defibrillator (AICD). The discussion of pacemakers in this unit has been reorganized so that the pacemaker components are discussed completely prior to the ECG assessment. The various types of temporary and permanent pacemakers are more clearly compared and contrasted. Information on temporary pacemakers has been updated to include transthoracic (transcutaneous) pacing and new diagrams on thoracic post-op pacing and the newer dual chamber pacing systems. Permanent pacemaker information has been updated to include more recent innovations/information such as rate-responsive pacing, pacemaker syndrome, and safety pacing. Information on non-committed and committed pacing has been rewritten for clarity with the focus on the now most commonly used DVI modified committed mode. Bibliographies have been updated in all of the units.

We continue to strongly recommend that readers of this text supplement their knowledge with a basic life support course provided by the American Heart Association. The topic of cardiopulmonary resuscitation is critically important in coronary care and is omitted from this text only because of the excellent training programs already established by the American Heart Association. Certain areas of this text may be useful for those interested in pursuing advanced life support training. With this purpose in mind, the units on drugs and arrhythmias have been correlated to the cardiac arrest setting.

We would like to acknowledge and thank Dr. Agustin "Tino" Castellanos, our teacher, philosopher, and friend, for his patience and encouragement, for always being available when we needed him, and for never complaining while proofing this text; Dr. Louis Lemberg, for his willingness to sponsor us in all our endeavors, for his dedication and commitment to coronary care nurse training, and for keeping us clinically oriented; Dr. Azucena Arcebal, for her unique ability to present complex material simply but accurately, for her willingness always to share her knowledge with us, and for treating us as peers; and The Florida Regional Medical Program and the Florida Heart Association, for giving us the opportunity to become involved in coronary care nurse training.

We would also like to acknowledge others who have taught and encouraged us during the past 10 years: Gloria Steffens, R.N., Dr. Joan Mayer, Dr. Robert Boucek, Dr. Ramanuja Iyengar, Dr. Ronald Fox, Dr. Charles Roeth, Shirley Mason, R.N., Judy Mercure, R.N., Dr. John Hildreth, Dr. Alvaro Martinez, Barouh Berkovits, Dr. Hooshang Balooki, Dr. R. Sung, Dr. Joseph Civetta, Tina Caruthers, R.N., Judy Hutson, R.N., Brenda Sanzobrino, R.N., Deborah Etter, R.N., Cheryl Hunneycutt, R.N., Judith Witmer, R.N., Virginia Stebbins, R.N., Marilyn Schactman, R.N., and Daree Gilliam, R.N., JoAnn Pillion, R.N., Donna Harbin, R.N., and our ever-skeptical graduate students (University of Miami School of Nursing). For their encouragement and overall assistance, we acknowledge our parents, Dr. and Mrs. Arturo C. Ortiz and Mrs. Harold Inglis, our husbands Hank and Jerry in addition to Tracy, Susan, and Sarah Spence.

Marielle Vinsant Crawford
Martha I. Spence

Contents

Priority Critical Care Assessment: Implications for Coronary Care

Critical care nursing is based on a dual challenge: (1) assessment of life maintenance priorities, and (2) implementation of a comprehensive, yet patient-centered approach to the care of the critically ill. This challenge can best be met by utilizing a systematic, scientifically based assessment process.

Patient responses to critical illness may be grouped into two categories: (1) patterned responses—both physiological and psychological—that are similar to those of other patients and (2) individual responses unique to each patient. Maslow's conceptual framework of basic needs provides a meaningful initial reference point for the assessment of the patterned responses. Selye's stress framework can also provide a reference point for less specific patterned responses (see Unit 6).

Maslow's framework is based on three principles highly applicable to critical care:

1. Both physiological and psychological needs may be patterned to some extent.
2. Physiological needs take first priority.
3. Complete satisfaction of physiological needs is not necessary for psychological needs to emerge as well.

Meeting physiological needs assumes first priority for both patient and nurse in life-threatening or crisis situations. This focus does not negate the existence or importance of psychological needs. Unmet needs generate the patient problems and responses that form the focal point of nursing care.

Although Maslow's original heading of *physiological needs* was divided into more spe-cific subcategories, priorities were not designated. Certain physiological needs assume priority over others in the critically ill patient. Comparison of these needs with Maslow's original list allows for modification of the original list with assignments of priorities. In this way a realistic system can be developed for the assessment of the physiological needs of the critically ill patient. A similar approach was recently suggested for use in general nursing practice in Campbell's textbook *Nursing Diagnosis and Intervention in Nursing Practice* (see Suggested Readings, p. 4).

It is our premise that *lack of oxygenation* is the most immediately life-threatening physiological problem. The two major systems providing for tissue oxygenation are the cardiovascular and pulmonary systems (see Unit 3). Thus assessment of these two major body systems must take priority in the management of the critically ill patient. The patient with coronary artery disease experiences a direct insult to the cardiovascular system. Assessment of this system therefore assumes the highest priority and is discussed in this text in great detail. *Fluid and chemical imbalances* also have life-threatening potential and exert a major influence on the cardiovascular and respiratory systems. Assessment of chemical imbalances thus assumes second priority. Subsequent physiological assessment, in decreasing priority, can include *metabolic* (nutritional) *imbalances;* alterations in body *defense mechanisms;* limitation in *struc-*

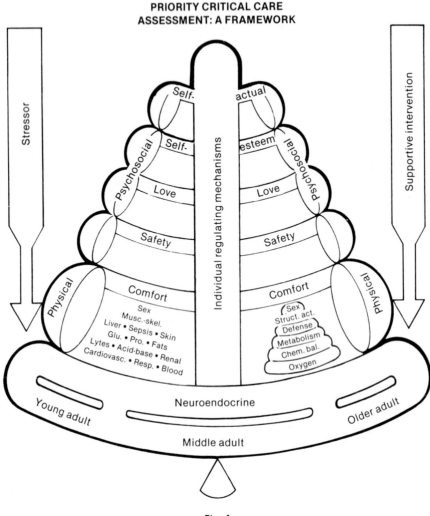

**PRIORITY CRITICAL CARE
ASSESSMENT: A FRAMEWORK**

Stressor

Supportive intervention

Individual regulating mechanisms

Self-actual

Psychosocial

Self-esteem

Psychosocial

Love

Love

Safety

Safety

Physical

Comfort

Comfort

Physical

Sex
Musc.-skel.
Liver • Sepsis • Skin
Glu. • Pro. • Fats
Lytes • Acid-base • Renal
Cardiovasc. • Resp. • Blood

Sex
Struct. act.
Defense
Metabolism
Chem. bal.
Oxygen

Young adult

Neuroendocrine

Older adult

Middle adult

Fig. 1

ture, *activity*, or *rest;* and alterations in *sexual activity* (Fig. 1). The neuroendocrine system integrates all these functions. Therefore assessment of *neuroendocrine function* is integrated within assessment of the cardiovascular and respiratory systems and fluid and chemical balances. It may be considered separately, as well, in the patient with a primary or secondary neurological disorder. Its exact priority level may be adjusted according to the specific clinical setting.

Maslow's *psychosocial* categories provide a framework for the assessment of the psychological needs and responses of the critically ill. *Safety* is regarded as the need for psychological order, consistency, and stability as well as protection from physical harm. The sense of safety may be disrupted by threats to either physical or psychological integrity, including pain, impending death, discomfort, and unfamiliar environments or routines.

Love or affiliation needs are regarded as needs for affection and attention from others as well as for interaction with others. Potential threats to meeting love needs include separation from family or significant persons and lack of attention from others, such as the nursing staff.

Self-esteem is Maslow's third psychosocial assessment level. Self-esteem may be regarded as the need for a sense of self-respect and personal worth. This sense of personal worth is derived from recognition by others, status, reputation, power, physical strength, mastery of skills or competence in selected peformance areas, independence, and a sense of control over one's physical and personal self. Potential threats to self-esteem include loss of physical strength, dependence on others for physical care or decision making, loss of control over one's behavior, repeated failure at performing tasks or overcoming obstacles, and verbal or nonverbal indications of lack of respect. Repeated criticism and lack of recognition (reinforcement) can further aggravate these threats.

Self-actualization is the last level in Maslow's assessment framework. Self-actualization includes the need to know and understand, to appreciate beauty and harmony, express creativity, and act spontaneously, and thus develop one's full potential as a human being. Most people probably exhibit certain aspects of these needs for at least short periods of time. (Examples are love of music and art, creative expression in hobbies, and enjoyment of favorite pastimes.) Emergence of self-actualization needs is particularly difficult for the patient with an acute myocardial infarction (MI) while he or she is in a coronary care unit, since so many basic needs are initially threatened. However, in the progressive care setting these needs may begin to emerge and may be utilized to release stress, promote relaxation, minimize boredom, and reduce the focus on the sick role.

Threats to psychological needs may be manifested by diffuse behavior patterns. In the patient with acute MI, the behavior patterns most commonly observed are overt anxiety, depression, and defense mechanisms. Temporary use of defense mechanisms can be a protective and often effective way to cope with the impact of multiple physiological and psychological threats. Denial is a commonly recognized defense mechanism used by the patient with an acute MI. This defense mechanism is crucial to the patient's well-being and should not be abruptly destroyed until the patient spontaneously expresses readiness or until the number of stressors have been reduced (as in a progressive care area). Although the specific cause of the behavior may be difficult to pinpoint, assessment of potential mechanisms (single or multiple) can remain systematic utilizing a framework such as Maslow's (see Unit 6, Table 7).

In addition to the patterned responses discussed so far, the critically ill patient will also exhibit unique responses based on individual background of resources, interactions, and experiences. This background can include such items as the patient's home, family, friends, occupation, past illnesses or experiences with hospitalization, stress patterns, diet, and elimination patterns. Specific tools can be developed to elicit this information. This core of individual resources and experiences influences the ability of the individual to deal with threats to his or her physiological and psychological needs. Threats or stressors may temporarily disturb the patient's inner balance. It is the nurse's role to investigate the patient's own resources as well as his or her potential needs so that the individual may be assisted in returning to a steady state of both physiological and psychological balance.

SUGGESTED READINGS

Buckley, W., editor: Modern systems research for the behavioral scientist, Chicago, 1968, Aldine Publishing Co.

Campbell, C.: Nursing diagnosis and intervention in nursing practice, New York, 1978, John Wiley & Sons, Inc.

Core curriculum for critical care nusing, Irvine, Calif., 1975, American Association of Critical Care Nurses.

Groër, M., and Shekleton, M.: Basic pathophysiology; a conceptual approach, ed. 2, St. Louis, 1982, The C.V. Mosby Co.

Hackett, T.P., and Cassem, N.H.: Psychological reactions to life-threatening illness. In Abram, H.S., editor: Psychological aspects of stress, Springfield, Ill., 1970, Charles C Thomas, Publisher.

Hudak, C.M., Gallo, B.M., and Lohr, T.: Holistic approach to critical care nursing. In Hudak, C.M., Gallo, B.M., and Lohr, T., editors: Critical care nursing, Philadelphia, 1973, J.B. Lippincott Co.

Maslow, A.H.: Toward a psychology of being, Princeton, N.J., 1968, D. Van Nostrand Co.

Maslow, A.H.: Motivation and personality, New York, 1970, Harper & Row, Publishers, Inc.

Maslow, A.H.: The farther reaches of human nature, New York, 1971, The Viking Press.

Maslow's terms and themes, Training HRD, March 1977, p. 48.

Mayer, G.G., and Peterson, C.W.: Theoretical framework for coronary care nursing education (pictorial), Am. J. Nurs. 78:1208, 1978.

McKay, R.: Theories, models, and systems for nursing, Nurs. Res. 23:10, 1974.

Riehl, J.P., and Callista, R.: Conceptual models for nursing practice, New York, 1974, Appelton-Century, Crofts.

Roberts, S.L.: Systems approach in assessing behavioral problems of critical-care patients, Heart Lung 4:593, 1974.

Undergraduate curriculum framework, Denver, 1976, University of Colorado School of Nursing.

Wilson, C.: New pathways in psychology: Maslow and the post-Freudian revolution, New York, 1972, Taplinger Publishing Co., Inc.

Young, O.R.: A survey of general systems theory, Gen. Syst. 9:61, 1974.

Anatomy and Physiology

1 The primary function of the heart is mechanical. It serves as a pump to deliver oxygenated blood to the body tissues in an attempt to meet their metabolic demands. The amount of blood put out by the heart *per minute* is known as the *cardiac output.*

2 Cardiac output is a product of *ventricular rate × stroke volume* (CO = VR × SV).
   Thus variations in cardiac output can be produced by altering the
   _____ _____ or the _____ _____.

   ventricular rate; stroke volume

3 The *heart rate* is determined primarily by the integrity of the heart's electrical system and the influence of the autonomic nervous system. The *stroke volume* is the amount of blood put out by the heart with *each beat.* It is determined primarily by the pumping efficiency of the cardiac muscle and the blood volume returning to the heart.

4 LET US REVIEW: In an attempt to meet the demands of the tissues, the heart pumps out a certain amount of oxygenated blood per minute. This amount of blood is known as the _____ _____.

   cardiac output

   Cardiac output is a product of _____ _____ and _____ _____.

   ventricular rate
   stroke volume

5 Normally the body compensates for rises and falls in stroke volume and heart rate so that as one increases the other decreases. Therefore when the trained athlete increases his cardiac muscle mass and thus his stroke volume, the heart rate *(increases/decreases).*

   decreases

6 If the body cannot compensate for a fall in heart rate by increasing the stroke volume or, conversely, for a fall in stroke volume by increasing the ventricular rate, the cardiac output then *(rises/falls).*

   falls

7 If the demands of the tissues for oxygen are not met because of this fall in cardiac output, the patient may begin to exhibit any of the

following symptoms:
1. Dizziness, fainting, or mental confusion
2. Cold clammy skin
3. Decreased urinary output

8 When *symptoms* develop because of a fall in heart rate, it is said that the patient is experiencing a _____ fall in cardiac output. The heart rate is too slow for this particular patient regardless of the exact number of beats per minute.

symptomatic

9 When the heart muscle has been damaged or injured, as in acute myocardial infarction resulting in heart failure, the stroke volume *(increases/decreases)*. The body compensates to maintain cardiac output by increasing the _____ _____.

decreases
heart rate

One of the earliest signs of heart failure is (fast/slow) heart rate.

fast

MECHANICAL STRUCTURES

10 The wall of the heart is composed of three major tissue layers (Fig. 1-1). The middle layer is the thickest layer and is composed of cardiac muscle (see Unit 4 for muscle structure). It is known as the *myocardium*. A thin layer of the endothelium lines the *interior* of the heart and is known as the _____.

endocardium

The endocardium is in direct contact with the blood pumped through the heart.

The outer myocardium is surrounded by a membranous sac known as the pericardium. This sac is composed of two layers—a fibrous layer and a smooth layer. The smooth layer has two separate linings. The visceral lining is in close contact with the myocardium. The parietal lining is in close contact with the outer fibrous layer. The visceral pericardium forms the third and outermost layer of the wall of the heart and is also referred to as the *epicardium*.

11 LET US REVIEW: The major portion of the wall of the heart is composed of _____ _____ and is known as the _____. It is lined by an inner layer of endothelium known as the _____ and an outer membranous layer known as the _____.

cardiac muscle
myocardium
endocardium
epicardium

The epicardium forms the innermost part of the two-layer sac surrounding the myocardium known as the _____. Between the epicardium and the parietal pericardium is a potential space. A small amount of fluid normally is contained within this space and provides protection against mechanical friction and excess movement of the heart with posture and thoracic pressure changes.

pericardium

12 The layer of myocardium just below the endocardium is referred to as the *subendocardium*. The layer of myocardium just below the epicardium is referred to as the *subepicardium*. The subendocardial layer of myocardium has a poorer blood supply than the subepicardium.

Myocardial infarction may be limited to only one area of the myocardium, such as the subendocardium or, more commonly, may affect the entire thickness of the myocardial wall. When the entire thickness of the myocardial wall is affected, the process is referred to as *transmural* (see Unit 6).

13 In summary:

LAYERS AND LININGS OF THE HEART WALL

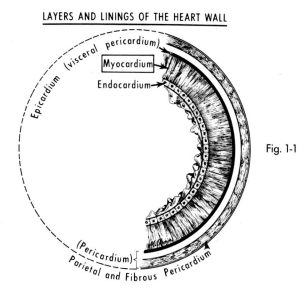

Fig. 1-1

14 The heart is divided into a right and left side by a muscular structure known as the *septum*.

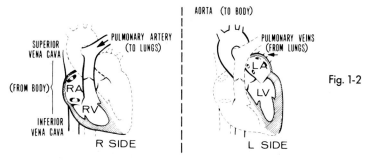

Fig. 1-2

The right and left sides of the heart *differ* in (1) function, (2) musculature, and (3) valvular structure.

15 The function of the right side of the heart is to deliver *unoxygenated* blood from the _____ to the _____. The function of the left side of the heart is to deliver oxygenated blood from the _____ to the _____.

body; lungs

lungs; body

16 Blood enters the right side of the heart via veins, the superior vena cava and the _____ _____ _____.

inferior vena cava

Blood leaves the right side of the heart via an artery, the _____ _____.

pulmonary artery

Blood enters the left side of the heart via four veins, the _____ _____.

pulmonary veins

Blood leaves the left side of the heart via an artery, the _____.

aorta

NOTE: Veins carry blood toward the heart.
Arteries carry blood away from the heart.

17 The right side of the heart has *thinner musculature* because it projects its volume against minimal resistance in the pulmonary circulation. The left side of the heart has *thicker musculature* because it projects its volume against *(greater/lesser)* resistance in the peripheral circulation.

greater

18 Each side of the heart has two sets of valves. Valves serve as separators and further divide each side of the heart into a receiving chamber, the *atrium,* and an ejecting chamber, the *ventricle.* Atrioventricular (AV) valves separate the atria from the _____.

Semilunar valves separate the ventricles from the vessels leaving them.

ventricles

19 The AV valve in the right side of the heart is the *tricuspid valve.* It separates the right atrium from the _____ _____. The AV valve in the left side of the heart is the mitral valve. It separates the left atrium from the _____ _____.

right ventricle

left ventricle

The AV valves on both sides of the heart are supported by rope-like structures known as *chordae tendineae,* which attach to papillary muscles. The chordae prevent movement of the valve cusps up into the atria with ventricular contraction.

The _____ muscles extending from the ventricular wall contract together with the ventricular muscle wall and _____ valves.

papillary

AV

20 The semilunar valve in the right side of the heart is the *pulmonary valve.* It separates the right ventricle from the vessel leaving it, the _____ _____.

pulmonary artery

Table 1. Comparison of right and left sides of the heart

Right ventricle	Left ventricle
A. Function	
1. Delivers unoxygenated blood from body to lungs	1. Delivers oxygenated blood from lungs to body
2. Projects its volume against minimal resistance—the lungs	2. Projects its volume against maximal resistance—the body
B. Musculature	
1. Thin walls	1. Thick walls
C. Valves	
1. AV valve; tricuspid	1. AV valve: mitral
2. Semilunar valve; pulmonary	2. Semilunar valve: aortic

21 The semilunar valve in the left side of the heart is the *aortic valve.* It separates the left ventricle from its outflow vessel, the
_____.

aorta

In Summary:

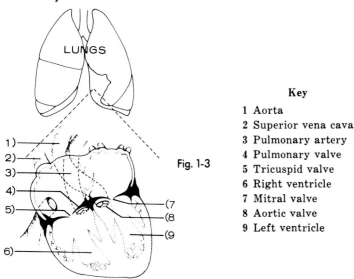

1) —
2) —
3) —
4) —
5) —
6) —

(7
(8
(9

Fig. 1-3

Key

1 Aorta
2 Superior vena cava
3 Pulmonary artery
4 Pulmonary valve
5 Tricuspid valve
6 Right ventricle
7 Mitral valve
8 Aortic valve
9 Left ventricle

Since more of the work of the heart is performed by the *(right/left)* ventricle, the major cardiac problems may be traced to the *(right/left)* ventricle. Myocardial infarction predominantly involves the *(right/left)* ventricle. The major valves affected in cardiac disease are the _____ and _____ valves, located on the *(right/left)*.

left
left
left

mitral; aortic; left

MECHANICAL ACTIVITY

22 The mechanical activity of the heart consists of a period of contrac-

tion known as *systole* and a period of relaxation and filling known as *diastole*. Atrial contraction may also be called atrial _____.   systole
Ventricular contraction may also be called ventricular
_____.   systole

NOTE: *Ventricular* systole corresponds to the apical pulse.

23 The right and left atria fill and contract together. For our purposes, then, they may be considered as a single functional unit. The right and left ventricles fill and contract together. They may also be considered as a single functional unit.

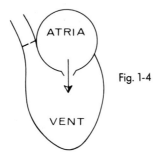

Fig. 1-4

24 The heart sounds serve as parameters for clinically outlining the mechanical events of the heart. Heart sounds are essentially produced by closure of the valves, although the exact mechanics involved in production of these sounds are more complex (see Unit 7).

25 During ventricular systole, the valves between the atria and the ventricles must close so that blood may be ejected into the blood vessels. Since ventricular systole is considered to be the first mechanical event, the sound produced by closure of these valves is known as the first heart sound, or _____. S_1

The "lubb" heard with a stethoscope is also representative of this event. S_1 is produced by closure of the _____ valves and   AV
marks the onset of ventricular *(systole/diastole)*.   systole

26 During ventricular diastole the semilunar valves are closed so that blood only enters the ventricles from the atria.

REMEMBER: The semilunar valves separate the ventricles from the
_____ leaving them. Since diastole is the second event of the   vessel
cardiac cycle, the sound produced by closure of these valves is known
as _____. S_2

The "dubb" heard with a stethoscope is also representative of this event. S_2 is produced by closure of the _____ valves   semilunar
and marks the onset of ventricular *(systole/diastole)*.   diastole

27 It is important to note that closure of the AV valves occurs not only as a result of ventricular contraction but also as a result of pressure

changes in the *ventricular chamber*.

Pressure increases in the ventricular chambers as they fill. As a result of this pressure the valves begin to close passively. When the ventricles contract, this mechanical event actively completes closure of the valves. Closure of the AV valves, then, is a result of both _____ and _____ mechanical activity.

active; passive

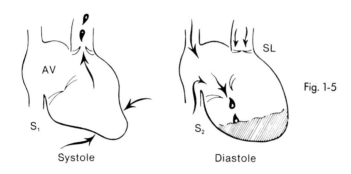

Fig. 1-5

Systole   Diastole

28 Atrial events also play a role during ventricular systole and diastole. Atrial systole occurs during ventricular diastole. It contributes the last boost of blood into the ventricles before ventricular systole.

29 In summary:

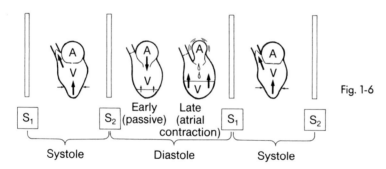

Fig. 1-6

Systole   Diastole   Systole

ELECTRICAL ACTIVITY

30 The heart has an intrinsic electrical system that allows for the origination and transmission of an electrical impulse. The electrical activity of the heart consists of (1) the *electrical stimulus* (the initiating factor), and (2) *depolarization* (the proliferating factor).

31 Essentially, this electrical activity *prepares* the heart to contract. The heart is prepared to contract by _____ activity.

electrical

The electrical activity of the heart may be recorded on paper. This record is known as the electrocardiogram, or ECG. Evidence of electrical activity, then, is manifested on the _____.

ECG

Relationship of electrical to mechanical activity

32 Electrical activity *precedes* mechanical activity. The *mechanical activity* consists of *contraction.* The heart can then function as a pump. The mechanical activity of the heart is noted by the presence of _____. Myocardial contraction results in the formation of a pulse. Evidence of mechanical activity, then, is manifested by the _____.

    Mechanical activity is more important than electrical activity because it is the assurance of actual _____ action.

    When there is electrical activity there is usually mechanical activity. For every beat on the ECG there is usually a corresponding _____. However, there can be beats on the ECG without a corresponding _____. This phenomenon is referred to as electromechanical dissociation and can occur in severe congestive heart failure (CHF) or cardiac tamponade. Clinically, then, the best evidence of mechanical activity is the _____.

contraction

pulse

pump

pulse

pulse

pulse

Cardiac cell properties

33 The heart cells have four main properties that allow for the integration of electrical and mechanical activity:
1. *Automaticity*—the ability to *initiate* an impulse of stimulus
2. *Excitability*—the ability to *respond* to an impulse or stimulus
3. *Conductivity*—the ability to *transmit* impulses to other areas
4. *Contractility*—the ability to *respond* to this electrical impulse with pump action

34 The heart can initiate its own impulse (_____), respond to this impulse (_____), and transmit this impulse (_____). These are *(electrical/mechanical)* properties.

automaticity

excitability

conductivity; electrical

35 *Contractility* is the _____ property of the heart.

mechanical

ELECTRICAL STRUCTURES

36 The conduction pathway normally begins in the *sinoatrial* (SA) *node.* The electrical stimulus is normally initiated in this area. Thus the _____ node is called the pacemaker of the heart.

sinoatrial

The SA node

37 The SA node is located in the right atrium close to the superior vena cava. It is a specialized piece of tissue that can periodically initiate its own impulses. The SA node is therefore said to have the property of _____.

automaticity

12

38 Normally, the SA node initiates its own impulses at a rate of 60 to 100 per minute.

NOTE: Other areas of the heart, such as the AV junctional tissue, lower portions of the atria, and the His-Purkinje system in the ventricles, also have the property of automaticity. The SA node is the normal pacemaker. It initiates impulses at a *(faster/slower)* rate than the other areas of the heart and therefore sets the _____ of the heart.

faster

pace

39 The SA node is innervated by the autonomic nervous system. Sympathetic stimulation can accelerate the SA node to a rate up to 150 *(sinus tachycardia)*. Parasympathetic stimulation can slow the heart rate to less than 60 *(sinus bradycardia)*. However, if the heart were separated from the body's nervous system, the SA node *(could/could not)* still initiate its own impulses.

could

40 Once an electrical impulse is originated, it spreads throughout the conduction system and the heart muscle. This is accomplished by a process known as *depolarization*. The pathway receiving the electrical stimulus is negatively charged *(polarized)*. It must be made positive so that the impulse may be conducted. The process by which these changes occur is known as _____.

depolarization

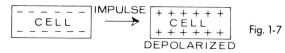

Fig. 1-7

These cells later recharge, or repolarize, in preparation for receiving the next electrical impulse.

41 When the impulse is released from the SA node, it travels through the specialized conduction tissue in the atria and causes them to contract.

NOTE: The specialized atrial conduction fibers, which lie between the SA node and the AV node, are known as the *internodal* tracts. One specialized conduction tract, known as Bachmann's bundle, branches off from the anterior internodal tract and carries the impulse be-

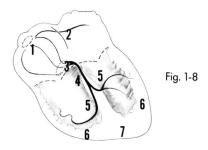

Fig. 1-8

tween the right and left atria. It is known as the *interatrial* tract. The existence of these specialized tracts is currently under dispute. Atrial impulses may spread along less well-defined pathways.

42 The normal sequence of activation in the heart is:

1. _____   SA node
2. _____   atria
3. _____   AV node
4. _____   bundle of His
5. _____   bundle branches
6. _____   Purkinje fibers
7. _____   ventricular musculature

AV junctional tissue

43 The AV node is located in the back of the right atrium close to the septal leaflet of the tricuspid valve. The AV node and the conduction tissue surrounding it, including the *bundle of His,* are known as the AV _____ tissue.   junctional

The bundle of His moves anteriorly, penetrating the septum. However, it is still located, for the most part, within the atria above the ventricles and is therefore regarded as supraventricular. AV junctional tissue, like the SA node, has the property of _____.   automaticity

44 Under normal conditions, the impulse from the SA node is released before the AV junctional tissue can be spontaneously depolarized. The SA node, therefore, normally *dominates* the AV junctional tissue and sets the _____ for the heart.   pace

If the SA node is unable to maintain its normal pace, the _____ _____ tissue can assume control as   AV; junctional
the dominant _____ of the heart.   pacemaker

45 Under normal conditions, the AV junctional tissue *(is/is not)* the pacemaker of the heart. It initiates impulses at a rate *(faster/slower)* than   is not
slower
the _____ node.   SA

If the SA node is injured or depressed, the _____   AV
_____ tissue can assume control. The rate of impulse formation in the AV junctional tissue is normally 40 to 70 per   junctional
minute. The rate of impulse discharge in the SA node is normally
_____ to _____ per minute.   60; 100

When the AV junctional tissue assumes the role of pacemaker of the heart, the heart rate will usually be *(faster/slower)* than when the   slower
heart is under the control of the _____ node.   SA

46 The heart's electrical impulse delays briefly at the _____   AV
junctional tissue. This delay allows for atrial contraction to precede

14

ventricular contraction. Thus the atria are able to provide the last boost of blood into the ventricles *before* ventricular contraction occurs. This *atrial component* contributes 20% to 30% of the cardiac output. In people with normal conduction, the atria contract *(before/after)* the ventricles and *(add to/subtract from)* cardiac output.

before

add to

His-Purkinje network (ventricular conduction tissue)

47 The conduction structures in the *ventricles* consist of the conduction structures *below* the bundle of His, also known as the His-Purkinje network. The ventricular conduction tissue, like the AV junctional tissue and the SA node, has the property of _____.

Under normal conditions, an impulse from the _____ node will occur before either the ventricular or AV junctional tissue is able to spontaneously depolarize.

The SA node therefore normally dominates both the AV junctional and _____ _____ tissues and functions as the _____ of the heart.

automaticity

SA

ventricular conduction

pacemaker

48 If both the SA node and the AV junctional tissue are unable to maintain control of the rhythm, the _____ assume control as the dominant _____ of the heart.

Under normal conditions, then, the ventricles *(are/are not)* the pacemakers of the heart.

REMEMBER: The ventricles initiate impulses at a rate *(faster/slower)* than either the _____ _____ or the _____ _____ _____.

If both the SA node and the AV junctional tissue are injured or depressed, the _____ conduction tissue can take over.

ventricles

pacemaker

are not

slower

SA node

AV junctional tissue

ventricular

49 LET US REVIEW: The normal pacemaker of the heart is the _____ _____.

If the SA node is injured or depressed, the _____ _____ _____ can assume control as pacemaker of the heart.

SA node

AV junctional tissue

50 The SA node, AV junctional tissue, and ventricular conduction tissue can all independently pace the heart because they all have the property of _____. The lower the pacemaker site in the heart, the *(faster/slower)* the heart rate.

automaticity

slower

51 More specifically, the ventricular conduction structures, also known as the _____ _____, consist of the bundle branches as well as the Purkinje fibers.

Two major bundle branches emerge from *below* the His bundle— the *right bundle branch,* which carries the electrical impulse to the right

His-Purkinje network

ventricle, and the *left bundle branch*, which carries the electrical impulse to the _____ ventricle. The main left bundle branch divides almost immediately into *two divisions*—an *anterosuperior division* and a *posteroinferior division* (Fig. 1-15). The Purkinje fibers emerge from the three ends of the bundle branches and carry the impulse through each ventricle.

left

PLANES OF THE HEART

52 A plane is an imaginary, flat, two-dimensional surface with four borders that can act as reference points for recording cardiac electricala nd mechanical activity. Planes slice through the body, providing cross-sectional views at different angles. Three planes may be used to record cardiac activity—the *frontal, sagittal,* and *horizontal* planes. The frontal and horizontal planes are referred to most frequently in the nursing assessment of the CCU patient.

53 The frontal plane slices through the body from side to side, separating the back of the body from the front. The frontal plane has two dimensions—height and width. The four *borders* of the *frontal plane* are labeled as superior, inferior, right and left. The heart within the body has similar borders formed by its outer surfaces. Electrodes placed on reference points reflecting the frontal plane borders may record events within the corresponding cardiac border. Movement of electrical activity toward these borders can also be recorded.

54 The borders of the frontal plane outline a view of a person seen from the *(side/front)*. Information recorded within the frontal plane is re-

front

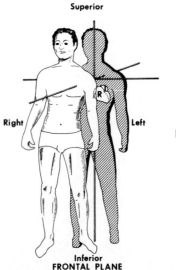

Superior

Right | Left

Fig. 1-9

Inferior
FRONTAL PLANE

corded from its _____.

borders

The front of the heart actually is *separated* from the back of the heart by the frontal plane. Therefore the front of the heart *(does/does not)* form a *border* of and is not contained within the frontal plane. The inferior portion of the heart *(does/does not)* form a border of the frontal plane. Thus the frontal plane is most accurate in recording events occurring in the *(anterior/inferior)* portion of the heart.

does not

does

inferior

55 The two dimensions of the sagittal plane are height and depth. The four borders of the *sagittal plane* outline a view of a person seen from the side. The sagittal plane separates the two sides of the body from each other, providing a cross-sectional view at another angle. The borders of the sagittal plane are _____, _____, _____, and _____.

superior

inferior; anterior; posterior

NOTE: The *left sagittal plane* is obtained by viewing the patient from the *left side.*

56 The two dimensions of the horizontal plane are _____ and _____. The four borders of the *horizontal plane* outline a view of a person seen horizontally, as if through a cros-sectional view. The borders of the horizontal plane are _____, _____, _____, and _____.

width

depth

anterior

posterior; right; left

The anterior portion of the heart *(does/does not)* form a border of the horizontal plane. The inferior border of the heart *(does/does not)* form a portion of the *horizontal plane.* It *(is/is not)* contained within the horizontal plane. Thus the horizontal plane is most accurate in recording events occurring in the *(anterior/inferior)* portion of the heart.

does

does not

is not

anterior

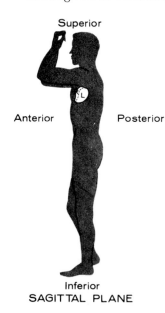

Fig. 1-10

SAGITTAL PLANE

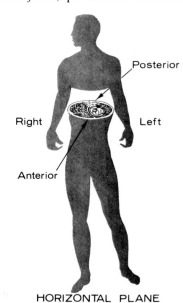

Fig. 1-11

HORIZONTAL PLANE

57 In summary:

The heart may be visualized in three planes. The borders of the frontal plane are (1) _____, (2) _____, (3) _____, and (4) _____.

The borders of the sagittal plane are (1) _____, (2) _____, (3) _____, and (4) _____.

The borders of the horizontal plane are (1) _____, (2) _____, (3) _____, and (4) _____.

left; right
superior; inferior
superior
inferior; anterior
posterior
left
right; anterior
posterior

POSITION OF THE HEART WITHIN THE CHEST

58 The heart is *rotated* and positioned on its side within the chest cavity. The right ventricle lies *anteriorly*, and the left ventricle lies *posteriorly*.

59 Let us now isolate the left ventricle within the chest cavity:

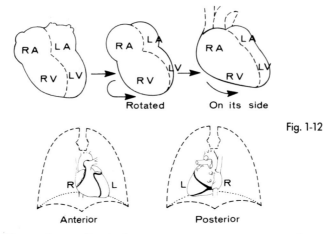

Fig. 1-12

This illustration reflects the _____ plane. The borders visualized are _____, _____, _____, and _____.

frontal
right; left
superior; inferior

60 In Fig. 1-13,

A represents the *anterior* portion of the left ventricle. Although the anterior surface is visible in this frontal plane view to which depth perception has been added, the anterior surface normally *(does/does not)* form a border of the frontal plane.

does not

B represents the *lateral* portion of the left ventricle. The lateral surface of the left ventricle *(does/does not)* form a border of the frontal plane.

does

C represents the *inferior* portion of the left ventricle. The inferior surface of the left ventricle *(does/does not)* form a border of the frontal plane.

does

18

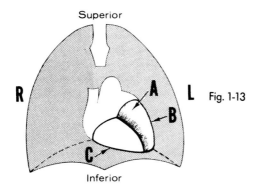

Superior

R   L   Fig. 1-13

Inferior

NOTE: The *inferior* surface of the left ventricle lies on the diaphragm. Therefore it may be called the _____ surface of the heart.

            diaphragmatic

61 An injury affecting area *A* of the left ventricle, then, would be called an _____ wall injury.

            anterior

     An injury affecting area *C* of the left ventricle would be called an _____ wall injury.

            inferior

62 The inferior surface of the heart may be better visualized in this sagittal plane view.

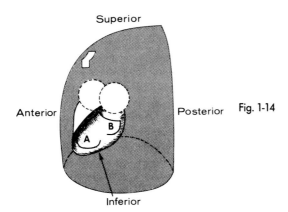

Superior

Anterior   Posterior   Fig. 1-14

Inferior

     A in this diagram represents the anterosuperior division of the left bundle branch.

     B in this diagram represents the postero- _____ division of the left bundle branch.

            inferior

CORONARY ARTERY SYSTEM

63 Like other organs in the body, the heart has its own rich blood supply. The heart receives blood for its own maintenance from *two coro-*

nary arteries, the *right* and the *left.* The coronary arteries are the first branches off the aorta. They originate from the cusps of the aortic valves in the *sinuses of Valsalva.*

The site of origin of the coronary arteries is the sinuses of _____ in the _____ cusps.

Valsalva; aortic

The coronary arteries exist from the aortic cusps and travel along the outer surface of the heart.

REMEMBER: The endocardial surface has a *(richer/poorer)* blood supply than the epicardial surface.

poorer

64 The coronary arteries provide blood for both the *electrical* and *mechanical* structures of the heart. The *electrical* structure of the heart are the structures of the *conduction system.* The major *mechanical* structure of the heart is the heart muscle, or *myocardium.* The heart's blood supply therefore provides blood to both the _____ system and the _____.

conduction
myocardium

The right coronary artery

65 Let us trace the pathway of each coronary artery and list the structures that each supplies:

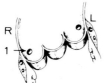 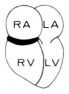 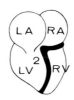

CROSS SECTION   ANTERIOR   POSTERIOR   Fig. 1-15
(AORTA)

The right coronary artery branches off from the _____ sinus of Valsalva. It then proceeds to the anterior surface of the heart and winds around to the right in the groove between the *right atrium* and the *right ventricle.*

right

NOTE: Before reaching the surface of the heart, a branch is emitted that supplies an important structure, the SA *node.*

66 The right coronary artery then winds around the back of the heart, dividing the right atrium and the right ventricle *(anteriorly/posteriorly).* An important branch is given off at this point, which descends posteriorly in the groove separating the right and left ventricles. The name of this branch is the *posterior descending branch.*

posteriorly

NOTE: The right coronary artery gives a branch to the AV node at about the same level as the origin of the posterior descending branch. The right coronary artery, then, supplies both the _____ and the _____ nodes.

SA
AV

67 As the right coronary artery winds around the back of the heart and descends, it emits a major branch known as the _____ _____ _____.

posterior descending branch

    The posterior descending branch also emits branches that perforate the *septum posteriorly*. These are called the *septal branches*. These branches supply a portion of the *bundle of His*, the *posterior third* of the septum, and a portion of the *inferoposterior division* of the *left bundle branch*.

68 The right coronary artery also supplies heart _____. The right coronary artery travels toward the (*right/left*) side of the heart, dividing the _____ _____ from the _____ _____.

muscle
right
right atrium
right ventricle

    The blood supply of the right _____ and right _____ is therefore provided by the _____ coronary artery.

atrium
ventricle; right

69 The right coronary artery also supplies a portion of the *left ventricular muscle*. The right coronary artery emits a posterior descending branch that separates the _____ ventricle from the left ventricle (*anteriorly/posteriorly*).

right
posteriorly

    The right coronary artery therefore supplies a portion of the left ventricle *posteriorly*.

70 Let us consider the left ventricle as it lies in the chest cavity:

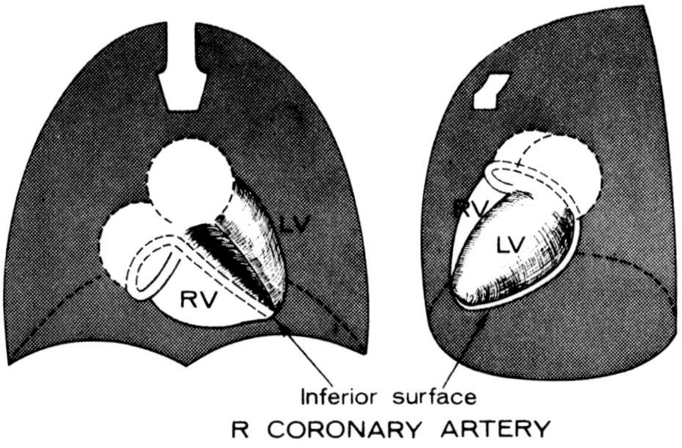

Fig. 1-16

Inferior surface
R CORONARY ARTERY

    NOTE: Most of the posterior portion of the heart as it lies rotated in the chest becomes the _____ or _____ surface. The right coronary artery is most significant for its blood supply to the _____ wall of the _____ ventricle.

inferior
diaphragmatic
inferoposterior
left

In summary:

The right coronary artery supplies the following:

1. SA node (55%)
2. AV node (90%)
3. Bundle of His (a portion)
4. Posteroinferior division of the left bundle (a portion)
5. Posterior third of the septum
6. Right atrial and ventricular muscle
7. Inferoposterior wall of the left ventricle

The left coronary artery

71 The left coronary artery branches off from the _____ sinus of Valsalva. It divides into two main branches as it reaches the surface of the heart—an *anterior descending branch* and a *lateral branch*.

left

72 The anteriorly descending branch is also called the _____ _____ coronary artery.

anterior descending

The *anterior* descending branch gives off perforating branches from the *(front/back)*, which supply the *anterior two thirds of the septum,* a major portion of the *right bundle branch,* and the *anterosuperior* division of the left bundle.

front

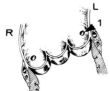

CROSS SECTION
(AORTA)   ANTERIOR   POSTERIOR

Fig. 1-17

73 The lateral branch, called the circumflex, winds around the *(right/left)* side, dividing the left atrium and left ventricle *anteriorly.* This branch then travels around the back of the heart, dividing the left atrium and left ventricle *(anteriorly/posteriorly).*

left

posteriorly

The circumflex *may* or *may not descend* posteriorly, depending on the individual. The circumflex supplies a portion of the *posteroinferior division* of the *left bundle.*

NOTE: The posteroinferior division has a dual blood supply—from both the *right* and the *left coronary arteries.*

74 The left coronary artery also supplies a portion of the cardiac _____.

muscle

The left coronary artery divides into two main branches, the _____ and the _____ _____.

circumflex; anterior descending

The circumflex travels toward the *(right/left),* supplying the lateral portion of the left atrium and left ventricle.

left

The anterior descending artery descends _____ anteriorly
to supply the _____ portion of the _____ anterior; left
ventricle.

The left coronary artery therefore supplies the _____ left
atrium and the _____ portion of the left ventricle. anterolateral

75 Let us again consider the left ventricle as it lies in the chest cavity:

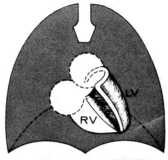

Fig. 1-18

L CORONARY ARTERY

The left coronary artery supplies a *(small/large)* portion of the left large
ventricle. The left coronary artery is most significant because it provides the blood supply to the _____ and _____ anterior; lateral
walls of the left ventricle.

In summary:

Table 2. Left coronary artery

Anterior descending	Circumflex
1. Anterior two thirds of septum	1. SA node (45%)
2. Right bundle branch (RBB) (major portion)	2. Posteroinferior division of left bundle (a portion)
3. Anterosuperior division of left bundle	3. Lateral wall of left ventricle
4. Anterior wall of left ventricle	

76 Let us observe the interrelationship of the coronary arteries:

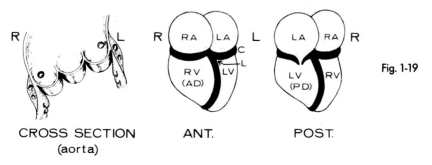

CROSS SECTION (aorta) ANT. POST. Fig. 1-19

The ventricles are divided in the front by the _____ anterior
descending branch of the _____ coronary artery. left

The ventricles are divided in the back by the _____ posterior
descending branch of the _____ coronary artery. right

The right atrium and the right ventricle are divided anteriorly
and posteriorly by the _____ coronary artery. right

The left atrium and left ventricle are divided anteriorly and posteriorly by the circumflex branch of the _____ coronary left
artery.

77 Let us again consider the left ventricle as it lies in the chest cavity:

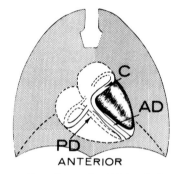

Fig. 1-20

78 The anterior descending branch *(AD)* of the _____ coro- left
nary artery supplies the _____ wall of the left ven- anterior
tricle.

The circumflex branch *(C)* of the _____ coronary artery left
supplies the _____ wall of the left ventricle. lateral

The left coronary artery as a whole supplies the
_____ surface of the left ventricle. anterolateral

79 The inferoposterior portion *(PD)* of the left ventricle is supplied by
the _____ _____ branch of the posterior descending
_____ coronary artery. right

The right coronary artery, then, supplies the _____ pos- infero
terior portion of the left ventricle.

CORONARY VEINS

80 The heart receives its oxygenated blood via the coronary artery system. Deoxygenated blood returns to the heart via the coronary veins.
Like deoxygenated blood from the body, deoxygenated blood from
the heart itself empties into the _____ atrium. right

81 The opening through which the coronary veins drain into the right
atrium is known as the *coronary sinus*. The opening is located in the
lower posterior portion of the right _____. atrium

82 **In summary:**

Table 3. Comparison of right and left coronary artery distribution

Right coronary artery supplies	Left coronary artery supplies
1. SA node (55%)	1. SA node (45%)
2. AV node	2. Anterosuperior division of left bundle
3. Bundle of His (a portion)	3. Right bundle branch (major portion)
4. Posterior one third of septum	4. Anterior two thirds of septum
5. Posteroinferior division of left bundle (a portion)	5. Posteroinferior division of left bundle (a portion)
6. Inferoposterior surface of left ventricle	6. Anterolateral surface of left ventricle

The coronary veins return deoxygenated blood to the right atrium through an opening known as the _____ _____.   coronary sinus

SUMMARY AND CORRELATION

83 The heart consists of a right side and a left side. The right and left sides of the heart differ in:

1. _____   function
2. _____   musculature
3. _____ structure   valvular

84 LET US REVIEW:

Table 4. Comparison of right and left ventricular function and structure

Right ventricle	Left ventricle	RV	LV
A. Function			
1. Delivers unoxygenated blood from the _____ to the _____.	1. Delivers _____ blood from the _____ to the _____.	body lungs	oxygenated lung body
2. Projects its volume against minimal resistance—the _____.	2. Projects its volume against maximal resistance—the _____.	lungs	body
B. Musculature			
1. _____ walls	1. _____ walls	thin	thick
C. Valvular structure			
1. AV valve: _____.	1. AV valve: _____.	tricuspid	mitral
2. Semilunar valve: _____.	2. Semilunar valve: _____.	pulmonary	aortic

85 Within the chest wall the heart is _____ and positioned on its _____. The right ventricle therefore becomes the *(anterior/posterior)* ventricle.   rotated
side; anterior

25

The left ventricle becomes the *(anterior/posterior)* ventricle.   posterior

Myocardial infarction occurs almost exclusively in the *(right/left)*   left
ventricle.

In the setting of coronary care, the primary concern is therefore
the *(right/left)* ventricle.   left

86 The heart has both _____ and   electrical
_____ activity.   mechanical

The electrical activity consists of:

1. An electrical _____ (the initiating factor)   stimulus
2. _____ (the proliferating factor)   Depolarization

The electrical *properties* of the heart consist of:

1. The ability to *initiate* an impulse (_____)   automaticity
2. The ability to *respond* to an impulse (_____)   excitability
3. The ability to *transmit* an impulse (_____)   conductivity

87 The electrical activity of the heart is detected by the _____.   ECG

Electrical activity of the heart begins in the _____ node,   SA
then continues on the _____, _____   atria; AV junctional tissue
_____ _____,
_____ _____   bundle of His
_____, _____ _____,   bundle branches
_____ _____, and   Purkinje fibers
_____.   ventricles

The function of the electrical activity is to prepare the heart for
_____ activity.   mechanical

88 The mechanical activity of the heart is known as
_____. The mechanical activity of the heart is best   contractility
detected by the _____. Mechanical activity of the heart be-   pulse
gins with a period of contraction, or _____, fol-   systole
lowed by a period of relaxation, or _____.   diastole

89 Mechanical activity enables the heart to function as a pump. The
amount of blood pumped from the heart is known as the cardiac
_____.   output

REMEMBER: Cardiac output is a product of _____   ventricular rate
_____ × _____ _____.   stroke volume

90 Electrical activity prepares the heart for _____ activ-   mechanical
ity. Mechanical activity is more important than electrical activity because it is the assurance of actual _____ action. For every   pump
beat on the ECG, there should be a corresponding _____.   pulse

91 Since normal heart function consists of normal
_____ and _____ activity, abnor-   electrical; mechanical

mal heart function will result in disturbances of either _____ activity, _____ activity, or both.   electrical; mechanical

Abnormal electrical activity will result in arrhythmias. Abnormal mechanical activity will result in heart failure or shock.

SUGGESTED READINGS

Anderson RH and Becker AE: Cardiac anatomy; an integrated text and colour atlas, New York, 1980, Cover Medical Publishing.

Anthony CP and Thibodeau GH: Textbook of anatomy and physiology, ed 11, St. Louis, 1983, The CV Mosby Co.

Conover MB: Understanding electrocardiography, ed. 4, St. Louis, 1984, The CV Mosby Co.

Darovic GO: Hemodynamic monitoring: invasive and noninvasive clinical application, Philadelphia, 1987, WB Saunders Co.

Guyton AC: Textbook of medical physiology, ed. 7, Philadelphia, 1986, WB Saunders Co.

Hurst JW and Logue RB, editors: The heart, arteries, and veins, ed. 6, New York, 1986, McGraw-Hill, Inc.

UNIT 2

Basic Electrophysiology

In Unit 1 it was stated that the heart has both electrical and mechanical properties. The heart has the electrical ability to (1) initiate electrical impulses (automaticity), (2) respond to electrical impulses (excitability), and (3) conduct electrical impulses (conduc-tivity). The heart also has the mechanical ability to respond to these impulses with pump action (contractility). Let us now consider each of the electrical properties in more detail.

ELECTRICAL PROPERTIES OF HEART CELLS
Automaticity

1 Certain areas of the heart normally have the ability to _____ electrical impulses. These areas include the SA node, the AV junctional tissue, and the His-Purkinje system in the _____. These areas act as natural pacemakers. Automaticity may be either enhanced or suppressed in the natural pacemaker areas by the autonomic nervous system, which innervates the heart.

    The autonomic nervous system is composed of the sympathetic and parasympathetic nerves. The sympathetic nerves innervate the entire myocardium and generally *enhance* automaticity. The parasympathetic nerves selectively innervate the structures within the *atrial* myocardium and generally *(enhance/suppress)* automaticity.

initiate

ventricles

suppress

2 The SA node fires at an inherent automatic rate of 60 to 100 beats per minute in the adult and is normally the dominant pacemaker of the heart. SA node activity may be enhanced by the _____ nervous system.

    Under sympathetic stimulation the heart rate may increase up to 150 beats per minute and yet remain under the control of the SA node. Beyond this point abnormal pacemakers often assume control of the rhythm. SA node activity may be suppressed by the _____ nervous system, resulting in heart rates of less than 60 beats per minute.

sympathetic

parasympathetic

3 The AV junction fires at an inherent rate of 40 to 70 beats per minute. AV junctional activity may be _____ by the sympathetic nervous system and _____ by the parasympathetic nervous system.

enhanced

suppressed

The ventricular (His-Purkinje) conduction system fires at an inherent rate of 20 to 40 beats per minute. Ventricular activity may be enhanced by the _____ system. However, ventricular activity is usually *not* affected by parasympathetic activity.

sympathetic

REMEMBER: The parasympathetic nerves selectively innervate the structures within the _____.

atria

4 The dominant pacemaker of the heart is the _____ _____. However, if this pacemaker fails, the _____ _____ tissue may assume control of the rhythm because it also has the natural property of _____. The heart rate then will be *(faster/slower)*. If the AV junctional tissue fails to release a stimulus, the _____ _____ tissue may assume control of the rhythm. However, the heart rate will be _____ to _____ beats per minute, which usually results in patient symptoms and may proceed to cardiac arrest.

SA node

AV junctional

automaticity; slower

ventricular conduction

20; 40

Excitability and conduction

5 All areas of the heart have the ability to _____ to and _____ electrical impulses. Cardiac cells respond to and transmit electrical impulses by the process of *depolarization*. At rest, cardiac cells are negatively charged on the inside with respect to the outside. In this state they are said to be *polarized*.

respond
transmit

In response to advancing electrical impulses, positive charges move into the cells. The inside of these cells become *(electropositive/electronegative)*. In this state the cells are said to be depolarized.

electropositive

6 This change in cell charge acts as a signal to normal adjacent cells. Thus the impulse is transmitted and spreads throughout the conduction tissue and myocardium.

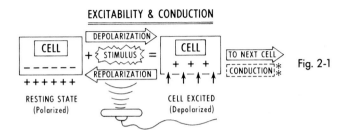

EXCITABILITY & CONDUCTION

Fig. 2-1

If adjacent cells are normal, the excitation process (depolarization) automatically results in conduction. Thus the term *depolarization* is often used synonymously with *conduction*.

7 The movement of positive charges into the myocardial cells causes them to become excited, or _____.

depolarized

Once depolarized the cell prepares for *another* electrical impulse by recharging, or _____. The impulse is transmitted, or conducted, to adjacent cells in response to _____.

repolarizing

depolarization

8 LET US REVIEW the normal sequence of conduction:

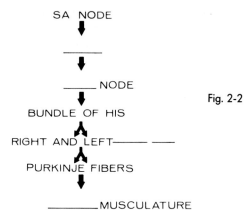

SA NODE

_____

_____ NODE

BUNDLE OF HIS

RIGHT AND LEFT——— ——

PURKINJE FIBERS

_____MUSCULATURE

Fig. 2-2

NOTE: The conduction system in the heart may be compared to a rapid transit system. It provides the most rapid means for the transmission of an electrical impulse. If there is a block in this system (for example, SA block, AV block, or bundle branch block), the heart can still be depolarized, but the process will occur more slowly.

ELECTROCARDIOGRAMS
Normal ECG complex

9 The wave of depolarization and repolarization spreading through the heart can be recorded on paper. This record is called the electrocardiogram, or ECG. The changes in cell charges occurring during depolarization and repolarization produce deflections on the recording paper, forming the ECG complex. Let us analyze the normal configuration of the ECG complex:

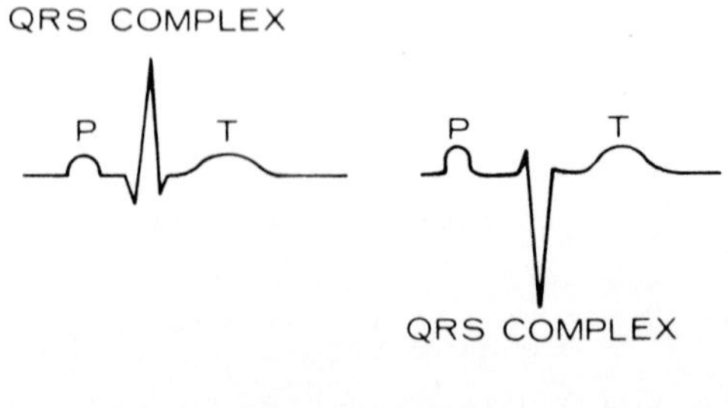

QRS COMPLEX

P   T   P   T

Fig. 2-3

QRS COMPLEX

10 The largest deflection in the ECG record is the QRS complex. The electrical impulses spreading through the ventricles produce the QRS complex. The QRS complex therefore represents depolarization of the _____. After depolarization has occurred, the heart must recover before it can receive another impulse. This process is known as _____.

ventricles

repolarization

Ventricular repolarization is represented on the ECG by the *T wave,* which follows the QRS complex. The T wave may not always be clearly visible following the QRS complex. However, if consecutive QRS complexes are seen, it can be assumed that T waves are present because depolarization cannot occur again without repolarization from previous impulses.

The electrical impulses spreading through the atria produce the *P wave,* which precedes the QRS complex. The P wave represents depolarization of the _____.

atria

Atrial repolarization is also represented by a T wave. However, this wave usually is not seen on the ECG because it is hidden within the QRS complex and is of low voltage.

NOTE: Identification of both the T wave and P wave may be facilitated by first identifying the large and more distinct QRS complex and using it as a guide.

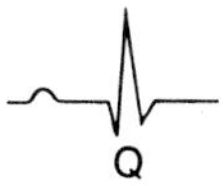

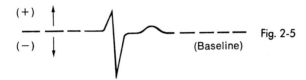

Fig. 2-4

Q

11 Let us consider the QRS complex in more detail. The *R wave* is defined as the first positive deflection in the QRS complex. A *Q wave* is defined as a negative deflection *preceding* the R wave.

In Fig. 2-4 there *(is/is not)* a Q wave.

is

An *S wave* is defined as a negative deflection *following* the R wave. A *completely negative* QRS complex is commonly referred to as a *QS complex.*

12 NOTE: A positive deflection is defined as one that points above the baseline. A negative deflection is defined as one that points _____ the baseline. The baseline may be determined by noting the beginning of the QRS complex.

below

(+)

(−)

(Baseline)   Fig. 2-5

13 Consider this QRS complex:

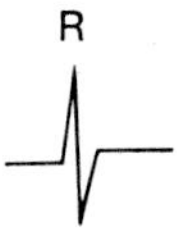

R

Fig. 2-6

The first deflection is *(positive/negative)*. It is called the
_____ wave. The second deflection is *(positive/negative)*. It is
called the _____ wave. In this complex, there *(is/is not)* a Q
wave.

positive
R; negative
S; is not

14 Not every QRS complex always has Q, R, and S waves. However, the
wave representing ventricular depolarization is collectively known as
the QRS complex, regardless of its configuration.
   (Every/Not every) QRS complex has Q, R, and S waves.
   All QRS complexes do reflect _____
depolarization.

Not every
ventricular

15 Each wave in the QRS complex may be described further according
to its size. A large wave would be denoted by a capital letter Q, R, or
S. A small wave would be denoted by a small letter q, r, or s.
   Label the following complexes:

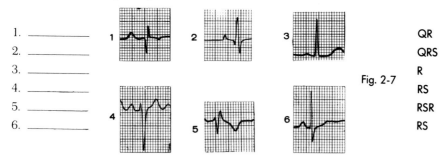

1. _____
2. _____
3. _____
4. _____
5. _____
6. _____

Fig. 2-7

QR
QRS
R
RS
RSR
RS

NOTE: In the fifth example of Fig. 2-7, there is a second positive
deflection. When this occurs, the wave is labeled R *prime* or R.
   REMEMBER: Q waves and S waves are always *(positive/negative)*. R
waves are always _____.

negative
positive

Intervals and segments of ECG complex

16 Certain intervals on the ECG also are significant. The first to be considered is the PR interval. It is measured from the beginning of the P
wave to the beginning of the QRS complex.

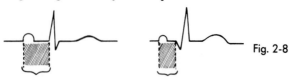

Fig. 2-8

PR interval

NOTE: In Fig. 2-8, the second interval is actually a pq interval. The
PR interval begins with atrial depolarization and ends with the beginning of _____ depolarization. It represents the de-
lay between atrial and ventricular depolarization, or the time that it
takes an impulse to travel from the _____ node to the

ventricular

SA

_____. This normal delay between atrial and ventricular conduction occurs within the AV conduction tissue (AV node, bundle of His, and bundle branches). The PR interval serves to correlate the electrical impulse of the atria with that of the ventricles and allows for detection of AV conduction blocks. The normal PR interval is from *0.12* to *0.20 second*. A PR interval of constant duration serves to establish a constant relationship between the _____ and _____.

This constant relationship implies _____ between the atria and _____ and allows time for atrial contraction before ventricular contraction. Atrial contraction occurs during ventricular *(systole/diastole)*, allowing an extra boost to cardiac output.

ventricles

atria
ventricles
conduction
ventricles

diastole

17 Another frequently measured interval in electrocardiography is the QT interval.

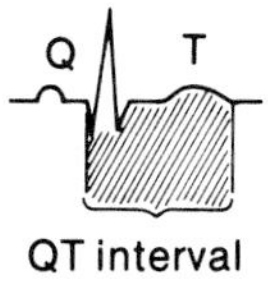

Fig. 2-9

QT interval

The QT interval includes ventricular depolarization (QRS complex) plus ventricular _____, or the _____ wave.

The QT interval thus may be altered by any change in ventricular electrical activity.

repolarization; T

18 Let us now consider a specific portion of the QT interval, the QRS duration. The QRS complex represents _____ _____. The QRS interval is measured from the beginning of the QRS complex to the end of the QRS complex. The normal QRS duration is from 0.08 to 0.10 second.

NOTE: If there is no Q wave present, the "QRS" is measured from the beginning of the first deflection in the complex.

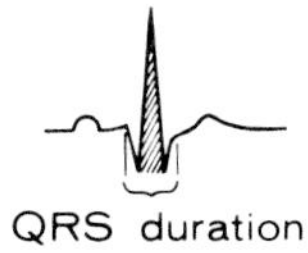

ventricular depolarization

Fig. 2-10

QRS duration

19 Another important portion of the QT interval is the ST segment. The *J*, or junction point, marks the beginning of the ST segment. The ST segment represents the heart's resting period between *(atrial/ventricular)* depolarization and repolarization.

ventricular

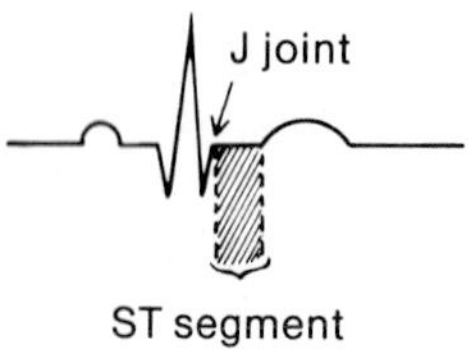

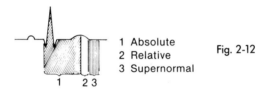

J joint

ST segment

Fig. 2-11

Refractory periods and vulnerable period

20 During repolarization, the individual cardiac cells gradually regain their normal excitability and during this process go through periods of varying excitability. These periods are known as the *refractory periods.*

REMEMBER: Excitability is the ability of the heart to _____ to an electrical impulse. The refractory periods of the heart are times during which the heart is unable to respond *normally* to a second electrical impulse.

respond

21 The refractory periods of the ventricles are represented by certain areas within the QT interval:

1 Absolute
2 Relative
3 Supernormal

Fig. 2-12

The absolute refractory period is that time during the cardiac cycle when the cardiac cells are unable to respond to a second stimulus, regardless of the strength of the stimulus. In the normal heart the *absolute* refractory period includes the QRS and part of the _____ segment. An electrical stimulus reaching the ventricles during the absolute refractory period *(will/will not)* cause a myocardial response. The *supernormal* period is that time during repolarization when a *weak stimulus* can cause a second response.

ST
will not

22 The refractory periods refer to *single* responses to electrical stimuli. However, at a critical point during repolarization, the heart may respond to a stimulus with more than one response. This period of *altered excitability* is known as the *vulnerable period.* The vulnerable period is that portion of the cardiac cycle when a stimulus may produce *repetitive firing,* also referred to as a chain reaction response.

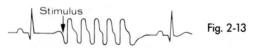

Stimulus

Fig. 2-13

23 During the absolute refractory period the heart *(will/will not)* respond to any stimulus. During the refractory period a *(weak/strong)* stimulus

will not
strong

34

may elicit a response. During the supernormal period a *(weak/strong)* stimulus may elicit a response. During the vulnerable period a stimulus may cause *(single/multiple)* responses, also known as _____ _____ or a _____ _____ response.

weak

multiple
repetitive firing; chain reaction

In the setting of acute myocardial infarction the vulnerable period occurs on the apex of the _____ wave.

T

RECORDING ELECTRICAL FORCES
Lead concept

24 A lead is an electrical system used to record electrical activity. Leads are used to record electrical activity in cardiac monitoring systems as well as in standard 12-lead ECG recording systems. A lead is composed of a *negative* and a *positive* electrode. These electrodes sense the *magnitude* and *direction* of electrical forces and record *surface information* from the cardiac borders.

25 The positive electrode is the most sensitive electrode. Electrical forces traveling toward a positive electrode produce a predominant positive deflection on the ECG monitor or record. Electrical forces traveling away from a positive electrode (or toward a negative electrode) produce a predominant _____ deflection on the ECG monitor or record.

negative

A lead is composed of a _____ electrode and a _____ electrode.

positive
negative

The limb leads

26 A standardized method of electrode placement was devised by Einthoven. In devising this method, he first utilized the frontal plane.

REMEMBER: The borders of the frontal plane are:

1. _____   right
2. _____   left
3. _____   superior
4. _____   inferior

27 Positions on the arms and legs are selected as potential electrode sites:

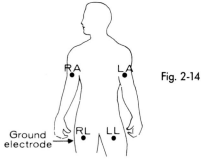

Fig. 2-14

NOTE: These limb positions border the _____   frontal
plane. With the use of two electrodes at a time, three *bipolar* leads are
derived. When the positive and negative electrodes are both located
on the body surface, this lead is referred to as a *bipolar lead.* An ECG
recorder is used with a recording cable attached. The cable endings
are then attached to monitoring electrodes placed in the designated
positions. The electrode placed at the right leg (RL) position functions as a ground, or neutralizing, electrode, allowing the electrode
placed at the left leg (LL) position to function as the major foot (F)
electrode.

28 In the two arm positions, the left arm (LA) is made positive and the
right arm (RA) is made negative. That is done by programming the
cable endings, which are marked RA and LA. The cable endings are
connected to _____ placed in the designated   electrodes
positions.

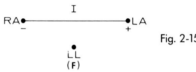

Fig. 2-15

29 This lead is known as lead I. In lead I the positive electrode is on the
_____ arm, and the negative electrode is on the   left
_____ arm.   right
    With the right arm position (RA) and the foot position (F) lead,
the right arm can be made negative and the foot made positive. This
lead is known as lead II.

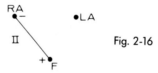

Fig. 2-16

30 In lead II the positive electrode is at the _____, and the   foot
negative electrode is on the _____ arm.   right
    With the LA and the F electrodes, the left arm is made negative
and the foot is made positive. This lead is known as lead III.

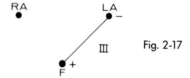

Fig. 2-17

    In lead III the positive electrode is at the _____, and the   foot
negative electrode is on the _____ arm.   left
    NOTE: The RL position serves as the _____   ground
for leads.

31 Fig. 2-18 summarizes the three bipolar leads.

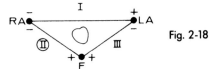

Fig. 2-18

The heart may be visualized as a central source of electricity within this triangle.

32 Three more leads may be derived from the frontal plane positions. Each position is designated separately as a positive electrode. The two other limb positions share the role of negative electrode to augment the voltage of the recorded forces (see Frame 33). Thus the negative electrode extends directly between the other two electrode positions. When only the positive electrode is actually on the body surface, the lead is called a _____ lead.   unipolar

33 Fig. 2-19 demonstrates a unipolar lead.

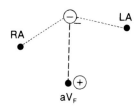

Fig. 2-19

Lead aV_F is created by making the foot electrode positive. The negative electrode extends in an imaginary direction _____ the two other electrode positions. The electri-   between cal forces recorded in a unipolar system are small and must use *augmented* voltage or extra electrical energy.

For this reason, this lead is known as the augmented voltage (aV) foot ($_F$) lead, or lead aV_F. In lead aV_F, the positive electrode is at the _____. *Lead* aV_F has *(one/two)* visible electrode(s) on the   foot; one body. It is therefore called a *(unipolar/bipolar)* lead.   unipolar

34 By the same principles the RA and LA electrodes were used to obtain leads aV_R and aV_L.

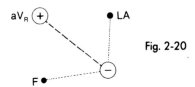

Fig. 2-20

In lead aV_R the positive electrode is on the right arm, and the negative electrode extends between _____ and _____.

aV_L; aV_F

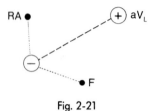

Fig. 2-21

35 Fig. 2-22 is a representation of all the limb leads.

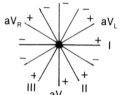

Fig. 2-22

Let us analyze how this diagram was derived.

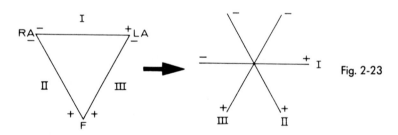

Fig. 2-23

The three *bipolar* limb leads are _____, _____, and _____. They may be moved to a center point so that they intersect. The heart may be pictured in the center as in Fig. 2-24.

I; II III

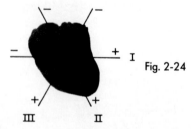

Fig. 2-24

36 Let us add the three unipolar limb leads: _____, _____, and _____.

aV_R
aV_L; aV_F

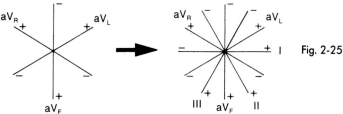

Fig. 2-25

Magnitude and direction of normal heart forces

37 Let us consider the forces of the heart in relationship to the leads. In the normal heart the *(right/left)* ventricle has the most muscle mass and the most electrical force. For this reason the sum *of all the electrical forces* traveling through the ventricles is usually represented by a force shifted slightly to the left.

left

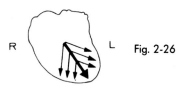

R   L   Fig. 2-26

38 In Fig. 2-26, the arrows represent both magnitude and direction of force. These arrows are known as vectors. The summation force (large arrow) is known as the summation _____, or axis. The ventricular, or QRS, axis in the normal heart is shifted toward the *(right/left)*. (For the more exact range of normal see Unit 8, frames 27-40)

vector

left

NOTE: An axis can also be derived for both the P wave and T wave. However, when discussing the axis of the heart, we are usually considering forces responsible for the production of the QRS complex. It is the ventricular axis, or ventricular summation vector, that is reflected on the ECG as the _____ complex.

QRS

39 LET US REVIEW: Electrical forces traveling toward a positive electrode produce a predominantly positive deflection on the ECG. Electrical forces traveling toward a negative electrode or away from a positive pole produce a _____ deflection on the ECG.

negative

Einthoven designated the polarity for lead I:

I

- •————————————————• +
RA   LA

Fig. 2-27

By superimposing the ventricular forces of a particular patient's heart over lead I, we can deduce the morphology of his QRS in this lead:

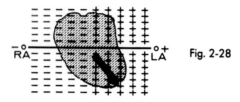

Fig. 2-28

The ventricular forces of the patient *(are/are not)* traveling in a normal direction.

are

40 The ventricular forces of this person's normal heart travel *(toward/ away from)* the positive electrode in lead I. Therefore it can be expected that a normal QRS complex in lead I will have a predominantly *(positive/negative)* deflection. Conversely, when a patient has a predominantly positive QRS complex in Lead I, it can be expected that the ventricular forces of this person travel *(toward/away)* the positive electrode in Lead I and thus could be normal.

toward

positive

toward

Lead I

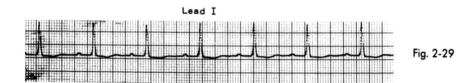

Fig. 2-29

41 This patient's ventricular forces also travel toward the positive electrode of lead II.

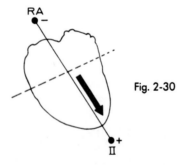

Fig. 2-30

Therefore the normal QRS in lead II will have a *(positive/negative)* deflection.

positive

42 REMEMBER: On the ECG, the P wave represents the atrial electrical forces, or the P wave axis. The normal forces of the atria also travel toward the positive electrode in lead II. In lead II, therefore, the P wave is also *(positive/negative)*. It can be expected that during normal conduction P waves will be upright and usually but not always best visible in lead _____.

positive

positive

43 Using these principles of electrophysiology, we can deduce the QRS morphology in all of the limb leads. Review Fig. 2-31 below. In lead aV$_R$, the normal QRS complex should be predominantly *(positive/negative)*.

negative

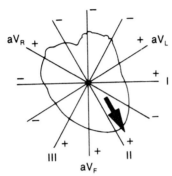

Fig. 2-31

The P wave in lead aV$_R$ is also negative because the atrial forces are moving *(toward/away from)* the positive electrode.

away from

REMEMBER: The normal P wave is always positive in lead _____ and always negative in lead _____. Therefore P waves are usually best identified in these two leads.

II; aV$_R$

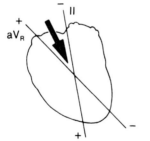

Figs. 2-32

44 Let us now examine the six-lead ECG and verify the configuration of all of the limb leads:

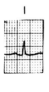 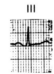

Figs. 2-33

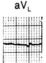 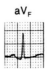

REMEMBER: The major direction of the QRS deflection is determined by the direction of the ventricular forces and with reference to the (negative/positive) electrode of each lead. When forces are traveling perpendicular to the lead, the QRS complex is smaller and is half positive and half negative as in Lead AVL (Fig. 2-33). This pattern is referred to as biphasic.

positive

The chest leads

45 The limb leads provide six views of the heart in the frontal plane. Other views of the heart's electrical activity can be obtained from the borders of the horizontal plane. This plane is obtained by slicing the body transversely, anterior to posterior.

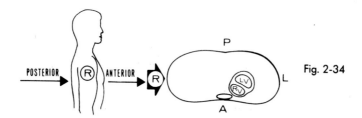

Fig. 2-34

The V leads, or chest leads, provide six possible views of the heart in the horizontal plane. The V leads are derived by using the principle of the unipolar leads. They also represent augmented voltage of vector forces and thus are known as V leads. In the V leads the positive electrode is placed on the chest wall, and the negative electrode extends posteriorly toward a central reference point created by the limb electrodes.

46 The positive electrode of V_1 is located just to the right of the sternum in the fourth intercostal space. The positive electrode is then moved along the chest wall toward the left to form leads V_2, V_3, V_4, V_5, and V_6.

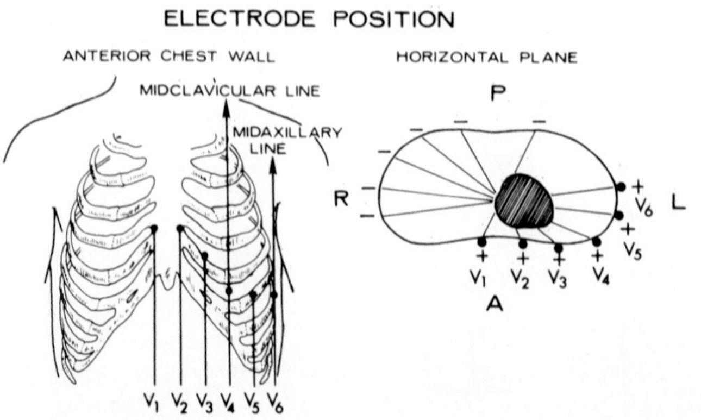

ELECTRODE POSITION

ANTERIOR CHEST WALL

MIDCLAVICULAR LINE

MIDAXILLARY LINE

HORIZONTAL PLANE

P

R

L

V_6

V_5

V_1 V_2 V_3 V_4

A

Fig. 2-35

V_1 V_2 V_3 V_4 V_5 V_6

The positive electrode in each of the chest leads is located on either the front or *side* of the chest. The negative electrodes extend toward the _____.

back

47 The forces of the QRS and normal axis travel toward the *(right/left)* ventricle

left

The left ventricle lies rotated posteriorly in the chest. Therefore the QRS forces in the horizontal plane travel *(anteriorly/posteriorly)*. Using this information, we can deduce the normal QRS direction in the chest leads.

posteriorly

In lead V_1, the ventricular forces travel *(toward/away from)* the positive electrode. Therefore the normal QRS in lead V_1 should be predominantly *(positive/negative)*.

away from
negative

48 NOTE: Leads V_2 to V_5 are a transition from the V_1 pattern to the V_6 pattern. The R wave becomes larger and the S wave smaller as the progression occurs. Let us examine the chest leads of the ECG in Fig. 2-36 to verify these configurations:

49 To complete a study of QRS configurations, we must consider the force created by depolarization of the septum. This force, although small, contributes to the QRS complex. The septum is the first por-

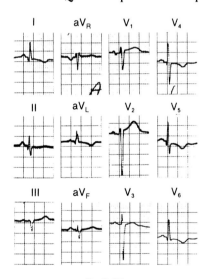

Fig 2-36

tion of the ventricle to be depolarized. Septal depolarization occurs from *left to right* and *posteriorly to anteriorly*.

REMEMBER: The ventricles are depolarized from right to _____ and _____ to posteriorly. Thus septal depolarization occurs in the *(same/opposite)* direction.

left; anteriorly
opposite

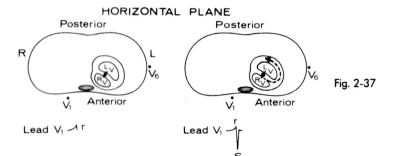

Fig. 2-37

50 In lead V_1 of Fig. 2-37 the initial, or septal, force is represented by a small r wave. It is caused by the wave of septal depolarization traveling toward the *(right/left)*.

The major ventricular forces travel in the *(same/opposite)* direction, toward the *(right/left)*. In lead V_1, this force is represented by a large *(R/S)* wave. In lead V_6 of Fig. 2-38, the initial, or septal, force is represented by a small q wave. This is caused by the wave of septal depolarization traveling *(toward/away from)* V_6.

The major ventricular forces travel in the *(same/opposite)* direction, producing a large *(R/S)* wave in lead V_6.

right

opposite
left
S

away from

opposite
R

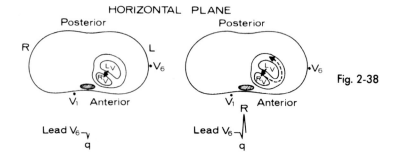

Fig. 2-38

Recording surface information

51 Let us now consider the surfaces of the left ventricle and correlate the leads with the surface they reflect.

REMEMBER: The most sensitive electrode is the _____ electrode. The foot electrode looks directly up toward the *(inferior/anterior)* surface of the left ventricle.

The leads that use the foot as a positive, or sensitive, electrode are leads _____, _____, and _____.

Leads II, III, and aV_F, then, reflect the electrical activity of the _____ surface of the left ventricle.

Therefore inferior wall myocardial infarctions (IWMI) can best be detected in leads _____, _____, and _____. Consider the relationship of these leads to the inferior wall (Fig. 2-39):

positive
inferior

II; III; aV_F

inferior

II; III
aV_F

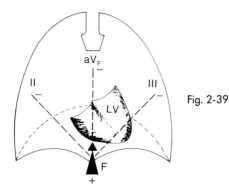

aV_F

II   III

LV

F
+

Fig. 2-39

52 Let us now discuss the anterior surface and the leads that reflect its electrical activity. The LA electrode in Fig. 2-40 looks directly at the _____ portion of the anterior surface of the left ventricle. The leads that use the left arm as the positive electrode are leads _____ and _____.

Leads I and aV_L, then, reflect the _____ surface of the left ventricle.

lateral

I; aV_L

lateral

53 The positive electrodes of the chest leads border the septal and lateral portion of the anterior surface of the left ventricle. Therefore leads I, aV_L, and V_1 to V_6 reflect the electrical activity of the entire_____ wall. It can then be expected that extensive anterior wall myocardial infarctions (AWMI) will be best seen in leads _____ and _____ and in the (*chest/limb*) leads.

Consider the anterior wall in Fig. 2-40:

anterior

I; aV_L; chest

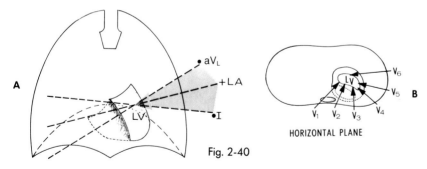

A

• aV_L

+LA

•I

LV

V_6

V_5

LV

V_1 V_2 V_3 V_4

B

HORIZONTAL PLANE

Fig. 2-40

NOTE: If an infarction is confined to the septal area of the anterior wall, it is best seen in leads V_1 through V_4. If an infarction is confined to the lateral portion of the anterior wall, it is best seen in leads I, aV_L, and V_4 to V_6.

54 An acute injury current in the lateral leads will produce opposite, or reciprocal, changes in the _____ leads within the same plane, which are _____, _____, and

inferior

II; III

45

_____. An acute injury current in the inferior leads will produce opposite, or reciprocal, changes in the _____ leads within the same plane, which are _____ and _____. An acute injury limited to the anteroseptal area will produce no reciprocal changes in any of the standard leads because there are no standard electrode positions directly opposite this surface within the same plane.

aV_F

lateral

I; aV_L

55 Let us now consider lead aV_R and its relationship to the left ventricle:

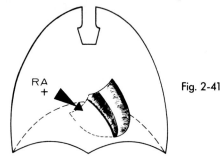

Fig. 2-41

Lead aV_R uses the RA as its *(positive/negative)* electrode. The RA electrode does not look directly at any surface of the left ventricle. This lead, however, does look at the inside of the heart. Lead aV_R reflects the *(outside/inside)* of the left ventricle. Lead aV_R is known as an intracavitary lead.

positive

inside

LEAD CONCEPTS APPLIED TO CARDIAC MONITORING

56 Cardiac monitoring systems usually require three major components: (1) *electrodes,* (2) *a monitoring cable,* and (3) *an oscilloscope display.* A bedside or central *recorder* is a critically important option in a coronary care unit. Another valuable option is an electronic or tape *memory* bank with the ability to play back a record of the *onset* of rhythm disturbances, ECG changes, or both.

Monitoring systems are available in the form of large bedside units or small portable units. The small units may be connected to radio transmitters (telemetry) or to recorders that are later connected to oscilloscope displays for playback (Holter monitoring). In the coronary care unit the larger, hardwire bedside units are most commonly used. The portable units are popular in convalescent (progressive care) cardiac units for diagnostic purposes.

All cardiac monitoring systems utilize lead concepts to obtain the ECG record or display. Knowledge of lead concept allows the nurse to select optimal electrode positions and facilitates problem solving.

57 A minimum of three electrodes is usually required to obtain an ECG record from a hardwire bedside unit. An external ground electrode may not be necessary with telemetry units, leaving two major electrodes.

REMEMBER: Cardiac electrical activity can be recorded by electrical systems known as _____.

Leads are composed of a _____ and _____ electrode and may also use a third electrode as a _____.

leads
positive
negative
ground

58 Three-electrode monitoring systems are popular in many coronary care units. The two-electrode systems used with telemetry units incorporate the same principles. These systems cost less and are less cumbersome than the four-electrode or five-electrode systems. However, to obtain their maximal efficiency, they require more ingenuity and adjustment from the nurses using them. In determining proper electrode position, nurses should first consider positions that most closely mimic the standard lead positions. Fig. 2-42 illustrates electrode positions mimicking the standard bipolar limb leads. The limb electrodes are moved in toward the chest to allow for patient movement with minimal muscle artifact. They are also placed on bony surfaces instead of muscle surfaces to minimize artifact (see Frame 66).

NOTE: The positive electrodes of leads II and III are usually placed lower on the chest wall than is indicated in the illustration above.

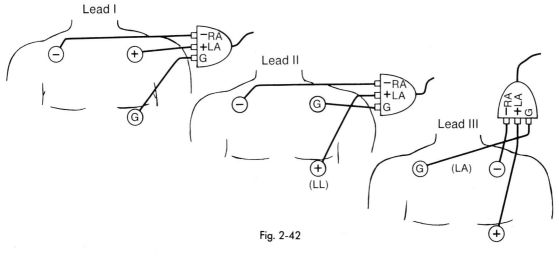

Fig. 2-42

REMEMBER: In *lead I* the positive electrode is on the _____ _____, and the negative electrode is on the _____ _____.

In *lead II* the positive electrode is on the _____ _____, and the negative electrode is on the _____ _____.

In *lead III* the positive electrode is on the _____

left arm
right arm
left leg
right arm

left leg

_____, and the negative electrode is on the _____   left arm
_____.

59 The negative and positive electrodes are usually identified by designations on the cable. These designations are far more useful in monitoring systems than the cable markings RA, LA, or LL, which are often best disregarded.

    NOTE: Once the cable ending that programs the _____ electrode is identified, it may be connected to   positive
electrodes placed in any limb position to obtain a *variety* of leads. A lead selector is not necessary. Systems recommending the RA, LA, and RL limb positions *require* moving the *positive electrode (LA)* to obtain leads other than lead I. Systems with the three major limb positions indicated on the cable (RA, LA, and LL) usually utilize a lead selector that automatically adjusts the positive and negative electrodes as required to obtain standard limb lead equivalents.

60 Chest lead equivalents also may be obtained from three-electrode monitoring systems.

    REMEMBER: The chest leads are *(unipolar/bipolar)* leads. Three-electrode monitoring systems function only as bipolar systems. Therefore the *chest lead* equivalents must be *modified (unipolar/bipolar) chest leads* and are referred to as MCL leads. The "CL" designation actually refers to "chest–left arm." These are the bipolar electrode positions used. The negative electrode is placed on the left arm. The positive electrode is placed in the appropriate "V," or chest, position and acts as the exploring or sensing electrode.

    REMEMBER: The most important electrode in a lead system is the *(negative/positive)* electrode. Fig. 2-43 illustrates the electrode positions   positive
mimicking standard leads V_1 and V_6. This modified chest lead system is referred to as _____ and _____. MCL_1; ; MCL_6

unipolar

bipolar

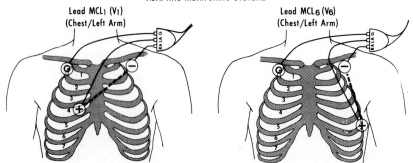

ADAPTING MONITORING SYSTEMS

Lead MCL_1 (V_1)
(Chest/Left Arm)

Lead MCL_6 (V_6)
(Chest/Left Arm)

Fig. 2-43

    NOTE: In monitoring systems without lead selection capabilities, the LA cable ending usually designates the positive electrode, and the RA cable ending usually designates the negative electrode. In systems

MCL lead equivalents is most easily accomplished by leaving the lead selector in the lead I position, thus designating the _____ cable ending as the positive electrode and the _____ cable ending as the negative electrode in a similar manner to the system previously described.

LA

RA

61 By obtaining equivalents of the standard ECG on the monitoring leads, we can initially detect many of the same changes on these leads and later verify them on a standard 12-lead ECG. This concept is particularly important because significant ECG changes are often transient and can be missed if not documented immediately. Whenever possible, a multilead record from the monitor is desirable (see Unit 7, Frames 184 to 187).

REMEMBER: The electrodes of lead systems sense the _____ and _____ of electrical forces and record _____ information.

magnitude; direction
surface

62 Multiple ECG views facilitate the interpretation of changes in the direction of electrical forces associated with such factors as bundle branch blocks, hemiblocks, and arrhythmias. Surface information is also significant because changes may indicate significant ischemia or infarct or both (see Unit 6). A record from each of the major surfaces should be obtained when a patient complains of chest pain.

REMEMBER: The inferior surface of the heart is reflected by leads _____, _____, and _____. The lateral surface of the heart is reflected by leads _____ and _____. The anteroseptal surface of the heart is reflected by leads _____ through _____, but especially V_2 and V_3.

II; III; aV_F

I

I; aV_L

V_1; V_4

63 The unipolar leads provide the most direct surface information. However, the bipolar equivalents are usually adequate in an emergency. Therefore, in a patient who has an acute MI or in a situation in which one needs to rule out a possible MI, electrodes should be kept in the LA (lead I-lateral position), LL (lead II-inferior position), and leads V_1 and V_2 or MCL_1 and MCL_2 (anterior position). When these patients complain of chest pain, a record should be obtained from each of these leads by adapting the cable endings to the appropriate electrode positions, as mentioned earlier.

64 A variety of other leads have also been adapted to facilitate a recording of specific ECG changes, for example, the Lewis lead for p waves. These leads are particularly popular for monitoring by telemetry in the convalescent period. However, these leads have the disadvantage of correlating less well with standard ECG records. *There is no single ideal monitoring lead for every patient.* For this reason, a multilead system

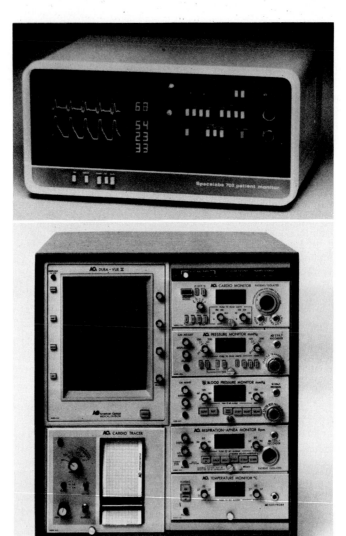

Fig. 2-44

is recommended. Although lead II usually records clear, upright p waves, lead V_2 may also record clear (although not necessarily upright) p waves in a given patient. Lead I often records less artifact in a mechanically ventilated patient than either V_1 or II because there is less movement of the positive electrode. Lead V_1 or its monitoring equivalent (MCL_1) often is helpful in detecting bundle branch blocks associated with acute AWMI (see Unit 6) or in detecting improper positioning of pacing catheters (see Unit 11). Acute myocardial injury requires multiple documentation. Thus the nurse is encouraged to use her own judgment in selecting the best monitoring lead for a given patient situation. This choice should be discussed with peers and the physician in charge of the patient.

65 LET US REVIEW: Cardiac monitoring systems require three major components: (1) _____, (2)_____ _____ and (3) _____ display.

electrodes; monitoring cables

oscilloscope

The oscilloscope dials in a monitoring system provide multiple options to facilitate arrhythmic diagnosis. Fig. 2-44 illustrates some of the most commonly available adjustments.

The *gain,* or *sensitivity,* dial adjusts the *amplitude* of the *trace.* The *position dial centers* the *trace.* The *rate meter* records an approximation of the *heart rate* and allows setting *high* and *low* alarms. The systole light allows for evaluation of monitor sensing. Modules for recording arterial and venous pressure and temperatures may also be added.

ECG ARTIFACTS

66 Electrical interference or poor electrical conduction can often distort the ECG trace. This distortion is referred to as *artifact.* A few examples of artifact are provided with corresponding corrective nursing action listed. To facilitate the listing or problem-solving steps, this information is not programmed.

Sixty-cycle interference artifact

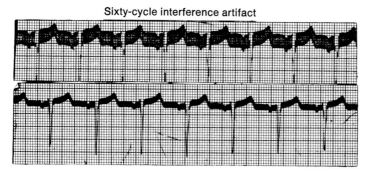

Fig. 2-45

NURSING ORDERS:

1. Check for crossing of cable wires with other electrical wires, such as calllight, bed-control, or transducer cables.
2. Check contact of cable with conductive parts of other electrical equipment, such as side rails of electrical beds or metal portions of ventilators.
3. Try momentarily pulling the plug of any other electrical equipment in contact with the patient.
4. Try turning the sensitivity (gain) control down to minimize the effect.
5. Check for loose connections at cable or electrode sites.
6. Try pressing on each electrode to temporarily improve contact. If baseline is corrected, change that electrode only. Check the positive electrode of each lead first.
7. If a wide baseline is present only on selected leads, solve the problem using the lead concept. For example, if the trace on leads II and III has a wide baseline but lead I does not, the faulty electrode or cable wire is designated by the LA cable ending.
8. Reapply new electrodes using a drying agent, such as alcohol, deodorant, or benzoin, if not previously used.
9. Rub the skin with a gauze pad or the abrasive tip on the disposable electrode, if not previously done, to lower skin resistance.
10. Needle electrodes can be tried.
11. Check for frayed or broken wires, and change the cable if indicated.
12. Try grounding electrical equipment with a ground wire.
13. If a five-lead cable is being used for three-lead monitoring, plug the cable's unused receptacles.
14. Remember when first connecting a patient to a monitor that has not been previously turned on, there may be a period of 60-cycle interference as the machine is "warming up."

MOVEMENT AND MUSCLE ACTIVITY ARTIFACT

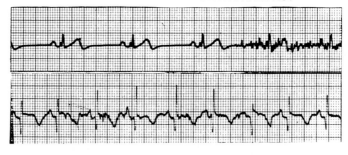

Fig. 2-46

NURSING ORDERS:

1. Check to see if the patient is moving or having tremors.
2. Prevent excessive cable movement by clipping the cable to the patient's clothing.
3. Ask the patient to hold still momentarily.
4. If artifact is still present, check to see whether the electrodes are positioned over skin folds, large muscle masses, large amounts of fatty tissue, or joints. If one is, move the electrode to another site.
5. Select another lead if necessary.
6. Do not attempt to diagnose atrial arrhythmias in the presence of this type of artifact.
7. For clues in differentiating ventricular arrhythmias, see Fig. 2-47.

ARTIFACT-MIMICKING VENTRICULAR ARRHYTHMIAS

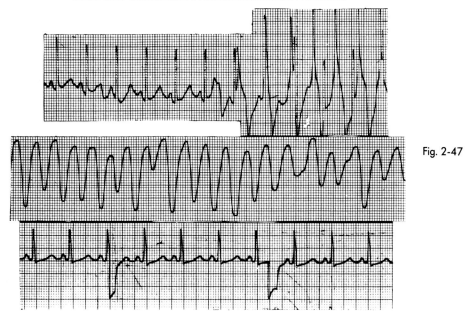

Fig. 2-47

NURSING ORDERS:

1. Never defibrillate from a tracing record before checking the patient for absence of pulse. Patient or cable movement artifact can mimic this pattern as well as tremors.
2. Premature ventricular contractions may be distinguished from artifactual QRS complexes if:
—They reset the natural QRS interval. Artifact does not.
—Sharp deflections coinciding with the QRS interval can be measured throughout the pattern change. (See trace in Fig. 2-48.)

WANDERING BASELINE ARTIFACTS

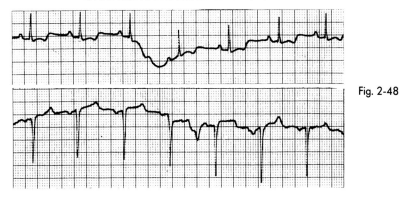

Fig. 2-48

1. Take measures to prevent excessive cable movement.
2. Note if the patient is moving.
3. Select another lead.
4. Select the monitoring rather than diagnostic mode on the monitor.
5. If the baseline is moving in a cyclic fashion, consider the possible effects of respiratory chest wall movement. Move the positive electrode away from the diaphragm (that is, higher) or change the lead.
6. Check to see if the electrodes are firmly attached to the skin. If not, reapply them with proper skin preparation.

RESPIRATORY ARTIFACT

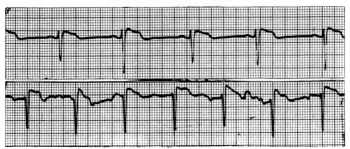

Fig. 2-49

NURSING ORDERS:

1. Differentiate these gradual ARS changes occurring with respiration from sudden, noncyclic QRS changes, which may indicate arrhythmias.
2. No action is indicated since this artifact is caused by normal movement of the heart with respiration. However, it usually can be abolished by switching to another lead.

SINUS RHYTHM DIAGNOSIS

67 A sinus rhythm is one that originates in the SA node.

LET US REVIEW the conduction of a sinus impulse (Fig. 2-50).

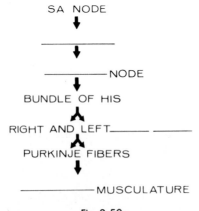

SA NODE

——————— NODE

BUNDLE OF HIS

RIGHT AND LEFT———— ————

PURKINJE FIBERS

——————— MUSCULATURE

Fig. 2-50

When interpreting rhythms, we suggest that the following systematic approach be used:
1. Analyze the QRS complex.
2. Analyze the P wave.
3. Analyze the relationship between the P wave and the QRS complex (PR interval).

68 Sinus rhythm is diagnosed according to the following criteria:
1. QRS complex—narrow and unchanging
2. P wave—visible preceding each QRS complex, upright (in lead II), no sudden irregularities in pp interval, P wave rate 150 or less
3. PR interval—a QRS complex following each P wave at constant intervals of normal duration
The most flexible of these criteria is the width of the QRS complex. Sinus rhythm can occur in the presence of an abnormal, or wide, QRS complex. Width merely implies that there is delay. A wide QRS complex occurring in a constant relationship with a normal P wave (as evidenced by a constant pr interval) means that the normal sinus impulse has been _____ in the ventricles. Sinus   **delayed**
rhythm can be diagnosed from a normal P wave alone because it implies that the impulse is of normal atrial origin (the SA node). A constant PR interval of normal duration serves primarily to verify that the sinus impulse is conducted normally.

69 LET US REVIEW: Sinus rhythm typically has a narrow and _____ QRS complex, a P wave that is *(positive/nega-*   **unchanging; positive**
tive) in lead II, and a PR interval that is constant and of
_____ duration. After the *origin* of a rhythm has   **normal**
been identified as sinus, it is further classified according to *discharge*
sequence, or _____ wave rate.   **P**

ATRIAL RATE

	ATRIAL RATE
NORMAL SINUS RHYTHM	60–100
SINUS BRADYCARDIA	LESS THAN 60
SINUS TACHYCARDIA	101 – 150

Fig. 2-51

In sinus rhythm, the atrial rate and the ventricular rate are usually the same, so the P wave rate will correspond to the more easily measured QRS rate.

70 Measurement of ventricular rate is made from one QRS complex to the next QRS complex.

NOTE: When measuring ventricular rate, we may use any component of the QRS complex as a reference point. However, the measurement must be made between two consistent points; that is, R to R, Q to Q, or S to S.

Let us now discuss the calculation of ventricular rates. ECG paper is divided by markings into intervals that represent spans of 3 seconds (Fig. 2-44). The ventricular rate for 1 minute may be estimated rapidly by counting the number of R waves occurring in a 6-second span and multiplying this number by 10. This figure will give the number of R waves occurring in 60 seconds, the _____ rate for 1 minute.

ventricular

The ventricular rate for 1 minute may also be obtained by multiplying the number of R waves occurring in one 3-second span by _____.

20

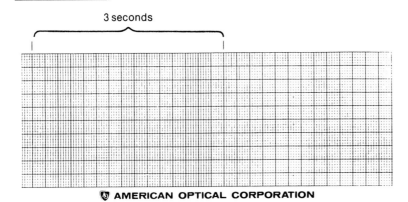

3 seconds

🛡 AMERICAN OPTICAL CORPORATION

Fig. 2-52

71 The ventricular rate in the following 6-second ECG strip is approximately _____.

70

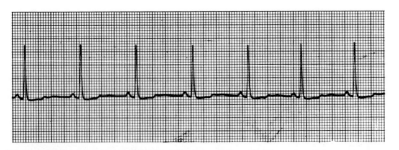

Fig. 2-53

72 A more accurate method for estimating rates also has been devised. We suggest that the student follow these steps when calculating rates: (1) obtain an ECG rhythm strip, and (2) look for an R wave that falls on a dark line or at the beginning of a larger box. The rate will be estimated from this point.

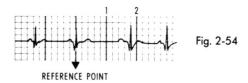

Fig. 2-54

REFERENCE POINT

Consider this R wave to be a reference point.

73 Each dark line occurring after the "R wave reference point" has been assigned a value. Therefore it is necessary for the student to memorize the values of each subsequent line:

Line	Value
1	300
2	150
3	100
4	75
5	60
6	50
7	43
8	37
9	33

74 Consider this ECG strip:

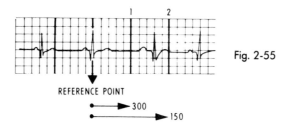

Fig. 2-55

REFERENCE POINT

→ 300

→ 150

NOTE: On an ECG recording at a standard paper speed of 25 mm per second, each large box (between two dark lines) = 0.20 second. Each small box (between two light-colored lines) = 0.04 second. Therefore, if a QRS complex occurs on every dark line, it means a ventricular impulse is occuring every 0.20 second, or 300 times per minute (60 sec/min ÷ 0.20 sec/beat).

75 The ventricular rate can be estimated as follows: if an R wave falls on the first dark line that occurs after the reference point, the value is 300, and the ventricular rate then equals _____ beats per minute. If an R wave falls on the second dark line occurring after the reference point, the value is _____, and the ventricular rate is then _____ beats per minute.

300

150

150

NOTE: Ventricular rate is measured between two points, or beats. The first is the "R wave reference point," and the second is the very next occurring beat.

76 Let us practice estimating ventricular rates. The ventricular rate in Fig. 2-56 is _____

100

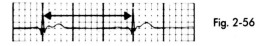

Fig. 2-56

The ventricular rate in Fig. 2-57 is _____.

75

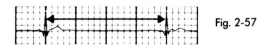

Fig. 2-57

77 NOTE: Each large box is composed of five smaller boxes. These smaller components must be considered when calculating rates that fall between the preassigned values.

Look at this example

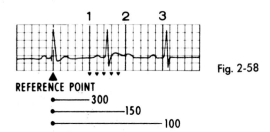

Fig. 2-58

78 The first complex that occurs after the reference point is located between line _____ and line _____.

1; 2

REMEMBER: Line 1 = 300 and line 2 = 150. Therefore the ventricular rate in this example falls between _____ and _____ beats per minute. The rate is *(less than/greater than)* 150, and is *(less than/greater than)* 300.

150

300; greater than
less than

79 To obtain the value of the space between these two lines, *subtraction* is used.

In Fig. 2-58:

Line 1	=	300
Line 2	=	150
		150

So there are 150 unit values between line 1 and line 2.

80 REMEMBER: There are five smaller boxes within each large box *or* between two dark lines. To obtain the value of each small box, division is used.

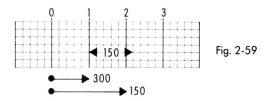

Fig. 2-59

In Fig. 2-59:

$$\frac{\text{Difference between lines 1 and 2}}{\text{Number of small boxes}} = \frac{150}{5} = 30$$

Each small box then equals _____.   30

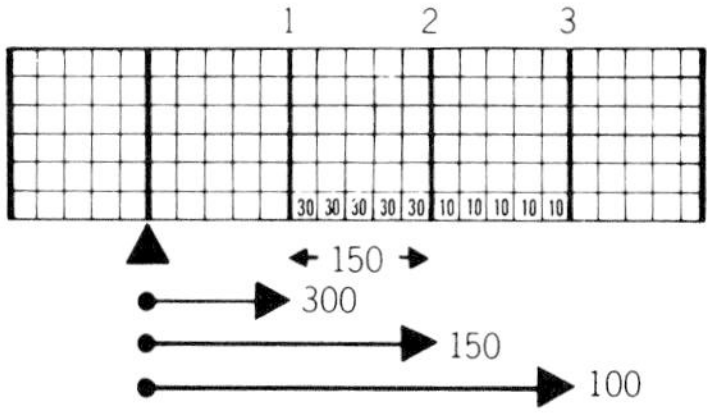

Fig. 2-60

Between lines 2 and 3 = $\underline{50}$ (rate difference) = 10
Number of small boxes = $\overline{5}$

81 Evaluate this practice strip:

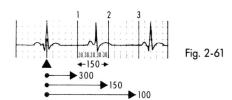

Fig. 2-61

The first complex after the reference point falls between lines 1 and 2. Therefore the rate must be between _____ and   150
_____ beats per minute. Each small square equals   300
_____.   30

82 The second complex falls on the second small box past 150. Therefore the rate would be *(greater than/less than)* 150 per minute.   greater than
Two small boxes = 2 × 30, or _____. Add this number   60
to the value of line 2.

$$\begin{array}{rl} \text{Line 2} & = 150 \\ \text{Small boxes} & = \underline{+60} \\ & 210 \end{array}$$

The ventricular rate, then, is _____ beats per minute.   210

83 When interpreting the ECG strip, we must also measure the *PR interval.*

The PR interval is measured from the beginning of the wave _____ to the beginning of the _____ _____.   P; QRS complex

REMEMBER: The PR interval extends from the beginning of _____ depolarization to the beginning of _____ depolarization.   atrial
ventricular

84 On graph paper, one large box equals *0.20 second.* Each large box is divided into five smaller boxes. Therefore each small box equals _____ second.   0.04

To determine the PR interval, the number of small boxes occurring during the period is multiplied by 0.04 second.

85 Look at this example:

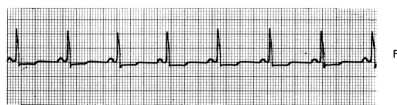

Fig. 2-62

Using the second complex from the end as clearest, we note that the number of small boxes in the PR interval equals three. The PR interval here equals _____ seconds.   0.12

NOTE: The normal PR interval is from 0.12 to 0.20 second.

The example in this trace may be diagnosed as normal sinus rhythm because the QRS complex is _____ and _____, the p wave is _____, upright and *(regular/irregular),* with a rate less than _____, and the pr interval is *(normal/abnormal).* For examples and discussion of sinus bradycardia and sinus tachycardia refer to Unit 7.

narrow
unchanging; visible
regular; 150
normal

SUGGESTED READINGS

Ambutas S: A teaching module: EKG interpretation in acute myocardial infarction, Crit Care Update 10(4):48, 1983.

Bryant M: Deciperhing the EKG's code, Nephrol Nurs, 2(6):297, 1985.

Caine R: Essentials of monitoring the electrocardiogram, Nurs Clin North Am 22(1):77, 1987.

Chase KM: Use vectors to round out an ECG, RN 49(3):18, 1986.

Cheung P: Cardiac monitoring at a distance, Nurs Times 82(1):51, 1986.

Conover MB: Understanding electrocardiography, ed 5, St. Louis, 1988, The CV Mosby Co.

Decker S: Continous EKG monitoring systems, Nurs Clin North Am 22(1):1, March 1987.

An Electrode Sampler, Am J Nurs 84(5):644E, May 1984.

Fought SG: Holter monitoring and electrophysiologic study, Crit Care Nurse 7(1):8, 1987.

Goldberg K., editor: Cardiac problems: Nurse Review, Springhouse, Pa, 1987, Springhouse Corp.

Hurst WJ and Logue RB, editors: The heart, arteries, and veins, ed. 6, New York, 1986, McGraw-Hill, Inc.

Hill NE and Goodman JS: Importance of accurate placement of precordial leads in the 12-lead electrocardiogram, Heart Lung 16(5):561, 1987.

Huang S et al: Coronary care nursing, Philadelphia, 1983, WB Saunders Co.

Jowett NI: Electrocardigraphic monitoring: I—static monitoring, Intensive Care Nurs 1(2):71, 1985.

Jowett NI et al: Electrocardiographic monitoring II—ambulatory monitoring, Intensive Care Nurs 1(3):123, 1986.

Krasover T: A Conceptual approach to the electrocardiogram, Crit Care Nurse 2(2):66-76, 1982.

Marriott HJ: Practical electrocardiography, ed. 7, Baltimore, 1983, William & Wilkins.

Nottingham A et al: Remote cardiac monitoring: nursing collaboration is the key, Dimens Crit Care Nurse 6(3):176, 1987.

Schamroth, L: An introduction to electrocardiography, ed 6, Edinburgh, 1982, Blackwell Scientific Publications, Inc.

Scheidt S: Basic electrocardiography: leads, axes, arrhythmias, Clin Symp, 35:2, 1982.

Sergeant LL: Tracking your outpatient's EKG with a Holter monitor, Nursing 16(10):47, 1986.

Suazo N: Is there a best lead system?, Crit Care Update 10(8):24-26, 1983.

Sumner SM: Guidelines for running a 12-lead ECG, Nursing 49(5):32, 1986.

West SW et al: Using monitors (nursing photobook), Horsham, Pa, 1981, Intermed Communications, Inc.

Oxygenation

TISSUE OXYGENATION

1 Tissue oxygenation depends on three factors: (1) the *oxygen demands* of the tissues, (2) the *blood supply* to the tissues each minute, and (3) the *oxygen supply* within that blood. The amount of oxygen used by the tissues each minute is also known as the *tissue O_2 consumption*. This amount directly reflects the oxygen demands that are determined by the cells' metabolic needs at the time. The terms "O_2 demand" and "O_2 consumption" are often used interchangeably. The available oxygen supply within the blood is determined by the integrity of the pulmonary system and hemoglobin (RBC) content of the blood.

2 REMEMBER: In an attempt to meet the demands of the tissues, the heart pumps out a certain amount of oxygenated blood each minute. This amount of blood that the heart puts out is known as the

_____ _____.

    Tissue O_2 consumption is directly dependent on the tissue O_2 _____ and indirectly dependent on the blood supply, or _____ _____, and the _____ supply within that blood.

    The cardiac output is determined by the integrity of the _____ system. The O_2 supply is maintained by the integrity of the _____ system. Inadequate tissue oxygenation in the patient with coronary artery disease can occur as a result of either decreased cardiac output or pulmonary congestion, or of _____ metabolic demands.

cardiac output

demands
cardiac output
O_2

cardiovascular
pulmonary

increased

Hypoxia and hypoxemia

3 Inadequate oxygenation is detected from signs and symptoms of either *hypoxia* or *hypoxemia*. The state in which there is a critically low Po_2 (that is, less than 60 mm Hg) and a potentially lowered O_2 content in the *blood* is known as *hypoxemia*. The state in which there is insufficient oxygen at the *tissue* level is known as *hypoxia* (Fig. 3-1).

    Hypoxemia is initially determined from alterations in the arterial Po_2 reported on an arterial blood gas sample. The arterial Po_2 is then correlated with the O_2 saturation levels as well as serum hemoglobin levels to determine the O_2 content. A critically low O_2 saturation is

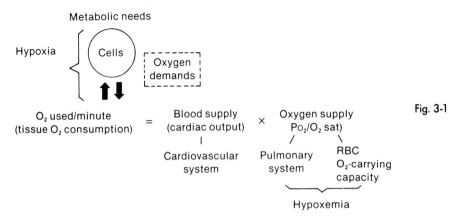

DETERMINANTS OF TISSUE OXYGENATION

Fig. 3-1

$$\begin{array}{c}
O_2 \text{ used/minute} \\
(\text{tissue } O_2 \text{ consumption})
\end{array} = \begin{array}{c}
\text{Blood supply} \\
(\text{cardiac output})
\end{array} \times \begin{array}{c}
\text{Oxygen supply} \\
(P_{O_2}/O_2 \text{ sat})
\end{array}$$

usually less than 90% (see Frame 22). Hypoxia is determined from the signs and symptoms of inadequate _____ tissue oxygenation.

4 Inadequate tissue oxygenation is manifested by cellular metabolic changes and cerebral symptoms. Significant tissue hypoxia will result in cellular metabolic changes leading to acidosis, which may be detected from the pH and bicarbonate values tested on either an arterial or venous blood gas sample (see Unit 5).

Tissue hypoxia also results in cerebral symptoms because of the sensitivity of the brain to lack of oxygen. These symptoms include restlessness, agitation, irritability, syncope, and alterations of consciousness. Dizziness, tremors, or convulsions may also occur. These cerebral symptoms may be referred to collectively as *sensorium changes*.

The alterations in consciousness may be divided into two categories: (1) alterations in mental function, such as confusion and disorientation; or (2) alterations in arousal, such as lethargy, stupor, and coma.

5 Alterations in consciousness, restlessness, agitation, dizziness, and confusion may be referred to collectively as _____ sensorium changes _____. These symptoms are associated with the cerebral effects of *(hypoxemia/hypoxia)*. hypoxia

Hypoxia is also detected by changes in the _____ and pH _____ values tested on blood gas samples. bicarbonate

6 Symptoms associated with reflex cardiovascular and respiratory responses may accompany either hypoxia or hypoxemia. These symptoms occur as the result of chemical stimulation of nerve receptor areas known as *chemoreceptors*.

The central chemoreceptors, located in the medullary area of the brain stem, respond to the changes in pH associated with *(hypoxia/hypoxemia)*. The peripheral chemoreceptors, located in the aorta and carotid arteries, respond to the changes in arterial P_{O_2} associated with *(hypoxia/hypoxemia)*.

hypoxia

hypoxemia

NOTE: The peripheral chemoreceptors also may respond to hypoxia resulting from severe drops in cardiac output (see Unit 4, Frames 39 to 42).

7 As the result of chemoreceptor stimulation, the sympathetic nervous system and the cardiovascular and respiratory centers are activated. The *cardiovascular* response includes an elevated blood pressure, tachycardia, cool and moist skin, and decreased urine output. The *respiratory* response includes increased respiratory rate and increased respiratory effort, evidenced by the individual's use of accessory muscles during inspiration and diaphragmatic muscles in forced expiration.

NOTE: Selective activation of the carotid chemoreceptors may cause a paradoxical bradycardia in ventilated patients.

8 When cardiovascular disorders that result in a fall in cardiac output cause the hypoxic state, it is said that the patient is experiencing a _____ _____ in cardiac output (see Unit 1, frames 7 and 8). The symptoms directly resulting from cardiovascular disturbance may differ slightly from those typically associated with hypoxia. The blood pressure, which indicates gross cardiovascular function, is more typically low, and the heart rate may be slow as well as fast because either may be the cause of the decreased cardiac output. The clinical state of hypoxia that results from inadequate cardiac output is also known as *shock* (see Unit 9, frames 117-150).

symptomatic fall

9 LET US REVIEW: Cardiovascular or respiratory symptoms or both may be associated with either hypoxemia or hypoxia. These symptoms occur as the result of _____ stimulation. The cardiovascular symptoms include _____ _____ _____, _____, _____ _____ _____, and _____ _____ _____. The respiratory symptoms include _____ _____ _____, _____ _____, and _____ _____.

chemoreceptor
increased blood pressure
tachycardia; cool moist skin
decreased urine output

increased respiratory rate
forced inspiration; forced
   expiration

Cardiovascular symptoms may also be associated with a direct cardiovascular disturbance. In this case the blood pressure is more typically *(high/low)*, and the heart rate may be either _____ or _____. Hypoxia that is caused by a direct cardiovascular disorder results in a _____ fall in _____ _____ and is also referred to as _____.

low; fast
slow
symptomatic; cardiac
   output

shock

Relationship of hypoxia to hypoxemia

10 Hypoxemia is defined as a lowered O_2 content in the
_____, as reflected by a critically low arterial
_____. Hypoxia is defined as insufficient oxygen at the
_____ level.

    Inadequate tissue oxygen may be caused by a decreased
_____ supply as well as a decreased O_2 supply. In
the patient who has an acute MI, hypoxia without hypoxemia is usually associated with a decreased *(blood/oxygen)* supply, or decreased
_____ output.

    Hypoxia in the absence of hypoxemia can also be associated with
an increase in tissue metabolism and thus in O_2 demands.

blood
P_{O_2}
tissue

blood

blood
cardiac

11 Hypoxia typically occurs as a consequence of hypoxemia. Hypoxemia
occurs in the presence of the pulmonary congestion associated with
congestive heart failure, which results in impaired pulmonary oxygen transport. The effectiveness of oxygen transport in the lungs is
best evaluated by assessing the arterial P_{O_2}. Hypoxemia related to
pulmonary congestion may lead to hypoxia in patients who have a
compromised myocardium because they are unable to compensate
for the decreased oxygen in the blood with an increase in cardiac output.

    The arterial P_{O_2} and O_2 saturation reflect the presence
of *(hypoxemia/hypoxia)*. The arterial P_{O_2} more specifically reflects _____ causes of hypoxemia. The P_{O_2} and O_2
saturation can be normal in the hypoxic patient if the
_____ _____ is low and the
lungs are *(normal/abnormal)*.

hypoxemia
pulmonary

cardiac output
normal

12 Hypoxia *(can/cannot)* occur in the absence of hypoxemia. Hypoxemia
(can/cannot) occur in the absence of hypoxia. However, in the patient
who has an acute MI, hypoxemia often leads to hypoxia because of an
inability to increase _____ _____.

can
can

cardiac output

EVALUATING OXYGEN TRANSPORT IN THE LUNGS: ROLE OF Pa_{O_2}

13 Although the arterial P_{O_2} (Pa_{O_2}) may be used as an indicator of adequate O_2 content based on an assumed correlation with the O_2 saturation, its major value is in evaluating altered O_2 transport in the
lungs as a potential cause of hypoxemia.

    The arterial P_{O_2} (Pa_{O_2}) reflects the _____ of the
oxygen dissolved in solution.

    The pressure of the dissolved oxygen in the arterial blood de-
pends on the pressure of O_2 gas delivered to the alveolus as well as
the integrity of the *alveolar capillary membrane.*

pressure

14 Room air is 21% oxygen. The *fraction* of the *inspired* air (100% or 1.00 gas) that is composed of oxygen gas is 0.21. A term that is frequently used clinically to express the inspired O_2 concentration is the FI_{O2} or *fraction of inspired oxygen.*

NOTE: The remainder of the gases in room air include nitrogen, water vapor, and *minimal* amounts of carbon dioxide. (At sea level, a gas that completely fills the atmosphere exerts a barometric pressure of 760 mm Hg)

The pressure of the oxygen delivered to the alveolus appears initially to be identical with the pressure corresponding with the FI_{O2}.

At room air the inspired O_2 pressure is 159 mm Hg (760 mm Hg × 0.21). However, CO_2 particles occupy the alveolar spaces, limiting the available space for oxygen. Carbon dioxide is generated as a byproduct of cellular metabolism and is carried to the lungs in the blood plasma. Because only minimal amounts of it are contained in the inspired air delivered to the alveolus, carbon dioxide diffuses out of the blood into the alveolar spaces.

REMEMBER: Diffusion is the movement of particles from an area of _____ concentration to an area of _____ concentration.

greater
lesser

15 The CO_2 particles in the alveolar gas exert a pressure of 40 mm Hg, and when combined with the water vapor pressure allow for only a little more than 100 mm Hg to be occupied by oxygen. In normal lungs this oxygen should diffuse into the capillary blood, fully saturating the hemoglobin and allowing the pressure of the particles in solution to equalize at a pressure of _____ mm Hg. Thus, at an FI_{O2} of 0.21 (21%), the alveolar P_{O2} (PA_{O2}) and expected arterial P_{O2} (Pa_{O2}) in the presence of normal lungs is _____ mm Hg.

100

100

OXYGEN TRANSPORT IN LUNGS
Role of Pa_{O_2}

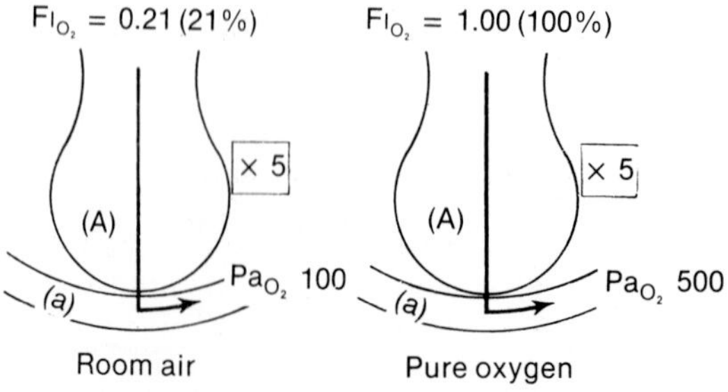

FI_{O_2} = 0.21 (21%) FI_{O_2} = 1.00 (100%)

× 5   × 5

(A)   (A)

(a)   (a)

Pa_{O_2} 100 Pa_{O_2} 500

Fig. 3-2

Room air   Pure oxygen

Alveolar-arterial oxygen difference
(A-aDO_2 or A-a gradient)

NOTE: The actual Pa_{O_2} is normally at 10 to 20 mm Hg less than the alveolar Po_2 due to normal disparities in the alveolar capillary membrane. Thus the normal Pa_{O_2} on room air ranges from 80-100 mm Hg.

16 At an $F_{I_{O_2}}$ of 1.00 (100%), O_2 particles completely fill the atmosphere. Therefore at sea level they should exert a pressure of _____. Only carbon dioxide and water vapor occupy the air passages, which limits the available space for oxygen. The CO_2 and water vapor particles combined exert a pressure of 87 mm Hg, which allows 673 mm Hg to be occupied by oxygen. In normal lungs, this oxygen should diffuse into the capillary blood, fully saturating the hemoglobin and allowing the pressure of the particles in solution to equalize at a pressure of _____ mm Hg. However, even in normal lungs some blood vessels completely bypass the alveoli and do not receive oxygen. Allowing for this normal limitation in gas exchange and the presence of minimal disease, the alveolar Po_2 (Pa_{O_2}) and expected Pa_{O_2} at an $F_{I_{O_2}}$ of 1.00 (100%) is at least 500 mm Hg (Fig. 3-2), or five times the $F_{I_{O_2}}$.

760 mm Hg

673

NOTE: The normal Pa_{O_2} of 100 mm Hg in room air is also at least five times the $F_{I_{O_2}}$ (0.21). Therefore it can be assumed that *at any* $F_{I_{O_2}}$ between room air and 1.00 (100%), the *expected* Pa_{O_2} *should be approximately five times the* $F_{I_{O_2}}$. (More accurate calculation processes verify this predicted correlation. However, this correlation is less accurate the higher the $F_{I_{O_2}}$ and is therefore only a gross initial assessment tool.)

17 The difference between the *alveolar* Po_2 (Pa_{O_2}) and the actual *arterial* Po_2 (P_{O_2}) is known as the *alveolar-arterial* O_2 *difference* (A-aD_{O_2}), or the *A-a gradient* (Fig. 3-2). This gradient is normally _____ mm Hg. The presence of an abnormal A-aD_{O_2} can be assumed in the presence of any Pa_{O_2} lower than expected for its corresponding $F_{I_{O_2}}$. Significant gradients can lead to hypoxemia.

10-20

18 LET US REVIEW: The Pa_{O_2} and Pa_{O_2} is predicted from the _____ and is then correlated with an actual Pa_{O_2}. The predicted normal Pa_{O_2} is _____ times the $F_{I_{O_2}}$. At an $F_{I_{O_2}}$ of 0.40 (40%), the expected Pa_{O_2} is _____. If the patient's actual arterial Po_2 is 100 mm Hg, interference with gas transport is present, resulting in an abnormal alveolar-arterial O_2 difference of approximately _____ mm Hg (i.e., 200 −100 mm Hg). At a lower $F_{I_{O_2}}$ hypoxemia (ie. Pa_{O_2} < 60 mm Hg) would actually be present.

$F_{I_{O_2}}$
five
200 mmHg

100 mmHg

The arterial Po_2 depends on the _____ of the oxygen delivered to the _____ and the presence or absence of airway obstruction as well as the integrity of the _____

concentration
alveoli
alveolar-capillary

_____ membrane. Thus an abnormally large A-a gradient is indicative of significant _____ pathology interfering with gas transport.

pulmonary

19 Alveolar-capillary changes contributing to a widened A-a gradient and hypoxia (Pa_{O_2} lower than expected for a given FI_{O_2}) include the following changes in pulmonary function: (1) alveolar collapse or compression; (2) alveolar congestion with mucus, fluid, or both; (3) interstitial fluid accumulation; (4) bronchospasm; (5) emboli; and (6) alterations in pulmonary blood flow associated with changes in cardiac output (see also frames 38-43).

Pulmonary edema caused by congestive heart failure (CHF) *(does/ does not)* interfere with O_2 transport across the alveolar-capillary membrane. Therefore in the presence of CHF with pulmonary edema the Pa_{O_2} is usually *(high/low/normal)*, and the A-a gradient is thus *(high/low/ normal)*. In the presence of alveolar-capillary changes O_2 transport is limited, and supplementary oxygen is often necessary to maintain the Pa_{O_2} at the minimal critical level of 60 mm Hg.

does

low; high

REMEMBER: A Pa_{O_2} of _____ mm Hg usually is necessary to adequately saturate the hemoglobin (O_2 saturation 90%).

60

20 Although a Pa_{O_2} of 60 mm Hg may be adequate for maintaining O_2 saturation and blood O_2 supply to the tissues, maintenance of a higher alveolar Po_2 (such as 80 to 100 mm Hg) may become necessary to prevent pulmonary vascular changes. The pulmonary capillary vessels constrict in the presence of low alveolar O_2 tensions in an attempt to redirect the blood flow away from poorly oxygenated areas. As a result of this constriction, the pulmonary vascular resistance *(increases/ decreases)*. Pulmonary artery pressures also *(increase/decrease)*, placing an increased load on the *(right/left)* side of the heart. This increased work load can affect the total myocardial oxygen consumption and cause or aggravate existing heart failure.

increases

increase

right

21 In patients who have acute MI, administration of supplementary oxygen is desirable, in concentrations sufficient to maintain the Pa_{O_2} at approximately 80 to 100 mm Hg.

Unnecessary administration of supplementary oxygen may present a potential hazard to the patient who has coronary artery disease. Coronary vasoconstriction has been reported in patients who have a Pa_{O_2} exceeding 100 mm Hg. For this reason some authors recommend routine analysis of the arterial blood gas (ABG) of all patients receiving oxygen in a coronary care unit.

In the patient with chronic obstructive pulmonary disease (COPD), whose respiratory drive depends on a low Pa_{O_2}, the level of 60 mm Hg is preferred.

MAINTAINING OXYGENATION
Oxygen therapy

22 Minimal amounts of supplementary oxygen are usually adequate in maintaining blood O_2 levels in the patient who has an acute MI, even in the presence of moderate CHF. Low-flow O_2 systems, such as nasal prongs (cannula), are relatively comfortable and provide an average $F_{I_{O_2}}$ range between 25% and 40%, depending on the patient's respiratory pattern. Irregular patterns may cause this amount to fluctuate from breath to breath.

Several factors should be considered when selecting appropriate modes of O_2 therapy. These include the following:
1. Degree of hypoxemia, pulmonary dysfunction, or both
2. The desired $F_{I_{O_2}}$
3. The need for a constant $F_{I_{O_2}}$
4. Patient comfort
5. Patient's respiratory pattern (whether breathing is regular, irregular, labored)
6. The need for concurrent moisture and respiratory support (in the absence of spontaneous respiration) as well as oxygen
7. The presence of a hypoxic respiratory drive because of chronic CO_2 retention
8. ABG response to previously used O_2 measures

Table 5 compares and contrasts the different modes of O_2 therapy that might be used in a coronary care unit.

23 As with any other drug, oxygen has the potential for being both therapeutic and toxic. The toxic actions of oxygen affect not only the lungs but also the liver, kidneys, myocardium, eyes, and red blood cells. In patients who have coronary artery disease, for example, unnecessary or excessive administration of oxygen may cause premature ventricular contractions (PVCs) because of constriction of the coronary arteries. Toxic pulmonary changes include atelectasis and increased capillary permeability with pulmonary edema. The amount of oxygen toxic to lung tissue remains controversial. *Significant* damage probably does not occur until inspired-O_2 concentrations of more than 50% with their corresponding high alveolar oxygen pressures have been delivered for periods longer than 24 hours. However, after sufficient oxygen has been delivered to saturate the hemoglobin maximally and result in a Pa_{O_2} of 80 to 100 mm Hg, the benefit obtained by extended exposure to larger inspired-O_2 concentrations is questionable. Exposure to 100% O_2 concentration can cause temporary atelectasis, which may further compromise oxygenation.

NOTE: Oxygen should never be withheld during a cardiac arrest for fear of either O_2 toxicity or respiratory depression.

24 LET US REVIEW: O_2 administration has both _____ and _____ effects.

therapeutic

toxic

The toxic actions of oxygen may affect the _____, _____, _____, myocardium, eyes, and _____ _____. In patients who have coronary artery disease, excessive O_2 administration may cause coronary _____ and _____.

lungs; kidney; liver

red blood cells

artery constriction

PVCs

The factors to be considered when selecting a mode of O_2 therapy for the patient in a coronary care unit include:

1. The need for constant _____

$F_{I_{O_2}}$

Table 5. Modes of oxygen administration in the patient without intubation or tracheotomy

O_2 system	Liter flow	$F_{I_{O_2}}$	Advantages	Potential disadvantages
1. Nasal cannula/prongs or nasal catheter	6 L	25% to 40%	Most comfortable, simplest	$F_{I_{O_2}}$ varies with respiratory pattern ($\downarrow$ with $\uparrow$ rate and depth)
2. Face masks	8-10 L	40% to 60%	Higher $F_{I_{O_2}}$	Less comfortable and falls off easier than cannula
3. Face tents	15 L	82% to 88%	Higher $F_{I_{O_2}}$; more comfortable than face mask; better tolerated; less variation with respiratory pattern	Can fall off
4. Mask with reservoir (partial rebreathing mask)	10-12 L	60% to 100%	High $F_{I_{O_2}}$	Less comfortable
5. Ventimask	4 L	24%, 35%, 28%, 40%	Less variation with respiratory pattern because of flow that fills lungs more completely; greater range of selection for $F_{I_{O_2}}$, especially in low ranges	$F_{I_{O_2}}$ may still vary slightly (for example, 21% to 23%); highly uncomfortable
6. Face mask with nebulizer at 100% setting	10 L	26% to 39% or 41% to 53% or 42% to 62%	Greater range of selection for $F_{I_{O_2}}$ especially in high ranges; provides particulate moisture as well as O_2	$F_{I_{O_2}}$ still varies with respiration (diluted with rate and depth)

2. Patient _____   comfort
3. The patient's _____ pattern   respiratory
4. _____ response to previously used O_2 measures   ABG

ROLE OF PULMONARY FUNCTION IN MAINTAINING OXYGENATION

25 The major function of the lungs is exchanging oxygen and carbon dioxide between the blood and the external environment. This process may be referred to as *external respiration*. The process of exchanging oxygen and carbon dioxide between the blood and the tissue cells is

Table 5. Modes of oxygen administration in the patient without intubation or tracheotomy—cont'd

O_2 system	Liter flow	FI_{O_2}	Advantages	Potential disadvantages
7. Face mask with nebulizer at 100% setting plus nasal prongs	15 L each	66% to 86%	Higher FI_{O_2}	FI_{O_2} still varies with respiration
Manual resuscitators				
8. Bag-valve mask resuscitator (Ambu/ Hope/Air-Shields) with O_2 reservoir cap over inlet	O_2 source at "flush"	90%-100%	No spontaneous respiration required; more aseptic for rescuer than mouth-to-mouth; extra O_2 can be provided to O_2 source	Difficult to obtain seal; tidal volume may be less than by mouth-to-mouth
9. O_2-powered mechanical resuscitator (Elder valve/Robert Shaw)	100 L/min	100%	Less effort required for rescuer	Rescuer unable to feel changes in resistance because of obstruction; can cause gastric distention; not recommended for less than age 12 because of inspiratory pressures (40 mm Hg)

referred to as *internal respiration*. The process of exchanging oxygen and carbon dioxide between the blood and the tissue cells is referred to as *internal respiration*. Internal respiration occurs as a consequence of external respiration (Fig. 3-3), and also is dependent upon cardiac function.

External respiration depends on the processes of: (1) *ventilation* (movement of air), (2) *perfusion* (movement of blood), and (3) *diffusion* (movement of gas particles between air and blood).

26 The pulmonary structures are composed of airways that serve mainly to transport the air (structures of _____) and airways that actually come into contact with the blood and participate in gas exchange (structures of _____). The structures of ventilation are also known as *conducting airways* because their major function is to _____ air.

ventilation

respiration

transport

These structures heat, humidify, and filter as well as transport the O_2-containing air. The structures of ventilation include the upper airways (nasopharynx) the larynx, the trachea, the bronchi, and the larger bronchioles. These airways subdivide into smaller airways, assuming a treelike appearance. The *last* level of bronchioles before gas exchange takes place is known as the *terminal* bronchiole level.

27 The gas-exchange, or *respiratory*, airways include the respiratory bronchioles, the alveolar ducts, and the alveolar sacs.

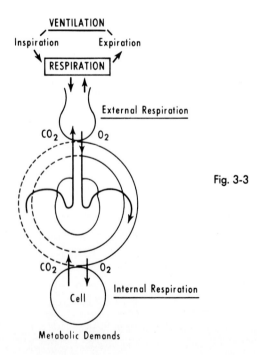

Fig. 3-3

REMEMBER: Respiration depends on _____ and _____. Therefore these airways *(are/are not)* in contact with the blood. Their cell membranes must also be permeable to gas particles so that movement of these particles, or _____, can take place (Fig. 3-4).

ventilation
perfusion; are

diffusion

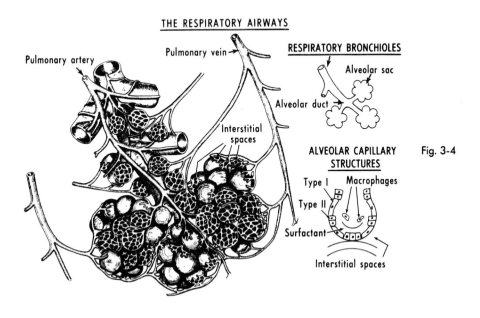

THE RESPIRATORY AIRWAYS

Pulmonary artery

Pulmonary vein

RESPIRATORY BRONCHIOLES

Alveolar sac

Alveolar duct

Interstitial spaces

ALVEOLAR CAPILLARY STRUCTURES

Type I Macrophages

Type II

Surfactant

Interstitial spaces

Fig. 3-4

The alveoli contain three types of cells. Types I and II, pneumocytes, alternate to form the alveolar lining. Macrophages act as scavengers, floating between alveoli to remove foreign substances that have not been filtered by the _____ airways. The *Type II penumocytes* secrete the substance *surfactant,* which forms a film that lines the inner surface of the alveoli. Surfactant lowers the surface tension of the alveoli, limiting their tendency to collapse at low volumes, that is, on *(inspiration/expiration).*

conducting

expiration

28 The alveoli and the respiratory bronchioles are wrapped by meshes of capillaries that come into contact with the lung cells at key sites (Fig. 3-9). In between these key contact points, large interstitial spaces exist, which may accumulate fluid. Thus the interstitial fluid spaces in the lung exist not only between the capillaries and the contact points with the alveolar surface but also between the capillaries themselves. The *lymphatic system* constantly drains this interstitial fluid space, exerting a *vacuum effect.*

The movement of gas particles across the alveolar-capillary membrane is limited by any fluid accumulation in this interstitial space, particularly in the small spaces between the alveolar and capillary contact surfaces. Diffusion of oxygen and carbon dioxide is also limited by the permeability of the alveolar-capillary membrane. This membrane permits carbon dioxide to diffuse more easily than oxygen. Therefore in the presence of pulmonary congestion interference with *(O$_2$/CO$_2$)* transport occurs first. Hypoxemia occurs before CO$_2$ retention and is usually severe when there is CO$_2$ retention. The presence of CO$_2$ retention in the patient who has pulmonary congestion caused by heart failure is usually an indicator of *(mild/severe)* congestion (see Unit 5, Frame 89).

O$_2$

severe

29 Like the heart the primary function of the lungs is *(electrical/mechanical)*. It serves as a pump to deliver oxygen to the blood and to remove carbon dioxide from it in an attempt to meet _____ demands.

mechanical

metabolic

30 The normal stimulus for respiration is the level of carbon dioxide in the blood and the cerebrospinal fluid. CO$_2$ levels are sensed by specialized chemically sensitive nerve cells located in the brain stem on either side of the medulla. These cells are known as *chemoreceptors* and are bathed by the cerebrospinal fluid. The chemoreceptors in the brain are sensitive to changes in the hydrogen ion (H$^+$) concentration as well as CO$_2$ levels. In the presence of an increased CO$_2$ level, nerve signals are transmitted from these cells to the inspiratory center in the medulla.

   The chemoreceptors are _____ sensitive cells in the brain that are stimulated by changes in _____ levels and _____ ion concentration.

chemically
CO$_2$
hydrogen

31 Chemically sensitive sensory nerve fibers that play a role in regulating respiration are also located *peripherally* in the carotid arteries and aorta. These areas are known as _____ chemoreceptors, in contrast to those in the brain, which are referred to as *central chemoreceptors*. The peripheral chemoreceptors are primarily sensitive to lack of oxygen. They respond by stimulating cardiovascular function and play a secondary role in regulating respiration.

peripheral

   Signals from the central and peripheral chemoreceptors are transmitted to the inspiratory center in the _____.

medulla

   Signals from the medulla descend within the spinal cord and stimulate the two sets of spinal nerves that innervate the thoracic cage. The *cervical spinal nerves* join together to form the phrenic nerve and innervate the diaphragm. The *intercostal nerves* exit from the thoracic region and innervate the intercostal muscles. The diaphragm and the intercostal muscles contract in resopnse to the nervous stimulation. As the chest wall expands, providing a greater potential space for air, the intrathoracic pressure becomes *negative*. This negative pressure acts as a vacuum, drawing air into the airways (Fig. 3-5).

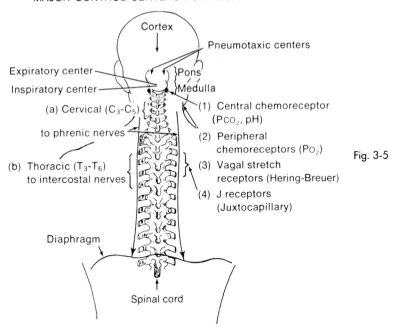

MAJOR CONTROL CENTERS FOR RESPIRATION

Cortex

Pneumotaxic centers

Expiratory center

Inspiratory center

Pons

Medulla

(a) Cervical (C_3-C_5)

to phrenic nerves

(b) Thoracic (T_3-T_6)
to intercostal nerves

(1) Central chemoreceptor
(P_{CO_2}, pH)

(2) Peripheral
chemoreceptors (P_{O_2})

(3) Vagal stretch
receptors (Hering-Breuer)

(4) J receptors
(Juxtocapillary)

Fig. 3-5

Diaphragm

Spinal cord

32 The normal process of inspiration is *(active/passive)*. During normal in-spiration, the intrathoracic pressure becomes more *(positve/negative)*.

   NOTE: The negative intrathoracic pressure draws blood toward the chest, (*(increasing/decreasing)* the venous return.

   Expansion of the alveoli with inspiration stimulates vagal stretch receptors, which send signals to the expiratory center in the medulla. The expiratory center of the medulla then stops active expansion of the chest, thus stopping _____ and beginning _____. This reflex is known as the Hering-Breuer reflex. This respiratory center may be influenced by other respiratory centers in the pons that further control the rate and regularity of both inspiration and expiration.

   During expiration the chest wall relaxes, allowing air to leave the lung passively. The intrathoracic pressure becomes less negative.

> active
> negative
>
> increasing
>
> inspiration
> expiration

33 The normal process of expiration is *(active/passive)*. Therefore the use of abdominal muscles during expiration indicates *(normal/forced)* expi-ration and is an early sign of respiratory distress in the patient who has CHF.

   During normal expiration the intrathoracic pressure becomes *(more negative/less negative/positive)*. However, during *forced* expiration the intrathoracic pressure becomes *positive*, compressing both normal and abnormal airways and limiting effective emptying of the lungs.

> passive
> forced
>
> less negative

Ineffective emptying of the lungs can limit filling of the lungs during inspiration. Forced expiration can be limited or prevented by such techniques as pursed-lip breathing, slow expiration, the use of inspirometers instead of blow bottles to reexpand atelectatic areas, temporary correction of hypoxemia with supplementary oxygen, and reversal of pulmonary congestion or obstruction.

34 LET US REVIEW: The normal stimulus for respiration is the level of _____ _____ in the blood and the cerebrospinal fluid. This chemical change is sensed by the *(central/peripheral)* _____ in the brain. Respiration may also be stimulated by changes in the blood _____ levels, which are sensed by the *(central/peripheral)* chemoreceptors.

carbon dioxide
central
chemoreceptors
O_2
peripheral

    The process of inspiration is *(active/passive)* and is regulated by the respiratory center in the *(medulla/pons)*. The process of expiration is *(active/passive)* and is primarily regulated by the respiratory center in the *(medulla/pons)* in response to the _____ reflex. During normal inspiration the intrathoracic pressure becomes *(negative/positive)*, causing *(increased/decreased)* venous return. During forced expiration the intrathoracic pressure becomes *(negative/positive)*, causing _____ of the airways.

active
medulla
passive
medulla; Hering-Breuer
negative
increased
positive
compression

35 Both inspiration and expiration may be influenced by factors other than the chemoreceptor response and the Hering-Breuer reflex. The cerebral cortex may exert an influence over the respiratory centers. Examples include the effects of biofeedback, pain, or stress on respiration. Juxtocapillary (J) receptors, which are sensitive to the effects of fluid and irritants, may also exist in the alveolar linings and cause stimulation of respiration.

36 The amount of air exchanged by the lungs in one minute is referred to as the _____ ventilation. Minute ventilation is a product of _____ rate and _____ _____.

minute
respiratory
tidal volume

    The tidal volume may be defined as the volume of air exchanged with every _____. The normal tidal volume is 10 ml/kg of normal body weight. The tidal volume is determined by the changes in airway resistance and compliance and by the integrity of the pleural linings and thoracic cage.

breath

    Airway resistance may be defined as interference to air flow occurring within the bronchial tubes. An increased airway resistance occurs in the presence of narrowing of or obstruction to the bronchial tubes. In the patient who has an acute MI, bronchial obstruction may occur in the presence of the fluid accumulation and bronchospasm that are associated with pulmonary edema.

Compliance is a natural property of the walls of healthy alveoli, bronchi, and bronchioles. Healthy lung tissue has the ability to stretch to accommodate the entering lung volume without a significant rise in pressure. In the presence of interstitial fluid accumulation caused by CHF the lung tissue becomes less compliant. For the same changes in volume, the airway pressure *(increases/decreases)*, which limits maximal filling of the airways.

increases

37 In the presence of an increase in airway resistance or a decrease in compliance, the tidal volume *(increases/decreases)*, or the inspiratory airway pressure *(increases/decreases)*, or both occur. As a result; gas exchange may be impaired.

decreases
increases

38 Not all of the normal inspiratory air volume participates in gas exchange due to both normal and abnormal ventilation (V)/perfusion (Q) relationships.

REMEMBER: Certain pulmonary structures function primarily to transport the air and are referred to as _____ airways. The air contained within these airways *(does/does not)* come into contact with the blood. Therefore this air does not participate in gas exchange and may be considered "wasted air." It is also referred to as *dead space*. The amount of normal (anatomical) dead space is approximately equal to a person's body weight in pounds (for example, 110 lb equals 110 cc dead space).

conducting
does not

Shallow breathing magnifies the influence of normal dead space. For example, in a patient with a normal tidal volume of 500 cc and a dead space of 110 cc, 390 cc of each inspiration (500 cc − 110 cc) is available to the respiratory airways for gas exchange. However, if that same patient is breathing at a tidal volume of 400 cc (shallow breathing), only _____ cc of each inspiration is available to the res-

290

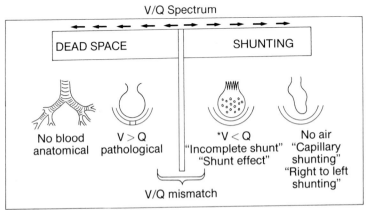

V/Q Spectrum

DEAD SPACE | SHUNTING

No blood   V > Q   *V < Q   No air
anatomical   pathological   "Incomplete shunt"   "Capillary
                      "Shunt effect"   shunting"
                                         "Right to left
                                         shunting"

V/Q mismatch

Fig. 3-6

*Most common cause of hypoxemia

piratory airways for gas exchange. When less volume is available to expand the respiratory airways, these airways may collapse (atelectasis), further limiting gas exchange. Occasional sighing, with larger tidal volumes, can reexpand these alveoli and may also stimulate surfactant production.

Additional dead space may be produced in pathological states. In contrast, this pathological dead space is usually produced within the respiratory airways. The most common clinical example of pathological dead space is pulmonary embolism. In pulmonary embolism, the blood flow to the _____ airways is occluded, allowing the air flow to these areas to be "wasted" because it cannot participate in _____ exchange.

respiratory

gas

39 Some of the *blood flow,* or _____, within the lungs is also wasted under both normal and pathological conditions. Wasted blood is referred to as *shunting.*

perfusion

When *no air* is available for gas exchange, a true capillary shunt exists. Certain blood vessels within the lungs completely bypass the respiratory airways and are responsible for a normal amount of shunting.

NOTE: Blood bypassing the lungs because of cardiac defects (for example, ventricular septal defect) is also referred to as shunting.

Additional pathological shunting may occur within the respiratory airways with disorders resulting in alveolar collapse (atelectasis), compression (pneumothorax), or occlusion (consolidation) (Fig. 3-6). These disorders include ARDS and pneumonia. The characteristic blood gas pattern is a significant decrease in Pa_{O_2} in spite of increases in FI_{O_2} up to 100%. The increased oxygen concentration does not penetrate a completely obstructed or collapsed alveolus, and, therefore does not reach the arterial blood. Only measures which reopen the alveoli restore the Pa_{O_2}.

These pulmonary changes *(do/do not)* typically occur in patients with acute myocardial infarction. They are also referred to as *right to left shunting* to distinguish them from the _____ to right shunting typical of cardiac mechanisms such as VSD. Cardiac shunting *(does/does not)* complicate acute myocardial infarction.

do not

left

does

40 When the airways are *partially obstructed* as with bronchospasm, pulmonary edema fluid, or mucus, *some air* reaches the alveoli (See Fig. 3-6). However, since the blood flow is not affected, the amount of ventilation to the airways *(does/does not)* match the amount of perfusion. This phenomenon is therefore described as *V/Q mismatch* and a *low V/Q unit* (V < Q), since the ventilation in *(more/less)* than the perfusion. It has also been more logically referred to as "incomplete shunt" or "shunt effect" since the major difference is that in a shunt the airways are *(partially/completely)* obstructed resulting in *(some/no)*

does not

less

completely; no

78

ventilation. The hypoxemia of V/Q mismatch is responsive to increases in the F_{IO_2} since some of the oxygen reaches the alveolus and capillary blood. These changes can occur in the patient with acute myocardial infarction complicated by congestive _____ _____. (See Unit 9).

heart failure

41 There is a built-in protective mechanism in the lung to prevent extreme wastage of blood traveling through poorly ventilated alveoli.

REMEMBER: The pulmonary capillary vessels constrict when there is low alveolar _____ tension, acidosis, or both, in an attempt to redirect the blood flow away from poorly ventilated areas. However, as a result of this constriction, the pulmonary vascular resistance *(increases/decreases)*. In the presence of moderate to severe pulmonary changes, however, this mechanism is only partially effective and can cause a severe strain on the right side of the heart.

O_2

increases

42 A further influence on V/Q mismatching in the lungs is the effect of gravity. Both gas and blood are influenced by gravity. A greater percentage of *both* normal ventilation and perfusion travels to the dependent areas in the lungs. However, because blood is heavier than air, there is a natural mismatching of ventilation *relative* to perfusion in the dependent and nondependent areas of the lung. In the dependent areas there is more perfusion relative to ventilation. In the nondependent areas there is more ventilation relative to perfusion.

During expiration the dependent airways empty more completely because of the effect of gravity on the airway pressures. For this reason they receive a greater portion of normal inspiratory volume. Because there is an excess of blood traveling to these areas, the net result is still wasted perfusion, or _____.

shunting

As the dependent airways empty, their radius decreases, the surface tension *(increases/decreases)*, and there is a greater tendency for these airways to collapse. Collapsed airways magnify the normal V/Q inequality of the dependent areas. Preventive measures include frequently changing position (rotating the dependent areas), sighing, coughing, and using incentive inspirometers.

increases

Pulmonary secretions are also gravity dependent and can magnify V/Q inequalities in dependent areas.

43 Mismatching of ventilation (V) and perfusion (Q) allows for areas of _____ _____ (wasted air) and _____ (wasted blood), and interferes with effective gas exchange. When there is interference with gas exchange in the lungs, *(O_2/CO_2) transport* is affected first and hypoxemia occurs. The most common causes of hypoxemia include: hypoventilation, diffusion defects, V/Q mismatch, and shunt. Of these, the most common is V/Q mismatch. This hypoxemia is associated with a wide A-a gradient

dead space
shunting

O_2

(See frames 17-19). Hypoxemia is more severe with (*V/Q mismatch/shunt*).   shunt

Respiratory failure exists when the lung fails to exchange either oxygen or CO_2 effectively. Therefore, either a Pa_{O_2} less than 50-60 mm Hg or a Pco_2 greater than 50 mm Hg may be considered a sign of _____ failure. Respiratory failure can occur sec-   respiratory
ondary to _____ failure in acute MI.   heart

AUSCULTATION OF THE LUNGS

44 Although auscultation is the most widely used respiratory assessment parameter in the CCU, the invaluable information gained by the *inspection* process cannot be minimized. Information gathered by inspection includes respiratory rate, effort, and symmetry. Evidence of

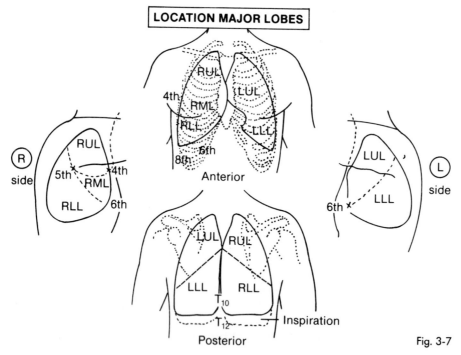

Fig. 3-7

shallow or forced respiration (as well as abnormal respiratory patterns, such as Cheyne-Stokes respirations, spontaneous coughing, and deep-breathing techniques) and sputum characteristics can be noted.

Both inspection and auscultation are aided by a knowledge of certain anatomical landmarks that outline the location of the lungs and its major lobes within the thoracic cavity (Fig. 3-7).

The sixth rib marks the lower rim of the right and left lung anteriorly. The _____ rib marks the lower rim laterally.   eighth

Posteriorly the lower border of the lung coincides with the _____ thoracic vertebrae on inspiration and the _____ vertebrae on expiration.

twelfth

tenth

45 Auscultation of the *posterior* chest wall primarily provides information about the _____ lobes of the lungs.

lower

Auscultation of the anterior chest wall provides information about all three lobes of the _____ lung and the _____ lobe of the _____ lung. The *fourth rib* marks the dividing point between the upper and middle lobes on the right.

right

upper; left

Auscultation of each chest wall *laterally* provides information about the _____ and _____ lobes.

upper; lower

A thorough auscultation of the lungs requires assessment of both the anterior and posterior chest walls and may be aided by assessing the lateral portions of the chest wall as well.

Characteristic breath sounds are produced within the alveoli and larger bronchial tubes. The normal *bronchial* sounds are tubular or hollow sounding with a prolonged expiration. They are best mimicked over the trachea. The normal alveolar sounds are soft and whispery sounding with a prolonged inspiration and short expiration. They are referred to as *vesicular* and are best heard over the major lung fields.

46 Auscultation of the lungs of patients who have heart failure may reveal areas of *decreased breath* sounds and the presence of *adventitious ("extra") sounds.* Bilateral, symmetrical decreased breath sounds may occur in the presence of decreased tidal volumes associated with shallow breathing or emphysema. Localized areas of decreased breath sounds may occur in the presence of pleural effusion associated with the interstitial fluid accumulation of CHF.

A pleural effusion may produce localized areas of _____ _____ _____.

decreased breath sounds

47 Abnormal breath sounds heard in a patient who has CHF include *crackles* (formerly referred to as *rales*) and *wheezes*. The movement of air through fluid in the terminal air passages, or alveoli, produces the noise known as a *crackle* (rale). The *quality* of crackles (rales) depends on their *origin*. The movement of air into fluid-filled alveoli produces fine crackling sounds. These sounds are heard best at the *end of inspiration* and do not disappear with coughing.

Fine-end inspiratory crackles (rales) indicate fluid in the _____.

alveoli

Fluid in the alveoli may be associated with _____ (see Unit 7).

CHF

48 The movement of air through narrowed bronchial tubes produces the noise known as a *wheeze*. The wheezes of CHF occur because of congestion and narrowing of the respiratory bronchiole and are heard first on *expiration*. The narrowed air passages expand with inspiration but return to their narrow state on expiration. Air moving out through these narrowed passages produces the sound known as a _____.

wheeze

> NOTE: With severe obstruction, wheezes may be heard throughout inspiration and expiration. Wheezes caused by CHF are usually associated with moderately dense crackles (rales).

49 The abnormal lung sounds of CHF may be distinguished, at times, from those of primary pulmonary disease or infection by differences in their onset, intensity, and timing in the respiratory cycle. The movement of air through the mucus in larger bronchial tubes produces the noise known as a *rhonchus,* which is related to the wheeze. Although these sounds are both referred to as either ronchi or wheezes by some authorities, a recent international symposium on lung sounds supports the separation of these adventitious sounds into separate categories in US nomenclature. The quality of the rhonchus is that of a coarse rumbling or snoring mingled with crackling and may at times sound very much like a coarse crackle (rale). However, these sounds are heard first on *expiration,* then *early* inspiration. The end of inspiration usually remains clear.

The respiratory *timing* is more critical than the quality of the sound in distinguishing its origin—eprhonchus: *(smaller/larger)* airways as opposed to crackle (rale): *(smaller/larger)* airways.

larger
smaller

50 In primary asthma, wheezes usually appear before the onset of any other abnormal sound. Later they are typically accompanied by rhonchi because of an increased mucus production in the same airways. In CHF, wheezes usually accompany crackles (rales).

Abnormal lung sounds (rhonchus and wheeze) that are caused by primary pulmonary disease usually begin during *(inspiration/expiration)* and eventually affect *(early/end)* inspiration.

expiration
early

> NOTE: This distinguishing characteristic is based on the ability of primary pulmonary disease to affect the bronchial tubes without necessarily affecting, or before affecting, the terminal airways.

Alveolar congestion caused by pulmonary disorders cannot be distinguished by auscultation from the alveolar congestion of CHF. It is also possible to have both small and large airway congestion and obstruction in the patient who has either cardiac or primary pulmonary disease. In these patients crackles (rales) often cannot be distinguished from rhonchi.

51 Changes in the *intensity* of the normal breath sounds may provide further distinguishing characteristics. Localized areas of *decreased* breath sounds may be associated with either the pleural effusion caused by CHF or a large area of atelectasis, or pneumothorax. However, areas of localized *increased* breath sounds are more typically associated with primary lung disease. Increased breath sounds indicate a complete occlusion (consolidation) or collapse (microatelectasis) of the terminal airways so that normal *(bronchial/vesicular)* sounds are lost. The louder, more hollow *(bronchial/vesicular)* sounds are no longer muffled.

vesicular

bronchial

REMEMBER: Bronchial sounds are normal in areas where larger tubes predominate, such as over the _____.

trachea

Additional characteristics of bronchial sounds include egophony ("e" to "a" changes) and whispered pectoriloquy (magnified transmission of whispered sounds). These sounds would be *(normal/abnormal)* if auscultated over lung areas where terminal airways such as alveoli should predominate.

abnormal

EVALUATING BLOOD OXYGEN CONTENT
Role of arterial Po_2 and oxygen saturation

Let us now consider the assessment of blood O_2 content and hypoxemia in more detail.

52 Oxygen is carried within the blood in two forms: (1) dissolved in solution and (2) bound to hemoglobin in the red blood cell for storage. The Po_2 reflects the pressure, or tension, exerted by the amount of oxygen in solution. The O_2 saturation reflects the amount of oxygen bound to hemoglobin.

Oxygen first enters the blood plasma as dissolved gas particles by the process of diffusion. Diffusion is defined as the movement of particles from a region of greater concentration to a region of lesser concentration. O_2 particles move from a region of _____ concentration in the alveolar air to a region of _____ concentration in the venous blood. Because gas particles exert pressure both in the atmosphere and in solution, a pressure gradient also exists across the alveolar capillary membrane, which facilitates the movement of oxygen into the blood.

greater

lesser

As the pressure of oxygen dissolved in the blood increases, some of the oxygen is pushed into the red blood cell for storage. Eventually the bulk of the oxygen in the blood is carried in the storage form. Therefore the greatest amount of information about the O_2 content in the blood is obtained from the *(Po_2/O_2 saturation)*.

O_2 saturation

Oxygen leaves the blood at the tissue level from the content dissolved in the plasma first. Oxygen moves from a region of greater concentration and pressure in the plasma to a region of _____ concentration and pressure in the tissue cells.

lesser

This process is known as _____. As the dissolved
oxygen is removed, it is replaced from the amount stored in the red
blood cells (Fig. 3-8).

diffusion

BLOOD OXYGEN-CARRYING CAPACITY

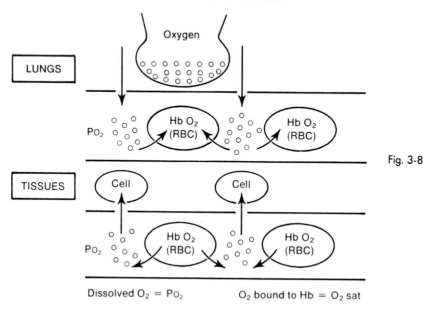

Fig. 3-8

Dissolved O_2 = Po_2 O_2 bound to Hb = O_2 sat

Total normal arterial capacity: 20 ml

53 The normal O_2-carrying capacity of the blood is 20 ml of oxygen per
each 100 ml of blood. Each gram of hemoglobin, fully saturated, has
the ability to store 1.34 to 1.39 ml of oxygen. A patient with 14 g of
hemoglobin has the capacity to carry 18.76 ml of oxygen bound to hemoglobin in each 100 ml of blood (that is, 14 g Hb $\times$ 1.34 ml O_2/g
Hb).

In contrast, each mm Hg of pressure exerted by the oxygen in solution represents only 0.003 ml of oxygen. If this same patient had an
arterial Po_2 of 100 mm Hg, the amount of oxygen represented by this
pressure would be only 0.3 ml of oxygen in each 100 ml of blood
(that is, Po_2 of 100 mm Hg $\times$ 0.003 ml O_2/mm Hg). Thus the amount
of oxygen in solution represents a (*large/small*) amount of oxygen exerting a large amount of pressure.

small

54 The *total O_2 content* of the blood equals the amount bound to hemoglobin (represented by the _____ _____ in
a blood gas sample) plus the amount of oxygen in solution (represented by the _____ in a blood gas sample). In the given patient example the amount of oxygen bound to hemoglobin when fully

O_2 saturation

Po_2

saturated is 18.76 ml, and the amount of oxygen in solution at a Po_2 of 100 mm Hg is 0.3 ml, which totals 19.06 ml.

About 98% of the blood O_2 content is represented by the *Po_2/O_2 saturation)*. Therefore, when evaluating blood O_2 content, clinicians often consider assessment of the O_2 saturation alone sufficient.

O_2 saturation

Accuracy of oxygen saturation

55 The percentage of O_2 saturation is determined by comparing the actual O_2 content of a patient's hemoglobin with the potential O_2 capacity of that hemoglobin. The O_2 saturation percentage can be calculated based on its relationship to a measured Po_2 (See frames 61-65) or can be more accurately measured directly with the use of an oximeter. Arterial pulse oximetry provides continuous O_2 saturation readings non-invasively using principles similar to those used with venous oximetry (see frames 72-75). For purposes of this discussion, the percentage of O_2 saturation signifies the percentage of available Hb sites that are actually filled by oxygen *in a given patient's blood*.

56 In the presence of anemia, fewer Hb sites are available. These sites become quickly filled with even small amounts of oxygen. Thus the O_2 saturation may be normal or high, even in the presence of a low O_2 supply.

In the presence of polycythemia, excess Hb sites are available. These excess sites become difficult to fill, even in the presence of adequate amounts of oxygen. Thus the O_2 saturation is _____, whereas the blood O_2 content is _____. In the presence of polycythemia the O_2 saturation is _____, whereas the blood O_2 content is _____.

normal
low
low
normal

57 The percentage of O_2 saturation, when measured directly, is highly dependent on the patient's serum *Hb level*. To assess the O_2 saturation accurately, the serum _____ level must also be noted.

Hb

58 The hematocrit value, or percent of blood that is composed of red blood cells, is often used interchangeably with the serum Hb level. When abnormal it often reflects the Hb content. However, to determine the exact O_2 content of the blood in milliliters, the exact Hb level is needed.

59 When at least 5 g of hemoglobin becomes unsaturated, *cyanosis* appears. In the presence of an elevated serum Hb level, asymptomatic cyanosis can appear. The blood O_2 content is likely to be _____. In the presence of a low serum Hb level, cyanosis may not appear, even though the blood O_2 content is low, until

normal

the hypoxemia is severe. The development of peripheral cyanosis is often related to vasoconstriction in response to cold.

Thus the presence of cyanosis *(is/is not)* an accurate sign of hypoxia. The presence of cyanosis *(is/is not)* an accurate sign of hypoxemia. The presence of cyanosis *(is/is not)* an accurate sign of the amount of oxygen bound to hemoglobin in the absence of peripheral vasoconstriction.

is not
is not
is

60 Ideally *the normal arterial O_2 saturation should be greater than 97%.* However, percentages above 90%, in the presence of a normal serum Hb level, are usually asymptomatically tolerated. The *normal venous O_2 saturation ranges between 60% and 75%.*

REMEMBER; As the dissolved oxygen is removed from the plasma at the tissue level, it is replaced from the amount stored in the _____ _____ _____. A large reserve of oxygen is stored in the red blood cell to accommodate increases in tissue demands or drops in cardiac output (see Frames 1, 2, and 10 to 12).

red blood cell

61 The amount of oxygen bound to hemoglobin is dependent to a great extent on the pressure exerted by the particles in solution *(the Po_2).* The pressure of these particles serves to push oxygen into the red blood cell where it can then bind with hemoglobin for storage.

NOTE: At a minimal Po_2 of 60 mm Hg, the expected O_2 saturation is 90%. It is for this reason the authors consider this the minimal O_2 saturation level. This relationship is illustrated in Fig. 3-9.

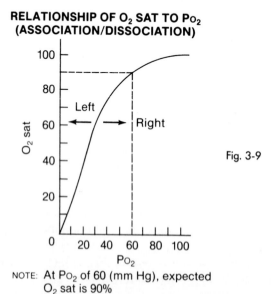

RELATIONSHIP OF O_2 SAT TO Po_2 (ASSOCIATION/DISSOCIATION)

Fig. 3-9

NOTE: At Po_2 of 60 (mm Hg), expected O_2 sat is 90%

62 Normally hemoglobin and oxygen bind together ("associate") tightly. However, certain factors may alter this relationship and cause oxygen and hemoglobin to dissociate from each other. These factors alter the expected O_2 saturation percentage associated with a given P_{O_2}. The graphic representation of this relationship, depicted in Fig. 3-9, is commonly referred to as the oxygen-hemoglobin _____ curve.

dissociation

Changes in pH, carbon dioxide pressure (P_{CO_2}), temperature, red blood cell (RBC) phpsphates, or all of these, can alter the hemoglobin-oxygen relationship. Hydrogen ions and carbon dioxide serve to push oxygen off hemoglobin and loosen the hemoglobin-oxygen relationship (Fig. 3-10).

CLINICAL FACTORS ALTERING Hb-O$_2$ BINDING

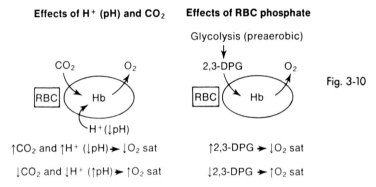

Fig. 3-10

Therefore, in the presence of decreased pH and increased carbon dioxide, the O_2 saturation should be *(higher/lower)* than expected (that is, P_{O_2} of 60 with O_2 saturation facilitates O_2 removal from the red blood cell and its delivery to the tissues, it impairs the uptake and storage of oxygen at the alveolar-capillary level.

lower

63 The RBC phosphate 2,3-diphosphoglycerate (2,3-DPG) also serves to push oxygen off hemoglobin. This phosphate, unlike other more commonly known cellular phosphates, such as adenosine triphosphate (ATP), accumulates during the preaerobic phase of glucose breakdown. Therefore, during hypoxia, 2,3-DPG continues to be produced and maintains a loose relationship between hemoglobin and oxygen, thus promoting O_2 delivery to the tissues (See Fig. 3-10). In the presence of hypoxia, the level of cellular 2,3-DPG *(increases/decreases)*, the O_2 saturation *(increases/decreases)*, and the O_2 delivery to the tissue is *(enhanced/inhibited)*. An increase in cellular temperature produces a similar effect on O_2-Hb binding in an attempt to facilitate the availability of oxygen for the increased metabolic demands.

increases
decreases
enhanced

NOTE: RBC phosphates deteriorate in stored blood because of the effects of storage and the preservatives added. In the presence of a decreased 2,3-DPG level, the O_2 saturation *(increases/decreases)*, but O_2 delivery to the tissues *(increases/decreases)*. Therefore administration of relatively fresh blood may be more desirable in patients with coronary artery disease.

increases
decreases

64 LET US REVIEW: In the presence of decreased pH, increased P_{CO_2}, increased temperature, or increased 2,3-DPG levels, hemoglobin and oxygen bind more *(tightly/loosely)*, and the arterial O_2 saturation is *(higher/lower)* than expected for a given P_{O_2}. Hypoxia is associated with *(increased/decreased)* pH. Therefore in hypoxic states *(increased/decreased)* O_2 saturationis expected.

loosely
lower
decreased; decreased

In the presence of inreased pH, decreased P_{CO_2}, decreased temperature, or decreased 2,3-DPG levels, the converse is true; the O_2 saturation will be *(higher/lower)* than expected. A high O_2 saturation facilitates O_2 uptake at the alveolar level but inhibits O_2 delivery at the cellular level.

higher

NOTE: Any extreme in pH, P_{CO_2}, temperature, or 2,3-DPG levels impairs O_2 transport at some level and should therefore be corrected as quickly as possible to promote efficiency of O_2 utilization.

65 These alterations in Hb-O_2 binding distort the level of _____ _____ corresponding with a given _____.

O_2 saturation
P_{O_2}

REMEMBER: The expected O_2 saturation at different levels of P_{O_2} can be represented in graphic form (see Fig. 3-9). Since the level of O_2 saturation depends on the degree of Hb-O_2 binding or association, as well as dissociation, this graph is also known as the *Hb-O_2 dissociation curve.* The decrease in O_2 saturation occurring with decreased pH, increased P_{CO_2}, increased temperature, and hypoxia is often referred to as a "shift to the right" in the Hb-O_2 dissociation curve. The increase in O_2 saturation occurring with increased pH, decreased P_{CO_2}, and decreased temperature is often referred to as a "shift to the left" in the Hb-O_2 dissociation curve.

EVALUATING TISSUE OXYGEN EXTRACTION AND CARDIAC OUTPUT: ROLE OF A-VDO_2/SV_{O_2}

66 The O_2 content of venous blood represents the amount of oxygen remaining in the blood after the tissues have extracted the amount they need.

REMEMBER: A large reserve of oxygen is stored in the red blood cells to accommodate increases in tissue demands or drops in _____ _____. If the amount of oxygen returning from the tissues (in the venous blood) is compared

cardiac output

with the amount of oxygen being delivered to the tissues (in the arterial blood), the difference should reflect the amount of oxygen _____ by the tissues for their use (Fig. 3-11). Comparison of the O_2 content difference between arterial and venous blood is referred to as the calculation of the A-Vo_2 difference, or A-VDo_2 and until recently was regarded as the best reflection of tissue oxygenation. However, the venous O_2 content alone, as reflected by the venous O_2 sat or Sv_{O_2}, has also been shown to accurately reflect tissue O_2 extraction/oxgenation and can be continuously monitored.

extracted

ARTERIAL-VENOUS O$_2$ DIFFERENCE (A-VDO$_2$)

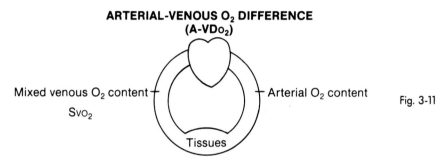

Mixed venous O$_2$ content + Sv_{O_2}

+ Arterial O$_2$ content

Tissues

Fig. 3-11

Arterial O$_2$ content—venous O$_2$ content (A-VDo$_2$) = O$_2$ extracted by tissues

To obtain an accurate reflection of the average tissue extraction from all parts of the body, a mixed venous sample is required. A mixed venous sample is best obtained from a catheter in the pulmonary artery, where the blood returning from all parts of the body has been optimally mixed before being oxygenated (see Unit 9).

67 The comparison of the O_2 content difference between arterial and venous blood is referred to as the assessment of _____ _____ or _____.

A-Vo$_2$ difference
A-VD$_{O_2}$

The A-Vo_2 difference indicates the amount of oxygen _____ by the _____ from each 100 ml of blood.

extracted; tissues

Tissue O_2 extraction may also be assessed from *(arterial/venous)* O_2 samples alone by determining *(Po$_2$/O$_2$ saturation)* of the sample. A continuous recording of tissue extraction can be obtained from *(A-VD$_{O_2}$ /Sv$_{O_2}$)* measurements.

venous
O$_2$ saturation
Sv$_{O_2}$

REMEMBER: The O_2 demands of the tissues each minute are known as the _____ _____ _____ (see Frame 1). Tissue oxygenation over a selected period depends on the tissue _____ _____, the blood supply or _____ _____, and the _____ extracted from the blood. The O_2 extracted depends on the arterial O_2 content or blood

tissue O$_2$ consumption

O$_2$ demands
cardiac output
O$_2$

_____ _____. When tissue O_2 con-

sumption increases or the cardiac output decreases, the tissues must extract a greater amount of oxygen from the blood O_2 reserve to meet O_2 needs. This principle is referred to as the Fick principle and is illustrated in Fig. 3-12. The venous O_2 sat and content decreases resulting in an increased A-Vo_2 difference.

Thus when the A-Vo_2 difference increases, (or the Sv_{O_2} decreases) as in Fig. 3-12, it can be assumed that either tissue O_2 demands have *(increased/decreased)* or that the cardiac output has *(increased/decreased)*.

increased; decreased

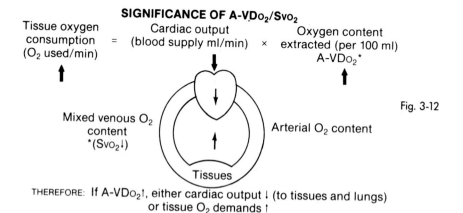

SIGNIFICANCE OF A-VDo$_2$/Svo$_2$

Tissue oxygen consumption (O_2 used/min) = Cardiac output (blood supply ml/min) × Oxygen content extracted (per 100 ml) A-VDo$_2$*

Mixed venous O_2 content *(Svo$_2$↓)

Arterial O_2 content

Tissues

Fig. 3-12

THEREFORE: If A-VDo$_2$↑, either cardiac output ↓ (to tissues and lungs) or tissue O_2 demands ↑

Normal persons can *triple* their cardiac output to meet increasing oxygen demands or compensate for decreases in arterial O_2 content. The critically ill cardiac patient may be unable to compensate by this mechanism due to a limited *cardiac reserve* of *heart failure*.

68 Calculation of the A-Vo_2 difference thus provides a means to estimate changes in cardiac output. Exact calculation of the cardiac output can only be determined if the tissue O_2 consumption per minute is actually measured concurrently. In the patient who has a severely damaged myocardium resulting from an acute MI, the cardiac output is usually *(high/low)*. The A-Vo_2 difference reflecting this change would be *(high/low)*.

low
high

If arterial oxygen content, hemoglobin, and oxygen demands are relatively stable and the AVDo$_2$ is increasing, then it can be assumed the _____ _____ is decreasing.

cardiac output

69 The O_2 content of the arterial and mixed venous blood samples is most accurately determined by calculating in each sample both the amount of oxygen bound to hemoglobin and the amount of oxygen in solution. However, since about 98% of the blood O_2 content is represented by the amount *(in solution/bound to hemoglobin)*, comparison of the *(Po$_2$/O$_2$ saturation)* alone in both samples is often considered sufficient.

bound to hemoglobin
O$_2$ saturation

70 LET US REVIEW: Each gram of hemoglobin *fully saturated* has the ability to store _____ ml of oxygen. A patient who has 14 g of hemoglobin has a potential arterial O$_2$ capacity of _____ in each 100 ml of blood (that is, 14 g Hb × 1.34 ml O$_2$/g Hb). If the arterial O$_2$ saturation of this patient's blood is 90%, his actual *arterial O$_2$ content* is 16.68 ml/100 ml blood (that is, 14 g Hb × 1.34 ml O$_2$/g Hb × 90% saturation). If the *venous O$_2$ content* is 9.38 ml/100 ml blood (that is, 14 g Hb × 1.34 ml O$_2$/g Hb × 50% saturation). The difference between the O$_2$ content of the arterial and venous samples is 7.30 ml O$_2$. *The normal arterial-venous O$_2$ difference is 5 ml.* Therefore in this patient the A-Vo$_2$ difference is *(high/low)*. The corresponding venous O$_2$ sat of 50% is *(high/low)*. An increase in the A-Vo$_2$ difference indicates that either tissue O$_2$ consumption has *(increased/decreased)* or the cardiac output has *(increased/decreased)*. Therefore this patient's cardiac output is very likely to be *(high/low)*.

1.34

18.76 ml

low; high

increased; decreased

low

71 Since it is the lowering of the *venous O$_2$ content* that makes the A-VDo$_2$ *increase,* then it follows that analysis of this value alone via the Svo$_2$ could provide a means of tracking cardiac output.

The Po$_2$ level is sometimes used clinically to evaluate O$_2$ content—arterial or venous—*based on an estimated corresponding level of O$_2$ saturation.*

The normal Pv$_{O_2}$vo$_2$ is 40 mm Hg, which corresponds with an O$_2$ sat of _____%.

70

However, a direct measurement of venous O$_2$ saturation is more accurate. This estimate is made assuming the presence of a normal serum Hb and pH values. Pco$_2$, and temperature. Thus these factors must still be taken into consideration.

A low venous Po$_2$ usually corresponds with a *(high/low)* venous O$_2$ saturation and for this reason may be used as an indirect indicator of an *(increased/decreased)* A-VD$_{O_2}$.

low

increased

Continuous monitoring of Sv$_{O_2}$ at the bedside

72 Although continuous monitoring of arterial and venous oxygen saturation with specialized catheters has been available for many years in the catheterization laboratory, bedside application of this technique has only recently been practical. The introduction of plastic fibers that can transmit light waves has allowed for the development of durable flexible catheters, which are suitable for long-term monitoring situations. The fibers that transmit light waves are known as *fiberoptics.*

Currently the most popular method for continuous monitoring of the mixed venous oxygen saturation (Sv_{O_2}) in the coronary care unit is with a specialized pulmonary artery thermodilution catheter. This catheter contains the usual hemodynamic lumens and, in addition, two fiberoptic channels capable of transmitting light waves. Because the fibers transmit *light waves* they are known as _____. (See Unit 9, Fig. 3-13, Frames 66-67).

fiberoptics

Analysis of oxygen saturation by fiberoptic light signals is based on the principle that oxygenated hemoglobin (oxyhemoglobin) (HbO_2)

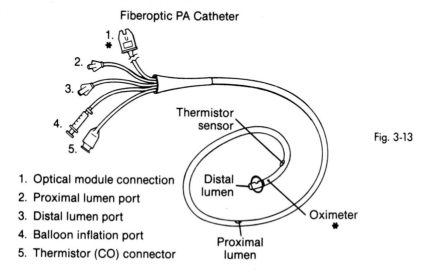

Fiberoptic PA Catheter

Thermistor sensor

Fig. 3-13

1. Optical module connection
2. Proximal lumen port
3. Distal lumen port
4. Balloon inflation port
5. Thermistor (CO) connector

Distal lumen

Oximeter

Proximal lumen

reflects a *different* wavelength of light than does unoxygenated hemoglobin (Hb). This method of analysis is known as *reflection spectrophotometry* and is a common method of analyzing unknown substances.

73 With this technique, light waves of different wavelengths are projected by an *optical module,* which is connected to the fiberoptic connecting part of the PA catheter. One fiberoptic channel transmits light waves to the catheter tip and *illuminates the blood* passing the *distal or pulmonary artery lumen* (See Fig. 3-14).

REMEMBER: The final pathway for all venous blood before oxygenation is the _____ _____.

pulmonary artery

The light *reflected* from the oxygenated hemoglobin (HbO_2) and unoxygenated hemoglobin (Hb) is transmitted back via a *second receiving fiberoptic* to the optical module and then a processor for analysis.

Similar non-invasive systems are also available using sensors, which attach to the earlobes or fingertips. However, these reflect arterial rather than venous saturation and thus *(do/do not)* reflect tissue oxygenation changes. They are useful primarily in monitoring pulmonary changes. The ratio of oxyhemoglobin (HbO_2) to total hemoglo-

do not

bin is calculated by the microprocessor, which provides the percent of hemoglobin saturated with oxygen in the mixed venous blood. (Sv_{O2}) Photoelectric devices, which measure the oxygen saturation of the blood using this principle, are known as *oximeters*.

74 LET US REVIEW: The method used to detect the Sv_{O2} with a fiberoptic pulmonary artery catheter is known as _____ _____.

    The fiberoptic light illuminates the _____ passing the catheter tip and the light is _____ back to the optical module and processor for analysis. _____ *Oxyhemoglobin* (Hbo_2)

reflection spectrophotometry

blood
reflected

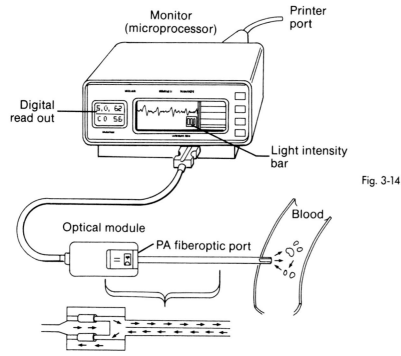

Monitor (microprocessor)

Printer port

Digital read out

Light intensity bar

Fig. 3-14

Optical module

PA fiberoptic port

Blood

reflects a different _____ of light than does _____.

wavelength
hemoglobin

    The ratio of oxyhemoglobin to total hemoglobin provides the percentage of hemoglobin saturated with oxygen.

    The fiberoptic catheter is *calibrated* against a controlled color reference prior to insertion or can be calibrated after insertion by comparison of the catheter readout with an actual PA blood sample sent from the blood gas lab.

75 The technological equipment involved in the delivery and analysis of the fiberoptical signals are an *optical module* and a *monitor*. The *optical module* emits the light and changes the light signals reflected from the blood cells into electrical signals to be analyzed by the processor.

The *monitor* contains a microprocessor, which computes the Sv_{O_2} data, displays the Sv_{O_2} in a monitor trace with a digital readout, and provides a retrievable hard copy record when attached to a printer. Some units can also be used to calculate multiple hemodynamic parameters. A *light intensity bar record* is also graphically displayed on the monitor trace and chart record (See Fig. 3-14 and 3-15). This allows the operator to evaluate the quality of the light signals being reflected and proceed with trouble shooting should the intensity be of poor quality.

76 Changes in the Sv_{O_2} usually precede critical changes in the patient's condition and thus alert the nurse to the risk of decompensation before it occurs. Any rise or fall in the Sv_{O_2} of *10% or greater* for ten minutes or longer should be considered significant and investigated within the context of the clinical situation. Time frames on the monitor trace or chart record can be condensed or expanded as desired (See Fig. 3-15).

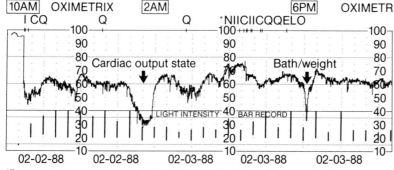

Fig. 3-15

*Event markers indicating designated nursing or medical interventions as entered

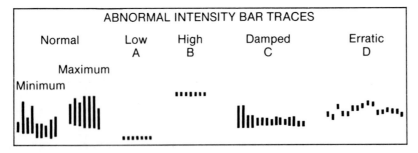

REMEMBER: The normal range for a venous O_2 saturation is _____ to _____%.

60; 80

77 A fall in the Sv_{O_2} may occur in the presence of factors which *decrease the cardiac output, decrease the arterial oxygen content,* or *increase oxygen demands* and thus compromise tissue oxygenation.

When tissue oxygenation is significantly compromised, lactic acidosis occurs potentiating cellular injury. This usually corresponds with a Sv_{O_2} recording of less than 35% for a sustained period of time (i.e. greater than 10 minutes). An Sv_{O2} *below 20%* may result in permanent cellular damage.

Factors that may *decrease the cardiac output* and thus potentially *decrease the Sv_{O2}* include: heart failure, hypovolemia, a decrease in inotropic support, a decrease in IABP support, an acute VSD, papillary muscle rupture, cardiac tamponade, and cardiac arrest.

78 Factors that may decrease *arterial oxygen content* include those that decrease hemoglobin levels or alter hemoglobin oxygen binding and those that impair pulmonary oxygen transport. The major factor that may decrease the hemoglobin level is acute blood loss as with hemmorhage. Carbon monoxide poisoning is a major factor that may alter hemoglobin oxygen binding.

Factors that may interfere with pulmonary oxygen transport include: unsuccessful weaning from a ventilator, pulmonary edema associated with CHF or ARDS, pulmonary thromboembolism, pneumonia, suctioning, and cardiopulmonary arrest.

79 Factors that *increase* _____ *demands* should also be considered when evaluating a *fall in Sv_{O2}* and include: hyperthermia, pain, shivering, and seizures.

    LET US REVIEW: A fall in Sv_{O_2} is considered significant when a drop of _____ % or greater occurs. This drop may indicate a _____ in cardiac output due to congestive _____ _____, cardiac tamponade or _____ volemia; a decrease in _____ O_2 content associated with altered _____ gas transport; and/or increased O_2 demands due to pain, shivering, or _____.

oxygen

10
decrease
heart failure
hypo
arterial
pulmonary
hyper

80 Although less commonly seen, an increase in Sv_{O2} may occur in the presence of *(increased/decreased)* cardiac output and *(increased/decreased)* oxygen demands.

increased; decreased

A pathological condition common in the critical care unit that may cause a dramatic increase in the cardiac output and O_2 demands and thus _____ the Sv_{O2} is *sepsis*. Excessive inotropic support could also result in a high cardiac output and high Sv_{O2}.

increase

81 Factors which *decrease tissue oxygen demands* and could potentially cause a rise in Sv_{O2} include: *(hyperthermia/hypothermia)* *(hyperthyroidism/hypothyroidism)* anesthesia, and pharmacologic paralysis.

hypothermia
hypothyroidism

An unusual condition that could potentially cause a high Sv_{O_2} *unrelated* to cardiac output or tissue oxygen demands is the *cyanide poisoning,* which is an unusual complication of sodium nitroprusside (Nipride) therapy (see Unit 10, frame 140). With this condition, the cells are unable to gain access to oxygen since it remains so closely bound to hemoglobin.

Decreased oxygenation of brain cells results in neurological symptoms, such as confusion and disorientation.

A wedged pulmonary artery catheter is another potential cause of a high Sv_{O_2}. When the catheter is wedged forward, flow of blood is obstructed and pooling of highly oxygenated retrograde flow results in the high Sv_{O_2}.

82 The intensity bar record allows the operator to evaluate the
_____ of the light signal to ensure accurate readings   quality
(See Fig. 3-15 and 3-14, frames 75 and 76).

A *low intensity* light signal reading may mean the catheter is kinked, the distal lumen is occluded, or the connection with the optical module is poor. A *high intensity* light signal reading may mean the catheter tip is against a vessel wall and needs repositioning.

A *damped intensity* may mean the catheter has become wedged or there is clotting over the tip of the catheter.

83 **In summary:**
Continuous Sv_{O_2} monitoring has proven valuable in the management of many types of critically ill patients to guide therapy. It is especially valuable to the nurse because it allows her to follow
_____ _____ and tissue oxygen   cardiac output
extraction minute to minute rather than episodically with cardiac profiles.
output   REMEMBER: There is a direct correlation between changes in venous O_2 sat (Sv_{O_2}) and *cardiac output.*
As the *cardiac output decreases* the Sv_{O_2} _____.   decreases
As the *cardiac output increases* the Sv_{O_2} _____.
As tissue *oxygen demands* and extraction decrease, the Sv_{O_2}
_____.   increases
As tissue oxygen demands and extraction increase, the Sv_{O_2}
_____.   decreases
Decreases in the Sv_{O_2} may also occur in the presence of
_____ hemoglobin or alterations in   decreased
_____ O_2 transport.   pulmonary
Management of patients with congestive heart failure, in cardiogenic shock, on the intraaortic balloon, ventilators, and/or complex intravenous drug therapy is enhanced with the ability to continuously monitor the Sv_{O_2}.

84 NURSING ORDERS: Sv_{O_2} Monitoring

1. Monitor for changes in the Sv_{O_2}:

    REMEMBER: a 10% increase or decrease for 10 inches or longer is a significant change.

    A. *Check the system:*
    1) Is the fiberoptic connector of the Swan plugged securely into the optical module?
    2) Is the quality of the *light intensity bars* okay? (See frame 75).
    3) Is the PA waveform of good amplitude and or normal contour?
        - Could there be a clot over the tip of the catheter?
        - Could the catheter be wedged?
        - Flush PA line or follow other guidelines for dealing with damped/wedged catheter.

    B. *Check the patient:*
    1) If the Sv_{O_2} *is decreasing:*
        a) Is the cardiac output decreasing?
            - Check urine output
            - Auscultate lungs for increased crackles (rales)
            - Auscultate for presence of new S3 gallop
            - Watch for decrease in inotropic support
            - Watch for change in IABP assist ratio
            - Check for possibility of new VSD, papillary muscle rupture, cardiac tamponade
            - Check wedge pressure
            - Validate with thermodilution C.O. measurement
        b) Is the arterial oxygen content falling?

        - Check to see if the hemoglobin level is normal—if there is any chance the patient may be bleeding
        - Check to see if there anything that could interfere with·hemoglobin binding and release to the tissue—carbon monoxide
        - Check to see if there a decrease in pulmonary O_2 transport—check for pulmonary edema, pneumonia, PTE, decrease in $F_{I_{O_2}}$, cardiopulmonary arrest, suctioning
        c) Are the tissue Oxygen demands increasing?
            - Check to see if the patient hyperthermic, shivering in pain, or having seizures
    2) If the Sv_{O_2} is increasing:
        a) Is the cardiac output increasing?
            - Check to see if the patient is septic—Is the C.O. increased and the SVR decreased
            - Check for excessive inotropic support
        b) Are tissue oxygen demands decreased?
            - Check to see if the patient is hypothermic, hypothyroid, on paralytic drugs, or has recently received anesthesia
        c) Is the patient receiving Nipride? Could he be experiencing cyanide poisoning? Are there any neurological symptoms that would indicate that this could be the problem?
        d) Is the PA catheter "wedged"?
            - Check PA pattern and notify physician if necessary

2. Advise use of the jugular approach for insertion of the catheter.
3. Infuse fluids through ports of fiberoptic P_A line at rates no greater than 100 cc per hour, and do not infuse blood due to the small size of the lumens.
4. When dressing the insertion site, do not tightly coil the catheter when applying the dressing.

SUMMARY: SYSTEMATIC APPROACH TO HYPOXEMIA AND HYPOXIA

85 The O_2 values reported on an ABG sample are the _____ and arterial _____. They reflect the presence of *(hypoxia/hypoxemia)*. Therefore systematic assessment of oxygenation from an ABG report begins with the assessment of potential *(hypoxia/hypoxemia)*. The following process is recommended:

> PaO_2, O_2; saturation
> hypoxemia
>
> hypoxemia

I. Analyze the Pa_{O_2} to determine critical hypoxemia and to evaluate O_2 _____ in the _____.

> transport; lungs

   A. Determine if critically low (i.e., is less than) _____ mm Hg). If so, provide supplementary O_2 immediately, unless a history of COPD is obtained.

> 60

   B. Determine if normal:

     1. Check the $F_{I_{O_2}}$ and determine the expected Pa_{O_2}.
     REMEMBER: The expected Pa_{O_2} at any $F_{I_{O_2}}$ should be _____.

> $5 \times F_{I_{0_2}}$

     2. Compare the actual Pa_{O_2} with the expected Pa_{O_2} to determine the _____ difference (gradient).

> A-a

   C. Correlate with the P_{CO_2} and, if available, the pulmonary artery pressure.
   REMEMBER: The pulmonary capillary vessels *(constrict/dilate)* in the presence of low alveolar tensions.

> constrict

   D. Determine potential causes
   REMEMBER: The presence of hypoxemia or increase in the A-aD_{O_2} gradient indicates the presence of interference in _____ O_2 transport. This interference with gas exchange may occur from abnormalities in ventilation _____ or _____ or combinations and mismatching of these. Pulmonary changes resulting in these abnormalities include pulmonary edema, bronchospasm, mucusal edema, excess mucus production, atelectasis, or changes in _____ blood flow. Wasted perfusion associated with abnormalities in ventilation is also known as _____. Wasted ventilation is also known as _____ _____. Auscultate the lungs to verify the presence of any of the above changes.

> lung
>
> perfusion; diffusion
>
> pulmonary
>
> shunt
> dead space

II. Analyze the arterial O_2 saturation to evaluate the blood _____ _____.

> oxygen content

A. Determine is critically low (i.e. less than) _____%).   90
B. Confirm arterial source-R/O contamination of sample with venous blood.
C. Verify the accuracy of the O_2 saturation as a reflection of the O_2 content by checking the serum _____   Hb
   levels.
D. Calculate the O_2 content (optional) or relate to reported value if available.
E. Check the relationship of the O_2 saturation with Pa_{O_2} and those factors that may alter this relationship; that is _____,   pH
   _____, patient's _____, or Pco_2; temperature
   administration of stored blood with deterioration of
   _____ _____.   RBC Phophates (2,3 DPG)

III. Correlate the signs of hypoxemia with potential signs of hypoxia.
A. Compare the arterial O_2 saturation with the Sv_{O_2} pattern, if available, or with a venous O_2 saturation of a mixed venous sample from a _____line to determine the P_A
   _____ difference.   A-Vo_2
   REMEMBER: An increase in the A-VDo_2 or decrease in the Svo_2 indicates that either the cardiac output has *(increased/decreased)*   decreased
   or tissue _____ _____ have O_2 demands
   increased. Thus the presence of impending *(hypoxemia/hypoxia)*   hypoxia
   may be detected. A low venous Po_2 may also be used as an indicator of an increased A-V$o_2$differencebecause it usually corresponds with a *(high/low)*venous saturation.   low
B. Correlate these with acid base changes reported on ABG sample.
C. Check for signs of altered cardiac output, such as CHF, arrhythmia, hypotension, and low urine output.
D. Note the presence of _____changes   sensorium

IV. Determine modes of *intervention*. Modes of intervention may include the following:
A. Administer therapy for CHF, shock, or both.
B. Administer pulmonary physical therapy, mechanical ventilation, or medications, such as bronchodilators or saline, to promote clearing of the lungs and O_2 transport.
C. Increase or decrease current amount of supplemental O_2 therapy, or change the mode of O_2 delivery.
D. Correct patient temperature or acid-base changes.
E. Administer blood in presence of severely low Hb levels; locate and provide therapy for bleeding sites; or administer iron supplements.

ABG examples reflecting changes combined in acid-base and oxygenation are provided at the end of Unit 5. Nursing orders may reflect both the ABG interpretation process and the modes of clinical assessment as well as suggested modes of intervention.

SUGGESTED READINGS

Ahrens TS: Concepts in the assessment of oxygenation, Focus Crit Care, 14(1):36, 1987.

Alspaco J and Williams, editors: Core curriculum for critical care nursing, ed. 3, 1985, WB Saunders Co.

Birman H et al: Continuous monitoring of mixed venous oxygen saturation in hemodynamically unstable patients, Chest 86(5):753, 1984.

Boutros AR et al: Value of continuous monitoring of mixed venous blood oxygen saturation in the management of critically ill patients, Crit Care Med 14(2):132, 198?.

Buehmann AA: Blood gases, Eur Heart J 6(Suppl C): 45, 1985.

Carnevale FA: Transcutaneous oxygen monitoring: assessment techniques, Dimens Crit Care Nurs 5(5):264, 1986.

D'Agustino J: Set your mind at ease on oxygen toxicity Nursing 13(7):55, 1983.

Darovic, GO: Hemodynamic monitoring: invasive and noninvasive clinical application, Philadelphia, 1987, WB Saunders Co.

Daily EF and Schoeder JS: Techniques in bedside hemodynamic monitoring, ed. 3, St. Louis, 1984, CV Mosby Co.

Davidson LJ et al: Continuous Svo$_2$ monitoring: a tool for analyzing hemodynamic status, heart Lung 15(3):287, 1986.

Davila F: Simplified bedside calculation of inspired and alveolar oxygen pressures, Crit Care Med 14(4):310, 1986.

Demling RH and Wilson RF: Decision making in surgical critical care, Philadelphia, 1988, BC Decker, Inc.

Fahey PJ, editor: Continuous measurement of blood oxygen saturation in the high risk patient: theory and practice in monitoring mixed venous oxygen saturation, vol. 2, Mountain View, Ca, 1985, Oximetrix, Inc.

Fuchs, PL: Getting the best out of oxygen delivery systems, Nursing 10(12):34-43, 1980.

Fulmer J and Snider G: Proceedings of American College of Chest Physicians National Heart, Lung, and Blood Institute National Conference on Oxygen Therapy, Heart Lung 13(5)550, 1984.

Gardner PE and Bopp-Laurent D: Continous Svo$_2$ monitoring, Prog Cardiovasc Nurs 2:9, 1987.

Gardner R: Pulse oximetry: is it monitoring's 'silver bullet'? J Cardiovasc Nurs 1(3):79, 1986.

Gore, JM: Use of continuous monitoring of mixed venous saturation in the coronary care unit, Chest 86(5):757, 1984.

Guyton AC: Textbook of medical physiology, Philadelphia, 1986, WB Saunders Co.

Hardy G: Svo$_2$ continous monitoring techniques, Dimens Crit Care Nurs 7(1):8, 1988.

Jaquith SM: Continous measurement of Svo$_2$: clinical applications and advantages for critical care nursing Crit Care Nurs 5(2):40, 1985.

Lehrer : Understanding lung sound, Philadelphia, 1984, WB Saunders Co.

Massaro D: Oxygen: toxicity and tolerance, Hosp Pract 21(7):95, 1986.

Mikani R et al: International Symposium on Lung Sounds, Chest 92(2):342, 1987.

Mims BC: The risks of oxygen therapy, RN 50(7):20, 1987.

Netter FH: Respiratory system (The CIBA collection of medical illustrations) Summit, N.J., 1979, Ciba-Geigy Corp.

Norton LC and Conforti C: The effects of body position on oxygenation, Heart Lung 14(1)45, 1985.

Pasterkamp H et al: Nomenclature used by health care professionals to describe breath sounds in Asthma, Chest 92(2):346, 1987.

Porth C: Pathophysiology, concepts of altered health, ed. 2, Philadelphia, 1986, J.B. Lippincott Co.

Relman AS: Blood gases: arterial or venous, (editorial), N Engl J Med 315(3):188, 1986.

Shapiro BA: Respiratory intensive care: State of the art vol 5, Chicago, 1984, Respiratory Care Seminars, Inc.

Shapiro BA et al: Clinical application of respiratory care, Chicago, 1984, Year Book Medical Publishers, Inc.

Shapiro BA: Clinical application of blood gases, ed. 3, Chicago, 1982, Year Book Publishers, Inc.

Standards and guidelines for cardiopulmonary resuscitation (CPR) and emergency cardiac care (ECC), JAMA 255(21):2905, 1986.

Textbook of advanced cardiac life support, Dallas, 1987, American Heart Association.

White K: Completing the hemodynamic picture: Svo$_2$, Heart Lung 14(3):272, 1985.

White K: Continous monitoring of mixed venous oxygen saturation (Svo$_2$: a new assessment tool in critical care nursing, Part I, Cardiovasc Nurs 23(1):1, 1987.

White K: Continuous monitoring of mixed venous oxygen nursing, Part II, Cardiovasc Nurs 23(2):7, 1987.

Wilkins RL et al: Lung sounds: a practical guide, St. Louis, 1988, The CV Mosby Co.

Yang SC et al: Oxygen delivery and consumption and p50 in patients with acute myocardial infarction, Circulation 73(6):1183, 1986.

Maintaining Fluid and Chemical Balance

DEFINITIONS AND DISTRIBUTION OF FLUID AND PARTICLES

1 The body's fluid is located within two major compartments. *Intracellular fluid (ICF)* is located *(inside/outside)* the cells. *Extracellular fluid (ECF)* is located *(inside/outside)* the cells. The extracellular fluid includes intravascular and interstitial fluids. Intravascular fluid *(IVF)* is the fluid located within the blood vessels and is synonymous with the blood plasma. It surrounds the blood cells. Interstitial fluid *(ISF)* is located between the cells and between cells and blood vessels. It surrounds the tissue cells.

inside
outside

2 Fluid may also accumulate, in pathological states, within spaces where normally only small amounts of fluid exist. These potential spaces include such areas as the spaces between the pleural, peritoneal, and pericardial linings. The term "third space" is used to refer to these potential spaces. The potential spaces are in close communication with the interstitial space. However, the term "third space" is also often used clinically to refer to fluid accumulation within the natural interstitial fluid compartment. Because of this dual yet closely related interpretation, this term's clinical usage requires careful scrutiny.

3 LET US REVIEW: There are two major fluid compartments of the body: the _____ and _____ fluid compartments.

Extracellular fluid is made up of _____ fluid and _____ fluid. The term "third space" may refer to either the natural _____ fluid compartment space or the _____ _____ in close communication with that compartment.

intracellular; extracellular

intravascular
interstitial
interstitial
potential spaces

4 Many types of particles are found within the body fluids and the fluid compartments. Many of these particles are electrically charged. The charged particles are known as *ions*.

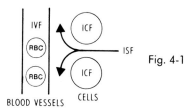

Fig. 4-1

An *anion* is a negatively charged particle. The four major anions in the body are chloride (Cl^-), bicarbonate (HCO_3^-), protein (PRO^-), and phosphate ($HPO_4^=$).

A *cation* is a positively charged particle. The four major cations in the body are potassium (K^+), sodium (Na^+), calcium (Ca^{++}), and magnesium (Mg^{++}).

5 An *electrolyte* is a combination of an anion and a cation in solution, which, when dissolved in water, will conduct an electrical current. However, the term "electrolyte' is often used loosely to refer to any charged particle, or _____.

ion

6 LET US REVIEW: Sodium (Na^+) is an example of a positively charged particle, or *(cation/anion)*, found within the body fluids. The other three major cations in body fluids are _____, _____, and _____. Chloride (Cl^-) is an example of a negatively charged particle, or *(cation/anion)*, found within the body fluids. The other three major anions in body fluids are _____, _____, and _____.

NaCl (cation + anion) in solution separates into the charged particles Na^+ and Cl^- and may thus conduct an electrical current. Each these charged particles may be loosely referred to as an _____.

cation

K^+ Ca^{++}; Mg^{++}
anion

HCO_3^-; PRO^-; $HPO_4^=$

electrolyte

7 The exact distribution of electrolytes varies between the body fluid compartments. The two major *cations* within the *intracellular* fluid compartment are K^+ and Mg^{++}. The two major *anions* within the intracellular fluid compartment are protein and phosphate. K^+ is located *primarily* but not exclusively within the _____ compartment.

intracellular

The two major *cations* within the *extracellular* fluid compartment are Na^+ and Ca^{++}. The two major *anions* within the *extracellular* fluid compartment are chloride and bicarbonate.

The distribution of electrolytes between the two extracellular fluid compartments (plasma and interstitial fluid) is identical, except for the presence of a greater amount of *protein* in the *plasma*. This protein inequality is the major factor responsible for fluid difference between the two extracellular fluid compartments (see Frames 61 to 70).

In summary:

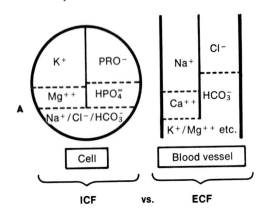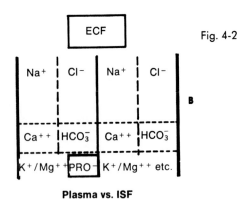

Fig. 4-2

MAJOR ROLES OF CHARGED PARTICLES

8 The major role of positively charged particles, or *(cations/anions)*, is to determine the electrical events of living cells, especially cardiac cells.

    cations

    The negatively charged particles, or *(cations/anions)*, play a major role in acid-base imbalances by either accepting or donating hydrogen ions (H^+) (see Unit 5, Frames 68 to 122).

    anions

ROUTINE SERUM ELECTROLYTE TESTS

9 *Serum electrolyte levels* reflect the ion concentrations in the *(intracellular/extracellular)* fluid compartment. The two cations measured on routine serum electrolyte tests are Na^+ and K^+.

    extracellular

    REMEMBER: Within the extracellular fluid compartment, there is a greater distribution of *(Na^+/K^+)*.

    Therefore the influence of Na^+ on serum concentration is greater than that of K^+.

10 The two anions measured on routine serum electrolyte tests are Cl^- and HCO_3^-. The HCO_3^- level is often reported as the *CO_2 content* and thus may not be as clearly apparent as the Cl^- level.

    Carbon dioxide is carried within the blood in three forms: (1) freely dissolved as a *gas,* (2) combined with water to form *carbonic acid,* and (3) converted to *bicarbonate* to facilitate acid excretion and buffering.

$$CO_2 + H_2O \leftrightarrows carbonic\ acid \leftrightarrows HCO_3^- + H^+$$

Thus the total CO_2 content of the blood is actually composed of not only free carbon dioxide, as the name suggests, but also carbonic acid and _____.

    HCO_3^-

Actually about 95% of the carbon dioxide is in the form of HCO_3^- instead of free carbon dioxide. Thus the measurement of *CO₂ content* essentially reflects _____ levels.

HCO_3^-

11 According to the law of electroneutrality, the total amount of positively and negatively charged particles in the serum must remain equal. However, not all charged particles in the blood are actually measured on a set of routine serum electrolyte tests.

LET US REVIEW: The positively charged particles measured on routine serum electrolyte tests are _____ and _____. The negatively charged particles measured on routine serum electrolyte tests are _____ and _____.

Na^+; K^+

Cl^-; HCO_3^-

12 The sum of the serum Cl^- and HCO_3^- levels does not normally balance the sum of the Na^+ and K^+ levels. There are *usually fewer negative charges* than positive charges. This gap of negative charges not accounted for (that is, not directly measured) in the determination of serum electrolytes is known as the *anion gap*. The normal anion gap is composed of small amounts of albumin and other proteins, phosphate, and organic acids such as ketoacids, lactic acid, and sulfuric acid, which are negatively charged.

REMEMBER: The negatively charged particles of the blood function in acid-base balance. When excess acids accumulate, this gap can become greater than normal. An example of this process occurs in hypoxia, which causes excess _____ acid production. Determination of the anion gap can thus be useful in assesing the mechanism of metabolic acidosis (see Unit 5, Frames 116 to 122).

lactic

HOMEOSTATIC MECHANISMS
Cellular level

13 Many interacting forces in the body combine to maintain physiological equilibrium, or *homeostasis*. Equilibrium of gas and fluid concentrations is maintained on a cellular level by processes that allow the movement of either *particles* or *fluid* across cell membranes.

14 *Diffusion* is the movement of particles from a region of greater concentration to a region of lesser concentration. An example of diffusion is the gaseous exchange in the lungs. Oxygen, in particles, moves from a region of _____ concentration (the air) to a region of _____ concentration (venous blood).

greater
lesser

REMEMBER: Since gas particles exert pressure both in the atmosphere and in solution, a _____ difference or gradient also exists, which facilitates the movement of oxygen into the blood (see Unit 3, Frame 13).

pressure

The process of diffusion is influenced not only by differences in concentration (concentration gradients) but also by *pressure* gradients and *electrical* gradients.

15 *Osmosis* is the movement of water from a region of lesser concentration (of dissolved particles) to a region of greater concentration (of dissolved particles). Within the body cells, semipermeable membranes limit the free movement of some particles. In this setting the movement of water by the process of _____ aids in stabilizing fluid concentration.

osmosis

16 **In summary:**

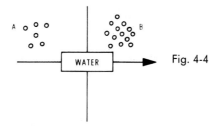

DIFFUSION	OSMOSIS
MOVEMENT OF PARTICLES	MOVEMENT OF WATER
GREATER TO LESSER CONCENTRATION	LESSER TO GREATER CONCENTRATION
EXAMPLE: GASEOUS EXCHANGE IN THE LUNGS	EXAMPLE: WATER TRANSPORT IN THE CELLS.

Fig. 4-3

17 Let us consider osmosis in more detail.

Fig. 4-4

REMEMBER: Osmosis is the movement of _____. In osmosis, movement occurs from a region of _____ concentration to a region of _____ concentration of dissolved particles. In Fig. 4-4, the less concentrated solution is *(solution A/solution B)*. Thus water moves from solution _____ to solution _____, where there are more particles but where there is less water. This process represents an effort to equalize the concentration of both solutions. Thus the process of osmosis is an attempt to maintain equilibrium or _____.

water
lesser
greater
solution A
A
B

homeostasis

18 Solutions having the same concentration in relation to each other are *isotonic*. A *hypertonic* solution is one with a greater concentration of dissolved particles in comparison with that of another solution. A *hypotonic* solution is one with a lesser concentration of dissolved particles in comparison with that of another solution.

19 In the human body, plasma changes in concentration often occur before either interstitial or intracellular changes occur. The plasma is also more easily accessible for fluid replacement therapy. Therefore let us focus on fluid movements and intracellular changes that result from changes in plasma concentration.

Consider solution B in Fig. 4-5 as the blood plasma (intravascular fluid compartment) and solution A as the fluid within the cell _____ fluid compartment).

intracellular

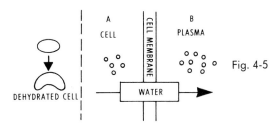

Fig. 4-5

In Fig. 4-5, the plasma is *(hypertonic/hypotonic)* in relation to the fluid within the cell.

hypertonic

Examples of hypertonic solutions or agents that may be introduced into the plasma include mannitol, albumin (25%), glucose solutions greater than 5% (as used in hyperalimentation and/or polarizing and glucose-insulin-potassium solutions), and 5% dextrose in 0.45 normal saline solution ($D_5\frac{1}{2}NS$). Clinical states that may result in hypertonicity of the plasma include diabetes and hypovolemia.

20 In the presence of a hypertonic plasma, water moves from the _____ into the _____. The cells become _____. Hypertonic solutions pull water *(into/out of)* the cells. These solutions have a similar effect on the interstitial fluid, probably before they affect intracellular fluid. The therapeutic significance of this interstitial effect may be greater than that of the intracellular effect.

cells; plasma
dehydrated; out of

Hypertonic agents should produce an immediate *(increase/ decrease)* in plasma and circulating blood volume. Thus in the presence of normal or minimally impaired renal function, these agents should produce an *(increase/decrease)* in fluid excretion, or a *diuretic* effect. Hypertonic solutions may be used n the cardiac patient to mobilize excess fluid from the interstitial and intracellular fluid compartments.

increase

increase

21 Now let us reverse the situaion. Consider solution A in Fig. 4-6 as the blood plasma (_____ fluid compartment) and solution B as the fluid within the cell (_____ fluid compartment).

intravascular
intracellular

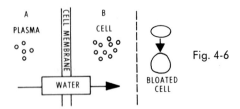

A PLASMA
CELL MEMBRANE
B CELL
WATER
BLOATED CELL

Fig. 4-6

In Fig. 4-6, the plasma is *(hypotonic/hypertonic)* in relation to the fluid within the cell.

Hypotonic solutions are potentially more hazardous to use than hypertonic solutions and are thus less commonly used clinically. The most common hypotonic solution, used in carefully selected patient situations, is ½NS. In contrast, clinical states resulting in hypotonic plasma concentrations are very common—especially in a coronary care unit (CCU). They include CHF, hepatic failure, and certain stages of renal failure.

hypotonic

22 In the presence of a hypotonic plasma, water moves from the _____ into the _____. The cells become _____.

plasma; cell bloated

Rapid administration of a hypotonic solution may push water *(into/out of)* blood cells and tissue cells, causing hemolysis and impaired cellular function, especially notable within brain cells. Plasma hypotonicity associated with clinical states such as CHF results in a similar change in the interstitial fluid compartment. This change occurs earlier than the effect on tissue cells. Fluid moves *(into/out of)* the interstitial space. In this setting the fluid movement occurs in response to other vascular changes as well as the changes in plasma tonicity (see Frames 61 to 70).

into

into

23 Both hypertonic and hypotonic solutions use the principles of *osmosis*. Another term for hypertonicity, then, is *hyperosmolality*. Another term for hypotonicity is _____. Normal serum osmolality is approximately 300 millisomols per liter (mOsm/L) and is determined to the greatest extent by the level of serum Na^+, although blood glucose and blood urea nitrogen levels also play significant roles.

hyposmolality

REMEMBER: Within the extracellular fluid compartment, there is a greater distribution of the electrolyte _____.

Na^+

NOTE: For purposes of simplicity and practicality, we are using the term "serum" synonymously with "plasma," as is often implied in serum electrolyte determinations. However, in strict usage of blood terminology, these terms are not identical.

24 Solutions having the *same concentration* in relation to each other are said to be _____.

isotonic

An isotonic solution administered into the body *(will/will not)* alter the osmotic concentratin. Examples of isotonic solutions (osmolality approximately 300 mOsm/L) include: normal saline, in water, and 5% dextrose in 25% sodium chloride ($D_5\frac{1}{4}NS$). 5% Dextrose in water (D5W) and lactated Ringer's solution (when all its particles, including the lactate, are taken into consideration) are examples of slightly hypotonic solutions. Although hypotonic solutions are not ideal for cardiac patients, solutions other than D5W may be undesirable because of their sodium and other electrolyte content *(K^+, lactate, Ca^{++})*. Thus D5W is usually the intravenous solution of choice.

will not

25 In summary:

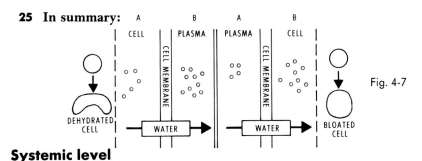

Fig. 4-7

Systemic level

26 Osmosis is one of the processes by which fluid balance is regulated at the cellular level. Fluid and electrolyte balance is also regulated systemically by special areas in the body known as *receptors*. These receptors are specialized cells or sensory nerve endings that send messages to the hormonal and cardiovascular centers in the brain.

27 Increases or decreases in intravascular fluid result in changes in plasma *concentration* (tonicity or osmolality). Special areas in the body known as *osmoreceptors* are sensitive to these changes in serum osmolality, or _____. The *osmoreceptors* are located in the *hypothalamus*.

concentration

28 Increases or decreases in body fluid also result in changes in blood volume, which may influence the *blood pressure*.
   Special areas in the body known as *pressoreceptors* are sensitive to these changes in _____. The pressoreceptors most directly affecting fluid balance are located in the walls of the aortic arch, the internal walls of the carotid arteries, and the juxtaglomerular apparatus in the kidneys. They are sensitive to the *pressure* exerted on the vascular walls as they are stretched by the *volume* of blood leaving the heart—the *cardiac output*. Thus the pressoreceptors are actually sensitive to changes in _____ _____.

pressure

cardiac output

29 Severe increases or decreases in body fluid may cause the cardiac output to drop enough to interfere with the supply of oxygen to the tissues (see Unit 3). Special areas in the body, known as *chemoreceptors,* are sensitive to these changes in the chemical oxygen. Oxygen-sensitive chemoreceptors are located in the walls of the aortic arch and carotid arteries. These receptors are sensitive to lack of oxygen.

30 LET US REVIEW: Fluid imbalances are detected systemically by _____ areas. The osmoreceptors are primarily sensitive to changes in serum _____. The pressoreceptors are sensitive to changes in _____ _____. The chemoreceptors are sensitive to severe changes in cardiac output that are associated with alterations in the blood chemical _____.

receptor
concentration
cardiac output

oxygen

31 Let us now consider each of these receptor areas in more detail. The *osmoreceptors* are cells located within the _____. These cells are bathed by the body's fluid. In the presence of plasma hypotonicity, or *(increased/decreased)* osmolality, the osmoreceptors *bloat* and in this way sense *(increased/decreased)* body fluid. In the presence of plasma hypertonicity, or *(increased/decreased)* osmolality, the osmoreceptors shrink and in this way sense *(increased/decreased)* body fluid.

hypothalamus

decreased
increased
increased
decreased

   The osmoreceptors send signals to the posterior pituitary gland to control the release of *antidiuretic hormone* (ADH). ADH inhibits excretion of water by the kidneys, thereby causing water conservation.

   THEREFORE: Inhibition of ADH secretion leads to *(diuresis/water reabsorption).* Increased ADH secretion leads to *(diuresis/water reabsorpotion)./*

diuresis
water reabsorption

32 **In summary:**

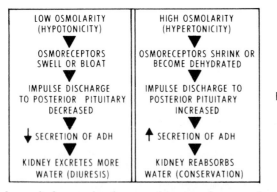

```
┌──────────────────────────┬──────────────────────────┐
│    LOW OSMOLARITY        │    HIGH OSMOLARITY        │
│    (HYPOTONICITY)        │    (HYPERTONICITY)        │
│           ▼              │           ▼               │
│    OSMORECEPTORS         │  OSMORECEPTORS SHRINK OR  │
│    SWELL OR BLOAT        │    BECOME DEHYDRATED       │
│           ▼              │           ▼               │
│  IMPULSE DISCHARGE       │   IMPULSE DISCHARGE TO     │
│  TO POSTERIOR PITUITARY  │   POSTERIOR PITUITARY      │
│      DECREASED           │      INCREASED            │
│           ▼              │           ▼               │
│  ↓ SECRETION OF ADH      │  ↑ SECRETION OF ADH       │
│           ▼              │           ▼               │
│  KIDNEY EXCRETES MORE    │   KIDNEY REABSORBS         │
│  WATER (DIURESIS)        │   WATER (CONSERVATION)     │
└──────────────────────────┴──────────────────────────┘
```

Fig. 4-8

33 The hypothalamus is also sensitive to *decreases* in *cardiac output.* In the presence of a decrease in cardiac output, the osmoreceptors are also stimulated, resulting in secretion of _____ and *(diuresis/water absorption).*

ADH; water absorption

34 The pressoreceptors (baroreceptors) are sensory nerve endings located in the walls of the _____ arch, in the internal walls of

aortic

the _____ arteries, and in specialized cells within the _____ apparatus in the kidneys. These areas are sensitive to pressure changes in the blood vessels that are associated with changes in _____ _____.

carotid

juxtaglomerular

cardiac output

Stimulation of the pressoreceptors ultimately results in both *hormonal* and *nervous* responses. The hormone controlled is *aldosterone*. Aldosterone is secreted by the adrenal cortex and causes the kidney to retain Na^+ and excrete K^+. Water is reabsorbed with the Na^+ retention. The nervous sytem affected is the *parasympathetic* nervous system via the vagus nerve. Vagal stimulation causes slowing of the heart and *(increases/decreases)* the cardiac output.

decreases

35 In the presence of an *increased cardiac output* the _____ nervous system is *(stimulated/inhibited)*, which causes _____ of the heart rate in an attempt to *(increase/decreae)* the cardiac output. The release of the hormone aldosterone is *(stimulated/inhibited)* so that additional Na^+ and water *are not* retained.

parasympathetic
stimulated; slowing
decrease
inhibited

In the presence of a *decreased cardiac output* the parasympathetic nervous sytem is *(stimulated/inhibited)*, causing a slight *(increase/decrease)* in the heart rate. Aldosterone release is *(stimulated/inhibited)*. Aldosterone causes _____, _____ reabsorption, and _____ excretion.

inhibited; increase
stimulated
Na^+; water
K^+

36 Secretion of aldosterone is stimulated by mechanisms involving both the brain and the kidney. Changes in cardiac output are sensed by the *(osmoreceptors/pressoreceptors)* in the aorta and carotid arteries, which send signals to the brain (hypothalamus). The hypothalamus, in turn, regulates the release of the hormone adrenocorticotropin (ACTH). This hormone stimulates the adrenal cortex to produce aldosterone.

pressoreceptors

ACTH is released in response to signals carried to the *(brain/kidney)* and stimulates the production of the hormone _____.

brain

aldosterone

37 Another mechanism that influences the release of aldosterone is found in the kidney. The renin-angiotensin mechanism is stimulated when the juxtaglomerular apparatus in the kidneys senses decreased pressure and ischemia.

Renin is released into the blood secondary to these pressure changes and acts as a catalyst in the synthesis of angiotensin I. Angiotensin I is carried by the circulating blood to the lungs, where an enzyme present in lung tissue converts it to angiotensin II. Angiotensin II causes *vasoconstriction* and *aldosterone secretion*.

Renin is released in response to changes sensed by the *(brain/kidneys)* and, after being converted to _____ _____, stimulates the release of the hormone _____.

kidneys
angiotensin II
aldosterone

NOTE: Secretion of aldosterone is stimulated not only by the renin-angiotensin mechanism and ACTH but also in response to (1) decreased Na^+ and increased K^+ in the extracellular fluid, (2) the effects of stress, and (3) the administration of certain steroids (see Unit 8).

38 In summary:

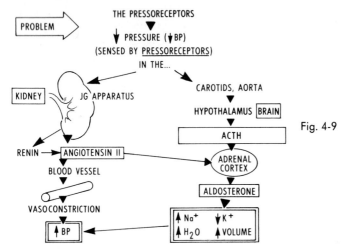

Fig. 4-9

39 Both the osmoreceptors and the pressoreceptors have been discussed in detail. Let us now consider the role of the *chemoreceptors* in fluid imbalances.

LET US REVIEW: The chemoreceptors are sensory nerve endings located in the walls of the _____ arch and at the bifurcation of the _____ arteries. These areas are primarily sensitive to lack of _____.

Oxygen-sensitive chemoreceptors are also located in the brain stem. However, these receptors are only *indirectly* sensitive to the lack of oxygen as it affects other chemicals, such as H^+. These receptors play a greater role in regulating the lungs rather than the heart. The brain chemoreceptors are referred to as *central* chemoreceptors, in contrast to those in the great vessels, called the *peripheral* chemoreceptors (see Unit 3, Frames 51 to 54).

aortic

carotid

oxygen

40 Lack of oxygen may be associated with either decreases in the oxygen dissolved in the blood or *severe drops in cardiac output* and systemic arterial pressure. When the arterial pressure drops to approximately 40 to 80 mm Hg, the influence of the peripheral chemoreceptors becomes more powerful than that of the pressoreceptors.

41 Stimulation of the chemoreceptors results simultaneously in both *hormonal and nervous* responses that support each other. The nervous system stimulated is the *sympathetic* nervous system. The hormones released are *epinephrine* and *norepinephrine,* which act as mediators for sympathetic activity (see Unit 10). These hormones are secreted by the adrenal medulla and cause stimulation of heart rate and contractility and constriction of the peripheral blood vessels.

42 In summary:

Fluid imbalances are regulated by _____ areas. The osmoreceptors are sensitive primarily to changes in _____. They are located in the _____ and regulate the release of the hormone _____, which causes _____ reabsorption.

receptor
osmolality/concentration
hypothalamus
ADH; water

When there is low extracellular fluid volume, the plasma is usually *(more concentrated/less concentrated)* than the intracellular fluid. It may thus be considered *(hypertonic/hypotonic).* In the presence of a hypertonic plasma there is an *(increase/decrease)* in the secretion of ADH in an attempt to conserve water.

more concentrated
hypertonic
increase

The osmoreceptors are also stimulated in the presence of a *(high/low)* cardiac output to release *(more/less)* ADH.

low
more

43 The *pressoreceptors* are sensitive primarily to changes in _____ _____. They are located in the walls of the _____ and _____ arteries and in the cells of the _____ apparatus in the *(brain/kidneys).* The pressoreceptors influence the _____ nervous system and the release of the hormone _____.

cardiac output
aorta; carotid
juxtaglomerular; kidneys
parasympathetic
aldosterone

REMEMBER: Stimulation of ADH may also be influenced by the action of the pressoreceptors.

In the presence of low extracellular fluid volume, the cardiac output is usually *(increased/decreased).* The parasympathetic nervous system is *(stimulated/inhibited),* causing a slight *(increase/decrease)* in the heart rate. Aldosterone release is *(stimulated/inhibited)* to cause _____ and _____ reabsorption and _____ excretion.

decreased
inhibited; increase
stimulated
Na$^+$; water
K$^+$

44 The *chemoreceptors* are sensitive primarily to the lack of _____ associated with severe drops in _____ _____. They are located in the _____ arch and at the bifurcation of the _____ arteries. The chemoreceptors regulate the _____ nervous system and the release of the hormones _____ and _____.

oxygen; cardiac output
aortic
carotid
sympathetic
epinephrine; norepinephrine

In the presence of severely low extracellular fluid volume, the cardiac output may drop enough to interfere with the delivery of _____. The sympathetic nervous system is then *(stimulated/inhibited)* and the release of the hormones epinephrine and norepinephrine *(increases/decreases),* causing stimulation of the heart

oxygen; stimulated

increases

_____, _____, and _____ of the peripheral blood vessels.

rate; contractility; constriction

45 In summary:

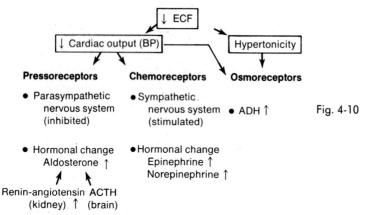

Fig. 4-10

FLUID IMBALANCES
Hypovolemia

46 Let us first consider the problem of *hypovolemia*. Hypovolemia is a condition in which there is a deficit of fluid in the extracellular fluid compartment. The most common cause of hypovolemia in the setting of a CCU is excessive diuresis.

47 With excessive diuresis both _____ and _____ are excreted.

Na^+; water

However, more water than Na^+ may be lost, and the serum (plasma) becomes *(hypertonic/hypotonic)*.

hypertonic

REMEMBER: Hypertonic serum (plasma) causes water to move *(into/ out of)* the cells. That results in *(bloated/dehydrated)* cells.

out of
dehydrated

With excessive diuresis there is also a(n) *(decrease/increase)* in blood volume and therefore a fall in cardiac output.

decrease

NOTE: Diuresis may also result in a disproportionate Na^+ loss and a *(hypertonic/hypotonic)* serum. In this case the symptoms of cellular dehydration may not be as pronounced.

hypotonic

48 In the presence of a change in either plasma concentration or cardiac output, systemic receptors are activated.

REMEMBER:Plasma hypertonicity is sensed by the *(osmoreceptors/pressoreceptors)*, causing an increase in the secretion of _____ in an attempt to conserve _____.

osmoreceptors
ADH
water

A fall in cardiac output is sensed by the *(pressoreceptors/osmoreceptors)*.

pressoreceptors

The pressoreceptors trigger a sequence of events that causes an increased production of the hormone _____ and loss of

aldosterone

(parasympathetic/sympathetic) system activation.

Aldosterone causes the reabsorption of _____ and _____ and the excretion of _____ by the kidneys.

Severe falls in cardiac output trigger a *(chemoreceptor/pressoreceptor)* response and *(parasympathetic/sympathetic)* system activation.

49 When volume losses exceed the ability of the receptors to compensate for them, *symptoms* appear, and supportive intervention is indicated.

The clinical symptoms associated with excessive diuresis are related to *hypertonicity, cellular dehydration,* and the *decrease* in *cardiac output.* Acute symptoms associated with dehydrated cells, or plasma hypertonicity, or both include thirst, an elevated temperature, and alterations in consciousness caused by the associated hypernatremia.

REMEMBER: Normal serum osmolality is determined to the greatest extent by the level of the serum _____.

Chronic symptoms of dehydration include dry mucous membranes and decreased skin turgor.

Symptoms associated with a decrease in cardiac output include decreased urinary output, hypotension, and decreased venous filling. Severe falls in cardiac output trigger a *(chemoreceptor/pressoreceptor)* response and are usually associated with inadequate tissue oxygenation, or *(hypoxemia/hypoxia).*

REMEMBER: The clinical syndrome of hypoxia associated with a fall in cardiac output is known as _____.

50 Laboratory assessment of volume imbalances includes analyses of (1) fluid intake and output, (2) hematocrit value, (3) blood urea nitrogen (BUN) and serum creatinine levels, (4) urine levels of Na^+ and K^+, (5) urine specific gravity, and (6) comparison of serum with urine osmolality.

Volume losses may be monitored by close observation of fluid intake and output, taking into acount an average 1000 ml of insensible fluid loss daily from the skin, lungs, and gastrointestinal tract. Serum concentration changes may be detected by alterations in hematocrit values, BUN levels, and serum osmolality. The remainder of the tests just noted assist in differentiating the causes of decreased urinary output. Decreased urinary output may be a sign of renal damage or merely a temporary alteration in renal function associated with a fall in cardiac output.

REMEMBER: In the presence of a fall in cardiac output the hormone _____ is released, causing conservation of _____ and _____ by the kidney cells and excretion of _____ in the urine. Therefore, in *low cardiac output states,* urine levels of Na^+ should be *low,* and urine levels of K^+ should be *high.*

parasympathetic

Na^+

water; K^+

chemoreceptor

sympathetic

Na^+

chemoreceptor

hypoxia

shock

aldosterone

Na^+; water

K^+

Damaged kidney cells are unable to conserve Na^+. Thus in the presence of a fall in urine output caused by renal damage, urine electrolyte levels of both Na^+ and K^+ will be high, and the urine Na^+-to-K^+ ratio will be equal.

51 Urine osmolality is a test of changes in urine concentration. It is a more sensitive test than the urine specific gravity test, although the latter is simpler and may be performed at the bedside. Normally, urine osmolality is approximately 2½ times greater than the serum osmolality (600 to 800 mOsm/L). In dehydration the serum osmolality is *(increased/decreased)*.

increased

In the absence of renal damage the kidneys conserve fluid. The urine osmolality may increase up to four times normal and remain significantly higher than the serum osmolality. However, if renal damage is present, the kidneys are unable to conserve fluid. The serum and urine concentrations become equal. Therefore comparison of the serum and urine concentrations, or _____, is a useful assessment tool for evaluating volume imbalances and renal function.

osmolality

52 The clinical symptoms of dehydration include _____ _____, _____, and alterations of _____. The clinical symptoms of a fall in cardiac output include a *(high/low)* urine output, *(high/low)* blood pressure, and _____

elevated temperature
thirst
consciousness
low; low
shock

The management of the dehydration and fall in cardiac output that are associated with hypovolemia is directed toward supporting the body's own homeostatic efforts by the administration of _____.

fluid

Hypervolemia

53 Let us now consider the problem of *hypervolemia*. Hypervolemia is a condition in which there is an excess of fluid volume in the extracellular fluid compartment.

REMEMBER: The extracellular fluid consists of the _____ fluid and the _____ fluid. Therefore in a state of hypervolemia there is an excess of fluid within the _____ _____ and between the _____.

intravascular
interstitial
blood vessels
cells

54 The most common cause of hypervolemia in the setting of a CCU is *congestive heart failure*. In CHF the heart is weakened and cardiac output *(increases/decreases)*.

decreases

This decrease in cardiac output results in a fall in blood pressure, which is sensed by the body's *(osmoreceptors/pressoreceptors)*.

pressoreceptors

The pressoreceptors trigger a sequence of events that causes an increased production of the hormone _____. In the pres-

aldosterone

ence of a fall in cardiac output, stimulation of the pressoreceptors or direct stimulation of the osmoreceptors causes an increased release of the hormone _____.

ADH

55 In response to the effects of aldosterone and ADH, Na^+ and water are retained. Retention of Na^+ and water by the kidneys leads to the development of a state of *(hypervolemia/hypovolemia)*.

hypervolemia

In CHF a state of hypervolemia imposes an increased strain on an already weakened myocardium. Thus the compensatory mechansims involved in this situation *potentiate* the underlying problem.

56 Although both Na^+ and water are retained in CHF, more water than Na^+ is retained. Thus the serum (plasma) becomes *(hypotonic/hypertonic)*.

hypotonic

REMEMBER: Although aldosterone controls the reabsorption of both Na^+ and water, ADH controls the reabsorption of *only water*.

In the presence of hypotonic plasma, fluid moves *(into/out of)* the interstitial fluid space and *(into/out of)* the cell. The cell and the interstitial fluid space become *(dehydrated/bloated)*. Because of the hypotonicity of the serum, the serum Na^+ is usually *(high/low)* in CHF. However, the total body Na^+ is *(high/low)* because of the effects of the hormone _____. This type of pseudohyponatremia is referred to as "dilutional hyponatremia" and should not be treated as a *true* low serum Na^+ condition.

into
into
bloated
low
high
aldosterone

57 The clinical symptoms associated with CHF are related to the *excess fluid* and *hypotonicity* of the extracellular fluid compartment and to the *decrease* in *cardiac output*. The excess fluid in the vascular compartment shifts first to the _____ space and eventually into the cell. The presence of fluid in the interstitial space produces the clinical symptom known as *edema* (see Frames 61 to 70). The edema of CHF may occur *systemically* or within the *pulmonary* vascular bed.

interstitial

The symptoms associated with the decrease in cardiac output mimic those of hypovolemic states and include a decrease in _____ output, *(high/low)* blood pressure, and, when severe, _____.

urine; low
shock

58 In the presence of hypervolemia caused by CHF the hematocrit value is usually *(high/low)*, and the serum osmolality is *(high/low)*. However, the urine specific gravity and urine osmolality are *(high/low)* because of the effects of *aldosterone* and ADH. Because of the action of aldosterone in response to the fall in cardiac output, the urine Na^+ level is *(high/low)*, and the urine K^+ level is *(high/low)*.

low; low
high

low; high

If renal damage has occurred, the serum and urine osmolality as well as the urine Na^+ and K^+ levels become _____.

equal

59 In the management of *hypervolemia* secondary to CHF, therapy is directed toward (1) decreasing pulmonary congestion, (2) decreasing the cardiac work load through diuresis, (3) stimulating myocardial contractility, and other measures. For a complete discussion of the therapy of CHF, refer to Unit 9.

60 **In summary:**

	HYPERVOLEMIA		HYPOVOLEMIA
CLINICAL EXAMPLE		CHF	Excessive Diuresis
PLASMA		Hypotonic	Hypertonic
CELL		Bloated	Dehydrated
CARDIAC OUTPUT		Decreased	Decreased
RECEPTOR RESPONSE	Response Potentiates Problem	Osmo — ▲ADH Presso — ▲Aldosterone Chemo — ▲Epinephrine Norepinephrine ▲Sympathetic	Response Insufficient to correct problem
SYMPTOMS	Edema (Pulmonary/Systemic) ▼Urine output Hypotension shock		Thirst ▲Temperature Alterations in Consciousness Dry Mucous Membranes ▼Skin Turgur ▼Urine output Hypotension Shock
LAB DATA	▼Hematocrit ▼Serum Osmolality ▼Serum Na$^+$	Intake/output Bun/Creatinine ▼Urine Na$^+$ ▲Urine K$^+$ Urine Osmolality > Serum Osmolality	▲Hematocrit ▲Serum Osmolality ▲Serum Na$^+$
THERAPY	Diuretics Decrease Workload Cardiac Stimulation		Fluid Administration

Monitor Cardiac Function

Fig. 4-11

MECHANISMS OF EDEMA: CAPILLARY DYNAMICS

61 Edema is strictly defined as excess fluid in the interstitial fluid compartment. However, the term is also used clinically to describe the accumulation of fluid inside the cell occurring as the result of cellular damage. The most familiar clinical example of this phenomenon is the intracellular accumulation of fluid in brain cells that is referred to as "cerebral edema." Cerebral edema as a result of cerebral hypoxia may occur in the patient with coronary artery disease.

Fluid accumulation occurring as the result of volume overload and circulatory changes should be distinguished from the intracellular and interstitial fluid accumulation associated with direct cellular damage. This second process is more commonly referred to as "inflammation" and is discussed in this section. Both processes occur in the patient who has an acute MI.

62 If volume overload is caused by CHF, a primary excess of interstitial fluid occurs, although secondary intracellular volume changes and cellular bloating may also occur.

LET US REVIEW: Plasma hypotonicity associated with clinical states such as CHF results in changes in the interstitial fluid compartment, which occur earlier than those in tissue cells. Fluid moves *(into/out of)*   **into** the interstitial space. In this example, the fluid movement occurs in response to vascular changes as well as to the changes in plasma tonicity.

63 An excess of interstitial fluid occurs when there are alterations in *capillary dynamics* as well as extracellular fluid excesses. This excess of interstitial fluid is known as _____. Four factors are in-   **edema** volved in capillary fluid movement:
1. Capillary pressure
2. Lymphatic action (negative interstitial fluid pressure)
3. Interstitial protein levels (interstitial fluid colloid osmotic pressure)
4. Serum protein levels (serum colloid osmotic pressure)

64 *Capillary pressure* is generated as a result of the pumping action of the *heart*. Capillary pressure tends to move fluid from the vascular

CAPILLARY DYNAMICS FAVORING EDEMA FORMATION

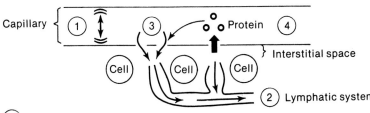

Fig. 4-12

(1) ⬆ Capillary pressure—pushes fluid out of the blood vessels into the interstitial space

(2) Lymphatic drainage—overloaded

(3) ⬆ Capillary permeability—proteins leak into interstitial space (interstitial colloid osmotic pressure)

(4) ⬇ Serum protein levels—less osmotic force (serum colloid osmotic pressure)

compartment to the interstitial space.

The negative *interstitial fluid pressure* is generated by the action of the lymphatic system, which drains interstitial spaces of fluid and small amounts of protein, thus creating a vacuum effect. Interstitial fluid pressure is another factor that tends to pull fluid out of the vascular compartment into the _____ spaces, although draining the interstitial space at the same time, which *prevents* fluid accumulation, or _____.

interstitial

edema

65 A third force favoring the movement of fluid into the interstitial space is the *interstitial fluid colloid osmotic pressure*. Interstitial fluid contains a small amount of protein that leaks from the capillaries into the interstitial spaces.

The presence of protein in the interstitial space exerts an osmotic pull, which favors fluid movement into the _____ space. This pull is known as the _____ _____ _____ _____ _____. In the presence of alterations in *capillary permeability* larger amounts of protein leak into the interstitial space, promoting edema formation.

interstitial
interstitial fluid colloid
osmotic pressure

66 One major force is responsible for holding fluid within the vascular compartment. This force is the *serum colloid osmotic pressure* (oncotic pressure). Oncotic pressure is the force exerted at the capillary membrane by the largely nondiffusible plasma proteins.

REMEMBER: The distribution of electrolytes between the plasma and the interstitial fluid compartments, or *(intracellular/extracellular)* fluid, is identical except for one major difference—the presence of a greater amount of protein in the _____ (see Frames 6 and 7). The protein primarily responsible for the plasma oncotic pressure is *albumin*. When serum albumin levels are low because of factors such as liver disease or stress, fluid will move more easily into the _____ compartment. Thus a lowered oncotic pressure *enhances* the potential for edema formation.

extracellular

plasma

interstitial

67 Factors predisposing to edema formation include the following:
1. Increases in capillary _____
2. Increases in _____ permeability
3. Decreases in plasma _____ levels
4. Inadequate _____ drainage

LET US REVIEW: In the presence of CHF, fluid movement and edema formation occur in response to _____ changes as well as plasma tonicity and volume changes.

In acute MI and left ventricular heart failure, pulmonary capillary pressure rises (see Unit 9). When the capillary pressure exceeds the plasma oncotic pressure, fluid moves *(into/out of)* the blood vessels and into the _____ spaces. Lymphatic drainage is *(in-*

pressure
capillary
albumin
lymphatic

vascular

out of
interstitial; increased

creased/decreased) in the body's efforts to minimize edema formation. The engorged lymphatic vessels can be seen in dependent areas on radiographic examination and are known as "Kerley's B lines."

68 Serum albumin levels may be lowered in the patient who has a coronary artery disease caused by the effects of stress. In response to corticosteroid release during stress, protein reserves are converted to glucose for energy, resulting in a protein deficit. Lowered serum albumin levels facilitate edema formation. Thus edema may occur at capillary pressures that are otherwise usually well tolerated.

In patients with cardiovascular disease, the serum albumin levels can be checked to determine whether this factor is contributing to the formation of edema. Supplementary albumin may be administered if hypoalbuminemia is present.

Accumulation of edema fluid in the interstitial spaces of the lungs eventually fills the alveolar spaces as well and interferes with gas exchange (see Unit 3).

69 Let us now consider the process of fluid accumulation occurring in response to direct cellular damage. This process is also referred to as *inflammation*. It is a patterned, nonspecific response to any type of cellular injury (see Unit 6, Frames 146 to 148).

Local damage to tissue cells results in a combination of intracellular and interstitial fluid accumulation. This process is also referred to as _____. The intracellular fluid accumulation [inflammation] occurs as the result of damage to the cell membranes, mitochondria, lysosomes, or all of these. The interstitial fluid accumulation—true edema—occurs as a result of an increase in vascular permeability.

REMEMBER: In the presence of alterations in capillary permeability, _____ leak from the plasma into the interstitial space, pro- [proteins] moting _____ formation. The increase in vascular perme- [edema] ability has been associated with histamine release from storage sites located in specialized cells embedded among most common tissue cells. Other vasoactive substances, such as bradykinin and serotonin, have also been implicated in myocardial injury.

70 In hypoxic cellular damage, intracellular fluid accumulation and swelling also occur as a result of inactivation of Na^+-K^+ pump caused by less available oxygen and ATP. As the Na^+-K^+ pump is inactivated, Na^+ and _____ accumulate within the cells. [water] For this reason intracellular fluid excess may exceed extracellular (interstitial) fluid excess in the hypoxic patient.

The intracellular cerebral swelling of hypoxia is often mislabeled "cerebral edema." This intracellular swelling also occurs in the myocardial cellular hypoxia and injury associated with acute MI and cardiogenic shock (see Units 6 and 9).

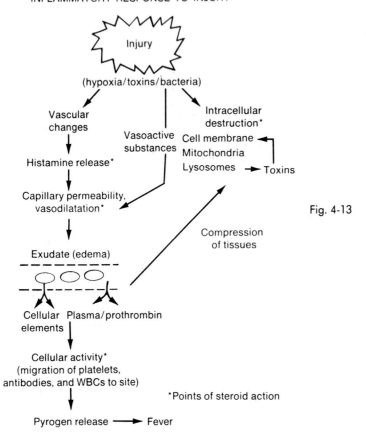

INFLAMMATORY RESPONSE TO INJURY

Fig. 4-13

ROLE OF ELECTROLYTES IN CONDUCTION OF ELECTRICAL IMPULSES

71 In the *polarized,* or resting, state, the inside of the cell is electrically *(negative/positive)* with respect to the outside. All of the body's charged particles, or *ions,* contribute to the cell's charge. However, the *(cations/anions)* play a more significant role in determining cell charge. During electrical events, changes in electrical activity occur because of the movement of these charged particles.

negative

cations

REMEMBER: Particles move by the process of *(osmosis/diffusion)* from an area of _____ concentration of particles to an area of _____ concentration of particles. Therefore, for movement of particles to occur, there must be a difference in concentration between two compartments.

diffusion

greater

lesser

72 To establish a difference in concentration across a cell membrane (a concentration gradient), active movement of particles is required. This active process requires energy and is known as *active transport.*

The Na^+-K^+ pump in living cells actively pumps Na^+ out of the cell and K^+ into the cells, establishing a _____ gradient for each ion. This pump requires energy in the form of ATP and represents a form of _____ transport. The Na^+-K^+ pump prepares the cells for electrical events and is necessary to allow the movement of particles responsible for charging the cell. However its actual contribution to cell charge in the normal cell is minimal. Most of the Na^+ pumped out is replaced by the equivalently charged K^+ pumped into the cell.

73 LET US REVIEW: Each ion is found both inside and outside of the cell. Therefore Na^+ and K^+ are found both _____ and _____ the cell. However, K^+ is found *primarily* inside the cell. Na^+ is found *primarily* _____ the cell. This difference in the actual distribution of these electrolytes is maintained by the _____ pump.

As a result of the Na^+-K^+ pump, there is more K^+ inside the cell than outside the cell. This difference in K^+ concentration inside the cell relative to the concentration outside the cell is known as a _____ gradient. This gradient allows for the movement of K^+ by the process of _____.

Free movement of charged particles across a concentration gradient in living cells is limited by permeability of the cell membrane.

74 Every ion (for example, Na^+, Cl^-, and PRO^-) inside and outside the cell has its own charge. In the *polarized,* or resting, state the cell has a net negative charge.

The inside of the cell is thus *(electronegative/electropositive)* with respect to the outside.

The major factors responsible for this electronegativity are:
1. The presence of *nondiffusible* intracellular proteins, which act as *anions.*
   REMEMBER: Anions are *(positively/negatively)* charged particles. The two major intracellular anions are phosphates and _____.
2. Enhanced membrane permeability to K^+, allowing for diffusion of K^+ *(into/out of)* the cell.
   REMEMBER: There is more K^+ _____ the cell than _____ the cell. If the cell membrane permits free diffusion, the K^+ particles will move from the area of *(greater/lesser)* concentration inside the cell to the area of *(greater/lesser)* concentration outside the cell.

As the positively charged K^+ particles leave the cell, the inside of the cell becomes more *(electropositive/electronegative)* with respect to the outside.

concentration

active

inside
outside
outside

Na^+-K^+

concentration
diffusion

electronegative

negatively

protein

out of
inside
outside
greater
lesser

electronegative

75 In the resting state, the cell membrane is 50 to 100 times more permeable to K^+ than to Na^+. Therefore *(Na⁺/K⁺)* diffuses more freely across the cell membrane. Thus the cell charge in the polarized or resting state is most dependent on the level of intracellular *(Na⁺/K⁺)*. The most important electrolyte in the polarized state is *(Na⁺/K⁺)*.

K^+

K^+

K^+

76 In summary:

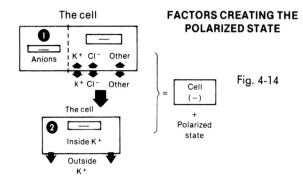

Fig. 4-14

77 Let us now consider the electrical response of cardiac cells to an impulse or stimulus.

REMEMBER: Excitation and conduction of electrical impulses in the heart depends on the process of *depolarization*. In response to advancing electrical impulses *(negatively/positively)* charged particles move into the cells. The inside of these cells becomes *(electropositive/electronegative)*, and the cells are said to be _____ (see Unit 2).

positively
electropositive
depolarized

Both Na^+ and Ca^{++} play major roles in the process of *depolarization*.

REMEMBER: Na^+ is a *(positively/negatively)* charged particle. The greatest concentration of Na^+ is found *(inside/outside)* the cell.

positively
outside

78 When an electrical impulse reaches a ventricular resting cell membrane, the permeability to K^+ decreases and the permeability to Na^+ suddenly increases. The Na^+ "gates" open. Sodium ions rush *(into/out of)* the cells by the process of *(osmosis/diffusion)*, upsetting the previous *(electronegativity/electropositivity)*.

into
diffusion
electronegativity

The inside of the cell loses its electronegativity and becomes *(electronegative/electropositive)* with respect to the outside. It is said to be _____. This local electrical response then acts as an electrical signal and stimulates adjacent cells, thus spreading the original electrical stimulus throughout the heart.

electropositive

depolarized

REMEMBER: The spread or transmission of electrical signals throughout the heart is known as _____.

conduction

Both excitation and conduction, then, depend on the process of _____.

depolarization

79 The cells of normal atrial and ventricular musculature and Purkinje fibers depolarize and conduct impulses rapidly. They are therefore referred to as *"fast* cells." Depolarization in fast cells is caused by the rapid influx of Na^+ and is referred to as "fast-channel electrical activity."

This rapid influx of Na^+ is followed by a secondary slower inward movement of Ca^{++}, which aids further in depolarization.

REMEMBER: Depolarization is caused by the movement of positively charged particles *(into/out of)* the cells upsetting the previous electronegativity. Like Na^+, Ca^{++} is a *(positively/negativly)* charged particle located primarily *(inside/outside)* the cell. The cell membrane permeability to Ca^{++} also changes when an electrical impulse reaches it, opening the Ca^{++} gates, usually *(before/after)* the Na^+ gates.

into
positively
outside

after

80 The slow, inward Ca^{++} movement during depolarization is logically referred to as _____-channel electrical activity. Slow-channel activity dominates in the normal SA and AV nodes. Therefore depolarization of the SA and AV nodes occurs *(rapidly/slowly)*, and these cells are logically referred to as _____ cells.

slow

slowly
slow

LET US REVIEW: Both excitation and conduction depend on the process of _____. Depending on the specific conduction structure, depolarization may involve either _____ or _____-channel activity or both. Fast-channel depolarization requires *(Na⁺/Ca⁺⁺)*. Slow-channel depolarization requires *(Na⁺/Ca⁺⁺)*.

depolarization
fast
slow
Na^+
Ca^{++}

81 To receive another impulse, the cells must return to their previous resting or _____ state. This process is known as *repolarization.*

polarized

During active repolarization the membrane permeability to both Na^+ and Ca^{++} decreases, and the permeability to K^+ increases. The Na^+ gates close, and the K^+ gates reopen.

REMEMBER: The greatest concentration of K^+ is found *(inside/outside)* the cell. Therefore, as the K^+ gates open, diffusion occurs, causing some of the intracellular K^+ to move *(into/out of)* the cell. Because of this loss of positive ions, the inside of the cell again becomes *(electropositive/electronegative)* with respect to the outside, and the cell is said to have been _____.

inside

out of

electronegative
repolarized

Thus the major influence of K^+ is manifested during the *(depolarization/repolarization)* phase of the cardiac cycle. The electrolyte K^+ is responsible for both the initial polarization and the subsequent repolarization of cardiac cells. The Ca^{++} gates remain open during early repolarization and then close, thus delaying active repolarization and extending the total period of repolarization, including the refractory periods.

repolarization

82 The Na^+ that enters the cell during depolarization is returned to its extracellular site by a pump exchange mechanism in preparation for the next impulse. Some of the K^+ that leaves the cell during repolarization is also returned to its _____ site to maintain the K^+ _____ gradient. The active pumping of Na^+ and K^+ requires work, or energy. The body's units of energy _____ are needed.

intracellular
concentration
ATP

The electrolyte Mg^{++} is important in the breakdown of ATP for energy. Therefore Mg^{++} is necessary for normal functioning of the Na^+-K^+ pump.

It is currently thought that the major role of the Na^+-K^+ pump is to return these electrolytes to their original location to maintain the _____ gradient. Its contribution to cell charge in the normal cell is thought to be negligible because for each Na^+ ion pumped out of the cell there is an almost equal replacement of a _____ ion back into the cell. A separate but closely related Ca^{++} pump returns the Ca^{++} to its extracellular site. This Ca^{++} pump also requires energy, or ATP.

concentration

K^+

83 In summary:

Depolarization and repolarization—roles of lytes

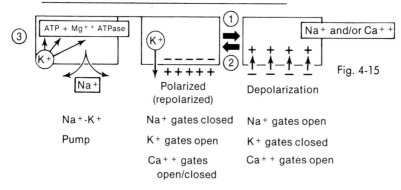

Fig. 4-15

Na+-K+ Pump	Polarized (repolarized)	Depolarization
	Na+ gates closed	Na+ gates open
	K+ gates open	K+ gates closed
	Ca++ gates open/closed	Ca++ gates open

84 An insult to the cell membrane, such as occurs in infarction, allows K^+ to leak in and out of the cell freely, thereby disturbing the resting electronegativity.

NOTE: Some have used these principles in formulating a mode of therapy in the management of acute MI. It has been theorized that if the electrical instability of infarction is affected by K^+ loss, replacement of this K^+ into the cell (in conjunction with glucose and insulin) should eliminate the electrical instability. Essentially a temporary substitute K^+ pump and cell membrane are created. This solution reportedly helps the injured cell to return to its previously polarized state. It is therefore known as a _____ solution. It is more commonly known as a glucose-insulin-potassium (GIK) solution. Us-

polarizing

ers claim fewer to no arrhythmias and accelerated healing. The use of polarizing solution in clinical practice, however, is still controversial. The potential benefits of the high glucose content to the ischemic myocardial cell are still under investigation (see Unit 6).

85 The electrolyte Ca^{++} plays both electrical and mechanical roles in cardiovascular cells. Ca^{++} plays a major primary and secondary role in *(depolarization/repolarization)*. A portion of the extracellular Ca^{++} also lines the Na^+ gates and decreases Na^+ permeability. The positively charged Ca^{++} repels some of the positively charged Na^+ and thus inhibit Na^+-dependent depolarization. AV block caused by bundle branch block has been associated with rapid calcium administration.

depolarization

As calcium moves *(into/out of)* the cell during depolarization and *(early/late)* repolarization, it also causes mobilization of the contractile proteins, resulting in _____ activity. Calcium thus acts as a link between electrical and mechanical activity, while maintaining separate, distinct roles in each.

into
early
mechanical

86 In summary:

Contractility is controlled by the electrolyte _____. Depolarization allows Ca^{++} to have this effect. Therefore Ca^{++} serves to correlate electrical activity with _____ activity. Calcium also plays a primary electrical role by controlling depolarization in *(fast/slow)* cells such as the _____ _____ and the _____ _____.

Ca^{++}

mechanical
slow
SA node
AV node

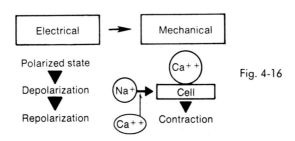

Fig. 4-16

ECG correlation

87 On the ECG the QRS complex represents ventricular depolarization. The ST segment immediately follows depolarization and precedes repolarization. The T wave represents ventricular _____. Na^+ may be said to affect *(depolarization/repolarization)* and therefore the *(QRS complex/T wave)*. K^+ may be said to affect *(depolarization/repolarization)* and therefore the *(QRS complex/T wave)*. Mg^{++} affects the level of intracellular K^+ by controlling the _____ pump. Therefore Mg^{++} also affects the *(QRS complex/T wave)*.

repolarization
depolarization
QRS complex;
  repolarization;
T wave; Na^+-K^+

T wave

ECG CORRELATION

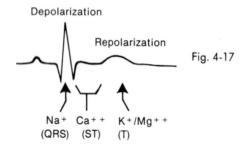

Depolarization

Repolarization

Fig. 4-17

Na+   Ca++   K+/Mg++
(QRS)   (ST)   (T)

The effect of Ca^{++} follows initial ventricular depolarization and extends into repolarization. During early repolarization its effects are unopposed by more significant movements of either Na^+ or K^+. Therefore Ca^{++} effects are most pronounced on the _____ segment, which corresponds with *(early/late)* repolarization.

ST; early

Action potential

88 In the resting, or polarized, state, the cardiac cell has the potential for electrical activation—a resting potential.

REMEMBER: In the resting state the inside of the cell is *(electronegative/electropositive)* with respect to the outside. The most important electrolyte in the polarized state is *(Na^+/K^+)*.

electronegative
K^+

As the electronegativity of a cell becomes greater, the resting membrane potential also becomes greater (more negative). Normal resting potential varies, depending on the type of cell. The atrial and ventricular muscle cells normally have a resting membrane potential of approximately -90 millivolts (mV). The level of the resting membrane potential depends on both the integrity of the cell membrane and its resting _____ to K^+.

permeability

89 The electrical characteristics of different types of cardiac cells vary. Let us first consider the electrical characteristics of the stable atrial and ventricular muscle cell. When a single cell is activated by a stimulus, local electrical changes occur that produce an action current or action potential. This action potential from a single cell can be recorded on graph paper, producing a pattern (Fig. 4-18).

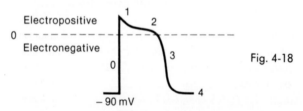

Electropositive

0

Electronegative

1

2

3

4

0

−90 mV

Fig. 4-18

90 The phase of electrical action denoted by 0 represents a change in cellular polarity from electronegative to _____. Therefore phase 0 represents the process of _____.

electropositive
depolarization

The phase of electrical action denoted by phases 1, 2, and 3 represents the return to electronegativity, or _____.

repolarization

91 The action potential represents the electrical activity of *(single/many)* cells. A surface ECG, recorded from the body surface, represents the electrical activity of *(single/many)* cardiac cells.

single

many

The surface ECG, then, records the effects of *(a single/many)* action potential(s). As a result, only a rough correlation may be drawn between the events of cellular action potentials and the events of the surface ECG.

many

92 LET US REVIEW:

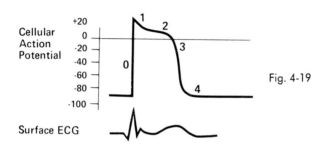

Fig. 4-19

93 Let us now correlate the phases of the action potential with the corresponding electrolyte movements.

Phase 0 of the action potential represents *(depolarization/repolarization)* and occurs because of the rapid influx of _____ and/or slower influx of _____. The effects of Na^+ subside im-

depolarization
Na^+
Ca^{++}

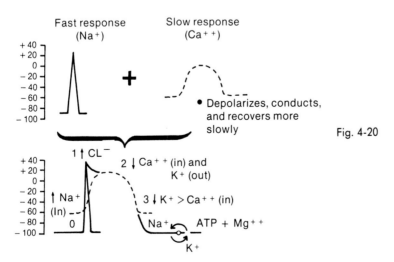

Fig. 4-20

mediately after phase 0, when the Na^+ gates close. In contrast, the effects of Ca^{++} extend into repolarization as the Ca^{++} gates remain open and then slowly close (see Fig. 4-20). In Na^+-dependent cells the effects of Na^+ and Ca^{++} overlap in phase 0 (see Fig. 4-20). At the end of phase 0 the inside of the cell is *(electropositive/electronegative)* with respect to the outside.

electropositive

Phases 1, 2, and 3 represent *(depolarization/repolarization)*, during which the cell returns to the _____ state.

repolarization

resting

94 *Phase 1* represents an early brief phase of repolarization. It is thought to be caused by movement of the negatively charged particle Cl^- into the cell.

NOTE: During this phase there is a small negative deflection on the action potential that corresponds with the inward movement of Cl^-. The inward flow of Na^+ is almost completely inactivated during phase 1.

Phase 2 in the repolarization process is a plateau period. This plateau occurs because of a persistent, slow, inward movement of Ca^{++} balanced by an early, outward movement of K^+. This plateau corresponds roughly to the absolute refractory period.

NOTE: Ca^{++} begins to move into the cell during phase _____ of electrical activity but continues into phase _____, where the effects of Na^+ stop, and the influence of Ca^{++} becomes more pronounced.

0

2

Phase 3 represents the rapid phase of repolarization, in which K^+ *(enters/leaves)* the cell, and the Na^+ and Ca^{++} currents are *totally inactivated*. The cell thus becomes progressively more electronegative. The active phase of repolarization is represented on the action potential by phase _____ and is due to loss of _____ from the cell.

leaves

3

K^+

95 *Phase 4* represents the return to maximum electronegativity or the resting _____ _____. It is during this phase that the Na^+-K^+ pump is most active, although Na^+-K^+ pump activity may occur throughout the repolarization process.

membrane potential

REMEMBER: Phase 4 is also known as the _____ state and represents complete repolarization of the cell. All the phases of electrical action (1, 2, and 3) may be collectively referred to as *electrical systole*. The resting phase (4) between electrical activity is known as *electrical diastole* and corresponds to the resting membrane potential, or _____ state.

resting

polarized

96 The level of resting membrane potential (phase 4) influences the rate of phase 0 or _____. Slow cells typically have a low resting membrane potential (RMP) of approximately -60mV. Cells that have a low RMP are *(more/less)* negative in the resting state than

depolarization

less

other cardiac cells. They may also be described as *(hypopolarized/hyperpolarized.)*

Hypopolarized cells depolarize slowly in response to electrical stimulation. Thus the upstroke of phase 0 is *(rapid/gradual)*, as depicted in Fig. 4-20.

The Ca^{++} gates open at a lower (less negative) membrane potential than do the Na^+ gates. Therefore Ca^{++} gates open *(before/after)* the Na^+ gates in fast cells, and hypopolarization favors *(Na^+ channel/Ca^{++} channel)* activity. Opening of the membrane Ca^{++} channel is usually triggered by the fast-channel depolarization or _____ states.

Hypopolarization also contributes to the property of automaticity or electrical instability (see Unit 7).

REMEMBER: Automaticity is a normal property of conduction structures such as the _____ node and _____ node (or AV junction). These structures are also *(slow/fast)* cells and are *(Na^+ dependent/Ca^{++} dependent)*. Slow cells typically *depolarize and repolarize (rapidly/slowly)*.

CALCIUM: CARDIOACTIVE VERSUS VASOACTIVE ROLES

97 The electrolyte Ca^{++} plays both _____ and _____ roles in living cells (including cardiovascular cells). The cardiovascular cells consist of (1) the *conduction structures*, (2) the *smooth muscle structures* in the coronary and peripheral arterial walls, and (3) the *cardiac muscle structures* in the myocardial walls.

The *cardioactive* roles of calcium refer to its effects on the conduction and cardiac muscle structures. The *vasoactive* roles of calcium refer to its effects on the _____ smooth muscle structures.

Cardiovascular electrical activity is controlled by the conduction structures and their autonomic innervation. Cardiovascular mechanical activity is controlled by the _____ and _____ muscle structures and their autonomic innervation. Ca^{++} acts as a mediator of this electrical and mechanical activity, performing distinct, key roles in each as well as serving as a _____ between them.

98 Cardiac and vascular smooth muscle differ from skeletal muscle with reference to their intracellular Ca^{++} stores. Cardiac and smooth muscle have minimal intracellular Ca^{++} stores and are thus more dependent on extracellular Ca^{++} levels for contraction. This extracellular Ca^{++} is transported into the cell through unclearly defined Ca^{++} channels. Blockade of these channels results primarily in decreased _____ and _____ muscle contraction. Skeletal muscle contraction *(is/is not)* significantly affected.

Margin answers:

hypopolarized

gradual

after
Ca^{++} channel

hypopolarized

SA; AV
slow
Ca^{++} dependent
slowly

electrical
mechanical

vascular (arterial)

cardiac; smooth

link

cardiac; smooth
is not

The specific characteritics of the cardiac versus smooth muscle calcium channels may differ, allowing them to be separately blocked. This may partially explain the selective cardioactive versus vasoactive actions of the calcium channel-blocking agents.

99 Cardiac and smooth muscle calcium channels differ significantly with respect to the effect of autonomic innervation. The heart and blood vessels are predominantly under the control of the sympathetic nervous system (see Unit 10, Frames 50 to 52). Beta-receptor stimuluation opens the calcium channels in cardiac muscle, thus facilitating contraction. However, beta-receptor stimulation inhibits the calcium channels in vascular smooth muscle, thus facilitating relaxation. Therefore the effects of autonomic (beta) blockade will be *(the same/different from)* those of calcium channel blockade. Calcium may also be mobilized to the interior of the cardiac or smooth muscle cell by voltage-dependent pathways as well as the previously mentioned receptor- dependent pathways. Other vasoactive factors that influence Ca^{++} flux into vascular smooth muscle include angiotensin, serotonin, prostaglandins, histamine, acidity, acetylcholine, $Mg+$, Na^+, and K^+.

different from

100 Cadiac muscle has a unique structure. It resembles *skeletal muscle* in its striped, or striated, appearance and in its mechanical function. However, it resembles *smooth muscle* in its electrical properties and in its single, centrally located nuclei. Like *skeletal muscle*, cardiac muscle is composed of contractile proteins arranged in parallel bands. The protein bands move inward by a sliding mechanism, causing shortening, or contraction, of the muscle fiber. These bands give cardiac and skeletal muscle its striated appearance. Like *smooth muscle*, cardiac muscle is autonomically innervated but does not require extrinsic innervation to contract.

Cardiac muscle also has unique properties of its own. A unique feature of cardiac muscle is the presence of intercalated discs separating each muscle cell. These discs allow for either facilitation or inhibition of electrical impulses (Fig. 4-21).

Another unique characteristic of cardiac muscle is its interconnecting, or branching, appearance (Fig. 4-21). Although smooth muscle cells may be tightly entwined and may have contact points, or bridges, between them, they are not clearly interconnected.

Cardiac muscle cells are _____ innervated, contract according to a _____ mechanism, form _____, _____ arrangements, and are separated by _____ discs. Contraction of cardiac muscle is primarily dependent on *(intracellular/extracellular)* Ca^{++} levels.

autonomically
sliding; interconnecting
branching
intercalated
extracellular

Skeletal muscle	Cardiac muscle	Smooth muscle	
	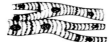	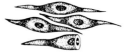	Fig. 4-21

- Striated
- Separate cells
- Multiple nuclei peripherally located
- Numerous mitochondria
- Somatic innervation (spinal nerves)

- Striated
- Cells interconnected with *branching appearance*
- Single nuclei centrally located
- Numerous mitochondria
- *Intercalated* discs
- Minimal ICF calcium stores

- Plain
- Cells entwined with close contact points
- Single nuclei, centrally located
- Fewer mitochondria
- Spindlelike appearance
- Minimal ICF calcium stores

Autonomic innervation
(Sympathetic/parasympathetic)

101 Both cardiac and smooth muscle contain the same contractile proteins—actin and myosin. However, these fibrils are arranged more loosely within the vascular smooth muscle. There are a few other differences as well (Fig. 4-21). Smooth muscle contains more actin and less myosin. Contraction of smooth muscle occurs by the interaction of Ca^{++} with the intermediary protein *calmodulin* on *myosin*-binding sites. For comparison with the determinants of cardiac muscle contraction see Frames 104 to 109. The tubular structure within the vascular smooth muscle is less well defined. Contraction of the arterial smooth muscle maintains normal and abnormal peripheral and _____ artery tone. Ca^{++}-channel blockade results in *(contraction/relaxation)* of the peripheral and coronary arteries. This concept has been applied to the pharmacological management of angina and hypertension.

coronary

relaxation

102 The structure of the cardiac muscle is more well defined and will be discussed in the next few paragraphs. However, there currently are fewer practical applictions for drug therapy, since the current major benefits of calcium blockade are related to its role either in the vascular smooth muscle or in electrical conduction structures. However, the role of calcium-channel blockade in the myocardium may have a future role in the preservation of ischemic myocardium and limitation of acute myocardial infarction (see Unit 10, Frames 224 and 226). The role of Ca^{++} in cardiac muscle is currently better correlated clinically to radionuclide studies and hemodynamic changes.

103 Within both cardiac and skeletal muscle cells are multiple inner cores of contractile proteins known as *myofibrils*. Each myofibril is wrapped by a meshlike tubular network that runs parallel with the muscle cell. These tubules are known as *longitudinal,* or L, *tubules*

MICROSTRUCTURE CARDIAC MUSCLE

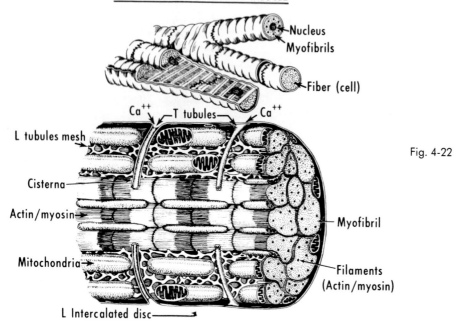

Fig. 4-22

(Fig. 4-22). The L tubules completely surround the muscle fibril and are, in turn, surrounded by a layer of mitochondria. Single tubules run perpendicular to the muscle cell. These tubules are called *transverse,* or T, *tubules* and serve to link the extracellular fluid with the interior of the cell. The points at which the L tubules contact the T tubules serve as storage sites for intracellular Ca^{++} and are called *cisternae.* The tubules serve to link electrical to mechanical activity.

104 LET US REVIEW: The ion that links electrical to mechanical activity is

_____. $\qquad$ Ca^{++}

The tubule that serves to store intracellular Ca^{++} is known as the (*L/T*) tubule. The tubule that links the intracellular with the extracellular fluid is the (*L/T*) tubule. Cardiac muscle contracts by a _____ mechanism involving contractile _____.

L

T

sliding; proteins

The contractile proteins are grouped together, forming long cores within the muscle fibers, referred to as _____. $\qquad$ bands

105 Let us now consider the activity of these proteins in more detail. Cardiac muscle contains contractile proteins known as actin and myosin. The proteins are also referred to as filaments. Small projections, known as crossbridges, emerge from the *thicker myosin* filaments within the muscle cell. These crossbridges serve as potential contact points between the contractile proteins. If a muscle fiber is overstretched so that optimal contact between the filaments is compromised, contractility may diminish.

    NOTE: This concept limits the effect of Starling's law of the heart (see Fig. 4-23 and Unit 9).

106 We can now describe the sequence of events that links cellular electrical and mechanical activities. When depolarization occurs, the electrical current, or action, potential travels to the interior of the cell via the T tubules.

    REMEMBER: The T tubules connect the interior of the cell with *(intracellular/extracellular)* fluid.

extracellular

    This electrical stimulus allows for contraction to be initiated in two ways:
1. It alters cellular permeability to Ca^{++} and thus allows Ca^{++} to flow into the cell from the extracellular fluid.
2. It causes Ca^{++} to be released from intracellular stores within the *(L/T)* tubules.

L

107 The electrical activity moves Ca^{++} from the _____ fluid and from inactive storage sites to active sites. Ca^{++} binds with the actin filament. This binding activates the crossbridges, which pull the actin toward the myosin, causing them to overlap. This sliding and overlapping of the protein filaments causes the muscle fiber to shorten. Shortening of muscle fibers is known as *contraction* (Fig. 4-23).

extracellular

MYOCARDIAL CONTRACTION

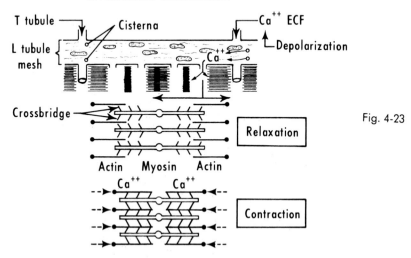

Fig. 4-23

108 The chemical energy required for sliding and shortening of the muscle protein units is obtained from the splitting of ATP produced in the muscle cell. When contraction is over, Ca^{++} is pumped out of the active areas, and relaxation occurs. This relaxation process also requires the body's ATP. ATP most effectively is produced by the breakdown of glucose in the presence of oxygen.

109 LET US REVIEW: Electrical activation causes Ca^{++} to move *(into/out of)* the muscle cell from the extracellular fluid via the _____ tubules. It also causes mobilizaion of the Ca^{++} stored inthe intracellular fluid of the _____ tubules. Ca^{++} then binds with the contractile protein _____ and acts as a trigger to cause overlapping of the actin and _____.

into

T

L

actin

myosin

Overlapping of actin and myosin causes *(shortening/elongation)* of the muscle fiber.

shortening

Shortening of muscle fibers is known as _____.

contraction

Both contraction and relaxation of cardiac muscle involve the splitting of _____ for energy.

ATP

In hypoxia, *(more/less)* ATP is produced. Thus both contraction and relaxation of hypoxic cardiac muscle cells will be *(more effective/less effective)*.

less

less effective

SUGGESTED READINGS

Beckwith N: Fundamentals of fluid resuscitation, Nurs Life 7(3):49, 1987

Berne RM and Levy MN: Physiology ed 2, St. Louis, 1988, The CV Mosby Co.

Cheveny B: Overview of fluid and electrolytes, Nurs Clin North Am 22(4): 749, 1987.

Collins RD: Illustrated manual of fluid and electrolyte disorders, ed. 2, Philadelphia, 1983, JB Lippincott Co.

Conover MB: Understanding electrocardiography ed. 5, St. Louis, 1988, The CV Mosby Co.

Demling R and Wilson R: Decision making in surgical critical care, Philadelphia, 1988, BC Decker Inc.

Cardiac arrythmias, Whippany, NJ, 1981, Knoll Pharmaceutical Co.

Guyton AC: Textbook of medical physiology, ed. 7, Philadelphia, 1986, WB Saunders Co.

Groer ME and Shekleton ME: Basic pathophysiology: a conceptual approach ed. 2, St. Louis, 1983, The CV Mosby Co.

Dyckner T and others: Salt and water balance in congestive heart failure, Acta Med Scand (Suppl) 707:27, 1986.

Hurst JW and Logue RB, editors: The heart, arteries, and veins, ed. 6, New York, 1986, McGraw-Hill Inc.

Hypovolemia—when to suspect it, how to stop it, RN December, 1986.

Keung E and Aronson R: Physiology of calcium current in cardiac muscle, Progress Cardiovasc Dis 25:279, 1983.

Lancaster LE: Renal and endocrine regulation of water and electrolyte balance, Nurs Clin North Am 22(4):761, 1987.

Laragh J: Atrial natriuretic hormone, the renin-aldosterone axis and blood pressure-electrolyte homeostasis, New Eng J Med 313(21):1330, 1985.

Lundemann JP and others: Potential biochemical mechanisms for regulation of the slow inward current: theoretical basis for drug action, Am Heart J 103:746, 1982.

Marriott HJL and Conover MH: Advanced concepts in arrythmias, St. Louis, 1983, The CV Mosby Co.

Martof M: Part I: Fluid Balance, J Nephrology Nursing 2(1):10, 1985.

Masiak M, Masiak N, and Duffin M: Fluid and

Electrolytes throughout the Life Cycle: Norwalk, Conn., 1985, Appleton-Century-Crofts.

Meola D and Walker V: Responding quickly to Tachyarrhythmias, Nursing 17(11):34, 1987.

Netheny N: Fluid and electrolyte balance: nursing considerations, Philadelphia, 1987, JB Lippincott Co.

Monitoring fluids and electrolytes precisely, Nursing Skillbooks ed 2, Springhouse, Pa. 1983, Springhouse Corp.

Movsessia M: Calcium physiology in smooth muscle, Prog Cardiovasc Dis 25:211, 1982.

Poyss AS: Assessment and nursing diagnosis in fluid and electrolyte disorders, Nurs Clin North Am 22(4):773, 1987.

Rose B: Clinical physiology of acid-base and electrolyte disorders, ed. 2, New York, 1984, McGraw-Hill Inc.

Singer D and others: Cellular electrophysiology of ventricular and other dysrhythmias: studies on diseased and ischemic hearts, Prog Cardiovasc Dis 24:97, 1981.

Sweetwood, HM: Clinical electrocardiography for nurses, Rockville, 1983, Aspen Publishers Inc.

Strout V et al, Fluid and lytes: a practical approach, Philadelphia, 1984, F.A. Davis Co.

Ten Eick RE and others: Ventricular dysrythmia: membrane basis of currents, channels, gates and cables, Prog Cardiovasc Disease 24:157, 1981.

Tilkian SM and others: Clinical implications of laboratory tests, ed. 3, St. Loius, 1983, The CV Mosby Co.

Watson JE; Fluid and electrolyte disorders in cardovascular patients, Nurs Clin North Am 22(4)797, 1987.

Wester PO and others: Intracellular electrolytes in cardiac failure, Acta Med Sand (Suppl) 707:33, 1986.

Witt AL and Rosen MR: Cellular electrophysiology of cardiac arrhythmias, Mod Concepts Cardiovasc Dis 50:1 1981.

Electrolyte Imbalances

1 The major role of the positively charged particles *(cations/anions)* in the plasma is to determine the electrical events of living cells (see Unit 4, Frames 8 to 12). The body's major cations are _____, _____, _____, and _____.

cations

Na^+; K^+; Ca^{++} Mg^{++}

In this discussion, we consider the electrolyte imbalances relating to K^+, Ca^{++}, and Mg^{++}. The Na^+ imbalances, in the setting of CCU, are usually directly associated with fluid imbalances, which are discussed in Unit 4, Frames 46 to 60.

POTASSIUM IMBALANCES

2 K^+ is the primary *(intracellular/extracellular)* cation.

REMEMBER: Potassium's major roles are in the process of *(depolarization/repolarization)* and the maintenance of the _____ state.

intracellular

repolarization

polarized

K^+ also plays a role in *acid-base* balance, cellular metabolism, aldosterone secretion, and the maintenance of intracellular osmolality. K^+ balance is especially significant in coronary care because of its key role in electrical events.

3 Let us now consider the role of K^+ in acid-base balance in more detail. The positively charged particles H^+ and K^+ are closely related. K^+ and H^+ have the ability to exchange with one another if there are excesses or deficits of either ion in the plasma. For example, if there are excess hydrogen ions in the plasma, K^+ will trade for the H^+ and move into the _____, allowing H^+ to leave and move *(into/out of)* the cell. Likewise, if there is an excess of K^+ or deficit of H^+ with high HCO_3^- levels in the plasma, some of the K^+ will shift into the cells in exchange for _____ (Fig. 5-1).

plasma
into

H^+

Thus the serum K^+ level will be *(high/low)* in the presence of an acidosis and *(high/low)* in the presence of an alkalosis.

high
low

4 K^+ is also needed for anabolic processes within the cells, which utilize *amino acids* and *glucose*. K^+ is transported into the cells with glucose and insulin.

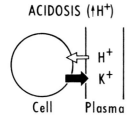
ACIDOSIS (↑H⁺)

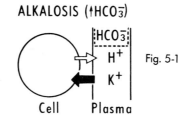
ALKALOSIS (↑HCO₃⁻)

Fig. 5-1

REMEMBER: To prepare for its electrical role, K⁺ is transported into the cell by the _____ pump.

Na⁺-K⁺

To prepare for its metabolic role, K⁺ is transported into the cell with _____ and _____. K⁺ is also needed for _____ _____ utilization. In addition to its electrical and metabolic roles, K⁺ plays a major role in intracellular osmolarity and _____ secretion.

glucose; insulin
amino acid

aldosterone

REMEMBER: The major intracellular cation is _____. The action of aldosterone is to retain Na⁺ and excrete _____.

K⁺
K⁺

Hypokalemia

5 Hypokalemia may occur as a result of increased K⁺ loss, decreased K⁺ intake, alkalosis, hormonal influences, or metabolic factors. In the setting of coronary care, hypokalemia most commonly occurs because of increased K⁺ loss with diuretic therapy. Loss of K⁺ may also occur with gastrointestinal (GI) suction or vomiting, diarrhea, intestinal drains, and excessive diaphoresis. Administration of potassium-free solutions or diets deficient in potassium may also result in hypokalemia.

6 The acid-base imbalance associated with *hypokalemia* is *(acidosis/alkalosis)*.

alkalosis

Hypokalemia may be either the cause of or the result of alkalosis and occurs because of the cation exchange relationship between K⁺ and H⁺ (see Frame 3). In alkalosis there is a deficit of H⁺ in the plasma. Hydrogen ions shift from the _____ to the _____. Potassium ions trade with these ions and shift back *(into/out of)* the cells to compensate for the loss of positive charges. Alkalosis thus results in hypokalemia.

cell
plasma
into

7 Any factor that results in increased release of aldosterone may potentially result in hypokalemia.

REMEMBER: Aldosterone causes the reabsoprtion of _____ and _____ and the excretion of _____ by the kidneys.

water; Na⁺
K⁺

Examples of disorders and therapeutic agents that enchance aldosterone secretion include Cushing's syndrome, stress, and the administration of selected steroids.

Consumption of extracellular K^+ occurs with _____ as glucose and amino acids are mobilized into the *(intracellular/extracellular)* fluid compartment. Therefore, when anabolism is promoted with hyperalimentation or other modes of protein or glucose supplementation, potassium must also be added, or *(hypokalemia/hyperkalemia)* may occur.

anabolism
intracellular

hypokalemia

8 LET US REVIEW: The most common cause of hypokalemia in coronary care is _____ therapy. Loss of K^+ may also occur secondary to GI causes, such as _____ or _____ suction. Hypokalemia and *(acidosis/alkalosis)* are related imbalances. That is because of the exchange relationship between K^+ and _____.

diuretic
vomiting
GI; alkalosis

H^+

9 Chronic stress or the administration of certain steroids may also result in _____. Anabolism results in loss of *(intracellular/extracellular)* K^+ because it is mobilized into the *(intracellular/extracellular)* fluid compartment.

hypokalemia; extracellular
intracellular

10 Let us now consider the clinical manifestations of hypokalemia. The signs and symptoms of hypokalemia may generally be divided into those relating to skeletal muscle, smooth muscle, and the heart.

The signs and symptoms of hypokalemia with regard to skeletal muscle are similar to those seen in hyperkalemia. The most common symptoms are generalized skeletal muscle weakness, aching, and tenderness, which may be perceived as muscle cramping. The weakness may progress to paralysis if the hypokalemia is severe.

The effects of hypokalemia on the smooth muscle of the GI tract are slightly more specific. Hypokalemia *decreases* smooth muscle tone in the GI tract and may result in atony of the bowel (paralytic ileus) and abdominal distention.

Hypokelamia may result in skeletal muscle _____, which may be perceived as _____ _____. GI manifestations of hypokalemia may include _____ of the bowel and abdominal _____.

weakness; muscle cramps

atony
distention

11 The adverse effects of hypokalemia on electrical activity in the heart are potentially life threatening.

REMEMBER: K^+ is necessary for maintenance of a stable polarized state. Therefore, hypokalemia may *(enhance/depress)* electrical instability and cause ventricular arrhythmias.

REMEMBER: Electrical instability is also referred to as *automaticity*. Automaticity is the ability of cardiac cells to *(initiate/conduct)* electrical impulses spontaneously.

enhance

initiate

12 Cardiac cells with unstable cell membranes possess natural automatic properties (see Unit 7, Frames 21 to 33). These cells are particularly sensitive to the effects of hypokalemia. Life-threatening ventricular arrhythmias may occur as a result of enhanced automaticity in the _____ fibers. Hypokalemia increases the sensitivity of the heart to digitalis. Therefore the potential for developing digitalis toxicity is enhanced in the presence of _____ (see Unit 10).

His-Purkinje

hypokalemia

It may also enhance ectopic impulse formation by its effects on *(depolarization/repolarization)*. Prolonged repolarization makes recovery and subsequent conduction in adjacent myocardial cells non-uniform and may allow for the development of ectopic impulses because of altered conduction or re-entry (see Unit 7, Frames 38 to 51).

repolarization

13 REMEMBER: K^+ affects the *(depolarization/repolarization)* phase of the cardiac cycle. Therefore hypokalemia initially affects the _____ wave on the ECG.

repolarization

T

In the presence of hypokalemia, repolarization is prolonged. There is a flattening of the T wave and the appearance of a prominent U wave, indicating delayed repolarization. The T and U waves fuse into one wave. TU wave fusion is an ECC sign of _____. TU wave fusion may be distinguished from normal U waves, which remain separated from their related T waves, and may appear for unknown reasons.

hypokalemia

14 We have noted in our own experience that early ECG changes caused by K^+ are most clearly detected on leads V_2 to V_4. These changes may be totally invisible on routine monitoring leads or on their standard lead equivalents, including V_1 and MCL_1. We have no explanation other than possibly the proximity of the heart to the chest wall in these leads. ECG evidence of hypokalemia is shown in Fig. 5-2.

The ECG sign of hypokalemia is the appearance of a prominent _____ wave with _____ _____ fusion. Hypokalemia may result in threatening arrhythmias because of enhancement of _____ in the _____.

U; TU wave

automaticity
ventricles

15 Potassium replacement therapy consists of administering potassium salts by oral and parenteral routes and increasing nutritional sources. Parenteral potassium should be administered with caution if more than 20 mEq/hr is required. It is advisable to obtain the approval of the pharmacist whenever greater concentrations are ordered. Monitoring on a lead V_2 equivalent is also recommended (see

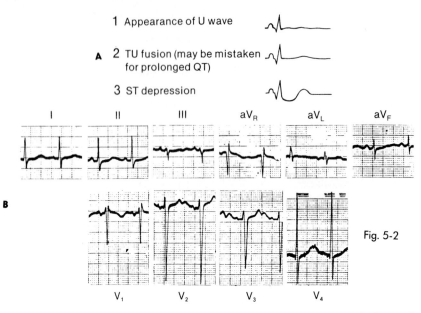

1 Appearance of U wave

A 2 TU fusion (may be mistaken for prolonged QT)

3 ST depression

I   II   III   aV$_R$ aV$_L$ aV$_F$

B

V$_1$ V$_2$ V$_3$ V$_4$

Fig. 5-2

Unit 2, Frame 60). Because parenteral potassium may irritate the blood vessels, it should be administered in large veins when high concentrations are used. Complaints of "burning" with parenteral admnistration should be reported so that flow rate concentration or dosages can be adjusted.

The dangers of parenteral potassium replacement include over-correction of the imbalance and _____ of the _____ _____.

irritation
blood vessels

16 Commonly administered oral potassium salts include: Kaon-Cl, Ka-ochlor Preps, K-Lyte/Cl, Slow-K, and Kay Ciel. Palatibility of the dissolvable oral preparations may be enhanced when given with fruit juice. Ulcerations of the stomach and small bowel have been reported with the use of some oral preparations.

There are many foods rich in K$^+$ in addition to the classically cited orange juice and bananas. Examples include prunes, raisins, fresh tomatoes, potatoes, and peas.

17 In summary:

↓ K$^+$ (hypokalemia)

Body	● Weakness ● Paralysis ● Atony of bowel
Heart	● ↑ Electrical instability (↑ automaticity) ● → Ventricular arrhythmias
ECG	● Appearance of U wave ● TU fusion
Treatment	● Replacement of K via IV or PO ● ST depression

Fig. 5-3

Hyperkalemia

18 Hyperkalemia may occur as a result of decreased K^+ excretion, acidosis, overzealous replacement therapy, or tissue trauma. The most common cause of hyperkalemia in coronary care is probably either (1) failure to discontinue potassium supplements when no longer necessary, or (2) parenteral replacement therapy without careful monitoring of serum K^+ levels and renal function.

REMEMBER: The primary route of excretion for K^+ is via the _____. Therefore careful monitoring of urinary output as well as serum creatinine and BUN levels is important during replacement therapy. *Renal failure* is a common cause of hyperkalemia.

kidneys

19 The *acid-based* imbalance associated with hyperkalemia is *(acidosis/alkalosis)*. Hyperkalemia may be the cause or result of acidosis because of the exchange relationship between _____ and _____.

acidosis

K^+

H^+

REMEMBER: In the presence of acidosis (excess H^+), H^+ shifts from the plasma (EC fluid) to the _____ fluid.

K^+ exchanges with the H^+ and shifts from the intracellular (IC) fluid to the _____. Thus acidosis causes *(hypokalemia/hyperkalemia)* (see Frame 3).

intracellular

plasma; hyperkalemia

20 K^+ is found primarily within the *(IC/EC) fluid.* Therefore, with destruction of cellular membranes, K^+ will be released into the *IC/EC)* fluid. Examples of conditions in which this loss may occur are crushing injuries, burns, and hemolysis associated with transfusion reactions. Local tissue ischemia with MI can cause the release of K^+ into the EC fluid within the injured zone. This K^+ increase is a type of "localized" hyperkalemia (see Unit 6, Frames 30 and 32).

IC

EC

21 LET US REVIEW: The primary route of excretion for K^+ is the _____. Therefore careful monitoring of serum K^+ levels as well as _____ and _____ levels are necessary with potassium replacement therapy. Monitoring blood gases for the presence of an _____ is also beneficial. Crushing injuries and burns may result in the release of IC K^+ into the _____.

kidneys

BUN; creatinine

acidosis

serum

22 The effects of hyperkalemia on skeletal muscle are similar to those of _____. Hyperkalemia also causes skeletal muscle weakness, which may progress to _____. The effects of hyperkalemia on the GI tract are more specific. Hyperkalemia increases smooth muscle tone or irritability in the GI tract. This increased irritability may result in intestinal cramping and diarrhea. It is difficult to distinguish K^+ imbalances on the basis of clinical

hypokalemia

paralysis

symptoms alone. Serum values and ECG evidence provide more information.

23 *Unlike* hypokalemia, hyperkalemia is an electrical *(stimulant/depressant)*.

    REMEMBER: K^+ affects the *(depolarization/repolarization)* phase of the cardiac cycle, or the _____ wave.

    Hyperkalemia alters electrical activity so that cardiac cells repolarize more rapidly *but* less effectively because they do not become as electronegative as they would be normally. The normal level of electronegativity (resting potential) is never reached (see Unit 4, Frames 88 to 96).

    Mild hyperkalemia may enhance automaticity and ectopic impulse formation. However, as the imbalance progresses, automaticity becomes rapidly *depressed,* an effect more commonly seen. End-stage hyperkalemia is associated with ectopy related to decreased conduction.

depressant
repolarization
T

24 If hypokalemia causes flattening of the T wave, then hyperkalemia should cause _____ of the T wave.

    The earliest ECG sign of hyperkalemia is peaking of the _____ wave.

    The peaked T waves of hyperkalemia are characteristically symmetrical and best visualized in leads V_2 to V_4 (Fig. 5-4, *B*). When repolarization is disturbed, the phase of depolarization may also become depressed. The next ECG sign of hyperkalemia is widening of the QRS complex. The last sign of hyperkalemia on the ECG is disappearance of the P wave (Fig. 5-4, *C*).

peaking

T

25 ECG evidence of hyperkalemia is shown in Fig. 5-4.

    It is important for nurses to be able to recognize the ECG manifestations of hyperkalemia because immediate treatment is indicated to correct the cardiac _____ and to prevent asystole.

    Therapy of acute hyperkalemia is directed toward counteracting the depressant effects on the heart and mobilizing the K^+ from the plasma (Fig. 5-5).

depression

26 Sodium and calcium may be given in hyperkalemia as cardiac *(stimulants/depressants)*. K^+ may be mobilized from the plasma into the cardiac cells, as well as into cells throughout the body, by the administration of *glucose* and *insulin*.

    REMEMBER: K^+ is transported *(into/out of)* the cells in the presence of glucose and insulin.

    The effects of hyperkalemia are caused by the excess of *(plasma/IC)* K^+ levels relative to IC levels. Bicarbonate administration pro-

stimulants

into

plasma

ECG evidence of hyperkalemia

1 Peaked T waves
 (note symmetry)

A

2 QRS widening

3 P wave disappearance

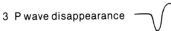

Early hyperkalemia

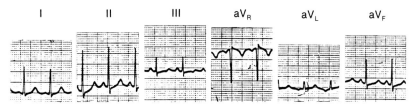

| I | II | III | aV$_R$ | aV$_L$ | aV$_F$ |

B

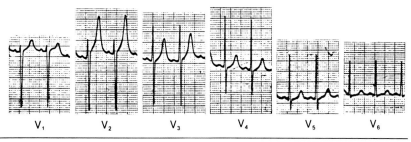

| V$_1$ | V$_2$ | V$_3$ | V$_4$ | V$_5$ | V$_6$ |

Fig. 5-4

Late hyperkalemia

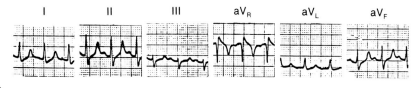

| I | II | III | aV$_R$ | aV$_L$ | aV$_F$ |

C

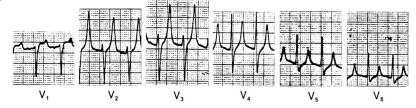

| V$_1$ | V$_2$ | V$_3$ | V$_4$ | V$_5$ | V$_6$ |

ACUTE SITUATION	• Na HCO$_3$ (SODIUM BICARBONATE) • GLUCOSE AND INSULIN • Ca^{++}
CHRONIC SITUATION	• ION EXCHANGE RESINS (KAYEXALATE) • DIALYSIS

Fig. 5-5

duces an alkalotic effect which also moves K$^+$ *(into/out of)* the cells in exchange for _____.

into
H$^+$

Therapy for chronic hyperkalemia is directed toward removing K$^+$ from the body, which may be accomplished with dialysis or cation exchange resins such as Kayexalate.

27 In summary:

	↓ K$^+$	↑ K$^+$
	Hypokalemia	Hyperkalemia
Body	o Weakness o Paralysis o Atony of bowel	o Weakness o Abdominal cramps
Heart	o↑ Electrical instability (automaticity) o Ventricular arrhythmias	o Cardiac depression o Asystole o Ventricular arrhythmias
ECG	o Appearance of U wave o TU fusion o ST depression	o Peaked T wave o QRS widening o Disappearance of P wave

Fig. 5-6

CALCIUM IMBALANCES

28 The calcium ion is important in the conduction of electrical impulses and in muscle contractility. Ca^{++} is also important in blood clotting and in the formation of bone matrix. The first two effects are the major considerations in coronary care.

REMEMBER: Ca^{++} affects *electrical* events by influencing (*Na$^+$/K$^+$*) permeability. Calcium ions line the pores of all cells and, by virtue of their positive charges, act to *repel* the *sodium* ion. Thus Ca^{++} partially controls the ability of Na$^+$ to enter the cell and initiate *(depolarization/repolarization)*.

Na$^+$

depolarization

In some types of cardiac cells, Ca^{++} is the *main ion responsible for depolarization* and thus actually participates in nerve impulse transmission (see Unit 4, Frames 79 to 86). Ca^{++} also enteres the muscle cell after electrical activation to trigger muscle _____ (see Unit 4, Frames 97 to 109).

contraction

29 Calcium is carried within the blood in two forms: (1) *free or ionized* and (2) *bound to serum proteins* (primarily albumin). The *ionized fraction* is the most important because it is the cause of virtually all of the physiological effects of calcium. When the serum protein levels are low, there is a resultant deficit of *(ionized/bound)* calcium. The amount of ionized calcium remains unchanged. Therefore symptoms of Ca^{++} deficit *(will/will not)* occur.

bound

will not

REMEMBER: The physiologic effects of calcium are determined by the *(ionized/bound)* portion.

ionized

About one-half of the total serum calcium is normally ionized. Commonly reported serum Ca^{++} levels usually reflect *total* serum Ca^{++} and do not differentiate between ionized and bound calcium. Newer methods are currently available for measuring ionized calcium levels in critical care areas and should allow for more complete analysis of Ca^{++} imbalances.

30 Let us now consider the hormonal regulation of Ca^{++} in more detail. The two hormones that primarily regulate Ca^{++} levels in the blood are parathormone, secreted by the parathyroid gland, and thyro calcitonin, secreted by the thyroid gland.

NOTE: Other hormones that may affect Ca^{++} balance include thyroxine, estrogen, steroids, and growth hormone.

31 *Parathormone* acts in three ways: (1) promoting Ca^{++} absorption from the GI tract, (2) promoting Ca^{++} release from bone stores, and (3) promoting Ca^{++} reabsorption in the renal tubules. Therefore parathormone *(raises/lowers)* the serum Ca^{++} level and thus protects against the development of *(hyper/hypo)* calcemia.

raises
hypo

There is a close relationship between Ca^{++} and phosphorus (phosphate) levels in the blood. The levels of these two related ions are primarily regulated by parathormone, which promotes Ca^{++} _____ and $HPO_4^=$ excretion in the _____ tubules. Generally, if Ca^{++} levels are increased, $HPO_4^=$ levels are *(increased/decreased)*. If $HPO_4^=$ levels are increased, Ca^{++} levels are *(increased/decreased)*.

reabsorption; renal
decreased

decreased

32 *Thyrocalcitonin* (calcitonin) protects against the development of hypercalcemia by *blocking* mobilization of Ca^{++} from bone stores when serum levels are elevated. Therefore calcitonin *(raises/lowers)* the serum Ca^{++} level.

lowers

LET US REVIEW: Parathormone protects against *(hypo/hyper)* calcemia. Thyrocalcitonin protects against *(hypo/hyper)* calcemia. The physiological effects of calcium are related to the *(ionized/bound)* portion. The regulation of Ca^{++} levels in the body is closely related to the levels of _____.

hypo
hyper
ionized

$HPO_4^=$

Hypocalcemia

33 Hypocalcemia may occur as a result of protein loss, alkalosis, renal failure, transfusions of stored blood, acute pancreatitis, or surgical resection of the parathyroid gland. The most common cause of hypocalcemia in coronary care is probably an underlying alkalosis. Alkalosis promotes the binding of calcium to serum proteins. The level of free, or _____, calcium then falls.

    REMEMBER: Most of the physiological effects of calcium are caused by *(ionized/bound)* calcium. Therefore, in *alkalosis,* symptoms of hypocalcemia *(will/will not)* apear.

    The total blood calcium level usually remains unchanged in alkalosis. Therefore the serum Ca^{++} level may appear normal unless the ionized portion is being separately measured.

ionized

ionized
will

34 Patients with chronic renal failure often have arteriosclerotic vascular disease involving the heart and may be seen in the CCU. In chronic renal failure, hypocalcemia results from decreased excretion of $HPO_4^=$ and decreased activation of vitamin D.

    REMEMBER: There is a close relationship between Ca^{++} and $HPO_4^=$. In the presence of hyperphosphatemia, calcium levels will *(increase/decrease).*

    Vitamin D is necessary for the absorption of calcium from the GI tract. Vitamin D is *activated* in the *kidneys.*

decrease

35 Hypocalcemia may be associated with the adminstration of stored blood or acute pancreatitis in any critical care saetting. Stored blood frequently contains *citrate* as a preservative. The administration of stored blood may be associated with the development of hypocalcemia because *citrate binds with* ionized calcium. Lipase, liberated in pancreatitis, emulsifies the fats of the omentum and mesentery into fatty acids. The fatty acids bind with calcium to form calcium salts or soaps. Glucagon release in pancreatitis may also aggravate the hypocalcemia by promoting calcitonin secretion.

    REMEMBER: Calcitonin protects against *(hypo/hyper)* calcemia by blocking the mobilization of Ca^{++} from _____ stores.

hyper
bone

36 LET US REVIEW: Alkalosis may result in hypocalcemia because of increased binding to _____ _____.

    Renal failure may result in hypocalcemia because _____ is activated in the _____ and is necessary for Ca^{++} _____. Hypocalcemia in renal failure may also occur because of decreased _____ excretion. Administration of stored blood result in hypocalcemia because _____ binds with _____.

    In acute pancreatitis, lipase is liberated and emulsifies the fats of the _____ and _____ into fatty

serum proteins

vitamin D; kidneys
absorption
$HPO_4^=$

citrate; ionized

omentum; mesentery

148

acids. Calcium binds with the _____ _____ to form calcium salts or soaps. Thus *(hypo/hyper)* calcemia may occur in acute pancreatitis. fatty acids
hypo

Surgical removal of the parathyroid glands may result in hypocalcemia because of the absence of _____ secretion. parathormone

37 Let us now consider the clinical manifestations of hypocalcemia. The signs and symptoms of hypocalcemia may generally be divided into those related to skeletal and smooth muscle and those related to cardiac muscle.

38 The effect of hypocalcemia on skeletal and smooth muscle is related to the ion's effect during depolarization, or *(electrical/mechanical)* activity. electrical

REMEMBER: Ca^{++} lines the pores of all cells and, by virtue of its charge, acts to _____ some of the _____ ions. repel; sodium

When serum Ca^{++} levels fall, there is *less* Ca^{++} available to repel Na^+ entry. As a result, repetitive depolarization of nerve cells occurs, resulting in increased motor neuron firing. This increase in neuromuscular irritability may result in the repetitive skeletal muscle contractions known as *tetany*. Therefore tetany represents a disturbance in _____ _____ firing secondary to loss of Ca^{++}. As serum Ca^{++} levels decrease, neuromuscular excitability *(increases/decreases)*. motor neuron

increases

39 In addition to tetany, the symptoms of this increased motor nerve discharge include skeletal muscle spasms, tingling and paresthesias of the fingers, and intestinal cramps. The skeletal muscle spasms may be manifested by the typical carpopedal spasm or by bronchospasm, laryngospasm, dyspnea, or difficulty in talking. Positive Chvostek's and Trousseau's signs are also associated with the skeletal muscle irritability of hypocalcemia. Twitching of the facial muscles in response to scratching of the cheek is referred to as a *positive Chvostek sign*. Carpopedal spasm precipitated by occlusion of blood flow to the hand with a blood pressure cuff is referred to as a *positive Trousseau sign*.

In addition to tetany, increased motor nerve discharge may result in _____ _____ spasms, _____, _____ of the extremities, and _____ cramps. skeletal muscle
tingling; paresthesias
intestinal
The increased skeletal muscle irritability is associated with postive _____ and _____ signs. Chvostek's; Trousseau's

40 In skeletal muscle, the EC (serum) CA^{++} does not directly cross the cell membrane following depolarization. It remains lining the mem-

149

brane pores. Contraction is dependent, primarily, on more static *IC* Ca^{++} stores. Therefore serum Ca^{++} level changes primarily alter *(electrical/mechanical)* activity. electrical

NOTE: The IC Ca^{++} stores are located in the ______________ or ______________ tubules (see Unit 4). cisterna; L

In the presence of hypocalcemia, electrical activity is *(stimulated/inhibited)*. Contractility remains normal or may appear augmented in response to the repetitive stimulation. stimulated

41 However, in cardiac muscle, the EC (ionized serum) Ca^{++} lining the pores enters the muscle cell from the T tubules immediately following depolarization. Contraction is *directly* and primarily dependent on this EC Ca^{++}. IC Ca^{++} stores are minimal (see Unit 4, Frame 95).

Thus the effects of hypocalcemia on cardiac muscle are primarily related to the role of the ion in contractility—that is, *(electrical/mechanical)* activity. When there is a decrease in ionized calcium, myocardial contractility *(increases/decreases)*. mechanical; decreases

Electrical effects may also be seen. In electrically unstable areas, spontaneous depolarization (automaticity) may occur and generate arrhythmias.

42 Ca^{++} has its effect on initiating contraction *between* depolarization and ______________ ______________, represented by phase ______________ of the action potential. This phase correlates with the ______________ segment on the ECG (see Unit 4, Frame 87). active repolarization; 2; ST

Therefore hypocalcemia affects the ______________ ______________ on the ECG. ST segment

In the presence of hypocalcemia, the ST segment is *prolonged*. This change is equally visible on all standard leads.

43 ECG evidence of hypocalcemia is shown in Fig. 5-7.

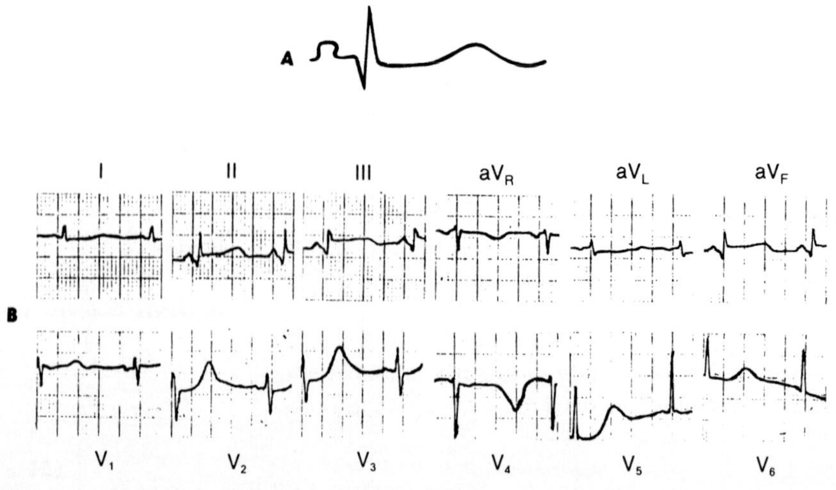

Fig. 5-7

44 Since the ST segment is contained with the QT interval, changes in the ST segment will also affect the QT interval.

45 Therapy for hypocalcemia consists of correcting the underlying problem and administering calcium salts. Evaluation of hypocalcemia must always be done in light of acid-base findings and protein analysis.

The calcium salts most commonly used for replacement therapy are calcium chloride and calcium gluconate. In the adult, calcium chloride is usually preferred because of its higher calcium content. Calcium should be administered by the intravenous (IV) route *slowly*, except in a cardiac arrest situation.

Therapy for hypocalcemia includes _____ of the underlying problem and administration of calcium _____ in the adult as well as assessment of _____ status and serum _____.

correction

chloride
acid-base; proteins

46 Calcium should *not* be administered intravenously in conjunction with sodium bicarbonate, because precipitation will occur. It should be noted that the actions of calcium and digitalis are synergistic. Thus calcium should be administered with caution in the presence of digitalis.

Hypercalcemia

47 Hypercalcemia occurs most commonly in the presence of malignancies and in conditions that promote release of Ca^{++} from bone stores. Disorders associated with bone demineralization and Ca^{++} release include hyperparathyroidism secondary to renal failure and immobility.

Hypercalcemia is *uncommon* in the CCU. However, hypercalcemia may occur in certain collagen diseases affecting the heart (for example, sarcoidosis) and in myocardial tumors. Both of these disorders are associated with increased serum protein, increased total serum calcium, and increased *(ionized/bound)* calcium.

bound

48 The effects of Ca^{++} on *skeletal* and *smooth muscle* are related to the effect of the ion during _____. This effect reflects the role of the Ca^{++} during *(electrical/mechanical)* activity.

The signs and symptoms of hypercalcemia are generally *opposite* to those of hypocalcemia. In hypercalcemia there is *(more/less)* Ca^{++} available to line pores of the cell and it _____ the Na ion. Therefore depolarization and neuromuscular activity are *(stimulated/depressed)*.

Signs of skeletal muscle depression include lethargy and muscle weakness. Signs of smooth muscle depression include constipation, nausea, and vomiting. Other related symptoms of neurological de-

depolarization
electrical

more
repels

depressed

pression include headache, apathy, and decreased levels of consciousness.

49 The effects of Ca^{++} on the *heart* muscle are related to the effect of the ion on _____. This effect reflects the role of Ca^{++} during *(electrical/mechanical)* activity. When there is an increase in ionized calcium, myocardial contractility *(increases/diminishes)*.

contractility
mechanical
increases

  Although mild increases in contractility may be beneficial, excess serum levels of Ca^{++} may result in extreme spastic contraction of the myocardium and interfere with relaxation. The cardiac signs and symptoms of hypercalcemia are generally *(the same as/opposite to)* those of hypocalcemia—Ca^{++} affects the _____ segment on the ECG. In the presence of *hypercalcemia* the ST segment is *(prolonged/shortened)* and disappears.

opposite to
ST
shortened

50 ECG evidence of hypercalcemia is shown in Fig. 5-8

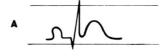

A

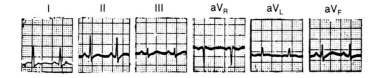

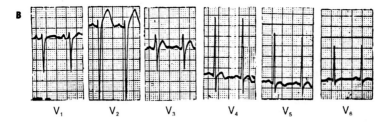

Fig. 5-8

NOTE: No space is visible between the QRS complex and T wave. However, hypercalcemia *(does/does not)* affect either the QRS complex or T wave.

does not

51 In the presence of hypercalcemia, Ca^{++} deposits may be evident in body tissues, especially within the *renal medulla*. An early sign of hypercalcemia is polyuria caused by impaired renal concentrating ability. Osteoporosis and pathological fractures may result from depletion of bone Ca^{++} stores in response to increased demands for Ca^{++}

release into the serum. This process is also referred to as bone _____.

demineralization

REMEMBER: Hyperparathyroidism may occur in the presence of renal failure, causing the eventual release of excess amounts of _____. This hormone raises the serum Ca^{++} level by promoting its reabsorption in the kidney and GI tract and stimualting its _____ from _____ stores.

parathormone

release; bone

52 Therapy for hypercalcemia consists of the following:
1. Correcting the underlying cause
2. Promoting Ca^{++} excretion by the kidneys
3. Binding excess ionized calcium
4. Counteracting the parathormone-like chemicals secreted by a variety of tumors

Direct suppression of serum Ca^{++} levels may be accomplished by the administration of *calcitonin* or *steroids* or both.

NOTE: Steroids promote the movement of Ca^{++} into the cells and competes with vitamin D to minimize GI reabsorption.

The elimination of Ca^{++} by the kidneys is facilitated by saline and diuretics. One method of binding excess ionized calcium is by the administration of sodium bicarbonate.

	↑Ca^{++}	↓Ca^{++}
	Hypercalcemia	Hypocalcemia
Body	Flaccid extremities	Spastic extremities
Heart	↑ Contractility	↓ Contractility
ECG	Shortened ST segment	Prolonged ST segment

Fig. 5-9

MAGNESIUM IMBALANCES

53 Mg^{++} is primarily an *(IC/EC)* cation. Therefore *serum* Mg^{++} levels are normally *(high/low)*. The normal serum Mg level is 1.5 to 2.5 mEq/L.

IC

low

Mg^{++} is closely related to other cations involved in electrical-mechanical activity and should be considered equally important.

REMEMBER: Mg^{++} is important in the breakdown of _____ for energy and in the normal function of the _____ pump, which requires ATP to function.

ATP

Na^+-K^+

The Na^+-K^+ pump is primarily important in cardiac *(electrical/mechanical)* activity.

electrical

Therefore the action of Mg^{++} on the Na^+-K^+ pump reflects a(n) *(electrical/mechanical)* role.

electrical

54 Mg^{++} is a necessary *activator* of the enzyme ATPase, which causes splitting of the ATP molecule with energy release. Splitting of ATP is required for *mechanical* activity as well as *electrical* activity. Energy from ATP breakdown is required to move the contractile proteins *actin* and *myosin*. Energy is also required for the transfer of Ca^{++} out of the myofibrils to allow for *muscle relaxation.*

55 By influencing ATP breakdown, Mg^{++} indirectly affects all energy-requiring processes in the body. The three major energy-requiring activities in the heart are (1) the _____ pump, (2) _____ _____, and (3) _____ _____.

Na^+-K^+
muscle contraction
muscle relaxation

56 Another action of Mg^{++} is to *inhibit acetylcholine* release in *smooth* and *skeletal muscles* and in the *central nervous system.* Electrical activity in these tissues is thus *(stimulated/inhibited).*

inhibited

Mg^{++} is also necessary for *parathormone* secretion and thus influences serum Ca^{++} levels. Both the electrical and mechanical effects of Ca^{++} are altered.

57 Mg^{++} is closely related to the other cations involved in electrical-mechanical activity. Mg^{++} controls the serum Ca^{++} levels by its action on _____. It controls serum K^+ levels by its action on _____. In the presence of hypomagnesemia *both* serum Ca^{++} and K^+ levels are *(high/low).*

parathormone
ATP
low

Hypomagnesemia

58 Mg^{++} deficits may occur as a result of deficient intake, increased loss, or decreased absorption. In the setting of coronary care the most common cause of decreased Mg^{++} levels is *diuretic therapy.* Mg^{++} is excreted by the kidneys and GI tract. With diuretic therapy, Mg^{++} loss generally parallels K^+ loss. It has been postulated that K^+ transport into the cells in the therapy for diuretic-induced hypokalemia may also require supplementary magnesium administration.

59 Hypomagnesemia may also be associated with GI losses from diarrhea, vomiting, intestinal drains, or the excessive use of laxatives commonly seen in the elderly. Hypomagnesemia is commonly seen in chronic alcoholism, probably resulting from a combination of predisposing factors, such as inadequate dietary sources (see Frame 64), impaired absorption or GI loss caused by associated GI disturbances, and renal losses associated with the diuretic effects of alcohol.

60 LET US REVIEW: Mg^{++} deficits occur as the result of losses from the _____ and _____ tract. The most common cause

kidneys; GI

of decreased Mg^{++} levels in the setting of coronary care is
_____.

diuresis

The elderly alcoholic patient receiving laxatives, diuretics, or both, may easily have an acute MI. At that time, this patient is at risk for developing the side effects of *hypomagnesemia* superimposed on and aggravating the complications of *acute MI.*

61 The signs and symptoms of hypomagnesemia are associated with neuromuscular irritability and instability. Increased smooth muscle, skeletal muscle, and central nervous system (CNS) irritability occur in response to related Ca^{++} deficits. Increased cardiac instability *(automaticity)* and chronic myopathies occur in response to related K^{+} deficits.

REMEMBER: Mg^{++} controls the serum Ca^{++} deficits by its action on _____. It controls K^{+} levels by its action on _____ and the _____ pump. One of the roles of the Na^{+}-K^{+} pump is to pump K^{+} *(into/out of)* the cell. When this pump is inactivated, intracellular K^{+} *(gains/losses)* occur.

parathormone
ATP; NA^{+}-K^{+}
into
losses

62 Skeletal muscle symptoms of hypomagnesemia include leg cramps, muscle spasms, twitching, tremors, and tetany. Low-magnesium tetany has been reported even in the presence of *normal* Ca^{++} levels. CNS symptoms include confusion, disorientation, coma, and seizures. Delirium tremens have been attributed to Mg^{++} deficits in some cases.

63 The most commonly cited cardiac symptoms are ventricular arrhythmias, leading to or potentiating ventricular fibrillation (VF). Magnesium therapy has been effective in selected cases of "refractory" VF and should at least be considered in such cases. The potential for developing digitalis toxicity is enhanced in the presence of hypomagnesemia. Hypomagnesemia enhances the myocardial uptake of *digitalis.*

The ECG effect of hypomagnesemia is similar to that seen in hypokalemia.

REMEMBER: Hypokalemia causes flattening of the _____ wave and the appearance of a _____ wave.

T
U

64 Therapy for Mg^{++} deficits consists of administration of magnesium sulfate by parenteral routes and dietary supplementation. The toxic effects of IV magnesium sulfate administration mimic hypermagnesemia (see Frames 65 to 67). The most marked are *hypotension* and *respiratory* arrest. Dietary sources include meat, nuts, green vegetables, and whole grains.

Hypermagnesemia

65 Hypermagnesemia is uncommon in the setting of coronary care. The most common causes of hypermagnesemia are renal failure and exogenous magnesium administration. The imabalance occurs in renal failure as a result of decreased excretion and the ingestion of magnesium-containing antacids. Hypermagnesemia may also result from excessive magnesium administration as in obstetrical settings or more recently where it has been used as an *antihypertensive* agent.

66 Increased Mg^{++} levels decrease neuromuscular irritability by inhibition of acetylcholine release.

REMEMBER: Mg^{++} inhibits acetylcholine release in the CNS, skeletal muscles, and smooth muscle. Hypermagnesemia may result in CNS depression, leading to respiratory arrest, loss of deep tendon reflexes, and hypotension. Mg^{++} also has a direct depressant effect on the heart, resulting in bradycardia.

67 The ECG effects of hypermagnesemia are similar to those seen in hyperkalemia.

REMEMBER: Hyperkalemia causes _____ of the T waves and _____ of the QRS. Therapy for hypermagnesemia is directed toward stopping the infusion or correcting the underlying cause. The depressant effects on muscle may be counteracted with a stimulant such as calcium.

peaking
widening

ACID-BASE BALANCE
Definitions

68 An *acid* is a proton (H^+) donor.

$$H_2CO_3 \leftrightharpoons H^+ + HCO_3^-$$
$$\quad A \qquad B \qquad C$$

In the above equation, a hydrogen ion (proton) is given up by the substanced labeled _____. Therefore this substance is known as a(n) *(acid/base)*.

A
acid

A *base* is a proton (H^+) acceptor. In the same equation, a hydrogen ion can be accepted by the substance labeled _____. Therefore this substance is known as a(n) *(acid/base)*.

C
base

69 Changes in the hydrogen ion concentration are measured by the *serum pH*. The pH is a mathematical representation of the H^+ concentration. It is not a direct measurement of the H^+ level in the blood. The pH reflects the H^+ concentration in an inverse, or reciprocal, manner.

THEREFORE: A decreased pH equals a(n) *(increased/decreased)* H^+ concentration. An increased pH equals a(n) *(increased/decreased)* H^+

increased
decreased

concentration. The regulation of the H^+ concentration is important because many cellular chemical reactions are pH dependent.

70 An *increased* H^+ concentration indicates the presence of an *acidosis*. Acidosis is an *acid-base* imbalance resulting from *increased acid* or *decreased base*.

A *decreased* H^+ concentration, or *(increased/decreased)* pH, indicates the presence of an *alkalosis*.

increased

Alkalosis is a state of *increased* base or *decreased* acid.

The normal pH of arterial blood is 7.35 to 7.45. A pH of 7.2 indicates *(acidosis/alkalosis)*. A pH of 7.6 indicates *(acidosis/alkalosis)*.

acidosis; alkalosis

Fig. 5-10

Mechanisms of normal acid-base balance

71 *Acids* are normally generated in the body as a result of cellular metabolism. The major by-product of cellular metabolism is *carbon dioxide,* which is excreted by the lungs as a *volatile* gas. Carbon dioxide may also combine with water to form *carbonic acid* and is thus potentially an *acid*. Since carbonic acid is formed from and may be reconverted into the volatile gas, CO_2, it is considered a *volatile acid*.

Noncarbonic acids are also produced as by-products of normal cellular metabolism. The noncarbonic metabolic acids are *nonvolatile* and are primarily excreted by the *kidneys*. These nonvolatile by-products are also known as *fixed acids*. Some examples of normal fixed acids are sulfuric acid, phosphoric acid, ketoacids, and lactic acid.

72 During normal cellular metabolism, two forms of acid are produced: _____ _____, also referred to as _____ _____, and _____ _____, also referred to as _____ _____. Although the source of all normal acids in the body is metabolic, these metabolic acids may be regulated by either respiratory or nonrespiratoy body mechanisms. In clinical usage, the term "metabolic" is reserved for *nonrespiratory mechanisms* or *imbalances*.

carbonic acid
volatile acid
noncarbonic acid
fixed acid

73 *Bases* are normally generated within the red blood cells (RBC), lower GI tract, and the kidneys. The primary base generated by the body is *bicarbonate*. Bicarbonate is generated from the breakdown of carbonic acid in the RBC and kidney tubules. Carbon dioxide (CO_2) not readily excreted by the lungs combine with water (H_2O) within the RBC and kidney tubules to form carbonic acid (H_2CO_3). The carbonic acid (H_2CO_3) is then broken down to produce free hydrogen ions (H^+) and the base *bicarbonate* (HCO_3^-). The H^+ is excreted in the urine. In the RBC, H^+ may attach to, and thus be absorbed by, the Hb molecule.

Bicarbonate may also act in the kidneys to promote excretion of the noncarbonic (fixed) acids. However, most of the bicarbonate enters the circulation to act as a plasma base. Intestinal bicarbonate may be formed within the intestinal or pancreatic cells or may be brought there by the circulation.

Base bicarbonate is produced in an attempt to absorb metabolic end products.

74 Other body bases include phosphates, hemoglobin, and ammonia, which may be obtained from protein breakdown. These bases are formed from substances contained in most foods, which are absorbed via the GI tract. Bases are excreted by the *kidneys* and *lower GI tract.*

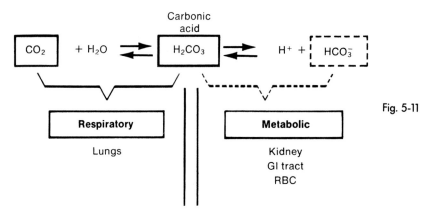

Fig. 5-11

75 LET US REVIEW: Acids are normally generated from _____ _____. Carbonic acid is excreted by the lungs in the form of _____. Carbonic acid may also be broken down and excreted by the _____.

NOTE: Carbonic acid (H_2CO_3) is broken down in a similar manner by the gastric mucosa and is excreted in the form of hydrochloric acid (HCl) in gastric secretions.

Noncarbonic metabolic acids are known as _____ acids and are primarily excreted by the _____.

Bases are normally generated within the _____, _____ _____, and _____. The primary base generated in the body is _____. Examples of other body bases include _____,

cellular
metabolism; CO_2
kidneys

fixed
kidneys
RBC
GI tract; kidneys
bicarbonate
phosphate

_____, and _____.   hemoglobin; ammonia
Bases are excreted by the _____ and _____   kidneys; GI
_____.   tract

    Acidosis is an acid-base imbalance resulting from *(increased/*   increased
decreased) acid or *(increased/decreased)* base.   decreased
    Alkalosis is an acid-base imbalance resulting from *(increased/*   decreased
decreased) acid or *(increased/decreased)* base.   increased
    In clinical usage the term *metabolic* is reserved for _____   nonrespiratory
regulating mechanisms or imbalances.

Role of buffers in the control of acid-base balance

76 Buffers are substances that can minimize or absorb the changes in
hydrogen ion concentration (pH) associated with excess acids or
bases. They act as "chemical sponges." Buffers may be single acids or
bases, a combination of an acid and its related base, or a substance
that can convert into either an acid or base as needed. Some of the
body's buffers include hemoglobin, which accepts H^+ and therefore
acts like a(n) *(acid/base)*; the carbonic acid-bicarbonate system; the   base
phosphoric acid-phosphate system; and proteins, which can convert
to an acid or base as needed.

77 Buffering is the body's first line of defense against changes in pH
caused by acid-base imbalance. The carbonic acid-bicarbonate buffer
system is the major buffer in the body because it is composed of the
major acid produced and its related _____.   base
    REMEMBER: H_2CO_3 may be broken down in the _____   RBC
and _____ tubules to produce free H^+ and   kidney
_____. HCO_3^-

    For the pH to be maintained within normal limits, the ratio of
HCO_3^- and H_2CO_3 must be in a balance of 20:1.

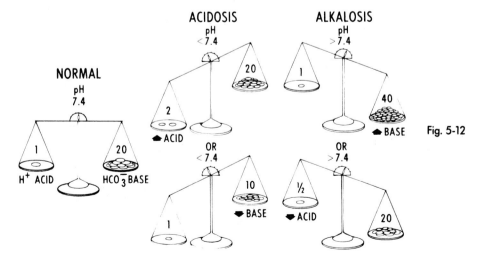

Fig. 5-12

78 LET US REVIEW: Buffer systems minimize or absorb changes in pH resulting from excess _____ and _____. The major buffer in the body is the _____ _____ _____ system.

> *acids; bases*
> *carbonic acid bicarbonate*

    REMEMBER: Bicarbonate is produced in an attempt to _____ acid metabolic by-products. When the pH is normal, the ratio of bicarbonate (HCO_3^-) to carbonic acid (H_2CO_3) is _____ to _____.

> *absorb*
>
> *20; 1*

RESPIRATORY AND METABOLIC ACID-BASE IMBALANCES
Respiratory imbalances

79 REMEMBER: Carbonic acid is a potentially volatile acid that is formed from and may be reconverted into the gas _____ _____. It is predominantly excreted by the respiratory system (lungs).

> *carbon*
> *dioxide*

    Respiratory disorders may interfere with the excretion of carbon dioxide in the lungs and produce disturbances in acid-base balance. When hypoventilation occurs, carbon dioxide is retained and _____ _____ accumulates. *Acidosis* resulting from respiratory disorders and _____ _____ accumulation is known as _____ acidosis.

> *carbonic acid*
> *carbonic*
> *acid*
> *respiratory*

    When hyperventilation occurs, there is excessive loss of carbon dioxide (CO_2) by the lungs, and carbonic acid (H_2CO_3) levels fall. This loss of acid results in an *(acidosis/alkalosis)*.

> *alkalosis*

    Alkalosis resulting from respiratory stimulation and _____ _____ deficit is known as _____ alkalosis.

> *carbonic acid*
> *respiratory*

    The *ABG values* most useful in the assessment of respiratory imbalances are the *pH* and the P_{CO_2}. The P_{CO_2} reflects the *pressure* of the dissolved CO_2 gas in solution within the plasma. Actual carbonic acid levels in the plasma are usually very small and thus are not separately measured clinically.

Metabolic imbalances

80 REMEMBER: In clinical usage the term *metabolic* is reserved for _____ regulating mechanisms or imbalances. Metabolic acidosis occurs from the accumulation of metabolic acids not readily excreted by the _____.

> *nonrespiratory*
>
> *lungs*

    REMEMBER: Acids not excreted by the lungs are referred to as *(nonvolatile/volatile)*, or _____, acids.

> *nonvolatile; fixed*

    Excess fixed acids may accumulate in abnormal metabolism or secondary to exogenous ingestion or impaired excretion.

    REMEMBER: Fixed acids are primarily eliminated by the _____.

> *kidneys*

Metabolic acidosis may also occur because of excessive loss of _____ via the lower GI tract.

Acidosis resulting from abnormal metabolism, impaired excretion of metabolic products by the kidneys, or loss of bicarbonate is known as _____ acidosis.

81 Excessive *elimination* of carbonic acids and fixed acids with compensatory retention of bicarbonate occurs in the presence of either excess gastric or renal excretion. Loss of acid or retention of base results in an *(acidosis/alkalosis)*.

Alkalosis resulting from excess elimination of metabolic acids via the kidneys or upper GI tract or accumulation of the base bicarbonate is known as _____ nonrespiratory alkalosis.

82 The *ABG values* most useful in the assessment of metabolic imbalances are the *pH, bicarbonate levels,* and *base excess* or *deficit.*

REMEMBER: Actual carbonic acid levels in the plasma are usually very small and are not routinely measured separately. Fixed acid levels are not routinely measured either. Their presence is implied by their effect on the *bicarbonate levels.*

Compensation

83 The respiratory system may assist the kidney in the regulation of metabolic acid-base imbalances. This assistance is known as the *compensatory* effort of the lungs. The respiratory system compensates for a metabolic acidosis by excreting _____ acid in the form of _____ _____. The respiratory system compensates for a metabolic alkalosis by _____ carbon dioxide. In acute situations the compensatory effort by the lungs represent a *secondary defense system* and is rarely completely effective in normalizing the pH. Compensatory efforts for metabolic alkalosis are limited by the effect of an increase in carbon dioxide on the respiratory centers.

REMEMBER: The normal stimulus for respiration is the level of _____ _____ in the blood and cerebrospinal fluid.

The kidneys also assist the lung in the regulation of respiratory *acid-base* imbalances. However, renal compensation for respiratory disorders is slow and is usually not seen in acute disorders.

84 *Arrhythmogenic* and *electrolyte effects of pH changes* in the H^+ level of the blood—high or low—may enhance cardiac automaticity and cause arrhythmias. Therefore arrhythmias may be associated with a(n) *(low pH/high pH/either high or low pH)*. Extremes in the pH may also decrease the effect of certain cardiac drugs, increase the sensitivity to toxic effects, or both. When acidosis exists, defibrillation is less effective because of the inevitable cardiac depression.

85 The three electrolytes directly affected by acid-base imbalances are K^+, Ca^{++}, and C^-. The serum levels of these electrolytes will all appear *high* in a state of *acidosis*. In contrast, serum levels of K^+, Ca^{++}, and Cl^- are all usually *low* in a state of _____.

    alkalosis

The total body levels of K^+ and Ca^{++} may be normal, but their *location* may be altered. K^+ may move from *IC* to *EC* fluid, and Ca^{++} may change from a state of *free* to *bound* (see Frames 6, 29, 102, and 113). The serum Cl^- level increases in selected forms of metabolic acidosis associated with increases in the level of HCl acid (see Frames 116 to 122). The serum Cl^- level decreases in metabolic alkalosis with the *(retention/excretion)* of HCl acid.

    excretion

86 **In summary:**

When an acid-base imbalance is triggered by a disturbance in the *respiratory* system, the disorder is classified as a _____ acid-base imbalance.

    respiratory

When an acid-base imbalance is triggered by a *metabolic*, renal, or GI disturbance, the disorder is classified as a _____ imbalance.

    metabolic

87 The ABG values most useful in the assessment of *respiratory* imbalances are the _____ and _____. The ABG values most useful in the assessment of *metabolic imbalances* are the _____, _____ _____, and _____ _____. Respiratory compensation for metabolic imbalances is *(immediate/delayed)*. Renal compensation for respiratory imbalances is *(immediate/delayed)*.

    pH; Pco_2

    pH; bicarbonate level
    base excess/deficit
    immediate
    delayed

88 Changes in the H^+ level of the blood may enhance cardiac _____ and cause _____. In the presence of an *acidosis*, serum levels of K^+, Ca^{++}, and Cl^- are usually *(high/low)*. In the presence of an *alkalosis*, serum levels of K^+, Ca^{++}, and Cl^- are usually *(high/low)*.

    automaticity; arrhythmias

    high
    low

Respiratory acidosis

89 Respiratory acidosis occurs when there is impaired excretion of carbon dioxide by the lungs.

REMEMBER: When carbon dioxide is retained, _____ _____ accumulates. Carbon dioxide may be retained when the *rate, depth,* or *effectiveness* of ventilation is *decreased*. Impaired ventilation occurs in the presence of the following:
1. Suppression in the respiratory centers
2. Obstruction or collapse of the airways

    carbonic acid

3. Compression of the airways by pneumothorax, hemothorax, or pleural effusion

90 Suppression of the respiratory centers may be associated with the effects of narcotic administration, post-cardiac arrest brain damage, or the chronic CO_2 retention associated with COPD. Patients with chronic bronchitis have severe V/Q mismatching, causing impaired CO_2 excretion and chronic _____ retention. Eventually the CO_2
central chemoreceptors lose their sensitivity to carbon dioxide. The *peripheral chemoreceptors* assume control of respiration.

REMEMBER: The peripheral chemoreceptors respond to lack of
_____. Administration of oxygen at high concentrations in O_2
these patients abolishes their respiratory drive and may cause excessive CO_2 retention or a respiratory arrest.

REMEMBER: It is important to consider that *not all patients with COPD* retain carbon dioxide. However, until the absence of CO_2 retention is confirmed, O_2 administration in a patient with COPD should be confined at low flow rates (1 to 2 L min) or low concentrations.

91 CO_2 retention may also occur as the result of *severe* obstruction or collapse of the conducting, or respiratory, airways. Obstruction of the airways may be caused by mucus, bronchospasm, or the fluid of pulmonary edema. Atelectasis, or collapse of the airways, may be caused by shallow breathing, the effects of anesthesia and cardiopulmonary bypass, or damage to the alveolar cells with loss of surfactant (see Unit 3).

92 In the early stages of pulmonary edema caused by CHF, the patient hyperventilates. Generally, this hyperventilation occurs in response to hypoxemia or hypoxia. Because carbon dioxide can still be excreted in the presence of minimally to moderately dense fluid, hyperexcretion of carbon dioxide occurs.

REMEMBER: Carbon dioxide diffuses across the alveolar-capillary membrane more easily than oxygen. Excess CO_2 excretion results in respiratory *(alkalosis/acidosis)*. As pulmonary congestion progresses in   alkalosis
the later stages of CHF, interference with diffusion of *both* oxygen and carbon dioxide occurs. As the cardiac output and pulmonary blood flow become markedly reduced, mismatching of poorly ventilated and underperfused areas, or V/Q imbalance, occurs, further limiting CO_2 excretion. At this stage respiratory *(acidosis/alkalosis)* is   acidosis
seen.

93 LET US REVIEW: In the presence of minimal to moderate obstruction of the airways, *(increased/decreased)* CO_2 excretion occurs. In the pres-   increased
ence of severe obstruction to the airways, *(increased/decreased)* CO_2 decreased

excretion occurs. Therefore respiratory acidosis occurs in the presence of the *(moderate/severe)* pulmonary edema of CHF. Respiratory acidosis also occurs when severe pulmonary edema complicates ARDS (adult respiratory distress syndrome).

94 Compression of the airways, which limits CO_2 excretion, may occur as the result of a *severe* pneumothorax or pleural effusion. The effect of this compression on the airways is also referred to as "compression atelectasis." Pleural effusion may occur in the setting of CHF because of the increased capillary pressure when the excess interstitial fluid exceeds the ability of the lymphatic system to drain the interstitial space.

    REMEMBER: The pleural space is one of the potential fluid spaces in the body, also known as a _____ space. The potential spaces are in close communication with the *(intravascular/interstitial)* space (see Unit 3).

    Excess fluid may accumulate in this space in the presence of interstitial fluid. The impairment of CO_2 excretion depends on the extent of the compression and the condition of the uninvolved airways. Pneumothorax may occur as a complication of aggressive cardiopulmonary resuscitation or subclavian catheter placement. If *severe,* the associated compression of the airways may lead to impaired CO_2 excretion and respiratory *(acidosis/alkalosis).*

95 LET US REVIEW: Impaired CO_2 excretion may occur in the presence of the following:
1. Suppression of the _____ _____
2. *Severe* _____ or _____ of the airways
3. *Severe* compression of airways by _____, _____, or _____.

    When carbon dioxide is retained, _____ _____ accumulates and respiratory *(acidosis/alkalosis)* is produced.

96 The *clinical signs* of respiratory acidosis are decreased rate and depth of respirations and sensorium changes. The patient's respirations represent the primary *cause* of the imbalance in respiratory acidosis rather than the _____ effort. The patient will experience sensorium changes because of the toxic effect of acidosis on the CNS. Generally, as the respiratory acidosis becomes more severe, the level of consciousness will decrease. The kidneys attempt to compensate for the imbalance by retaining base in the form of _____. However, renal compensation for respiratory disorders is slow and is usually not seen in acute disorders.

	severe
	third
	interstitial
	acidosis
	respiratory centers
	obstruction; collapse
	pneumothorax
	hemothorax; pleural effusion
	carbonic acid
	acidosis
	compensatory
	bicarbonate

97 The ABG values most useful in the assessment of acid-base changes caused by respiratory disorders are the _____ and _____. The ABG values diagnostic of a *respiratory acidosis* are:

pH
Pco2

  1. *(Increased/decreased)* pH

decreased

  2. *(Increased/decreased)*Pco$_2$

increased

98 Aggressiveness of *intervention* is dependent on the pH rather than the CO$_2$ level, taking into consideration any attempts at compensation. *Therapy* may include the following:

  1. Treatment of the CHF, including specific measures to decrease pulmonary congestion (for example, high Fowler's position with legs dangling and rotating tourniquets)
  2. Chest physical therapy (moisture, saline instillation, postural drainage, percussion or vibration, bronchodilators, incentive inspirometers, coughing techniques, and so forth) or suctioning to mobilize secretions and relieve atelectasis or bronchospasm
  3. Mechanical ventilation with airway-splinting measures to reverse atelectasis
  4. Drainage of air or fluid

Respiratory alkalosis

99 Respiratory alkalosis occurs when there is an increased excretion of carbon dioxide by the lungs.

  REMEMBER: When carbon dioxide is lost, a deficit of _____ _____ occurs. Carbon dioxide is lost when the respiratory *rate* or *depth* is increased. Conditions in which respiratory rate or depth may be increased include the following:

carbonic acid

  1. Pain
  2. Anxiety
  3. Flail chest
  4. Respiratory therapy
  5. *Early phases* of pulmonary edema and other acute respiratory conditions mentioned earlier

100 In the early phases of pulmonary edema caused by CHF or other acute respiratory conditions, such as asthma, pneumonia, pulmonary emboli, pneumothorax, or adult respiratory distress syndrome, CO$_2$ excretion may continue in the absence of effective O$_2$ transport because _____ _____ diffuses more easily than oxygen. When the respiratory rate and depth are stimulated in response to hypoxemia or hypoxia, hyperexcretion of carbon dioxide occurs. Excess excretion of carbon dioxide results in respiratory *(alkalosis/acidosis)*.

carbon dioxide

alkalosis

NOTE: Hyperventilation may also result from stimulation of vagal receptors in the lungs, independent of the aortic chemoreceptors. These juxtapulmonary capillary receptors in the alveolar wall are stimulated by increased interstitial fluid. They also are stimulated by histamine, serotonin release, or both from degradation of additional platelets and thrombin, which accumulate on the surface of emboli.

The presence of a flail chest is usually not associated with severe ventilatory impairment. Respiratory alkalosis rather than acidosis is therefore more commonly seen.

101 The CNS exerts a stimulating effect on the respiratory center in the presence of stress associated with pain or anxiety. Respiratory alkalosis has been reported in patients in CCUs in the absence of hypoxemia or hypoxia. The presence of chest pain, anxiety, or both is currently thought to be the mechanism. Anxiety associated with the effects of mechanical ventilation exerts a similar influence.

102 The *clinical signs* of respiratory alkalosis are deep, rapid respirations and tremors, tetany, or convulsions caused by the effect of decreased Ca^{++}. The dep, rapid respirations are the *cause* of the imbalance. Alkalosis causes an increase in bound Ca^{++} and thus a(n) *(increase/decrease)* in free Ca^{++}. This will result in symptoms of *(hypocalcemia/hypercalcemia)*.

decrease

hypocalcemia

REMEMBER: Calcium occurs in two forms—free (ionized) and bound-to-plasma protein (albumin). The systemic effects of Ca^{++} are related to the levels of _____ _____ calcium. Bound calcium may be considered to be inactive calcium because it is in a stored form. The serum Ca^{++} level reflects *(ionized/bound/total)* calcium. Alkalosis causes a shift in the amount of ionized, as opposed to bound, calcium but does not affect the total serum Ca^{++} level. Therefore calcium changes caused by alkalosis *(will/will not)* be reflected on routine serum calcium tests. Newer techniques for measuring ionized calcium levels are currently available but are not widely used at this time.

free (ionized)

total

will not

103 The ABG values most useful in the assessment of acid-base changes caused by respiratory disorders are the _____ and _____. The ABG values diagnostic of a *respiratory alkalosis* are the following:
1. *(Increased/decreased)* pH
2. *(Increased/decreased)* P_{CO_2}

pH
P_{CO_2}

increased
decreased

Fig. 5-13

RESPIRATORY

	pH	P_{CO_2}
ACIDOSIS	↓	↑
ALKALOSIS	↑	↓

$(H^+) + HCO_3 \longleftrightarrow H_2CO_3 \longleftrightarrow CO_2 + H_2O$

104 *Therapy* or *intervention* in this imbalance may include the following:
1. Relief of pain
2. Relief of hypoxemia by positioning the patient for optimal chest expansion and ventilation (that is, semi-Fowler's position without pressure on diaphragm) and by administering supplementary oxygen as indicated (see Unit 3)
3. Treatment of CHF, including specific measures to decrease pulmonary congestion (see Unit 7)
4. Selection of more comfortable modes of O_2 therapy (see Unit 3)
5. Chest physical therapy techniques, as with respiratory acidosis (see Frame 98)
6. Airway-splinting measure or drainage of air or fluid, as with respiratory acidosis (see Frame 98)
7. In the setting of suspected pulmonary emboli, anticoagulation preventing further clot accumulation and degradation, which may result in irritation of J receptors

Metabolic acidosis

105 Metabolic acidosis may result from increased levels of fixed (nonvolatile) acids or decreased levels of _____ (bicarbonate). The acid accumulation may occur as a result of abnormal metabolism, decreased excretion of fixed acid by the _____, or exogenous ingestion. Loss of bicarbonate (base) from selected GI disturbances or bicarbonate deficits associated with drug therapy may also result in a _____ acidosis.

base

kidneys

metabolic

106 Metabolic acidosis caused by abnormal metabolism may occur with diabetes and shock. In diabetes, fats may be preferentially metabolized for energy because there is not sufficient insulin available to metabolize glucose. The increased breakdown of fats releases an excess of ketoacids. When acidosis is associated with an excess of ketoacids in the diabetic patient, it is referred to as _____ acidosis.

keto

Ketoacidosis is a form of *(metabolic/respiratory)* acidosis. In shock, metabolism takes place in the absence of sufficient oxygen. This anaerobic metabolism results in the accumulation of *lactic acid*. The acidosis associated with shock may also be referred to as _____ acidosis. Metabolic acidosis caused by decreased excretion of fixed acids occurs in *renal failure*.

metabolic

lactic

REMEMBER: The primary route of excretion of fixed acid is the *kidneys*.

107 Metabolic acidosis can also occur because of decreased levels of _____ _____. Decreased levels of bicarbonate can occur with either direct loss or decreased formation. Clinical examples of these factors include diarrhea and admin-

base bicarbonate

istration of acetazolamide (Diamox). Diarrhea results in loss of lower GI secretions rich in bicarbonate. Administration of the commonly used diuretic Diamox results in the inhibition of bicarbonate formation from the breakdown of carbonic acid. Thus in the presence of Diamox, not only is bicarbonate not formed, but also acid is not eliminated, and *(acidosis/alkalosis)* therefore occurs. If H^+ (acid) is not excreted, Na^+ may be excreted as an exchange product to maintain electrical equilibrium, thus allowing for Diamox's diuretic effect.

acidosis

108 The clinical signs of metabolic acidosis are *sensorium changes* and *deep, rapid respirations*. The sensorium changes are a manifestation of the toxic effect of acidic substances on the CNS.

REMEMBER: Alterations in consciousness, restlessness, agitation, dizziness, and confusion may be referred to collectively as _____ _____. The symptoms are associated with the cerebral effects of *(acidosis/alkalosis)*.

sensorium changes
acidosis

The deep, rapid respirations seen in metabolic acidosis represent the *effort* of the *respiratory system* (lungs) to assist the kidneys in excreting acid. This symptom is an example of the *efforts of the lungs*. These respirations are more commonly known as Kussmaul's respirations.

The respiratory system compensates for a metabolic acidosis by excreting acid in the form of _____ _____. In acute situations this effort represents a *secondary defense system* and is rarely completely effective in normalizing the pH.

carbon
dioxide

109 The ABG values most useful in the assessment of metabolic imbalances are the _____, _____, and _____. The ABG values diagnostic of a *metabolic acidosis* are the following:
1. *(Increased/decreased)* pH
1. *(Increased/decreased)* bicarbonate and base excess (deficit)

pH; bicarbonate
base excess/deficit

decreased
decreased

110 The *therapy* for metabolic acidosis is partly dependent on the degree of pH alteration. Aggressive sodium bicarbonate administration may overcorrect the problem. It may result in a pH shift too rapid for the brain to adjust to or create a metabolic alkalosis, which is far more difficult to correct. Thus sodium bicarbonate is most safely administered in small amounts when the drop in pH is severe (for example, pH < 7.2). Bicarbonate administration should be followed by tests on blood gas samples to verify its effectiveness. When the pH is greater than 7.2, therapy consists of correcting the underlying cause. Supplementary oxygen along with modes of cardiovascular support is beneficial in the CCU patient with a lactic acidosis caused by hypoxia.

Metabolic alkalosis

111 Metabolic alkalosis results from *increased* levels of *base* (bicarbonate) or *excess loss* of *nonvolatile acid,* or both. The bicarbonate accumulation may occur as a result of exogenous ingestion and parenteral administration, or, secondary to the loss of fixed (nonvolatile) acids, it may occur with vomiting or mechanical removal of upper GI secretions. Some common conditions that may result in metabolic alkalosis are excessive ingestion of antacids containing bicarbonate, overzealous correction of an acidosis with IV sodium bicarbonate, loss of acid and chloride secondary to diuresis, vomiting, or GI suction. When chloride (an anion) is lost from the body, bicarbonate is retained by the kidneys to maintain the body's electroneutrality. Accumulation of bicarbonate secondary to chloride loss may result in a *(metabolic/respiratory)* alkalosis.

metabolic

112 The clinical signs of metabolic alkalosis are slow, shallow respirations and symptoms of decreased calcium effect. The slow, shallow respirations represent the *effort* of the *respiratory system* to assist the kidneys in *conserving acid.* This respiratory change reflects the compensatory effort of the respiratory system. The hypoventilation is an attempt to compensate for the metabolic alkalosis by retaining acid in the form of _____ _____. This compensatory effort is limited because of the immediate effects of the rising Pa_{CO_2} on the central respiratory center, which limits hypoventilation.

carbonic acid

113 The symptoms of decreased calcium become manifest in the presence of an alkalosis because of the effect of pH on bound and free calcium levels (see Frame 102).

REMEMBER: Alkalosis causes increased binding of calcium and decreased levels of *(free/bound)* calcium. Therefore the nurse can expect to see symptoms of *(hypo/hyper)* calcemia in the presence of alkalosis.

free

hypo

114 The ABG values most useful in the assessment of *metabolic* imbalances are the _____, _____, and _____ _____. The ABG values diagnostic of a *metabolic alkalosis* are the following:
1. *(Increased/decreased)* pH
2. *(Increased/decreased)* bicarbonate and base excess (deficit)

pH; bicarbonate; base excess/deficit

increased
increased

	METABOLIC	
	pH	HCO$_3$
ACIDOSIS	↓	↓
ALKALOSIS	↑	↑

Fig. 5-14

115 *Therapy* or *intervention* in metabolic alkalosis imbalance includes the following:
1. Cessation of diuretics
2. Replacement of chlorides in the form of KCl in renal losses or NaCl in GI losses
3. Administration of acetazolamide (Diamox) to promote conservation of acid and restore H^+ equilibrium by the kidneys (see Frames 105 to 107)
4. Implementation of seizure precautions

Direct administration of dilute hydrochloric acid solutions or use of acidifying agents such as ammonium chloride may also be employed to correct severe metabolic alkalosis. However, these agents are usually not necessary in coronary care. This imbalance is the most difficult to correct and is most effectively managed by prevention.

The anion gap: role in assessing metabolic acidosis

116 Not all the charged particles in the blood are actually measured on a set of routine serum electrolyte tests.

REMEMBER: The two cations measured on routine serum electrolyte tests are _____ and _____. The two anions measured on routine serum electrolyte tests are _____ and _____.

Na^+; K^+

Cl^-

HCO_3^-

The bicarbonate is often measured and reported as the _____ _____ (see Unit 3).

CO_2 content

117 According to the law of _____, the total number of positively and negatively charged particles in the serum must remain equal. However, the sum of the CL^- and HCO_3^- levels does not normally balance the sum of the Na^+ and K^+ levels. There are usually *fewer* _____ charges than _____ charges. This gap of negative charges not directly measured in the determination of routine serum electrolytes is known as the _____ _____.

electroneutrality

negative; positive

anion gap

The normal anion gap is 8 to 12 mEq/L. It is composed of small amounts of albumin and other proteins, $HPO_4^=$, and *organic acids,* such as _____, _____ _____, and _____ _____. When excess acids accumulate, as in hypoxia, this gap can become greater than normal. Thus the acidosis may be detected in a set of routine serum electrolyte tests as well as in ABG samples. The electrolyte changes may be noted before ABG changes and suggest the possible importance of an ABG sample. They may also be useful in between ABG samples for assessment of acid-base improvement or deterioration.

ketoacids; lactic acid
sulfuric acid

118 The causes of metabolic acidosis can be grouped into two categories: (1) those associated with *high serum Cl^-* levels caused by the accumulation of acid in the form of HCl, and (2) those with *normal serum Cl^-* levels caused by accumulation of acids other than HCl (see Frame 120).

The acids other than HCl are negatively charged and usually represent excess amounts of the normal organic acids. However, exogenous acids such as acetylsalicylic acids (ASA) may also carry a negative charge and add to amounts of nonmeasured particles. The presence of such particles may contribute to an anion gap that is *(greater/less)* than normal.   greater

The CO_2 content (bicarbonate) is usually *(high/low)* in the presence of a metabolic acidosis.   low

As the low CO_2 content in the serum is replaced by the negatively charged acids, an abnormally large _____ gap becomes apparent.   anion

119 Let us consider the following example:

Na^+	147 mEq/L
K^+	4.6 mEq/L
Cl^-	105 mEq/L
CO_2^-	18 mEq/L

The normal CO_2 content is 24 to 30 mEq/L. The CO_2 content in this example is *(high/low)*, indicating the presence of   low
_____ _____. The sum of the se-   metabolic acidosis
rum anions (CL^- and CO_2) equals _____. The sum   123 mEq/L.
of the serum cations is 141 mEq/L. However, the serum K^+ levels are so small that they are usually not considered.

NOTE: *If* the K^+ level is considered, the normal anion gap level must be extended to 8 to 16 mEq/L.

The sum of anions does not equal the serum Na^+ level. There is a gap of _____ mEq/L (147 − 128 mEq/L.) This difference   24
(is/is not) a normal anion gap.   is not

120 This gap is *(greater/less)* than normal. An abnormally large anion gap   greater
may indicate the presence of excess _____ acids,   organic
such as _____ _____,   lactic acid
_____, or uremic acids. The presence of exoge-   ketoacids
nous acids, such as _____ and _____ may also   ASA; alcohol
contribute. In the patient with an acute MI, the *most common causes* of an abnormal anion gap is *lactic acidosis*.

NOTE: The serum Cl^- level typically remains normal because acids other than HCl are responsible for this change.

121 When HCl accumulates, causing metabolic acidosis, the serum Cl^- level is *(high/low/normal)*. This change usually compensates for the drop in CO_2 content, and the gap remains normal or may appear small.

high

Causes of metabolic acidosis with a normal anion gap include diarrhea or excessive intestinal drainage; renal tubular acidosis; adrenal insufficiency; administration of certain drugs, such as acetazolamide (Diamox) and mafenide (Sulfamylon); and administration of certain types of hyperalimentation fluid. These causes of metabolic acidosis are not commonly seen in the CCU and thus, when found, eliminate more commonly associated complications.

122 A systematic approach to the assessment of anion gap on routine serum electrolyte tests includes the following steps:

1. Determine the presence of a _____ acidosis by checking the _____ content. (Calculating anion gap in the absence of an acidosis can produce spurious findings of no significance.)

metabolic
CO_2

2. Screen other electrolytes for abnormalities. (Check _____, _____, and _____. This factor can distort the anion gap.)

Na^+; K^+; Cl^-

3. Calculate the anion gap by comparing the _____ and _____ content with the _____ level.

Cl^-
CO_2; Na^+

4. Determine potential mechanisms and intervention.

An abnormally small anion gap may indicate either low serum levels of *anions,* such as albumin, or high serum levels of *cations,* such as Ca^{++} or Mg^{++}.

PRACTICAL APPLICATION: CORRELATION OF ABG VALUES WITH OXYGENATION

123 When analyzing a set of ABG values, we find it is easier initially to consider the acid-base and oxygen values separately. Alterations in acid-base balance may not necessarily be associated with states of inadequate oxygenation.

124 Let us first consider the normal values that have been assigned to the acid-base parameters.

pH	7.35-7.45
P_{CO_2}	35-45 mm Hg
HCO_3^-	22-26 mEq/L

NOTE: These levels apply to a normal adult who is breathing room air. The values may vary in different institutional settings.

When analyzing the acid-base component of ABG values, follow these steps:

Step 1. Check the pH. Is the value above or below normal? The pH will indicate whether the major problem is acidosis or alkalosis. REMEMBER: Decreased pH = acidosis; increased pH = alkalosis

Step 2. Check the values that reflect the respiratory side of the equation. Is the Pco_2 normal, increased, or decreased?

Step 3. Check the value that reflects the metabolic side of the equation. Is HCO_3^- level normal, increased or decreased?

	RESPIRATORY		METABOLIC		
	pH	P_{CO_2}	pH	HCO_3	
ACIDOSIS	↓	↑	↓	↓	Fig. 5-15
ALKALOSIS	↑	↓	↑	↑	

125 *Step 4.* Make a diagnosis based on the fact that the pH will most likely indicate the primary disorder (Fig. 5-15).

Step 5. Determine whether any compensatory mechanisms are involved by checking the other values for abnormalities.

Step 6. Evaluate why the patient's blood gas values are abnormal, and decide on the nursing action to be taken.

126 Now apply the following value to a set of ABGs.

pH	7.6
Pco_2	18 mm Hg
HCO_3^-	16 mEq/L

127 According to the data given in Frame 127:

The pH is *(increased/decreased/normal)*.   increased

The pH indicates a(n) _____.   alkalosis

The Pco_2 is *(increased/decreased/normal)*.   decreased

The Pco_2 indicates respiratory *(acidosis/alkalosis)*.   alkalosis

The HCO_3^- level is *(increased/decreased/normal)*.   decreased

The level of HCO_3^- indicates metabolic *(acidosis/alkalosis)*.   acidosis

The pH indicates that the primary disorder is most likely the _____ _____ imbalance.   respiratory alkalosis

The other changes most likely reflect the body's attempts at _____.   compensation

128 When analyzing the oxygenation component of blood gas values, follow the systematic approach presented in Unit 3.

LET US REVIEW:

Step 1. Analyze the Pa_{O_2} to determine O_2 _____ in the _____.   transport; lungs

Step 2. Analyze the O_2 saturation to determine the O_2 content

content

Step 3. Correlate the signs of hypoxemia with signs of hypoxia.

Step 4. Determine modes of intervention.

129 Now apply these steps to the following complete blood gas report, which reflects changes more commonly seen in a coronary care unit:

pH	7.20
P_{CO_2}	60 mm Hg
HCO_3^-	18 mEq/L
Pa_{O_2}	50 mm Hg
O_2 saturation	70%
$F_{I_{O_2}}$	approximately 0.6 (60%); manual resuscitator (Ambu)
Hg	14.2 g/dl

The pH is *(increased/decreased/normal)*.   decreased
The pH indicates a(n) _____.   acidosis
The P_{CO_2} is *(increased/decreased/normal)*.   increased
The P_{CO_2} indicates respiratory *(acidosis/alkalosis)*.   acidosis
The HCO_3^- level is *(increased/decreased/normal)*.   decreased
The HCO_3^- level indicates metabolic *(acidosis/alkalosis)*. acidosis
The pH indicates a *combined* disorder (see Frame 134).

130 The critically low Pa_{O_2} (less than _____) reflects the presence of *(hypoxemia/hypoxia)*. The low O_2 saturation reflects a corresponding deficit in _____ _____.

60 mm Hg
hypoxemia
O_2 content

REMEMBER: To verify the accuracy of the O_2 saturation, check the serum _____. The low Pa_{O_2} reflects a deficit in _____ _____. The extent of this deficit can be further evaluated by comparing the $F_{I_{O_2}}$ with the Pa_{O_2}.

hemoglobin
O_2 transport

131 REMEMBER: At an $F_{I_{O_2}}$ of 0.6 (60%), the expected Pa_{O_2} should be approximately _____. Therefore this patient's Pa_{O_2} represents a *(mild/severe)* defect in pulmonary O_2 transport.

300 mm Hg
severe

132 The low pH assists in confirming the presence of *hypoxia* when correlated with typical patient symptoms (see Unit 3, Frames 4 to 9).

REMEMBER: Hypoxia typically occurs as a consequence of hypoxemia. Because of its effect on Hb-O_2 binding (O_2 saturation), the low pH facilitates O_2 delivery to the tissues; however, it inhibits the uptake of oxygen in the lungs.

Hydrogen ions and carbon dioxide serve to push the oxygen off the hemoglobin and loosen the O_2-Hb relationship. Therefore the O_2 saturation appears *(higher/lower)* for a given P_{O_2}. Correction of

lower

the pH can stabilize both O_2 uptake and O_2 delivery and maximize tissue oxygenation.

133 The complete interpretation of these blood gases indicates a combined _____ and _____ acidosis   respiratory; metabolic
with severe hypoxemia caused by impaired pulmonary O_2 transport. Two major conditions that may result in this clinical picture are cardiopulmonary arrest or severe pulmonary edema caused by left ventricular failure.

    Nursing action is directed toward improving ventilation and cardiac output (see Unit 9). Medical orders for bicarbonate therapy should also be requested.

134 Analyze the following complete blood gas values using a systematic approach:

pH	7.31
P_{CO_2}	72 mm Hg$_3^-$
HCO_3^-	37 mEq/L
Base excess	+ 10
Pa_{O_2}	55
O_2 saturation	85%
Hg	24 g/dl
$F_{I_{O_2}}$	0.55 (55%)

The pH is *(increased/decrease/normal)*.   decreased
The pH indicates a(n) _____.   acidosis
The P_{CO_2} is *(increased/decreased/normal)*.   increased
This P_{CO_2} indicates respiratory _____.   acidosis
The HCO_3^- level is *(increased/decreased/normal)*.   increased
The HCO_3^- level indicates metabolic *(acidosis/alkalosis)*.   alkalosis

135 REMEMBER: The primary disorder is indicated by the _____.   pH
In this patient the *(respiratory/metabolic)* component correlates with   respiratory
the pH. Thus the patient's primary problem is
_____ _____.   respiratory; acidosis

    The metabolic changes may be best described as
_____.   compensatory

    The presence of metabolic compensation indicates a(n) *(acute/*   chronic
chronic) respiratory disorder.

    REMEMBER: Renal compensation is *(immediate/delayed)*.   delayed

136 The critically low Pa_{O_2} and O_2 saturation indicate the presence of *hypoxemia*. The low O_2 saturation reflects an apparent deficit in
_____ _____. However, this patient's se- O_2 content
rum Hb level is *(high/low/normal)*.   high

REMEMBER: In the presence of polycythemia _____ Hb
sites are available. These excess sites become difficult to fill even if
there are adequate amounts of oxygen. Thus this O_2 saturation
(does/does not) actually represent an inadequate O_2 supply.

excess

does not

137 The low Pa_{O_2} reflects a deficit in _____
_____. The extent of this deficit can be further
evaluated by comparing the _____ with the Pa_{O_2}.
REMEMBER: At an $F_{I_{O_2}}$ of 0.55 (55%), the expected Pa_{O_2} should be
approximately _____ mm Hg. Therefore this patient's
Pa_{O_2} represents a *(mild/severe)* defect in O_2 transport. However,
symptoms of hypoxia may not be apparent because of the comensa-
tion provided by the high Hb content. The compensatory efforts of
the cardiovascular system may be impaired in the patient with an
acute MI and chronic respiratory disease.

O_2 transport

$F_{I_{O_2}}$

275
severe

138 The complete interpretation of these blood gas values indicates
chronic respiratory acidosis with impaired O_2 transport. A major disorder that may result in this clinical picture is chronic bronchitis
(COPD). Nursing action is directed toward measures improving ventilation (see Frame 98).

SUGGESTED READINGS
General

Collins RD: Illustrated manual of fluid and elctrolyte disorders ed. 2, Philadelphia, 1983, JB Lippincott Co.

Demling RH and Wilson RF: Decision making in surgical critical care, Philadelphia, 1988, BC Decker Inc.

Guyton AC: Textbook of medical physiology, ed 7, Philadelphia, 1986, WB Saunders Co.

Huang S et al: Coronary care nursing, Philadelphia, 1983, WB Saunders Co.

Lancaster LE: Core curriculum for nephrology nursing, ed. 1, 1987, American Nephrology Nurses Association.

Masiak M, Masiak N, and Duffin M: Fluid and electrolytes throughout the life cycle, Norwalk, Conn. 1985, Appleton-Century-Crofts.

Metheny N: Fluid and electrolyte balance: nursing considerations, Philadelphia, 1987, JB Lippincott Co.

Rose BD: Clinical physiology of acid-base and electrolyte disorders ed 2, New York, 1984, McGraw-Hill Inc.

Strout V and others: Fluid and electrolytes: a practical approach, Philadelphia, 1984, FA Davis Co.

Monitoring fluid and electrolytes precisely, Nursing Skillbooks, ed 2, Springhouse, PA, 1983, Springhouse Corp.

The electrolyte imbalances: potassium, calcium and magnesium

Barta MA: Correcting electrolyte imbalance, RN 50(2):30, 1987.

Bidani A: Electrolyte and acid-base disorder, Med Clin North Am 70(5):1013, 1986.

Calloway C: When the problem involves magnesium, calcium, or phosphate, RN 50(5):30, 1987.

Caralis PV and others: Electrolyte abnormalities and ventricular arrhythmias, Drugs (Suppl) 31(4):85, 1986.

Chipperfield B and Chipperfield JR: Magnesium and the heart, Am Heart J 93:679, 1977.

Dickerson R and Brown R: Hypomagnesemia in hospitalized patients receiving nutritional support, Heart Lung 14(6):561, 1985.

Huerta B and Lemberg L: Potassium imbalance in the coronary care unit, Heart Lung 14(2):193, 1985.

Hurst JW and Logue RB, editors: The heart, arteries, and veins, ed 6, New York, 1986, McGraw-Hill Inc.

Martof M: Electrolyte balance: part II, J Nephrol Nurs 2(2):49, 1985.

McCormack A and others: Master care plan: preventing electrolyte imbalances, RN 47(11):32, 1984.

McFadden E and Zaloga P: Calcium regulation, CCQ 6(3):12, 1983.

McFadden E and others: Hypocalcemia: a medical emergency, Am J Nurs 83:227, 1983.

Polyss AS: Assessment and nursing diagnoses in fluid and electrolyte disorders, Nurs Clin North Am 22(4):773, 1987.

Quinlan M: Solving the mysteries of calcium imbalance: an action guide, RN 45:50, 1982.

Quinlan M: Would you recognize this (magnesoum) dangerous electrolyte imbalance, RN 48:51, 1983.

Sweetwood HM: Clinical electrocardiography for nurses, Rockville, 1983, Aspen Publishers Inc.

Toto K: When the patient has hyperkalemia, RN 50(4):34, 1987.

Valladares B: Catecholamines, potassium, and beta-blockade, Heart Lung 15(1):105, 1986.

Watson JE: Fluid and electrolyte disorders in cardiovascular patients, Nurs Clin North Am 22(4):797, 1987.

Zaloga GP and Chernow B: Magnesium metabolism in critical illness, CCQ 6(3):22, 1983.

Acid-base balance and blood gas analysis

Alspach J and Williams S, editors: Core curriculum for critical care nursing, ed 3, Philadelphia, 1985, WB Saunders Co.

Buckingham AK: Arterial blood gases made simple, Nurs Life 5(6):48, 1985.

Buehmaan AA: Blood gases, Eur Heart J (C):45, 6(Suppl) 1985.

Burton J: Respiratory care update. Part III. Acid/base balance, Crit Care Update p. 23, Oct. 1982.

Burton J: Respiratory care updated. Part IV. Compensation of acid/base disturbance, Crit Care Update p. 15, Nov. 1982.

Glass LB and Jenkins CA: The ups and downs of serum pH, Nursing 13(9):34, 1983.

Guyton AC: Textbook of Medical Physiology, ed. 7, Philadelphia, 1986, WB Saunders Co.

Janusek LW: Metabolic acidosis: physiology, signs, and symptoms, Nursing 14(7):44, 1984.

Janusek LW: Metabolic alkalosis: Physiology, signs, symptoms, Nursing 14(8):60, 1984.

Kenner CV and others: Crit care nurs: body-mind-spirit, ed 2, Boston, 1985, Little, Brown & Co. Inc.

Pfister S and others: Interpreting arterial blood gas values, Crit Care Nurse 6(4):9-14, 1986.

Porth C: Pathophysiology, concepts of altered health, ed 2, Philadelphia, 1986, JB Lippincott.

Raffin TA: Indications for arterial blood gas analysis, Ann Intern Med 105(3):390, 1986.

Relman AS: Blood gases: arterial or venous, New Engl J Med 315(3):188, 1986.

Romanski S: Interpreting ABG's in four easy steps, Nursing 16(9):58, 1986.

Shapiro BA: Clinical application of blood gases, ed 3, Chicago, 1982, Year Book Publishers Inc.

Shapiro BA: Respiratory intensive care: state of the art vol 5, Chicago, 1984, Respiratory Care Seminars Inc.

Taylor DL: Respiratory alkalosis: physiology, signs, symptoms, Nursing 14(11):44, 1984.

Taylor DL: Respiratory acidosis: physiology, signs, and symptoms, Nursing 14(10):44, 1984.

Ventriglia WJ: Arterial blood gases, Emerg Med Clin North Am 4(2):235, 1986.

Weaver T: ABG's: taking the sample, interpreting the results, RN 46:64, 1983.

The electrolyte imbalances: potassium, calcium, and magnesium

Iseri LT and French JH: Magnesium: nature's physiologic calcium blocker, Am Heart J 108:188, 1984.

Oster JR: Magnesium, South Med J 9:1111, 1985.

Valle G and Lemberg L: Electrolyte imbalances in cardiovascular disease: the forgotten factor, Heart Lung 17(3):324, 1988.

Wills MR: Potassium and magnesium metabolism: an overview with regard to diuretics and the heart, CV Review and Reports (Suppl)6(7):7, 1985.

Diagnosis of Coronary Artery Disease

1 Coronary artery disease is manifested by two closely related syndromes—angina and acute myocardial infarction as well as by their associated complications.

Myocardial infarction (MI) is death, or necrosis, of a section of the cardiac muscle resulting from an interrupted or severely diminished supply of oxygenated blood. Myocardial infarction occurs secondary to coronary artery changes and is associated with periods of severe, sustained myocardial hypoxia.

REMEMBER: The heart muscle receives its blood supply from two coronary arteries, the _____ and the _____.

right; left

2 Angina is a syndrome characterized by chest pain resulting from a transient myocardial O_2 imbalance and hypoxia. It *(is/is not)* typically associated with death of tissue. Angina occurs secondary to the same coronary artery changes that are associated with acute MI. However, these changes are *(more/less)* severe.

is not

less

Angina can occur either at rest or during exertion and is typically triggered by increased O_2 demands, coronary spasm, or both. Rest angina is more typically associated with coronary spasm. Effort, or exertional, angina is more typically associated with increased O_2 _____.

demands

The pain of effort angina is usually relieved rapidly by rest or by the administration of sublingual nitroglycerin. The pain of rest angina is also relieved by sublingual nitroglycerin or by the long-term administration of calcium channel blocking agents (see Unit 10).

3 Mixed angina is the most common form of angina and refers to a mixture of spasm and fixed coronary disease as contributing factors. Patients with mixed angina may have a _____ of angina at _____ and during _____. Chronic stable angina is usually either an effort angina or a mixed angina syndrome.

mixture
rest; exertion

Angina is not necessarily followed by acute MI. However, acute MI is usually preceded by at least one or more episodes of angina, which can act as warning signs. An increase in the frequency, severity, or duration of anginal attacks may indicate that acute MI is imminent. The term *unstable angina* has been used to describe the signs and symptoms suggestive of impending infarction (see Frame 8).

4 Coronary artery disease has key structural, functional, and metabolic components (Fig. 6-1). The structural coronary changes occurring in acute MI and angina are the *(same/different)*. Coronary blood   same
supply is diminished and/or interrupted in the patient with acute MI or angina because of a process of coronary narrowing, or
_____. This process ultimately results in coronary   stenosis
occlusion. Occlusion is more typically associated with acute MI.

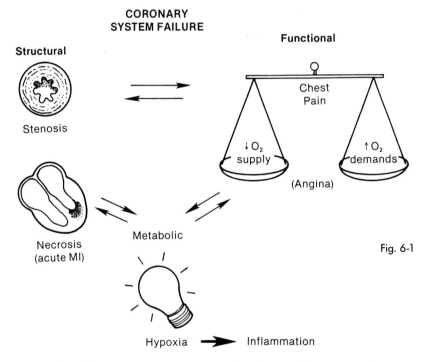

Fig. 6-1

The three most common mechanisms of large-vessel coronary stenosis are the following:
1. Lipid infiltration (atherosclerosis)
2. Thrombosis (platelet/fibrin)
3. Coronary spasm

5 The majority of cases of acute coronary stenosis or occlusion occur as a result of atherosclerotic heart disease. Atherosclerosis is characterized by thickening of the intima of the artery, which occurs as a result of intimal stress and fatty atheroma deposits. Atherosclerosis triggers platelet aggregation and eventual fibrosis and calcification.

Severe coronary stenosis and decreased blood flow is associated with fibrin deposition. Fibrin thrombus formation is often the final event resulting in complete or significant occlusion. Necrosis and hemorrhage may also occur. These intimal changes lead to *narrowing* or occlusion of the coronary arteries. Fig. 6-2 shows how atherosclerosis narrows the channel of the artery and decreases or occludes the free flow of blood. Atherosclerotic lesions are also highly sensitive to the effects of coronary spasm, which further narrows the lumen. Coronary spasm is thought to be triggered by increased sympathetic activity closely related to stress.

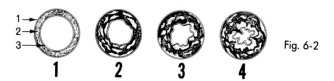

Fig. 6-2

As a result of inadequate blood and O_2 supply, cellular metabolic changes occur that irritate pain receptors, alter cellular function, and cause the death of cells. These changes may be temporary, as in _____, or permanent, as in _____.

angina
acute MI

6 The presence of collateral, or accessory, circulation may minimize the detrimental effects of coronary vessel _____ or occlusion. Because of these collateral vessels as well as individual variations in O_2 demand and work load tolerance, the degree of stenosis does not always correlate well with the functional or metabolic impact of the disease (Fig. 6-3). For this reason, separate as well as integrated assessment of _____, _____, and _____ components provides a more thorough viewpoint of the disease.

narrowing

structural
functional; metabolic

7 Angina and MI differ in their functional and metabolic impact.

However, the structural coronary changes occurring in angina and acute MI are the *(same/different)*. Therefore the initial clinical presentation of both may be similar.

same

The characteristic presenting symptom or *history* of both angina and acute MI is *chest pain*. The chest pain may be accompanied by nausea or diaphoresis, depending on the subjectively perceived severity of the pain and the related stress response (see Frame 146).

8 Chest pain is a symptom of myocardial _____ and the resulting metabolic compromise. This metabolic compromise can lead to immediate and delayed electrical and mechanical alterations and complications. (Fig. 6-3).

hypoxia

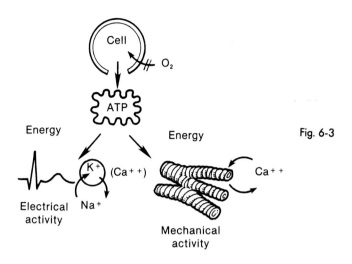

Fig. 6-3

Invasive and noninvasive diagnostic tests currently detect and evaluate the structural, functional, and _____ components of coronary artery disease. These tests can also evaluate the _____ and _____ complications of this disease. The major invasive test is cardiac catheterization, which is considered the standard for detecting structural coronary disease and mechanical dysfunction. Examples of major noninvasive tests are radionuclide studies, echocardiography, and stress testing.

metabolic

electrical; mechanical

The detection of acute MI requires other diagnostic information, which can be readily obtained with the patient at rest.

DIAGNOSIS OF ACUTE MI

9 The medical diagnosis of acute MI is based on three major parameters: history, serum enzymes, and ECG changes. When the results of two out of these three are positive, the diagnosis of acute MI is made. When either the history, serum enzymes, or ECG changes typical of acute MI accompany angina pectoris, the diagnosis of unstable angina may be made. These patients should be monitored in coronary care units (CCUs). They should be clinically regarded as if MI has occurred until their condition stabilizes.

The ECG and serum enzymes are readily available diagnostic tests that can be performed _____ with the patient _____ _____. They provide information sufficiently accurate to guide initial intervention. Although serum enzymes reflect death of tissue or _____ more accurately than do ECG changes, the results are not as immediately available. Therefore the ECG assumes a greater initial practical importance.

immediately

at rest

infarction

Table 6. Differential diagnosis of chest pain

Question	MI pain	Angina	Pericarditis	Pulmonary embolus
Where do you feel the pain? (location)	Retrosternal, but may radiate to back, neck, arm, and jaw	Same	Located over the precordial area and radiates to the back; may also radiate to jaw and arms	Usually over lung fields, to the side and the back
What is the pain like? (quality)	Pressure, choking, burning, tightness, viselike, usually *severe*	Similar in description to MI	Sharp ache in the chest, not necessarily severe but annoying	Similar to pericarditis, except to the side and the back
How long did it last? (duration)	At least 30 minutes	Relief usually in 15 minutes or less	Continuous; may last for days	Continuous for hours
Did you have any nausea? Did you feel short of breath Did you feel weak or dizzy? Did you have cold sweats? (accompanying symptoms)	*May have* nausea, dyspnea, weakness, diaphoresis, and dizziness	Usually *not* accompanied by diaphoresis or nausea	Usually *not* accompanied by these symptoms	Accompanied by *acute* shortness of breath, tachycardia, and apprehension (most characteristic—bloody sputum)
Was the pain relieved when you took a deep breath? (effects of respirations)	Not affected by respirations		Increased pain on inspiration	Increased pain on inspiration
Did you feel better when you sat up? (change of position)	Not relieved by change in position	May be only slightly relieved by change in position	Pain decreased on sitting up and increased when on *left* side	Decreased on sitting up
Was the pain relieved by anything?	Usually requires narcotics for relief	Relieved by rest when associated with *exertion*; relieved by NTG	Continuous soreness usually relieved somewhat by ASA or Tylenol	May be relieved by narcotics

HISTORY

10 A *positive* history from a patient who has acute MI will usually include a description of characteristic *chest pain* and accompanying symptoms. *Pain* is the presenting symptom in most patients with acute MI and will usually follow a characteristic pattern. Patients who have acute MI may also present with signs of peripheral vascular collapse, nausea or vomiting, diaphoresis, dyspnea and pulmonary congestion, and apprehension.

11 A complaint of chest pain must be assessed within the clinical setting in which it occurs. Because chest pain may be caused by many different conditions, it is important that other causes be ruled out. We will briefly consider three disorders commonly seen in a CCU in which the history may mimic acute MI: angina pectoris, pericarditis, and pulmonary embolus.

12 See Table 6 for differential diagnosis.

13 NURSING ORDERS: The patient with chest pain

REMEMBER: A *positive* history from a patient who presents with acute MI will usually include a description of characteristic *chest pain*.

1. Evaluate chest pain according to:
   —Location
   —Quality
   —Its association with respiration and change of position
   —Accompanying symptoms (shortness of breath, dizziness, cold clammy skin, and nausea or vomiting)
   —Precipitating factors and mode of relief
2. Obtain vital signs and note any alterations in the following:
   —Blood pressure
   —Pulse rate
   —Respiratory rate
   NOTE: An increase in blood pressure is an expected response to pain. Wait until the pain is relieved and take blood pressure again.
3. Obtain a sample ECG tracing in the *inferior, lateral,* and *anteroseptal* monitoring leads. Analyze the ECG tracing and report the following:
   —Arrhythmias
   —Displacement of the ST segment or changes in the T waves
   —Abnormalities in the QRS morphology
   —Changes in the polarity of the QRS complex
4. Relieve the patient's pain, a priority for any cardiac patient, as follows:
   —Prompt medication

—Recording mode of relief (rest, administration of nitroglycerin or morphine)
5. Report immediately any chest pain that is:
—Different from that which has occurred before
—Accompanied by different symptoms
—Accompanied by change in the ECG or vital signs
—Increasing in frequency or severity or both

Serum enzymes

14 Enzymes are proteins that change the speed of chemical reactions. Thus enzymes are located wherever chemical reactions take place. The chemical reactions of the body occur in three major sites: (1) within the *plasma*, (2) within the *cells*, and (3) within the *GI tract*. The plasma contains a mixture of the enzymes required for plasma functions such as coagulation, the GI enzymes that are transported by the plasma, and small amounts of the intracellular enzymes that leak out through the normal membrane pores. In the presence of cellular membrane damage, large amounts of intracellular enzymes are released into the bloodstream. Thus the serum levels of these enzymes *(increase/decrease)*.

Therefore an elevation in serum enzymes that are normally intracellular indicates cellular _____ _____.

increase

membrane damage

15 Characteristic enzymes are present in different types of cells. The major enzymes that are present in high concentrations within *cardiac cells* are: (1) creatine phosphokinase (CPK), now referred to as *creatine kinase* (CK); (2) lactic dehydrogenase (LDH); and (3) serume glutamic oxaloacetic transaminase (SGOT).

In the presence of cardiac necrosis there will usually be elevations in serum levels of the enzymes _____, _____, and _____. Levels of these enzymes may become elevated in the presence of any myocardial injury. MI, countershock, cardiac massage, and cardiopulmonary bypass can all *(elevate/decrease)* these enzymes levels.

CPK; LDH
SGOT

elevate

16 Each of the cardiac enzymes is also present in other body tissues. CPK is also found in the tissues of the brain, lung, and skeletal muscle. Increased serum CPK levels are highly specific for myocardial injury when abnormalities in the _____ muscle and _____ can be ruled out. It is also a highly sensitive enzyme because even small amounts of myocardial injury will cause it to become elevated. Both LDGH and SGOT may be released from many tissues other than the heart. Therefore both LDH and SGOT levels are highly *nonspecific*. Conditions that may elevate the serum

skeletal

brain

levels of both of these enzymes include muscle trauma, pulmonary infarction, liver disease, and CHF.

17 Following MI, the serum levels of the major cardiac enzymes seem to follow a characteristic pattern.

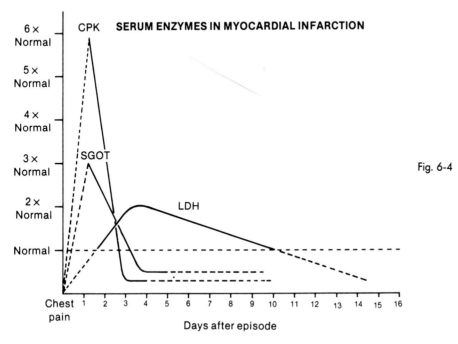

Fig. 6-4

NOTE: Because of the delayed onset and decline of LDH elevation, this enzyme is particularly useful in patients who delay reporting the signs of acute MI for a period of days.

Isoenzymes

18 Each of the routinely measured enzymes actually reflects the activity of a *group* of enzymes that, having only slight molecular differences, influence the same metabolic reactions. The different forms of a particular enzyme are known as its isoenzymes. CPK has three currently recognized isoenzyme forms. LDH has five currently recognized isoenzyme forms. Separation of total enzyme activity into its separate components allows for more accurate identification of enzyme elevations indicative of MI.

19 LET US REVIEW: The different forms of a particular enzyme are known as its _____. All forms of the same enzyme influence the same _____ _____. The isoenzymes of CPK and LDH allow for more accurate identifi-

isoenzymes
metabolic reactions

cation of enzyme elevations caused by _____. Thus, the
isoenzymes are *(more/less) specific* for acute MI than their corresponding total enzyme activity.

MI

more

20 CPK has _____ currently recognized isoenzyme forms.
These isoenzymes form three separately colored *bands* on acetate paper with electrophoresis. The CPK contained primarily within *skeletal muscle* is referred to as *CPK₃ (MM band)*. This enzyme is released
following muscle trauma, during convulsions, following surgical procedures and IV cutdowns, in the presence of alcoholic myopathy or
shock states, or following intramuscular injections. CPK-MM is also
found within cardiac muscle and may become elevated following myocardial trauma or infarction.

three

    The CPK contained within the *brain* is referred to as *CPK₁ (BB
band)*. However, in the presence of CNS disorders, it is unusual to
see elevations in CPK-BB, since it does not cross the blood-brain barrier. CPK elevations in these settings are usually associated with accompanying release from skeletal muscle and are thus of the
_____ type. CPK-BB is also found in the lungs,
bladder, and bowel.

CPK-MM

21 The third isoenzyme of CPK is found selectively within *cardiac muscle*. This isoenzyme form is referred to as *CPK₂ (MB band)*. CPK-MB
is highly specific for myocardial necrosis and begins to rise at 2 to 4
hours. It may not always differentiate damage resulting from acute
MI from that associated with surgical myocardial trauma or severe
myocardial ischemia (that is, severe unstable angina). However, a patient with a suspect history and positive CPK-MB activity should be
given the benefit of the doubt and treated as if he or she has sustained an acute MI. CPK-MB is a highly specific and sensitive enzyme for MI. Minimal amounts to none of this isoenzyme form (3%
to 5%) are present in the plasma of normal subjects. Any recorded
activity over 5% is considered abnormal. Serial CPK-MB have been
correlated with infarct size, arrhythmic complications, ventricular
performance, and prognosis.

22 LET US REVIEW: The CPK isoenzymes separate into _____
during electrophoresis. CPK-MM is found primarily in
_____ muscle but also in _____
muscle. CPK-BB is found in the _____, _____,
bladder, and bowel. CPK-MB is found almost exclusively within
_____ muscle.

    In the presence of acute MI there *(will/will not)* be a rise in total
CPK activity. This rise occurs *(early/late)* in the progress of an acute MI
and is composed of two CPK isoenzymes, _____ and

bands

skeletal; cardiac
brain; lungs

cardiac
will
early
CPK-MM

_____. The most specific CPK isoenzyme for acute   CPK-MB
MI is _____.   CPK-MB

23 LDH is another useful cardiac enzyme with recognized isoenzyme forms.

REMEMBER: LDH has _____ currently recognized isoen-   five
zyme forms.

LDH and LDH_2 are concentrated within the heart, kidneys, and RBCs. LDH_4 and LDH_5 are concentrated within the liver and skeletal muscle and become elevated in the presence of CHF with acute MI. Serum LDH_2 activity usually exceeds LDH_1 activity in the normal individual. In the presence of acute MI, LDH_1 activity exceeds LDH_2 activity. This pattern is referred to as a *flipped* LDH pattern.

LDH ISOENZYME PATTERN

Normal

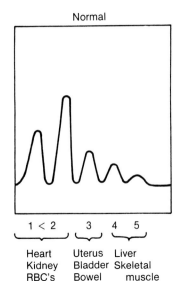

1 < 2   3   4   5

Heart   Uterus   Liver
Kidney   Bladder   Skeletal
RBC's   Bowel   muscle
Brain

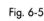

Fig. 6-5

"Flipped" pattern

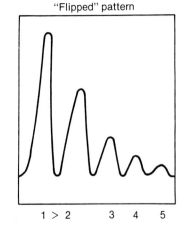

1 > 2   3   4   5

The combination of CPK-MB levels in the serum and a _____ LDH isoenzyme pattern is currently diag-   flipped
nostic for acute MI.

NOTE: The assessment of hydroxybutyrate dehydrogenase (HBD) is used in some institutions as a rough estimate of LDH_1 and LDH_2 values but does not reveal the flipped pattern.

24 Nurses should consider the following points when serum enzymes are being evaluated:
1. Avoid hemolysis of blood specimens.

REMEMBER: LDH_1 and LDH_2 are released from damaged _____ _____ cells.

red; blood

2. Look for the flipped LDH pattern as well as levels of LDH_1 and LDH_2.
3. Check CPK-*(MB/MM/BB)* activity.

MB

4. In the presence of CPK-MB activity greater than 5% and a flipped LDH pattern, the patient shoud be treated as if he or she had sustained acute MI.
5. Note the use of countershock, including number of times and voltage used.

ECG in acute myocardial infarction

25 The ECH changes reflect the electrical activity of the surfaces of the heart as recorded from the body surface. Before discussing specific ECG manifestations of acute MI, let us consider the layers of the heart wall that are involved in MI. MI may be limited to only one area of the heart wall.

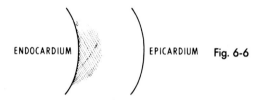

ENDOCARDIUM   EPICARDIUM   **Fig. 6-6**

An infarction limited to the endocardium and the layer of muscle adjacent to the endocardium is known as a *subendocardial infarction*.

26 Most infarctions are not limited to one area of the muscle but extend across the entire wall of the heart, from the endocardium to the epicardium. An MI that extends from the endocardium to the epicardium is known as a *transmural* (across the wall) *infarction*.

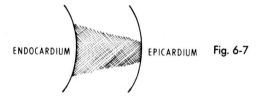

ENDOCARDIUM   EPICARDIUM   **Fig. 6-7**

NOTE: There is *always* more damage in the endocardial area than in the epicardial area in a transmural infarction.

REMEMBER: The endocardium is a *(richer/poorer)* blood supply than the epicardium and is therefore *(more/less)* vulnerable to a decrease in blood supply or oxygenation.

poorer

more

27 LET US REVIEW: An infarction limited to the layer of muscle below the endocardium is known as a _____ infarction. An

subendocardial

infarction that *extends across* the heart wall, from the endocardium to the epicardium, is known as a _____ infarction.

transmural

The following discussion will focus on the *transmural infarction* because it is the type most frequently diagnosed.

28 In this section the terms *ischemia, injury,* and *necrosis* are used to describe *electrical* events as seen on the ECG. These terms should not necessarily be equated with the physiological phenomena they usually describe.

REMEMBER: The term *myocardial infarction* means *physiological death,* or necrosis, of cardiac muscle tissue.

The electrical manifestation of necrosis, the abnormal Q wave, indicates that the cells are electrically dead but does not necessarily indicate that the cells are mechanically dead, because documented abnormal Q waves are known to disappear.

REMEMBER: The ECG is merely one of the parameters used in the clinical diagnosis of the MI syndrome.

29 The earliest sign of MI is the appearance of subendocardial ischemia and subendocardial injury. The peaked T waves of subendocardial ischemia are related to local Na^+-K^+ shifts and are often referred to as *hyperacute T wave changes*. These early signs are usually rapidly masked by more significant changes and thus are often missed on the ECG.

30 The *first stage* in the ECG evolution of a *transmural* MI is ST *segment elevation* in the leads, reflecting the *injured epicardial area*. This sign is usually the first ECG manifestation of acute MI and corresponds with the physiologic process of inflammation. In this stage some of the injured cells may respond poorly to the activation process. As a result, there is also a decrease in the amplitude of the R *waves* in the leads overlying the *injured area*.

The next stage in the ECG evolution of an MI is the appearance of *abnormal Q waves* referred to as *necrosis*. Abnormal Q waves indicate electrical death, or the inability to transmit electrical impulses, temporarily or permanently. An abnormal Q wave is one that is wider than 0.02 second, is deeper than a fourth (¼) of the R wave, is associated with a loss in the amplitude of the R wave, and simultaneously appears in several leads. (For example, in inferior wall infarction, abnormal Q waves will appear in leads II, III, and a V_F.) In this stage there is still evidence of myocardial injury because a zone of injury always surrounds an area of necrosis.

The last stage is that of *ischemia. Symmetrical inversion of the T wave* denotes electrical ischemia. Ischemia appears as the injury or _____ subsides. Ischemia may precede or follow Q wave formation. Thus T wave inversion may be seen in conjunction

inflammation

with _____ elevation and abnormal _____ waves.   ST; Q

31 ECG changes in acute MI are shown in Fig. 6-8.

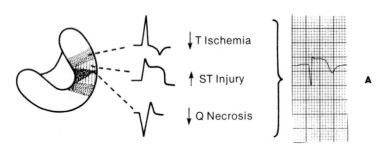

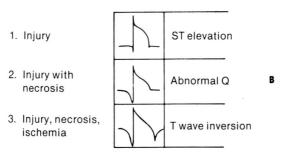

Fig. 6-8

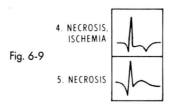

1. Injury   ST elevation

2. Injury with   Abnormal Q   B
   necrosis

3. Injury, necrosis,   T wave inversion
   ischemia

In the recovery stage the current of injury subsides, but the necrosis and ischemia are still present.

REMEMBER: Abnormal _____ waves denote myocardial   Q
necrosis. Symmetrical inversion of the _____ waves de-   T
notes myocardial _____.   ischemia

4. NECROSIS,
   ISCHEMIA

Fig. 6-9

5. NECROSIS

The ischemic may then subside. The only ECG manifestation of
infarction that then remains is the abnormal _____ wave.   Q
In some patients the abnormal Q wave may subsequently disappear.

NOTE: The duration of each stage of infarction will vary from patient to patient.

32 The ECG changes described occur in the leads directly reflecting the
area of infarction. *Indirect* ECG evidence of myocardial injury may
be obtained from leads that are *opposite* the *injured area* and within
the same plane.

REMEMBER: Myocardial injury produces ST segment _____ in the leads overlying the injured area. In the leads opposite the injured area, *opposite*, or *reciprocal*, changes will be seen. These changes are a mirror image of the ECG changes associated with the injury current. Thus reciprocal changes are manifested on the ECG as ST segment *(elevation/depression)* in the leads directly _____ the injured area and within the same plane.

elevation

depression
opposite

In the setting of acute MI, ST segment elevation in the inferior leads will produce ST segment _____ in the lateral leads. ST segment elevation in the lateral leads will produce ST segment _____ in the inferior leads.

depression

depression

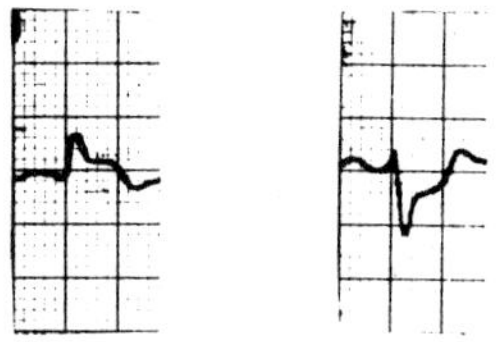

aV~L~   aV~F~

Fig. 6-10

33 LET US REVIEW: The stage of *ischemia* is characterized on the ECG by symmetrical abnormalities in the _____ waves. The stage of *injury* is characterized by abnormal displacement of the _____ segment. The stage of *necrosis* is characterized by the appearance of abnormal _____ waves.

T

ST
Q

The first ECG manifestation of acute MI is usually _____ _____ elevation in the leads overlying the injured area. The appearance of abnormal Q waves indicates that there is an area of electrical _____. Symmetrical *inversion* of the T wave denotes myocardial _____.

ST
segment

necrosis
ischemia

During the stage of injury, the disturbance in cellular metabolism is accompanied by cell *membrane damage*. Therefore the cells in the injured area as well as in the ischemic area are *electrically unstable*. Ventricular arrhythmias may occur as a manifestation of this electrical instability. Because some of the cells in an area of injury may respond poorly to the activation process, there may also be *decreased contractility* in an *injured area*.

Infarction sites

34 Knowledge of the anatomic location of an infarction enables us to anticipate the types of complications that are likely to occur. In this discuss we will consider the following four surfaces of the *left ventricle:* (1) the anterior wall, (2) the lateral wall, (3) the inferior wall, and (4) the posterior wall.

REMEMBER: The blood supply to the left ventricle is from both the _____ and _____ coronary arteries.

right; left

LET US REVIEW: The right coronary artery primarily supplies the *(inferoposterior/anterolateral)* surface of the left ventricle. The left coronary artery primarily supplies the *(inferoposterior/anterolateral)* surface of the left ventricle. The left coronary artery has two main branches:

1. The left anterior _____ branch
2. The left _____ branch

The anterior descending branch primarily supplies the _____ surface of the left ventricle. The circumflex branch *primarily* supplies the _____ surface of the left ventricle.

NOTE: When discussing acute MI, it is important to consider the location of the occlusion in the coronary artery tree. Occlusions that occur high in the tree will produce more extensive damage than those in the smaller branches.

inferoposterior
anterolateral

descending
circumflex

anterior
lateral

Extensive anterior wall myocardial infarction

35 Let us first consider infarctions that occur as a result of *left* coronary artery pathology.

REMEMBER: The left coronary artery has two main branches. If an occlusion occurs in the *main trunk* of the left coronary artery, an infarction may occur in both the septal and lateral areas of the _____ wall of the left ventricle.

anterior

EXTENSIVE ANTERIOR WALL MI

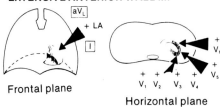

Frontal plane

Horizontal plane

Fig. 6-11

36 The leads that reflect the electrical activity of the *septal* and *lateral* areas of the left ventricle are leads 1 and _____ and V_1 through _____. Therefore massive infarctions of the anterior wall may produce changes in these leads (Fig. 6-12).

NOTE: The ST segment elevation occurs in the V leads and in leads I and aV_L. The reciprocal changes are in the inferior leads. The inferior lead changes are reciprocal to the changes in the *(anterior/lateral)* leads.

aV_L
V_6

lateral

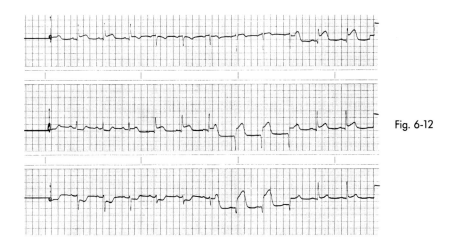

Fig. 6-12

Anteroseptal wall myocardial infarction

37 REMEMBER: The left coronary artery has two main branches: the left _____ _____ and the left _____ branches.

Occlusion of the left anterior descending branch will usually produce infarction of the septal area of the anterior wall. This is commonly referred to as *anteroseptal wall* MI.

anterior descending
circumflex

ANTEROSEPTAL MI

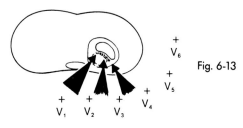

Fig. 6-13

Horizontal plane

The leads that reflect the electrical activity of the anteroseptal wall of the left ventricle are leads V_1 through _____. Therefore infarctions of the anteroseptal wall will produce changes in these leads.

NOTE: Leads V_2 and V_3 lie directly over the septum (Fig. 6-14).

The ST segment elevation occurs in leads V_1 through V_4.

There are no posterior positions on the six standard chest leads. Therefore reciprocal changes reflecting anteroseptal injury *(are/are not)* usually seen in the standard leads.

V_4

are not

193

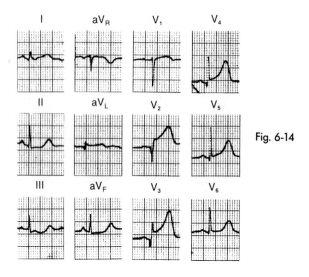

Fig. 6-14

Lateral wall myocardial infarction

38 Occlusion of the circumflex branch of the left coronary artery will produce infarction of the lateral area of the anterior wall.

LATERAL WALL MI

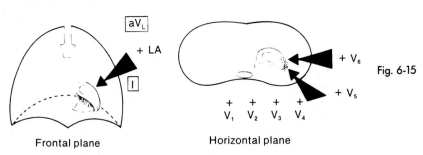

Frontal plane   Horizontal plane

Fig. 6-15

    REMEMBER: The electrode that looks directly toward the lateral surface of the left ventricle is the _____ arm electrode. **left**
The leads that use the LA electrode as their positive electrode are leads _____ and _____. **I; aV_L**

    Therefore these leads are used in the diagnosis of lateral wall MI. Leads V_4, V_5 and V_6 are *also* used when diagnosing lateral wall MI. However, these leads reflect the lower lateral rather than the upper lateral left ventricular surface and usually indicate involvement of the left ventricular apex.

    NOTE: The ST segment elevation occurs in leads I, aV_L, V_4, V_5, and V_6, and the reciprocal changes occur in the inferior leads.

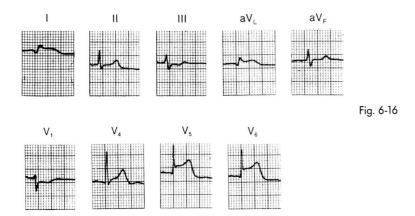

I II III aV_L aV_F

Fig. 6-16

V_1 V_4 V_5 V_6

39 In addition to supplying a *large portion* of the *muscle mass* of the left ventricle, the left coronary artery also supplies the following structures:

1. The _____ bundle branch (major portion) right
2. The _____ division of the left branch anterosuperior
3. The _____ division of the left branch (a portion) posteroinferior
4. The anterior two-thirds of the ventricular septum

   With this information we can anticipate the types of problems that will occur as a result of left coronary artery pathology.

40 Left coronary occlusion commonly produces necrosis of large areas of left ventricular musculature. Therefore it may be exected that patients with anterior wall MI will frequently present with *pump failure* more severe than that which accompanies right coronary artery pathology.

   Therefore patients with left coronary artery pathology are prone to the development of _____ _____ and heart failure
its accompanying arrhythmias.

   The arrhythmias that classically occur as a manifestation of heart failure are the following: (1) sinus tachycardia and (2) rapid atrial arrhythmias. Therefore these arrhythmias are frequently seen in the presence of anterior wall MI.

41 It is also stated that the left coronary artery supplies important structures of the intraventricular conduction system: (1) the right _____ _____, (2) the antero bundle branch
_____ division of the left branch, and (3) a portion superior
of the postero-_____ division of the left branch. inferior
Therefore it can be expected that intraventricular conduction disturbances will frequently accompany *left* coronary artery pathology (see Unit 8). The arrhythmia that occurs as a result of blocks in the

intraventricular conduction system is Type II, or Mobitz, block (see Unit 7).

42 LET US REVIEW: The left coronary artery has two main branches: (1) the left _____ _____ and (2) the left _____ branches. Occlusion of the main trunk of the left coronary artery usually produces extensive _____ wall MI.

anterior descending
circumflex

anterior

The leads used in the diagnosis of extensive anterior wall MI are leads _____ and _____, and _____ through _____. Occlusion of the anterior descending branch of the left coronary artery usually produces _____ wall MI.

I; aV$_L$; V$_1$
V$_6$

anteroseptal

The leads used in the diagnosis of anteroseptal wall MI are _____ through _____. Occlusion of the circumflex branch of the left coronary artery usually produces _____ wall MI.

V$_1$; V$_4$

lateral

The leads that reflect the electrical activity of the lateral wall are leads _____ and _____, and V$_4$, _____, and _____. It can be expected that patients who have left coronary artery occlusion will frequently present with (1) heart _____ and (2) _____ conduction disturbances.

I; aV$_L$; V$_5$
V$_6$

failure; intraventricular

43 NURSING ORDERS: For the patient with left coronary artery occlusion
1. Anticipate the development of heart failure.
   —Check lungs for rales.
   —Auscultate heart for gallops.
   —Check fluid balance and CVP or wedge readings.
   REMEMBER: The arrhythmias commonly associated with heart failure are sinus _____ and rapid _____ arrhythmias.

tachycardia
atrial

2. Monitor the patient for the development of intraventricular conduction disturbances and AV blocks, or Type II Mobitz block and its precursors (see Unit 8).

Inferoposterior wall myocardial infarction

44 Let us now consider infarctions that occur as a result of right coronary artery pathology.

REMEMBER: The *right* coronary artery primarily supplies the *(anterolateral/inferoposterior)* wall of the left ventricle. Although it is relatively common for *infarction* to extend across the entire inferoposterior wall, it is common for these two walls to be *injured* simultaneously. Most frequently infarction is limited to the inferior wall, and the injury current extends to the posterior wall. As the infarction evolves, the posterior wall injury often subsides.

inferoposterior

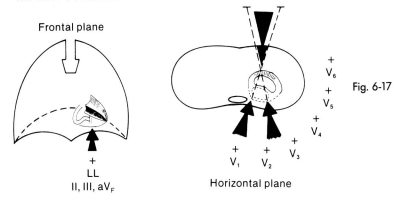

INFEROPOSTERIOR WALL MI

Frontal plane

+
LL
II, III, aV$_F$

+ V$_6$
+ V$_5$
+ V$_4$
+ V$_3$
+ V$_1$ + V$_2$

Fig. 6-17

Horizontal plane

45 The foot electrode looks directly toward the inferior surface of the _____ ventricle. The leads that use the foot electrode as their positive electrode are _____, _____, and _____.

left
II; III
aV$_F$

   Leads II, III, and aV$_F$ are used in the diagnosis of _____ wall MI. There is no electrode that looks directly up toward the posterior surface of the left ventricle. Therefore, to detect the electrical activity in the posterior wall, we must consider the leads located directly opposite this area. Leads V$_1$ and V$_2$ are thus used in the diagnosis of _____ wall MI.

inferior

posterior

   REMEMBER: Injury is manifested by ST segment *(elevation/ depression)* in the leads reflecting the injured area. Therefore, in the leads opposite the injured area, we would expect to see ST segment _____.

elevation

depression

46 Posterior wall injury is thus reflected in leads V$_1$ and V$_2$ by ST segment *(elevation/depression)*. Electrical death, or necrosis, is represented by an abnormal Q wave in the leads reflecting the area of necrosis. Therefore, in the leads *opposite* an *area of necrosis*, we would expect to see *(Q waves/R waves)*. Thus, in the presence of posterior wall necrosis, there is an increase in the amplitude of R waves in leads _____ and _____.

depression

R waves

V$_1$; V$_2$

   NOTE: The ST segment elevation occurs in leads II, III, and aV$_F$, and the ST segment depression occurs in leads V$_1$ and V$_2$. There are also reciprocal changes in leads I and aV$_L$.

47 In addition to supplying the inferoposterior surface of the left ventricle, the right coronary artery usually also supplies the following structures:
1. The _____ note
2. The _____ _____ tissue
3. Bundle of His

SA
AV junctional

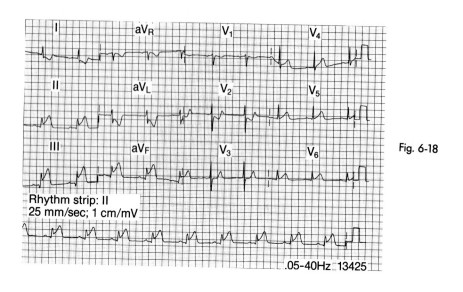

I aVR V₁ V₄

II aVL V₂ V₅

III aVF V₃ V₆

Fig. 6-18

Rhythm strip: II
25 mm/sec; 1 cm/mV

.05-40Hz 13425

4. Posterior one-third of the _____   septum

5. Posteroinferior division of the _____ branch (a portion)   left

6. Right atrium and right ventricle

   With this information, we can anticipate the types of problems
that will occur as a result of right coronary artery pathology.

48 Right coronary artery occlusion commonly causes ischemia to the SA
node, AV junctional tissue, and the parasympathetic (vagal) fibers
supplying these structures. As a result of this ischemia, *bradyarrhythmias,* or slow rates, occur. The specific bradyarrhythmias commonly
associated with right coronary artery occlusion are (1) sinus bradycardia and (2) Type I or Wenckebach, block.

49 LET US REVIEW: The right coronary artery primarily supplies the *(infe-*   inferior
rior/anterior) surface of the left ventricle. Occlusion of the right coronary artery commonly produces _____ wall MI.   inferior

   The leads used in the diagnosis of inferior wall MI are leads
_____, _____, and _____. It can be ex-   II; III; aVf
pected that the patients who have right coronary artery occlusion
will frequently present with *(bradyarrhythmias/tachyarrhythmias).* Less   bradyarrhythmias
commonly, occlusion of the right coronary artery may result in right
ventricular infarction.

   REMEMBER: The right coronary artery supplies most of the right
atrium and _____ _____. Logically RV   right ventricle
infarction may appear in combination with _____   inferoposterior
MI and results in significant hemodynamic compromise. The ECG
diagnosis is confirmed by obtaining an ECG with *"reversed"* chest
leads—i.e., V leads obtained on the *right* side of the chest labeled as
V_1R - V_6R. (see Fig 6-19, *A* and *B*) (see Unit 9).

Standard ECG

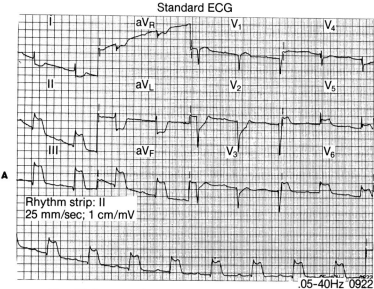

NOTE: The ECG shows ST elevation in leads II, III, aV$_F$, V$_5$, and V$_6$, which suggests acute inferoapical injury/infarction. ST depression in I, aV$_L$ represents a reciprocal change. ST depression in leads V$_1$ and V$_2$ is suggestive of posterior wall injury. Note rhythm is 2° AV block with 2:1 conduction.

Fig. 6-19

Reverse ECG

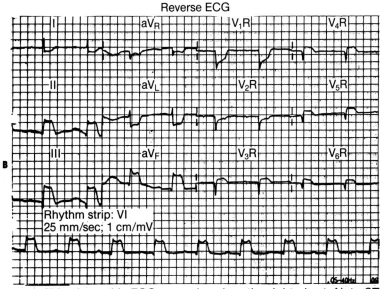

NOTE: V leads on this ECG were placed on the right chest. Note ST elevation in leads V$_3$R through V$_6$R suggestive of right ventricular injury/infarction. The limb leads are positioned normally.

50 NURSING ORDERS: For the patient with right coronary artery occlusion
1. Anticipate bradyarrhythmias
   —Sinus bradycardia
   —First-degree AV block
   —Type I, or Wenckebach, second-degree AV blocks
2. Watch for arrhythmias that may break through in the presence of slow rates (see Unit 7).
3. Have atropine at the bedside.
4. Be cautious with the administration of depressive drugs such as morphine or with vagal stimulation such as taking rectal temperatures.
5. Assess the patient for hemodynamic signs of right ventricular infarction (see Unit 9). If present, use nitrates and diuretics with extreme caution.

Posterior wall myocardial infarction

51 Let us now consider infarctions confined to the posterior wall of the left ventricle. Formerly the terms *inferior* and *posterior* were used synonymously. Although frequently injured simultaneously, these two areas have now been identified as two *separate surfaces* of the left ventricle.

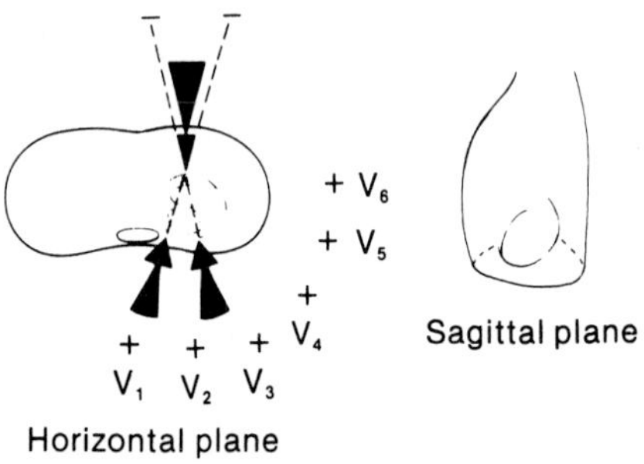

Fig. 6-20

The *inferior surface* of the left ventricle is that resting against the diaphragm. The "true" *posterior surface* of the left ventricle is that lying closer to the atria.

52 Infarctions limited to the true posterior wall of the left ventricle usually occur as a result of occlusion of the circumflex branch of the left coronary artery.
   Infarctions of the posterior wall frequently occur in *conjunction* with infarctions of the inferior wall. However, inferoposterin infarctions occur as a result of right coronary artery occlusions.

53 REMEMBER: Leads V_1 and V_2 are used in the diagnosis of _____ wall MI. In the presence of posterior wall MI there is an increase in the amplitude of the R waves in leads V_1 and V_2.

posterior

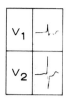

Fig. 6-21

Pericarditis

54 A more diffuse form of myocardial injury is that occurring with pericarditis.

REMEMBER: The pericardium is a two-layered membrane _____ that surrounds the myocardium on the *(inside/ outside)* of the heart.

Inflammation of the pericadrium is known as *pericarditis*.

sac; outside

55 The pericardium surrounds the entire heart. Inflammation of the pericardium therefore produces a *(localized/diffuse)* injury. Inflammation produces pain. Inflammation of the pericardium produces chest pain. Therefore the clinical picture of pericarditis *(may/may not)* confuse the differential diagnosis of acute MI.

Both pericarditis and MI produce _____ pain. Pericarditis differs from MI, however, because it represents a *(localized/ diffuse)* myocardial injury.

diffuse

may

chest
diffuse

56 Pericarditis may not be related to coronary artery disease. However, it may occur in the setting of MI because the myocardial injury extends to the epicardium and therefore the _____.

pericardium

57 Myocardial injury is reflected on the ECG by _____ _____ elevation.

ST
segment

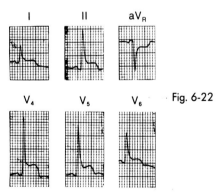

Fig. 6-22

Pericarditis produces *(localized/diffuse)* myocardial injury. The ECG changes produced will also be diffuse. In the presence of pericarditis, ST segment elevation is seen in *all* the epicardial leads. Re-

diffuse

ciprocal changes will be seen only in the endocardial lead, lead
_____.

aV_R

NOTE: When pericarditis is superimposed on MI, the former reciprocal ST segment depression associated with the infarction will either disappear or become elevated.

Subendocardial infarction (incomplete/nontransmural)

58 Completed myocardial infarctions usually extend transmurally across the entire wall of the heart from the _____ to the _____.

endocardium
epicardium

Myocardial infarctions may be initially limited, however, to the subendocardial layer and involve less than a third of the thickness of the heart wall.

REMEMBER: The subendocardial layer is especially vulnerable because of a *(richer/poorer)* blood supply. Blood flow to this layer is further compromised with the force of normal systole and in the presence of abnormally high filling (diastolic) pressures (see Unit 9).

poorer

59 Recent studies have suggested that some endocardial infarctions are more accurately characterized as "incomplete" because of the possibility for extension transmurally.

These seemingly minor infarcts are now viewed more cautiously in light of data describing a 1-year mortality as high as that associated with transmural MI. The high risk of extension suggests that the patient with subendocardial infarction should probably be observed closely for at least 2 weeks after the initial attack.

60 Infarctions confined to the subendocardial layer are classically associated with more subtle symptomatology and ECG changes.

The ECG changes associated with subendocardial injury may be localized or diffuse, depending on the extent of the injury.

REMEMBER: Injury is recorded on the ECG as _____ _____. However, the majority of the standard epicardial leads reflect only the *(endocardial/epicardial)* surface. Therefore the standard leads reflect and record the opposite or _____ change, that is, ST _____. Only the endocardial lead _____ records ST elevation.

ST
elevation
epicardial

reciprocal; depression
aV_R

NOTE: Leads V₁ and aV_L may also act at times as endocardial leads, depending on the cardiac position, and may thus also record ST elevation.

61 ECG evidence of diffuse endocardial infarction is shown in Figs. 6-23 and 6-24.

Diffuse subendocardial injury is detected by noting similar ST changes in normally reciprocal epicardial leads (for example, leads I

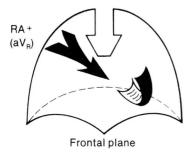

**SUBENDOCARDIAL
INFARCTION**

RA +
(aV$_R$)

Fig. 6-23

Frontal plane

**DIFFUSE SUBENDOCARDIAL
INJURY**

I

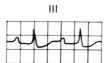

V$_1$

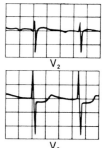

II

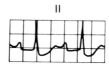

V$_2$

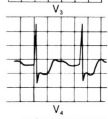

III

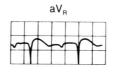

V$_3$

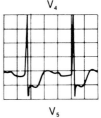

aV$_R$

Fig. 6-24

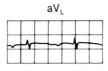

V$_4$

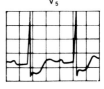

aV$_L$

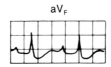

V$_5$

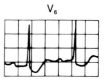

aV$_F$

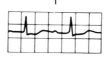

V$_6$

203

and II) and then confirming the change by checking the endocardial leads.

62 When these ECG changes are sustained, they are compatible with the severe decreases in blood supply accompanying acute _____. A history of typical chest pain and a serum enzyme elevation are often needed to confirm the diagnosis.   MI

    If these ECG changes are *transient*, they are compatible with the less severe decreases in blood supply accompanying _____ pectoris. Therefore, in this setting, these changes are often referred to as *ischemic* changes, although in electrical terminology they actually represent _____.   angina

    injury

63 Electrical ischemia, that is, T wave _____, may also accompany the ST changes (Fig. 6-25). However, necrosis is rarely seen.   inversion

ECG CHANGES IN SUBENDOCARDIAL MI

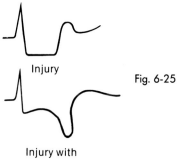

Injury

Fig. 6-25

Injury with ischemic changes

64 *Localized* subendocardial injury may also occur in patients with symptomatic coronary artery disease. This type of injury is suspected with the following ECG evidence: (1) ST depression on selected epicardial leads; (2) absence of reciprocal changes on the epicardial leads; and (3) ST elevation on leads aV_R, V_1, or aV_L. These local injury changes are far more difficult to recognize and interpret. They may mimic other acute or chronic disease changes, such as the patterns of left ventricular or right ventricular strain and acute posterior wall MI.

Cardiac catheterization: diagnostic versus therapeutic role

65 Cardiac catheterization is an invasive procedure that involves the introduction of a catheter into the right or left side of the heart and coronary artery system. It utilizes the concept of *angiography*. Angiography involves the visualization of blood flow through the chambers or blood vessels through use of a radiopaque dye or nuclear tracer (see Frames 99 to 125). Visualization of blood flow in cardiac catheterization is accomplished with a *radiopaque dye*.

Ventriculography is a form of angiography limited to visualization of the _____. *Coronary arteriography* is a form of angiography limited to visualization of the _____
_____.

ventricles

coronary
arteries

During cardiac catheterization both ventriculography and coronary arteriography are commonly performed. These studies are recorded on video film. Intracardiac pressures and chamber oxygen saturations are also assessed during the catheterization procedure.

66 Cardiac catheterization can be used to detect and evaluate disorders of cardiac *(electrical/mechanical)* activity and coronary artery structure. It is primarily a diagnostic procedure, which is also currently used therapeutically to a lesser extent because of its access to the coronary circulation. It is the best diagnostic tool for determining the pressure and severity of coronary artery disease (CAD) and serves as the standard against which all methods of assessing CAD are measured. Cardiac catheterization is also regarded as the standard for assessing the parameters of mechanical dysfunction.

mechanical

67 Generally cardiac catheterization is indicated when a precise diagnosis is critical to the selection of appropriate medical or surgical therapy. It is most commonly used to exclude the presence of surgically treatable disease and/or to define the cardiac anatomy preoperatively. Cardiac catheterization may also be used to assess the effectiveness of medical therapy, the progress of disease, and graft patency.

Cardiac catheterization should be performed only when similar noninvasive tests cannot provide sufficient diagnostic information to guide therapy. A limitation of cardiac catheterization as a diagnostic tool is its inability to determine functional impact of the coronary artery structural changes without the concurrent use of pacing or exercise.

68 Cardiac catheterization usually involves assessment of both right-sided and left-sided *(electrical/mechanical)* function. Right-sided heart access is accomplished via the brachiocephalic or femoral vein. A cutdown in the right antecubital area allows for catheter insertion in the _____ vein. Percutaneous catheter insertion via the *femoral vein* is currently a more common route of access to the right side of the heart.

mechanical

brachiocephalic

Passage of the catheter into the superior or inferior vena cava and right heart is facilitated by the use of fluoroscopy and physical maneuvers such as deep breathing, coughing, and position change. A flow-directed, balloon-tipped catheter is most commonly used (see Unit 9).

69 Right-sided heart catheterization allows for assessment of right-sided structures and pressures, as well as the presence of intracardiac shunts, pulmonary hypertension, and cardiac output.

Right-sided ventriculography is not done routinely. However, if pressure findings indicate the probability of a structural or functional abnormality, right _____ will be performed.

REMEMBER: Ventriculography involves the injection of a _____ dye to assess the *(electrical/mechanical)* function of the ventricle. A right ventricular pacer may be inserted prophylactically following the right-sided heart catheterization in patients at high risk for developing conduction abnormalities during the catheterization procedure.

ventriculography

radiopaque; mechanical

70 Left-sided heart catheterization is accomplished by *(antegrade/ retrograde)* insertion of the catheter through an *(artery/vein)* to the *aorta*.

The patient is heparinized systemically before catheter insertion to reduce the change of _____ formation on the catheter tip with subsequent embolization. With left-sided heart catheterization the catheter is inserted into either the brachial artery (Sones technique) or femoral artery (Judkins technique). The brachial artery insertion technique (Sones) involves a cutdown and arteriotomy to reach the vessel. Advantages of this technique include requirement of only one catheter, close proximity to the aortic root, and easier catheter manipulation. Disadvantages include the potential for median nerve damage and increased risk of thrombus formation caused by vessel size.

retrograde
artery

thrombus

71 The femoral artery catheter insertion is done percutaneously, with a guide wire in the right _____ _____. The catheter is advanced *(antegradely/retrogradely)* through the aorta, guided by fluoroscopic imaging. The percutaneous femoral artery technique has the advantage of being easier to learn and is associated with decreased risk of complications.

femoral
artery
retrogradely

72 Catheterization of the left ventricle allows for pressure measurement, oxygen sampling, and assessment of left-sided structural and functional abnormalities.

The left atrium is *not* routinely catheterized unless pressure abnormalities indicate severe *(mitral/tricuspid)* disease.

Left ventriculography with a _____ dye is commonly performed to allow for assessment of such mechanical parameters as regional wall motion abnormalities and ejection fraction (see Frame 118).

mitral

radiopaque

73 Selective right and left coronary arteriography (angiography) is ac-

206

complished by insertion of the catheter(s) into the coronary orifices and injection of a small amount of _____ dye.

REMEMBER: The coronary arteries originate behind the aortic valve cusps in the _____ of _____.

Nitroglycerin may be given sublingually before dye injection to maximize visualization and prevent vessel spasm caused by mechanical catheter irritation. Introcoronary nitroglycerin may also be indicated if severe spasm is induced during the procedure. Other coronary vasodilators, such as the Ca^{++}-blocking drug nifedipine (Procardia), may also be used precatheterization and postcatheterization to minimize vessel spasm.

In selected patients a provocative test that induces spasm may be employed to ascertain the role of spasm in *(rest/effort)* angina.

74 During coronary arteriography the patient is rotated from side to side so that visualization of the coronary arteries is maximized. The views, or projections imaged are similar to those used with radionuclide angiography. After each dye injection the patient may be asked to cough to clear residual dye from the coronary circulation.

Visualization of the coronary arteries allows for assessment of *(structural/functional)* evidence of coronary artery disease. Coronary arteriography can identify the site and severity of stenotic lesions and also general characteristics of the vessels in term of size, collateral flow, distal runoff, and mass of myocardium served. Cardiac drugs, exercise, and pacing may be used in conjunction with cardiac catheterization to attempt to assess the *(structural/functional)* impact of coronary artery disease.

75 On completion of the catheterization procedure, a special embolectomy catheter may be passed antegradely and retrogradely at the insertion site to prevent thrombus formation and subsequent embolization.

Complications occurring *during* the catherization procedure are primarily related to catheter manipulation and dye injection. Right-sided catheterization may cause a vasovagal reaction by irritation of nerve endings in the right-sided conduction structures. Arrhythmias may also occur as the catheter is manipulated thorugh the right cardiac chambers. The arrhythmias are most commonly (1) bradycardia caused by *(increased/decreased)* vagal tone and (2) ventricular arrhythmias caused by mechanical irritation of the _____ from catheter manipulation.

Rarely *(pulmonary/cerebral)* embolus may occur caused by thrombus formation on the catheter tip.

76 Left-sided heart catheterization may also produce arrhythmias due to mechanical irritation of the _____ from _____ manipulation.

radiopaque

sinuses; Valsalva

rest

structural

functional

increased
ventricles

pulmonary

ventricles
catheters

Systemic heparinization has reduced the risk of *(pulmonary/ cerebral)* embolization with left-sided heart catheterization. Vessel spasm may complicate *coronary arteriography* during a left-sided catheterization.

cerebral

REMEMBER: Medications such as _____ and _____ are used to prevent and treat coronary spasm. Rarely embolization *within* a *coronary artery* caused by thrombus or plaque disruption may also complicate this procedure and could result in _____ infarction. Sensitivity reactions to the iodine-based radiopaque dye may occur during _____ and coronary _____. These reactions may range from a mild urticaria to a severe anaphylactic reaction. With careful screening and premedication before catheterization, anaphylactic reactions are rare.

nitroglycerin
nifedipine

myocardial

ventriculography; arteriography

Patient discomfort or distress may also complicate the catheterization procedure. However, with appropriate precatheterization instruction, premedication, and reassurance during the procedure, this problem is usually averted or minimized.

77 Postcatheterization complications relate primarily to *access site trauma,* which can result in bleeding or ischemia in the involved limb.

Close observation for overt bleeding and hematoma formation or expansion at the insertion site is crucial in the first 2 to 4 hours after catheterization. Maintenance of prescribed pressure dressings and/ or sandbags and limb immobility is also important.

Circulation checks of the involved limb with documentation of pulses, color, temperature, and sensation will facilitate detection of any signs of thrombolic or embolic occlusion of a vessel.

Therapeutic roles

78 Cardiac catheterization is now also used therapeutically in the management of *structural* coronary artery disease.

REMEMBER: Structural coronary artery changes occurring in acute MI and angina are the same *(same/different)*. Coronary blood supply is diminished and/or interrupted because of the process of coronary narrowing or occlusion. This narrowing, or stenosis, results from three interrelated pathological processes: (1) lipid _____ (atherosclerosis), which results in thickening of the vessel wall and plaque formation; (2) thrombus formation initially due to _____ aggregation and later associated with _____ deposition; and (3) coronary spasm. Therapeutic application of cardiac catheterization is currently directed to ward these three mechanisms in an attempt to prevent mycardial infarction.

same

infiltration

platelet
fibrin

79 Two pharmacological agents, nitroglycerin and streptokinase, may be injected directly into the coronary circulation when the patient has signs and symptoms of acute infarction. The patient with suspected infarction is taken directly to the catheterization laboratory. Following coronary arteriography and documentation of vessel occlusion, nitroglycerin is usually the initial drug infused. Nitroglycerin, a *(vasodilator/vasoconstrictor),* relaxes the smooth muscle of the vessel wall and may re-establish flow by reversing spasm. Failure to re-establish flow after nitroglycerin infusion justifies the use of the more potent thrombolytic agent, streptokinase.

vasodilator

80 Intracoronary streptokinase may lyse an acute _____ resulting from fibrin deposition. An acute thrombus may be the final event, resulting in coronary artery _____. Maximal benefits from intracoronary nitroglycerin or streptokinase in acute MI is achieved when this mode of therapy is instituted the first 2 to 4 hours after the onset of acute symptoms. The use of intracoronary streptokinase is rapidly being replaced by the use of IV thombolytic agents. (see Unit 10).

thrombus

occlusion

81 Another procedure used both acutely and electively to alter structural changes contributing to coronary stenosis is known as percutaneous transluminal coronary angioplasty, or PTCA. This procedure requires direct access to the coronary circulation and is performed in the catheterization laboratory.

82 PTCA is directed towards the atheromatous plaque and involves the controlled compression and disruption of the plaque with a specially designed balloon catheter. Compression is accomplished by introducing the catheter into the coronary artery across the stenotic area and intermittently inflating the balloon. This controlled intimal disruption results in expansion of the _____ lumen and improved flow.

arterial

83 Before PTCA, coronary _____ is performed to define the anatomy and determine the suitability of the lesion for angioplasty. Measuring the drop in pressure across the lesion at this time verifies the extent of the arterial narrowing and allows for subsequent assessment of the results of the angioplasty. The drop in pressure across the lesion is known as the pressure gradient. Generally the larger the pressure change, or _____, the more severe the narrowing, or _____.

arteriography

gradient

stenosis

84 PTCA is considered as an alternative to coronary bypass surgery. Both single and multiple-vessel angioplasty have been successfully performed in many institutions. PTCA is also performed acutely in selected patients having signs and symptoms of acute MI. Intracoro-

BALLOON DILATATION CATHETER

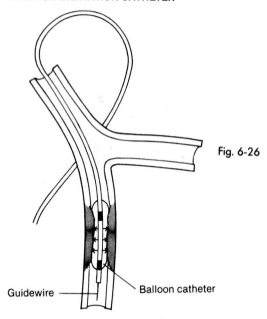

Fig. 6-26

Guidewire ——— Balloon catheter

nary streptokinase and/or nitroglycerin may be implemented before or in conjunction with PTCA. More commonly, angioplasty is performed electively following coronary arteriography when it is determined that the vessel and lesion characteristics are suitable for the procedure.

85 Accessibility of the lesion is of prime importance with PTCA so that the dilating catheter can reach the site. The guiding catheter is curved to facilitate vessel access. However, the more distal the lesion and the more tortuous and angulated the vessel, the *(more/less)* appropriate it is for angioplasty.

less

86 Older lesions are frequently fibrotic and calcified and thus noncompressible and therefore also _____ suitable for angioplasty. Size and configuration of the stenotic area are also considered. The ideal lesion for angioplasty is less than 2 cm in length, subtotal, and concentric in configuration. Patients with diffuse multivessel disease or irreversible wall motion abnormalities *(are/are not)* considered candidates for PTCA.

not

are not

87 PTCA is associated with the usual risks and complications of cardiac catheterization as well as having its own unique risks.

REMEMBER: Complications occurring *during* the catheterization procedure are primarily related to catheter manipulation and dye injection. Examples of these complications include vessel

_____, allergic reactions to the iodine-based _____, and arrhythmias. Rarely a *(pulmonary/cerebral)* embolus may occur, caused by thrombus formation on the catheter _____.

spasm

dye; cerebral

tip

88 Premedication with vasodilators such as _____ and _____ _____ reduce the risk of coronary artery _____. Severe spasm is so commonly associated with lesions in the main trunk of the left coronary artery that patients with single, critical lesions in this area are not considered candidates for PTCA and require bypass surgery.

nitroglycerin

Ca^{++} blockers

spasm

89 The use of anticoagulants such as _____ reduce the risk of thrombus formation with subsequent embolization. The use of prophylactic antiarrhythmic medications reduces the risk of life-threatening _____ arrhythmias.

heparin

ventricular

90 Complications after cardiac catheterization primarily relate to access site trauma, which can result in _____ or ischemia in the involved _____.

bleeding

limb

Close observation for overt bleeding and hematoma formation or expansion at the insertion site is crucial in the first _____ to _____ hours after angioplasty. Maintenance of prescribed _____ dressings and/or _____ for limb _____ is also important.

2

4

pressure; sandbags

immobility

Circulation checks of the involved limb with documentation of _____, color, _____, and sensation facilitate detection of thrombotic or embolic occlusion of a vessel.

pulses; temperature

91 NOTE: After PTCA the catheter introducer is commonly left in place a few hours to allow for resolution of the effects of anticoagulants used during the procedure. Thrombotic occlusion of the femoral artery is less common after PTCA than after cardiac catheterization because of the greater use of anticoagulants.

92 Complications unique to PTCA relate to the actual performance of the procedure.

Arterial dissection leading to coronary occlusion and myocardial infarction may occur during the angioplasty procedure. If this occurs, emergency coronary artery bypass surgery will be required. Release of thrombogenic factors with plaque compression and disruption may also precipitate myocardial infarction by promoting _____ formation.

thrombus

The administration of antiplatelet agents before, during, and after PTCA decrease the probability of _____ formation.

thrombus

The antiplatelet agent, low-molecular weight dextran (LMD) may be infused the first 4 hours after PTCA in some institutions to protect against _____ formation.

thrombus

Aspirin or other antiplatelet or antithrombin drugs may be used the first few months after PTCA to reduce the chance of thrombus formation or restenosis (see Unit 10).

93 Patient preparation for PTCA is complex. The patient must be advised of the risks involved and consent to coronary artery bypass surgery should complications occur. A surgical team is on call at the time of the procedure should they be needed. Preparation for pre-angioplasty and postangioplasty testing is also part of the teaching protocol. Coronary artery disease screening tests are commonly performed before and after angioplasty (see Echocardiography, Radionuclide Studies, and so forth, Frames 99 to 130).

94 After angioplasty the gradient across the involved lesion is reassessed to determine the effects of the procedure.

REMEMBER: A *(decrease/increase)* in the pressure gradient should occur with successful angioplasty, indicating *(increased/decreased)* flow across the stenotic area. Arteriograms of the involved vessels immediately after angioplasty are also performed. These initial films will show a fuzzy appearance at the site of the procedure because of the intimal disruption. Follow-up arteriograms several weeks later *(will/ will not)* show this fuzzy appearance, since the increased blood flow allows for healing of the endothelial injury.

decrease
increased

will not

95 Postangioplasty nursing care is similar to that following _____ _____.

cardiac catheterization

After PTCA *report any chest pain.* Prompt treatment and reporting of chest pain assumes critical importance. Chest pain in this setting may indicate vessel _____ or stenosis.

spasm

96 NURSING ORDERS: Before cardiac catheterization
1. Verify the patient's understanding of procedure and obtain his or her informed consent.
2. Remind the patient that food will be withheld before the catheterization.
3. Encourage hydration before catheterization to facilitate dye excretion after catheterization and to prevent inaccurate readings caused by hypovolemia (see Postcatheterization nursing orders).
4. Check with the patient regarding history of iodine allergies or any previous reactions to radiopaque dyes.
REMEMBER: Most radiopaque dyes are _____ based and may induce an allergic re-

iodine

action. Patients with known iodine sensitivity may be premedicated with antihistamine and/or steroids.

5. Remind the patient that he or she may feel a transient, hot, flushing sensation or nausea with the dye injection.
6. Document the circulation status of extremities, including pulses, temperature, color, and sensation, to serve as a baseline for postcatheterization assessment.
7. Check for recent vital signs and ECG documented in chart record.
8. Premedicate the patient, and remind the patient to void before catheterization.
9. Continue with usual medications unless otherwise specified.

97 NURSING ORDERS: After cardiac catheterization

1. Monitor pressure bags and/or dressings over access sites. Determine activity restrictions with the physician.
2. Check dressing/access site every 30 minutes for the first 2 to 4 hours for hematoma formation, expansion, or overt bleeding.
3. Assess circulation in limbs, especially those distal to the insertion site, every 30 minutes for the first 3 to 4 hours after catheterization. Check pulses, sensation, color, and temperature.

   REMEMBER: Any loss of sensation or decrease in pulse amplitude may indicate leg ischemia resulting from _____   thrombotic
   or _____ occlusion of the involved artery. Notify the   embolic
   physician immediately if any change in circulation is noted.
4. Watch for signs and symptoms of delayed reactions to radiopaque dye: urticaria, hives, or, rarely, decreased urine formation secondary to _____ failure.   renal
5. Encourage voiding as soon as possible after catheterization. Radiopaque dyes act as an osmotic diuretic, which will *(increase/decrease)* intravascular volume and, subsequently, urine   increase
   flow. Prompt excretion of the dye decreases the chance of a delayed sensitivity reaction and volume overload.
6. Discourage smoking after catheterization. Nicotine may aggravate coronary artery spasm, especially after vessel manipulation.

Radionuclide studies

98 Radionuclide studies are a noninvasive method for assessing cardiac function and involve the injection of a radioactive chemical into the circulation. These chemicals are absorbed by the blood cells or the heart muscle and are called *radionuclides*, or *isotopes*.

Radionuclide substances emit particles that sparkle and flash; these are known as *scintillations*. These scintillations can be detected by a special camera, and the picture or *image* visualized is known as a *scintigraphic* image. Since the camera recording the image moves across the body at different angles, this procedure is also referred to as a *scan*.

99 Radionuclide imaging can be used to study the mechanical function of the heart as well as assess the metabolic impact of coronary artery disease. There are three major types of nuclear studies in common use in coronary artery disease: thallium-201 imaging, technetium-99m-pyrophosphate imaging, and radionuclide angiography (also known as gated blood pool studies).

Thallium-201 and technetium-99m-pyrophosphate imaging are closely related, since they both involve the use of tissue cell traces, in contrast to the gated blood pool studies, which use blood cell tracers.

100 Radioactive cell tracers are absorbed by either normal or abnormal myocardial cells providing a contrast between them. Thallium-201 (thallous chloride) imaging provides contrast between normal and is-chemic or infarcted myocardium. Serial thallium-201 imaging can assist in further differentiating between ischemic and infarcted myo-cardium. Technetium-99m-pyrophosphate imaging provides only a contrast between normal and infarcted tissue.

Both ischemic and infarcted tissue are associated with metabolic changes.

REMEMBER: Radionuclides may be used to study the mechanical function of the heart as well as to assess the _____ impact of coronary artery disease. | **metabolic**

If the radioactive cell tracer is absorbed only by normal myocar-dium, the infarcted or ischemic tissue shows up as a blank area (re-ferred to as a "cold spot," or negative image). If the radioactive cell tracer is absorbed only by infarcted tissue, this tissue shows up as a "hot spot," or _____ image. | **positive**

Thallium-201 imaging

101 Thallium-201 (thallous chloride) is the radioactive chemical used with cold spot imaging. Thus thallium-201 serves as a cell tracer for *(healthy/infarcted)* tissue. With this type of imaging ischemic or in-farcted tissue will show up as a blank spot, or _____ image (see Fig. 6-28). | **healthy** **negative**

The absorption of radioactive indicators with cold spot imaging depends on myocardial blood flow and intracellular potassium (K^+) shifts. Thallium-201 is a radioactive analog of, or chemical similar to, potassium (K^+) and thus moves as K^+ does into and out of myocar-dial cells.

REMEMBER: In a healthy myocardium there is more K^+ _____ the cell than _____ the cell. The difference in K^+ concentration is maintained by the action of the _____ pump, which requires energy in the | **inside; outside** **Na^+-K^+**

214

form of _____. The diffusion out of the cell across this concentration gradient is limited by the permeability of the _____ _____. In the presence of ischemia, infarction, or both, inactivation of the Na^+-K^+ pump occurs with alteration in cell membrane permeability. Both of these factors contribute to *(gains/losses)* of intracellular K^+ in the affected areas only. Thus impairment of K^+ uptake occurs in areas of _____ and _____.

ATP

cell; membrane

losses

ischemia; infarction

102 Since thallium-201 is an analog or chemical similar to _____ it *(would/would not)* be also taken up in areas of ischemica or infarction. The infarcted or ischemic area would thus show up as a blank spot referred to as a _____ image (Fig. 6-18). Thallium-201 scans can be used early in the detection of myocardial ischemia or infarction. They are particularly useful in detecting small infarctions associated with only small incrases in serum enzymes. Thallium-201 scans are also helpful in detecting ischemia or infarction in patients with abnormal ventricular conduction patterns, such as LBBB, pacer rhythm, and preexcitation, which can mask the classic ECG signs of infarction.

potassium (K^+); would not

negative

THALLIUM-201 IMAGING

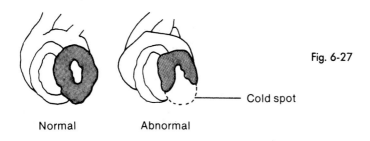

Fig. 6-27

Cold spot

Normal   Abnormal

103 An initial drawback of thallium-201 scans was the inability to distinguish between ischemic and infarcted tissue. This drawback is overcome by obtaining serial images with a usual *delay* between images of 2 to 4 hours.

This delay allows time for resolution of acute ischemia. Any defect remaining on the second image may be assumed to be a permanent metabolic change—most typically *(necrosis/ischemia)*. Any defect resolving or disappearing between the initial and delayed image may be assumed to be a temporary metabolic change or _____.

necrosis

ischemia

Occasionally the effects of a severe ischemic response may persist long enough that a defect is present even on a 3-hour to 4-hour delayed image. If the physician feels that this is a possibility, a repeat scan may be ordered in 24 hours to verify the findings.

104 Multiple projections or views are necessary to localize the ischemic and/or infarcted area. Common projections used are anterior, left anterior oblique (LAO), and left lateral (LL) (Fig. 6-29). The anterior view is best for localizing lateral wall abnormalities of the left ventricle. The LAO view is best for localizing anteroseptal or inferoapical changes. The left lateral projection is best for inferoposterior wall changes.

COMMON PROJECTION: RADIONUCLIDE STUDIES

 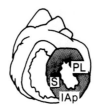 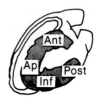

Fig. 6-28

| Anterior (best for lateral wall) | LAO (best for anteroseptal and inferoapical walls) | Left lateral (best for inferoposterior wall) |

NOTE: Inferior wall changes are the most difficult to verify because of uptake of thallium-201 by subdiaphragmatic organs.

105 Thallium-201 imaging also has wide application as the adjunct to exercise stress testing.

With dynamic exercise, myocardial oxygen demands are *(increased/decreased)*. Thus the functional or metabolic significance of any coronary artery narrowing will become apparent in this setting. Thallium defects apparent with exercise images that disappear on a delayed image 2 to 4 hours later represent an area of myocardium metabolically compromised because of *(ischemia/infarction)*.

increased

ischemia

106 Thallium-201 exercise stress testing is indicated to assess the functional significance of suspicious or borderline lesions, to verify equivocal or uncertain exercise test results, and to assess the patency of coronary artery bypass grafts. The use of thallium-201 imaging in conjunction with stress testing increases the accuracy of the stress test results.

With stress testing, thallium-201 is injected at the peak of exercise, and the exercise is continued for 1 minute to allow the chemical to circulate and be absorbed. Imaging is then done immediately to verify the presence or absence of an ischemic response.

A delayed image is then obtained 2 to 4 hours later to serve as a "rest," or baseline, image for comparison.

107 LET US REVIEW: Thallium-201 is an analog of _____ and serves as a tracer for *(normal/abnormal)* myocardium.

potassium (K$^+$)

normal

A thallium-201 defect on a single scan could represent either _____ or _____ tissue. The presence of a defect on both an initial and a delayed scan would indicate myocardial _____.

ischemic; infarcted

infarction (necrosis)

A defect on an initial *exercise* scan that resolves or disappears on a delayed scan probably indicates myocardial _____ occurring secondary to increased myocardial oxygen demands. This defect would thus confirm that the coronary narrowing was _____ significant.

ischemia

functionally

Technetium-99m-pyrophosphate imaging

108 Technetium-99m-pyrophosphate may also be used to assess the _____ consequences of coronary artery disease.

metabolic

REMEMBER: Unlike thallium-201, technetium-99m-pyrophosphate is taken up by *(healthy/infarcted)* tissue. Technetium-99m-pyrophosphate imaging can thus provide a contrast between normal and _____ tissue.

infarcted

infarcted

Technetium-99m-pyrophosphate utilizes the principle of hot spot, or _____, imaging.

positive

Major uses of technetium-99m-pyrophosphate imaging are to detect infarction when ECG and enzyme data are unclear or when a new MI is suspected in an area of old infarction.

109 The major mechanism by which technetium-99m-pyrophosphate is taken up by infarcted tissue is by binding with calcium. Absorption of this chemical is thus dependent on deposition of significant calcium wastes within the mitochondria of *(infarcted/ischemic)* tissue. This process occurs about 8 to 12 hours after MI and is associated with irreversible myocardial cell death, or _____. The maximal sensitivity for technetium-99m-pyrophosphate imaging is 24 to 72 hours after myocardial infarction, since the calcium in necrotic tissue is eventually reabsorbed.

infarcted

necrosis

NOTE: Calcium fluxes into myocardial cells have also been documented with reperfusion to an area following an ischemic episode. Thus reperfusion calcium ion shifts could potentially produce a false positive technetium-99m-pyrophosphate scan if the scan is performed too early.

110 Technetium-99m-pyrophosphate also binds readily with calcium complexes in the bone matrix of the overlying ribs and sternum (see Fig. 6-30). This may make interpretation of test results difficult, especially in IWMI, if the infarcted surface is aligned with an overlying rib.

The usefulness of the technetium-99m-pyrophosphate scan remains in doubt because the diagnosis of MI via ECG and enzyme values is in most cases complete by the time a pyrophosphate scan is

TECHNETIUM-99M-PYROPHOSPHATE IMAGING

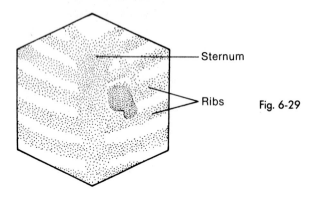

Fig. 6-29

NOTE: Pyrophosphate is absorbed by
bony structures, sternum and ribs,
and infarcted tissues.

indicated. Technetium-99m-pyrophosphate uptake after scar formation is poor, so that images taken even 2 weeks after MI may not
show signs of infarction.

REMEMBER: The calcium in necrotic tissue is eventually
_____.

        reabsorbed

Technetium-99m-pyrophosphate imaging is probably most useful in assessing intraoperative myocardial damage after bypass surgery. In this setting differentiation of chest wall pain versus coronary chest pain is particularly difficult because serum enzymes may
be elevated as a result of surgery alone. It may also be helpful in patients who delay reporting atypical chest pain. Technetium-99m-py-
rophosphate imaging will probably not have widespread application
in guiding therapy in coronary artery disease.

111 LET US REVIEW: Technetium-99m-pyrophosphate is a cell tracer taken
up by *(ischemic/infarcted)* tissue.

        infarcted

The mechanism of uptake is binding with _____
deposits in irreversibly injured tissue.

        calcium

Technetium-99m-pyrophosphate is also readily taken up by
_____ structures, rendering test interpretation difficult.

        bony

Technetium-99m-pyrophosphate imaging is probably most useful in detecting myocardial damage after _____
surgery.

        bypass

Uptake of the cell trace technetium-99m-pyrophosphate is probably most optimal _____ to _____ hours after MI.

        24; 72

Radionuclide angiography, or gated blood pool scans

112 Radionuclide angiography, or gated blood pool scans, provide a

non-invasive means of assessing cardiac _____ mechanical
function.

REMEMBER: The term *radionuclide* is used to refer to a mildly
_____ chemical. Angiography is a picture or image   radioactive
of the blood flow through a vessel or the heart.

113 With radionuclide angiography an image, or _____,   picture
of the blood flow through the heart is obtained by labeling the
_____ cells with the radioactive chemical techne-   blood
tium pyrophosphate. This labeling may be accomplished outside the
body (in vitro) by removing some of the patient's blood and then rein-
jecting it for the test. Labeling of the blood pool is more commonly
done within the body (in vivo) by first injecting stannous pyrophosphate and then, 30 minutes later, injecting technetium-99m-pertech-
netate to complete the labeling. The properties of this radionuclide
are such that it remains evenly mixed for several hours after
injection.

114 As the labeled blood cells, or blood _____, circu-   pool
lates, radioactive particles are emitted from the blood cells.

REMEMBER: These particles, which sparkle and flash, are known as
_____. They can be detected by a special camera   scintillations
and the picture, or _____, visualized is known as a   image
_____ image.   scintigraphic

Radionuclide angiography is accomplished by placing the patient
in a supine position beneath the camera and obtaining multiple serial images as the radioactive blood pool circulates through the
heart. These images are synchronized with the phases of the cardiac
cycle (systole and diastole) via the electrocardiogram.

The ECG serves as the physiological trigger, or "gate," which
marks the time relationship of the scintillation data with the cardiac
cycle (see Fig. 6-30). For this reason this test is also referred to as a
_____ blood pool scan.   gated

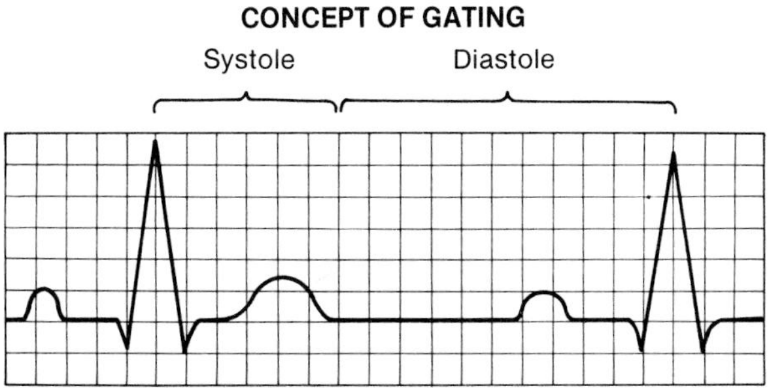

CONCEPT OF GATING

Systole   Diastole

Fig. 6-30

115 Each cardiac cycle is actually divided into many segments so that each phase of systole and diastole can be analyzed by the computer. The accumulated data from multiple images are computer analyzed and displayed as an endless-loop movie so the beating heart can be visualized.

Radioactivity in the cardiac chambers with systole and diastole reflects ventricular volume. Measurement of systolic and diastolic dimension becomes possible when images of radioactivity are recorded.

Parameters most commonly analyzed with gated blood pool scans are right and left ventricular wall motion and ejection fraction. Gated blood pool studies may also be used for measurement of ventricular size, ventricular volumes, septal thickness, septal motion, and valve regurgitation.

116 Detection of wall motion abnormalities allows identification of possible ischemic or infarcted areas but does not allow for differentiation between the two unless exercise scans are used as comparison (see Frame 216).

REMEMBER: Serial thallium-201 imaging allows for differentiation between ischemic and _____ tissue.　　　　　　　　*infarcted*

Aneurysms may also be detected by wall motion analysis. Regional wall motion is commonly scored on a point scale, so that relative differences in motion or kinetics can be quantified. Kinetic terms commonly used to describe wall motion are the following: "hypokinetic" (decreased motion), "hyperkinetic" (increased motion), "akinetic" (without motion), and "dyskinetic" (asymchronous motion).

117 *Ejection fraction* is the percentage of diastolic volume ejected with each systolic event; it serves as another parameter to evaluate mechanical performance.

Comparison of systolic and diastolic images may be used to estimate ejection fraction abnormalities. Ejection fraction may be more accurately calculated by measuring radioactivity emitted by the blood pool with systole and diastole.

REMEMBER: Radioactivity in the cardiac chambers with systole and diastole reflects ventricular _____.　　　　　　　　*volume*

Good correlations have been reported between the left ventricular ejection fraction determined by radionuclide techniques and by contrast left ventriculography (cardiac catheterization).

Projections commonly used in radionuclide imaging are 45-degree right anterior oblique (RAO), anterior, and 45-degree left anterior oblique (LAO) (see Frame 105).

118 The patient may be exercised during the gated blood pool scan to assess mechanical function with exercise.

REMEMBER: Adding exercise can help to differentiate between _____ and _____ and to evaluate _____ significance.

ischemia; infarction
functional

The bicycle ergometer is used for this procedure. The patient is placed at a 45-degree angle for comfort, and parameters normally monitored during stress testing, such as heart rate, BP, and ECG changes, as well as other signs and symptoms, are assessed. A physician, nurse, and emergency equipment should be on hand during this procedure.

Gated blood pool images obtained at rest and exercise can be displayed side by side as endless-loop movies.

119 Comparison of wall motion and ejection fractions with exercise and rest allows for further evaluation of the functional consequences of cardiac disease. For example, the normal response to dynamic exercise is to raise the ejection fraction. Failure to increase the _____ _____ with exercise is a sign of severe (*electrical/mechanical*) dysfunction.

ejection fraction
mechanical

A new regional wall motion abnormality induced with exercise has been shown to be a very specific indicator of the presence of coronary artery disease.

120 Exercise radionuclide angiography has been shown to be more sensitive for the detection of coronary artery disease than exercise electrocardiographic studies are. This is probably because electrical changes occur at a higher ischemic threshold than do contractile changes.

Successful gated blood pool studies depend on a constant heart rate or the computer's ability to select only those in a given range. The ability of the computer to subtract background data may also affect test results.

121 LET US REVIEW: Radionuclide angiography, or _____ blood pool scans, are used primarily to assess the _____ function of the heart.

gated

mechanical

With radionuclide angiography the _____ cells are labeled with _____ _____.

blood
technetium-99m-
pyrophosphate

Images are recorded as the labeled blood pool circulates. The images synchronized with the _____, so that the phases of _____ and _____ can be analyzed.

ECG
systole; diastole

Continuous-loop movies of the beating heart projected visually by the computer allow for analysis of regional _____ _____ abnormalities.

wall motion

Wall motion abnormalities detected on exercise scans but not present on rest scans may indicate myocardial _____.

ischemia

Ejection fraction calculated by radionuclide angiography is based on the radioactivity recorded with _____ and _____.

systole

diastole

First-pass radionuclide angiography

122 First-pass radionuclide scans are similar to gated blood pool scans in that a radionuclide is injected intravenously and traced as it passes through the heart and great vessels. However, unlike gated studies, which record multiple images, first-pass scans show only the initial pass of the isotope through the cardiac chambers. If another image is required, the isotope must be reinjected. The test may be performed separately or as the first step of a combination of first-pass and gated pool studies. However, combined studies are not commonly done, since gated pool studies alone are adequate tests of left ventricular function.

Parameters of both right and left mechanical function, such as ejection _____ and wall _____, can also be evaluated with a first-pass scan. The time it takes the radionuclide to move, or transit, from the right side of the heart through the _____ to the left side also allows for evaluation of many cardiac structural and functional abnormalities.

fraction; motion

lungs

A delay in tracer movement, or _____ time, may be the result of factors such as changes in cardiac output, chamber size, and pulmonary blood volume.

transit

The best use of first-pass studies is for the assessment of (RV/LV) function. A right anterior oblique projection allows clear separation of right-sided and left-sided structures.

RV

First-pass studies can be done at rest and with exercise. Exercise scans are done with the patient in the upright positin using a bicycle ergometer. Comparison of rest and exercise images allows for assessment of the functional impact of heart disease and increases the validity of the findings.

123 LET US REVIEW: First-pass radionuclide scans image the _____ pass of the isotope through the heart and great vessels.

initial

Evaluation of tracer _____ time allows for the calculation of _____ output as well as assessment of structural and _____ abnormalities.

transit

cardiac

functional

Best use of first-pass studies is for the assessment of _____ ventricular function.

right

124 NURSING ORDERS: Radionuclide imaging
Thallium-201 imaging
  1. Record factors affecting K^+ shifts that may distort test results.
    —administration of energy subtrates; e.g. glucose and insulin

—administration of drugs that is, diuretics, dopamine, epinephrine, and laxative preparations

—pH shifts

2. Do not schedule barium enemas or glucose tolerance tests with thallium-201 imaging.
3. Explain the purpose of serial images.

   NOTE: Patients are usually allowed only nondairy liquids between the initial image and the 3-hour to 4-hour delayed images, to prevent energy subtrates from altering the test results. If the initial image is negative, the repeat scan will usually be cancelled. If the initial and 3-hour to 4-hour delayed scans are both positive, some physicians may order a repeat scan 24 hours later to validate those findings.

4. Prepare patient for thallium-201 injection at peak exercise with stress testing and rapid transfer for imaging.
5. Do not schedule other nuclear tests with thallium-201 imaging.
6. If the thallium-201 image is positive, care for the patient as an acute cardiac patient.

Technetium-99m-pyrophosphate imaging

1. Do not obtain a scan until 90 to 120 minutes after the IV injection.

   REMEMBER: Technetium-99m-pyrophosphate scans are most sensitive _____ to _____ hours after MI.   24; 72

2. If the technetium-99m-pyrophosphate image is positive, care for the patient as an acute MI patient.

Radionuclide angiography

1. Do not schedule with other nuclear tests.
2. Explain blood cell labeling procedure to patient.
3. If an exercise scan is done, remember that a physician, a nurse, and emergency equipment should be on hand.

Other diagnostic tests

125 Echocardiography is another major noninvasive test that can be used to evaluate various forms of mechanical dysfunction or complications associated with coronary artery disease. Examples of two other noninvasive tests reflecting mechanical dysfunction are phonocardiography and the chest x-ray film.

Electrical dysfunction may be evaluated by invasive electrophysiological studies, including His bundle studies, or by noninvasive methods, such as serial 12-lead ECGs, vectorcardiography, Holter monitoring, or stress testing.

126 Echocardiography involves beaming painless, high-frequency (ultrasonic) sound waves into the chest and recording reflected vibrations, or *echoes*. These sound waves are transmitted, received, and translated into electrical signals on an oscilloscope by a pencil-like device referred to as a *transducer*.

NOTE: A transducer is an instrument capable of changing, or _____, one form of energy into another form of energy.   translating

The vibrations are reflected by the chest wall and solid structures of the heart. Thus this procedure allows for the examination of the size, shape, and motion of the cardiac structures to detect *(electrical/ mechanical)* dysfunction. A simultaneous ECG trace is recorded for reference only. The major structures visualized are the four cardiac valves, RV and LV walls and chambers, and pericardial sac. Major abnormalities detected include valvular stenosis or insufficiency, septal defects, hypertrophy, aneurysms, mural thrombi, asynchronous or ineffective left ventricular contraction, and pericardial effusion.   mechanical

127 Coronary artery disease is detected primarily by the presence of regional wall motion abnormalities or *(synchronous/asynchronous)* LV contraction.   asynchronous

REMEMBER: Abnormalities in LV wall movements occur during _____ or following _____ _____. These movements may be _____ kinetic (decreased) or _____ kinetic (paradoxical).   angina; acute MI
                                                                        hypo
                                                                        dys

Hemodynamically significant coronary artery disease may also be confirmed and quantified from evidence of decreased or ineffective LV _____. The effectiveness of LV contraction is determined from measurements of ejection fraction.   contraction

REMEMBER: Ejection fraction is the percentage of the diastolic volume that is ejected during _____. Ejection fraction can be estimated from changes in the LV chamber _____ during diastole and systole. Echocardiographic determinations are comparable to those obtained during radionuclide studies (see Frame 118). Accuracy can be further increased by combining this procedure with exercise. Actual visualization of the coronary artery system has been accomplished but is not very accurate at this time.   systole

                                                                        diameter

128 The diagnosis of complications following acute MI may also be facilitated by echocardiography. Sudden systolic murmurs caused by ventricular septal rupture versus papillary muscle rupture may be differentiated. The pericardial effusion associated with cardiac tamponade is easily detected and may allow it to be differentiated from right ventricular infarction, especially in the context of the similar hemodynamic patterns (see Unit 9).

Confirmation of the presence or absence of a mural thrombus can facilitate the decision whether to anticoagulate after MI.

129 Echocardiography may be performed with either a narrow-angle or a wide-angle beam. The older narrow-beam method is known as M-mode, or motion mode. In the newer, wide-angle method the sound beams sweep like an arc over a broader cross section of the heart, allowing more of a two-dimensional view. This method, although also a motion ode, is referred to by comparison, as two-dimensional (2-D) echocardiography. Two-dimensional echocardiography allows for a life-like view of the cardiac structures, making it easier to detect most of the major abnormalities. The major advantage of M-mode is its ability to detect rapidly occurring changes better, since the pictures are more simply and rapidly obtained. Pericardial effusion may also be more easily seen on an M-mode view.

There are no special patient preparations required for echocardiography. Patients should be told that it is painless. No sedation is necessary, and no drugs should be withheld. Patients may eat and drink normally before the test.

130 Electrocardiographic monitoring and/or invasive testing provide information related to either rhythm disturbances (arrhythmias) or changes in the ECG pattern (QRS-ST-T wave complex). This information can facilitate the detection, evaluation, and follow-up therapy of these disorders. Invasive ECG testing is most extensively indicated in patients with *(rhythm disturbances/ECG pattern changes)*. These include patients with (1) unexplained palpitations or syncope; (2) exercise-related palpitations; (3) documented life-threatening arrhythmias (VT or SVT); (4) implanted pacemakers; or (5) complex ventricular arrhythmias in the setting of chronic coronary artery disease.

rhythm disturbances

Although chronic ventricular and supraventricular arrhythmias are common in the general population, both at rest and during exercise, certain patterns are more suggestive of coronary artery disease, especially in patients in high-risk categories (see Frames 161 to 175). Arrhythmias occurring in the setting of coronary artery disease—especially ventricular—are generally more serious and should be more carefully monitored and treated. Arrhythmias have also been implicated in reports of sudden death in patients with noncoronary cardiac syndromes, such as mitral prolapse, idiopathic hypertrophic subaortic stenosis (IHSS), and Wolff-Parkinson-White (WPW) syndrome.

131 Rhythm disturbances are best detected and monitored initially by noninvasive means such as telemetry, Holter monitoring, or stress testing. Transtelephonic ECG transmission is also useful and is very popular in patients with implanted pacemakers. Long-term ECG recording, or _____ monitoring, is the most sensitive

Holter

method of detecting the frequency and character of arrhythmias whether at rest or correlated with various forms of activity or symptoms. Invasive electrophysiological testing should be reserved for the follow-up evaluation of more complex, hard-to-control arrhythmias.

NURSING DIAGNOSIS AND PLANNING

132 Nursing assessment, often referred to as *nursing diagnosis*, focuses on identifying problems that reflect the *effects* of the pathological damage on the patient, family, and their life-style rather than on the identification or correction of the pathological process itself. The nursing focus is thus functional rather than _____.   pathological
These concepts are supported by the general ANA definition of nursing diagnosis. However, the nurses have an obligation to support the medical diagnostic process while still establishing their own focuses. The medical diagnosis or the medical diagnostic tools may also be used by nurses to guide their assessment processes. The medical and nursing diagnostic processes should ideally complement each other, becoming interdependent rather than isolated, independent processes.

NOTE: More specifically the term "nursing diagnosis" is used to refer to either the functional classification of problem statements or a cluster of signs and symptoms rather than to a single preliminary sign or symptom. In its strictest sense, it can refer to the exclusive use of only NANDA (North American Nursing Diagnosis Association)-approved diagnostic labels.

To minimize confusion and multiple interpretations, the authors prefer to avoid the term "nursing diagnosis" and focus on the statement and considerations of patient problems compatible with the more generally defined ANA focus, which can in turn interface with medical diagnostic process and therapy. The NANDA-approved diagnostic labels are used only as a resource.

133 The patient diagnosed as having an acute MI, unstable angina, or suspected MI usually has a pathological process involving his or her _____ system.   coronary
The coronary arteries supply both the _____ and   electrical
_____ structures of the heart. They provide an adequate blood and O_2 supply to meet cellular _____   mechanical
needs. The effects of acute coronary artery disease on the patient include the following: metabolic

1. *Chest pain* due to toxins released in the presence of abnormal
_____   metabolism
2. *Arrhythmias* due to alterations in the _____   electrical
structures

226

3. *Congestive heart failure* or *cardiogenic shock* due to alterations in the _____ structures. These forms of cardiovascular system failure are jointly manifested in the patient as pulmonary congestion or the cluster: "impaired oxygenation."   mechanical

4. *Stress* due to the physical insult and psychosocial impact (see Table 7).

Nursing assessment and planning should take into consideration at least these potential patient problems. Other less specific potential problems include electrolyte, acid-base, and volume imbalances, as well as the toxic effects of drug therapy.

134 The plan of care can be made more specific when the medical diagnosis of IWMI, as opposed to AWMI, is made.

REMEMBER: In an IWMI, *(right/left)* coronary artery is usually   right
involved. The specific conduction structures affected are the
_____ and _____ nodes; this predisposes the pa-   SA; AV
tient to *(bradyarrhythmias/tachyarrhythmias)* and an increased sensitivity   bradyarrhythmias
to vagal simulation such as rectal temperatures, straining, and morphine therapy.

In an AWMI the *(right/left)* coronary artery is usually in-   left
volved. The specific conduction structures affected are the
_____ _____; this predisposes the   bundle branches
patient to _____ _____ blocks   bundle branch
and more serious forms of _____ blocks.   AV

135 Individual psychological reactions or psychosocial problems may be assessed by the use of a framework such as Maslow's. The psychological problems may be identified by their general behavioral manifestation, for example, denial, fear, restlessness, anger, or depression, or by the hypothesized mechanisms, such as threat to safety, loss of self-esteen, or lack of knowledge about self-care measures. Examples of threats to safety include unfamiliar surroundings, sensations, language, or procedures, as well as disturbances of sleep and activity patterns. Examples of threats to love or inclusion needs are separation from family and friends and lack of attention. Examples of threats to self-esteem are inactivity, inability to care for oneself or make decisions for oneself, loss of strength, and failure to accomplish tasks (without recurring symptoms). Self-actualization needs (knowledge, understanding, and goal-setting) usually emerge after the acute stage, when denial begins to subside. These needs are thus more commonly seen in progressive or intermediate care units.

A sample care plan is provided in Table 7. Specific patient outcomes are indicated. Nursing assessment parameters are included in the nursing actions.

Text continued on p. 233.

Table 7 Care plan: the patient with an acute MI

Patient problems	Expected outcomes	Nursing action
1. Chest pain related to: —Metabolic changes in ischemic areas (usually within first 24°) —Angina associated with other diseased vessels —Extension of infarction or new infarction (usually if after first 24°) —Postresuscitation trauma —Pulmonary emboli	1. Reports onset of new chest pain to nursing staff 2. Reports symptoms suggestive of coronary ischemia that may not be readily identified as pain: —Burning —Pressure —Numbness in upper extremities —Other:_____ 3. Expresses relief of pain following medication 4. Expresses at least partial relief of pain following positioning and/or medication 5. BP and/or heart rate will return to baseline following the relief of pain (Circle appropriate outcome or outcomes)	1. Immediately obtain tracing from monitoring leads reflecting multiple surfaces—at least lead I (lateral), lead II (inferior), lead V_1 or MCL_1 and MCL_2 (anterior) *Report and document:* —Displacement of the ST segment —T wave peaking or inversion —Changes in QRS morphology (width and polarity) —Arrhythmias associated with the pain *or* occurring immediately before it *Later, compare* any suspected change with former tracing and verify by obtaining a standard 12-lead ECG record 2. Obtain vital signs and document any alterations in: —BP (↑ or ↓) —Pulse rate (↑ or ↓) —Respiratory rate ( ) —PAEDP (wedge pressure) If BP is elevated, wait until pain is relieved and take BP again Auscultate for presence of S_4 gallop 3. Evaluate chest pain quickly according to: —Location —Quality —Duration —Precipitating factor, such as activity, meals, visitors, expressed anxiety, change in routines, or multiple procedures —Effects of respirations, change of position, movement of extremities, or local pressure Note accompanying symptoms: shortness of breath, dizziness, nausea or vomiting, or cold clammy skin

Table 7 Care plan: the patient with an acute MI—cont'd

Patient problems	Expected outcomes	Nursing action
		4. Medicate *promptly* with: —Nitroglycerin gr. _____ —Morphine sulfate _____ may repeat × 1 _____ —Other _____ (Circle as per physician order) Document mode of relief with dosage Document *other* modes of relief, i.e., sitting up, antacids, rest 5. Consider the effects of drugs that may ↑ demand for O_2 (digitalis) 6. Provide for O_2 administration 7. Instruct patient to report any new pain 8. Instruct patient to report signs and symptoms that may indicate coronary ischemia and not be recognized as pain 9. Look for nonverbal communication of pain 10. Explain the intended effects of pain medication 11. Reassure the patient that pain will subside 12. Ask the patient what makes him or her the most comfortable 13. Monitor serum enzymes and isoenzymes
2. Arrhythmias—potential aggravation related to: —Ischemic ventricular areas —Hypoxemia and hypoxia —K+ or Mg+ —Acidosis or alkalosis —Stress —Heart failure —Drug toxicity —Pericarditis —Conduction defects associated with specific location of the MI —Increased serum FFA levels	1. Absence of VF 2. Immediate correction of VF 3. VR <100 4. Absence of sustained symptomatic bradycardia 5. Demonstrates hemodynamic stability during arrhythmias as evidenced by absence of: —Diaphoresis —Respiratory depression —Altered mental status —Cool skin temperature —Hypotension (Circle one or more outcomes)	1. ECG observation and documentation —Monitor rhythm continuously —Document rhythm interpretation with trace at least q 2-4h —Obtain direct ECG record of any arrhythmia and memory record for previous precipitating changes —Note changes in lead or size/gain in rhythm tracing 2. Arrhythmia prevention: —Monitor blood gases —Monitor serum electrolytes

Continued.

229

Table 7 Care plan: the patient with an acute MI—cont'd

Patient problems	Expected outcomes	Nursing action
		—Maintain supplementary O_2 —Watch for signs of CHF (see problem 3) —Reduce psychological stressors (see problem 4) —Keep environments calm —Monitor FFA levels —Substitute caffeine-free coffee 3. Keep atropine and Xylocaine at the bedside 4. When an arrhythmia occurs, document and report any of the following symptoms: —Dizziness or altered levels of consciousness —Cold clammy skin —Rales, S_3 gallop —Changes in rate or character of respirations 5. Maintain patient IV 6. Make sure cardioverter or defibrillator is in working order 7. Have equipment for emergency pacemaker insertion available 8. In the presence of VF open airway, confirm the absence of pulse, then defibrillate (for indicated intervention with specific arrhythmias see Units 7 and 10)
3. Pulmonary congestion; impaired oxygenation related to: —heart failure —cardiogenic shock	1. Respiratory rate <_____ 2. Absence of use of accessory muscles on inspiration or expiration 3. Lungs clear 4. Heart rate <100 5. Absence of S_3 gallop 6. Absence of PACs 7. Skin warm and dry 8. BP> _____ but < _____ 9. Urine output > _____ 10. Absence of serious hemodynamic imbalance as indicated by:	1. Elevate head of bed 2. Monitor vital signs at least q 2° first 24°, then q 4° or as ordered 3. Auscultate heart and lungs with each set of vital signs, and note abnormal respiratory pattern 4. Decrease O_2 demands: —Assisting with activities of daily living —Bedside commode —Scheduled rest periods —Refraining from performing nonessential procedures —Maintaining comfortable room temperature

Table 7 Care plan: the patient with an acute MI—cont'd

Patient problems	Expected outcomes	Nursing action
	—Wedge pressure <18 mm Hg —Cardiac index >2.2 L/M^3 —SVR _____ —A-Vo$_2$ difference <5-6 ml O$_2$ 11. Related lab findings within normal limits: —Hematocrit —Urine electrolytes —Serum Na+ (Circle appropriate outcome or outcomes)	—Anticipating needs —Reduce psychological stressors (see problem 5) 5. Maintain accurate I and O 6. Monitor for PACs or sinus tachycardia 7. Monitor hematocrit, urine electrolytes, and serum Na+ 8. Offer relaxation techniques —Back rub/massage —Breathing exercises —Biofeedback —Meditation, etc. 9. Administer diuretics, vasodilators, and inotropic agents as ordered 10. Have on hand for severe pulmonary congestion: —Rotating tourniquets —Phlebotomy (phoresis) bags —Nebulizer 11. If Swan-Ganz in place, monitor wedge, PA, RA, cardiac output, SVR, and A-Vo$_2$ differences 12. Instruct the patient on the effects of therapy
4. Predisposition to stress ulcer	1. Absence of nausea or vomiting 2. Absence of heartburn or abdominal pain 3. Stools and emesis hematest negative 4. Normal RBC, hemoglobin, and hematocrit values 5. Gastric pH >4.5	1. Provide milk with medications 2. Administer antacids as ordered 3. Administer anticholinergic drugs, histamines, and antagonists, as ordered 4. Hematest stools and emesis 5. Monitor blood studies: RBC, hemoglobin, and hematocrit 6. Check pH of gastric contents 7. Reduce psychological stressors (see problem 5) 8. Document and report patient complaints of burning or abdominal pain; note if triggered by any specific events
5. Depression related to: —Threats to self-esteem —Fear of death or bodily harm	1. Expresses positive feelings about self 2. Participates in self-care 3. Verbalizes feelings about	1. Assess psychological threats that may potentiate the depressive state: —Disturbing conversation topics,

Continued.

Table 7 Care plan: the patient with an acute MI—cont'd

Patient problems	Expected outcomes	Nursing action
—Unfamiliar surroundings, routine, or sensations —Separation from family or significant persons —Disturbances in sleep and rest patterns —Lack of physical comfort	death and loss 4. Relaxed facial expression when sleeping 5. Absence of startled responses to normal stimuli 6. Calm speech pattern 7. Calm breathing pattern 8. Absence or decreased use of distressing mannerisms (twitches, grimacing, frequent use of call light, tremors, _____) 9. Makes decision regarding activities 10. Initiates conversations with staff or family 11. Responds positively to staff and family 12. Makes plans for immediate future 13. Requests information about self, environment, and routine 14. Cooperates with plan of care 15. Expresses confidence in survival (Circle appropriate outcome or outcomes)	unfamiliar equipment or routines, visitors, family, or staff —Abnormal perceptions, delusions, misinformation about self and others, fixed ideas 2. Assess normal values that are important to the person (manhood, motherhood, physical strength) and personality: —Strengths and weaknesses —Former pleasurable interests —Verbally validate our perceptions of his or her feelings 3. Utilize supportive measures: —Support patient's coping mechanisms, such as limited denial —Stress patient's strengths —Utilize patient's support systems (family, friends, religion); allow flexible visiting hours for supportive visitors —Arrange a pleasant physical environment —Maintain usual rituals of daily living —Provide consistent nursing personnel —Initiate contact with cardiac rehabilitation system in hospital 4. Initiate relief measures: —Encourage expression of feelings —Respond immediately when called —Terminate emotionally threatening conversations —Inform patients of signs of progress (i.e., vital signs, rhythm stability, activity) —Provide diversional activities —Provide for physical comfort —Restrict unwanted visitors —Communicate optimistic future outlook (return to work, survival status, return to normal activity level, return to usual sexual activity) —Limit nonessential activities

136 Discharge planning begins during the acute phase with short explanations of procedures and identification of educational and activity levels as well as defense mechanisms. The patient is encouraged to verbalize, but defense mechanisms are not destroyed, to prevent too rapid a release of anxieties.

REMEMBER: In acute stress, the blood pressure *(increases/decreases)*, heart rate *(increases/decreases)*, and _____ may occur.

increases
increases; arrhythmias

Intermediate care goals include increasing the patient's self-care actvities; providing gradually increasing physical activity; and teaching the patient about the disease process, control of risk factors, diet, medications, and which symptoms to report.

Teaching the patient to become aware of his or her cardiac response to stress can allow the patient to limit this response through relaxation and biofeedback. Concerns over sexual activity, role changes, physical activity, and the threat of recurrent heart attacks should be anticipated and discussed with the patient and his or her family. Treadmill tests can be used to evaluate and determine an activity program (see Frames 176 to 223).

METABOLIC ASSESSMENT: EFFECTS OF CORONARY IS-CHEMIA

137 The word *metabolism* refers to the chemical processes involving *energy release* and *energy use* by the body. The major chemicals used by the heart as an energy source are *free fatty acids.* Under normal conditions, myocardial cells, unlike other cells in the body, use free fatty acids in preference to glucose, although glucose remains a secondary energy source. Fats are thus a key substance in myocardial metabolism. Proteins are a less significant energy source.

138 Fats (lipids) are carried within the plasma in two forms:
1. *Free fatty acids* bound to albumin
2. Large lipid-protein compound known as *lipoproteins*

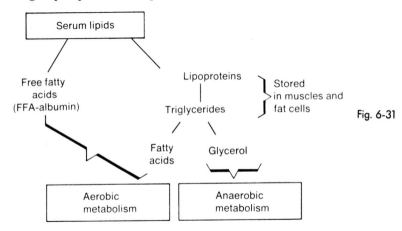

Fig. 6-31

The free fatty acids are readily available as an energy source via *aerobic* pathways (Fig. 6-31).

To act as an energy source fatty acids thus require the presence of *oxygen*. The lipoproteins are either transported to muscle and fat tissue for storage or may also be used as energy sources via both aerobic and anaerobic pathways. Lipoproteins contain smaller fatty acid–glycerol compounds known as triglycerides. Lipoproteins and triglycerides may be broken down into fatty acids and glycerol by enzymes known as lipoprotei liposes. The fatty acids enter the *(aerobic/ anaerobic)* metabolic pathways. The glycerol may enter the less effective anaerobic pathways for energy production.

aerobic

139   LET US REVIEW: The major energy source used by myocardial cells is *(glucose/fat/protein)*.

Fats are carried within the plasma in the form of _____ _____ _____ and _____. The most readily available fat energy sources are the _____ _____ _____.

fat
free
  fatty acids;
lipoprotein
free
  fatty acids

140   In the presence of myocardial ischemia and hypoxia, alterations in free fatty acids (FFA) metabolism occur.

REMEMBER: FFA enters *(aerobic/anaerobic)* metabolic pathways. During hypoxia, *(aerobic/anaerobic)* metabolism occurs. Thus in hypoxia the utilization of FFA is inhibited, causing serum levels to *(rise/fall)*.

aerobic
anaerobic
rise

During episodes of chest pain, levels of FFA have been shown to rise sharply. Increased serum FFA levels have been associated with increased myocardial O_2 consumption, decreased contractility, and increased ventricular arrhythmias. The release of epinephrine as part of the stress response further increases FFA levels by promoting their release from storage sites.

141   In the absence of FFA as an energy source, the heart must rely on its secondary energy source, _____.

glucose

Glucose is released from glycogen stores within the myocardium and liver. The released glucose enters the anaerobic energy pathways (glycolysis) in addition to the impaired aerobic pathways, thus providing temporary support to critically ischemic tissues.

Insulin plays a key role in FFA metabolism as well as in glucose metabolism. Insulin prevents the release of FFA from lipoprotein and triglyceride stores. Insulin also inhibits myocardial uptake of these fatty acids while facilitating the uptake and metabolism of glucose. Chest pain and stress appear to inhibit serum insulin release, thus *(increasing/decreasing)* FFA levels and impairing glucose transport and metabolism.

increasing

142   K^+ leakage from hypoxic myocardial cells adds to the arrhythmogenic effects of increased FFA levels and contributes to the ECG

changes associated with acute MI.

REMEMBER: K$^+$ is located predominantly *(inside/outside)* the cell and is reponsible for _____ and _____. K$^+$ is pumped into the cell by the action of the _____ pump in the presence of _____. The movement of K$^+$ out of the cell is limited by the permeability of the _____ _____.

inside
polarization; repolarization
Na$^+$-K$^+$
ATP
cell membrane

In the presence of hypoxia the permeability of the cell membrane increases. The action of the Na$^+$-K$^+$ pump is suppressed because of less available ATP.

143 In the first hour after acute MI, the following local metabolic changes occur:
1. Swelling of mitochondria with *severe* ATP depletion
2. Intracellular K$^+$ *loss* and increased extracellular K$^+$
3. *Increased* levels of *FFA*
4. *Reduced* myocardial *glycogen stores*
5. *Increased* lactic acid levels caused by anaerobic metabolism
6. *Decreased insulin* levels
7. *Increased* intracellular Na$^+$ and water

Continuous intravenous administration of GIK solution containing glucose, insulin, and potassium may limit or reverse many of these changes. The theorized benefits of GIK solution include the following: (1) supplemental glucose for anaerobic metabolism in critically ischemic areas, (2) lowering of plasma FFA levels, and (3) replacement of intracellular K$^+$.

REMEMBER: Insulin facilitates the _____ and _____ of glucose and *(raises/lowers)* FFA levels because of its effects on lipid _____ and _____. The movement of K$^+$ into the cells is *(facilitated/suppressed)* by glucose and insulin (see Unit 4). Replacement of K$^+$ into the cell restores the _____ gradient necessary for the maintenance of a stable _____ state (see Unit 4).

transport
metabolism; lowers
breakdown
storage; facilitated

concentration
polarized

GIK solution was first used by its originator, Sodi-Pallares, because of this effect. For this reason, it was first referred to as *polarizing solution.*

Reported clinical benefits of GIK solution include improved ventricular function with lowering of wedge pressures (see Unit 9), reduction of infarction size, rapid reversal of ECG changes, and fewer ventricular arrhythmias. Although the results of research in the early 1980's regarding these effects appeared promising, this solution is used rarely in the United States at this time. However, it is the belief of these authors that this could again change in the future. The two major reported side effects are hyperglycemia and hyperkalemia. These effects can be detected by frequent laboratory assessments and can be controlled by adjusting the rate of infusion, adding supplementary insulin, or, in rare cases, administering Kayex-alate.

144 Knowledge of the metabolic substrates used by the myocardium and coronary vessels as well as the metabolic changes following acute MI allows the nurse to more completely assess the needs of the patient and plan his or her care.

Metabolic assessment can include the following:
1. Effectively assisting with diagnostic procedures (nuclear imaging, enzymes, and serum lipids) and interepreting these procedures to the patient
2. Documentation of significant findings during chest pain, such as the hyperacute T wave changes occuring with _____ release

K^+

3. Recognition of potential arrhythmogenic effects in acidosis, increased _____ levels, and recent onset of ischemic chest pain

FFA

4. Patient teaching for control of lipid levels and related risk factors

Protein *(is/is not)* a key metabolic substance used by the myocardium. However, protein deficits are associated with stress and can contribute to the formation of pulmonary edema once heart failure occurs (see Units 4 and 7). Therefore assessment of protein deficits and nutritional replacement should also be a part of the nursing plan of care for patients with acute MI—particularly those with signs of pulmonary edema.

STRESS AND STRESS RESPONSE: ASSESSMENT AND PATIENT TEACHING/DISCHARGE PLANNING IMPLICATIONS

145 Many of the presenting symptoms associated with acute MI represent a manifestation of the stress response. Prolonged excessive stress is also a long-term risk factor for coronary artery disease. The concept of stress is based on the theory of a *patterned* physiological response to factors that upset either physiological or psychological balance. This response may be triggered by a variety of factors (stimuli). The response is *nonspecific,* that is, not characteristically associated with a certain type of stimulus. Factors potentially triggering a stress respnse are referred to as *stressors.*

Minimal, short-term stress can provide healthy challenges that make life more interesting and satisfying. However, severe or long-term stress can trigger potentially harmful stress responses, or *distress.* Unfortunately, the latter is more commonly recognized. Harmful stress responses are typically triggered when normal compensatory mechanisms have been exceeded or exhausted.

146 Patterned, nonspecific responses may be either *local* (inflammation) or *systemic.* The local response, often referred to as the *local adapta-*

tion syndrome (LAS), is discussed in Unit 4. The systemic response was first described by Selye, who referred to it as the *general adaptation syndrome* (GAS). This response occurs in three stages: (1) the alarm *reaction,* (2) the stage of *resistance,* and (3) the stage of *exhaustion.* The alarm reaction signals the cerebral cortex and hypothalamus to trigger a dual autonomic and adrenocortical response. Balance is restored during the stage of resistance. When balance cannot be restored, the stage of exhaustion is reached.

147 LET US REVIEW: Factors potentially triggering a stress response are referred to as _____. stressors

The physiological response to a stressor is nonspecific and _____. The systemic response to stress is known patterned
as the _____ _____ syndrome and con- general adaptation
sists of _____ stages. The stage of alarm triggers an three
_____ and _____ response. autonomic; adrenocortical

148 Let us consider the *alarm reaction* in more detail. In the alarm reaction, signals are first transmitted to the cerebral _____ cortex
and _____. hypothalamus

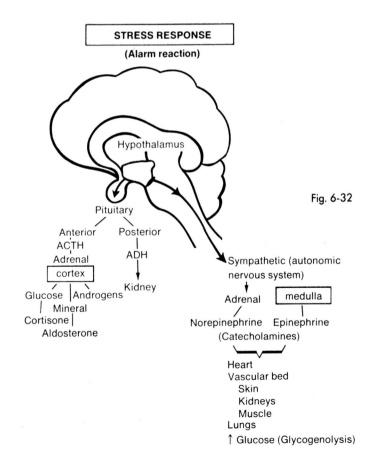

STRESS RESPONSE
(Alarm reaction)

Hypothalamus

Fig. 6-32

Pituitary

Anterior   Posterior
ACTH
Adrenal   ADH
cortex   Kidney
Glucose │Androgens
│ Mineral
Cortisone│
Aldosterone

Sympathetic (autonomic nervous system)

Adrenal   medulla
Norepinephrine   Epinephrine
(Catecholamines)

Heart
Vascular bed
Skin
Kidneys
Muscle
Lungs
↑ Glucose (Glycogenolysis)

The hypothalamus is in direct communication with the pituitary gland and is the site of origin of the autonomic nervous sytem (Fig. 6-33). The autonomic nervous system is composed of the _____ and _____ nervous systems.

sympathetic; parasympathetic

149 The initial response to acute stress is stimulation of the sympathetic nervous system. The response to sympathetic stimulation is dual: (1) increased discharge of sympathetic nerve fiber endings throughout the body and (2) stimulation of the adrenal medulla to release hormones that act as chemical *mediators* for sympathetic activity.

REMEMBER: The hormones _____ and _____ act as mediators for sympathetic activity (see Unit 4, Frame 41, and Unit 10). These chemicals are also referred to as catecholamines because of their common catechol rings.

epinephrine
norepinephrine

150 The key end organs of sympathetic activation are the heart, blood vessels, lungs, and liver (Fig. 6-24). In the presence of sympathetic stimulation, heart rate and contractility *(increase/decrease)*. Thus cardiac output *(increases/decreases)*.

increase
increases

The cardiac output may exceed the amount necessary for meeting O_2 demands at the expense of an increase in myocardial work and O_2 consumption (see Unit 9). Ischemia may become more pronounced, resulting in recurring angina or extension of the infarcted area. Arrhythmias may also occur because of the direct effects of the sympathetic chemicals.

151 In response to sympathetic stimulation, the blood vessels of the skin, kidneys muscle, and GI tract *(constrict/dilate)*. The vascular resistance *(increases/decreases)*. Blood pressure is determined by both the cardiac output and peripheral vascular resistance. Therefore blood pressure also *(rises/falls)*, placing an even greater work load on the heart.

constrict
increases

rises

152 Also in response to sympathetic stimulation, the bronchioles of the lungs dilate, providing a beneficial effect. The liver is stimulated to convert glycogen stores into free glucose to meet extra energy demands. This process is known as glycolysis. However, at the same time, the action of insulin is inhibited, which produces the paradox of an *(increase/decrease)* in blood glucose with cellular starvation. In borderline diabetes this change may produce more severe, labile hyperglycemia with its accompanying side effects. For this reason, diabetic patients are often given regular insulin therapy in the period immediately following an MI.

increase

153 LET US REVIEW: The initial response to stress is stimulation of the _____ nervous system. In response to this stimulation, the heart rate, blood pressure, and serum glucose level *(in-*

sympathetic
increase

crease/decrease). The effects of insulin are *(augmented/inhibited).* Arrhythmias may also occur because of the effects of the chemicals _____ and _____. For the most part, sympathetic stimulation accompanying severe stress is *(beneficial/harmful)* to the patient with acute MI.

inhibited

epinephrine; norepinephrine

harmful

154 During the alarm reaction, stress signals from the hypothalamus also stimulate both the anterior and posterior pituitary gland to cause the release of specific hormones (Fig. 6-24). Stimulation of the posterior pituitary gland causes the release of ADH (vasopressin).

REMEMBER: ADH acts on the _____ to cause the reabsorption of _____ and thus *(augments/depletes)* the circulating blood volume (see Unit 4).

kidneys

water; augments

155 Stimulation of the anterior pituitary gland causes the release of ACTH, which in turn stimulates the adrenal *cortex* to release the glucocorticoid, *cortisone,* and the mineral corticoid, *aldosterone.*

The *effects of cortisone* include the following:
1. Increased blood glucose level from protein and fat breakdown (glyconeogenesis)
2. Decreased local inflammatory responses by a variety of mechanisms, such as stabilization of cell membranes, lysosomes, and mitochondria; inhibited histamine release; decreased capillary permeability; and decreased migration of platelets, antibodies, and WBCs. Alterations in the blood cells may also occur, including an increase in RBCs and hemoglobin, increased neutrophils with decreased levels of other WBCs, and platelets.

The *effects of aldosterone* include increased absorption of _____ with increased excretion of _____ (see Unit 4).

Na^+

water

Gastric and duodenal ulcers also occur in response to the cortisone release during stress.

156 LET US REVIEW: During the alarm reaction to stress, _____ is released from the posterior pituitary gland, and _____ is released from the anterior pituitary gland. In response to ACTH, _____ and _____ are released from the adrenal *(cortex/medulla),* causing *(increase/decrease)* in blood glucose and *(increase/decrease)* in serum protein levels. Serum _____ and serum _____ levels *(increase/decrease)* in the inflammatory response, and alterations in the blood cells (_____, _____, and _____) may also occur.

ADH

ACTH

cortisone; aldosterone

cortex; increase

decrease; Na^+

K^+; decrease

WBC

RBC; platelet

During the stage of *resistance,* hormone levels subside and the body adapts to the stressor.

157 Stressors may be either physiological or psychological.

REMEMBER: Factors potentially triggering a stress response are referred to as _____. Pain is a key stressor in the

stressors

acute phase of MI. This key stressor has both physiological and psychological components. Pain—especially chest pain—represents a threat to both physiological and psychological integrity. Sudden sensations of severe chest discomfort accompany feelings of instability, helplessness, and impending death.

158 In response to pain, the patient with acute MI experiences stimulation of the _____ nervous system. Blood pressure, heart rate, and serum _____ levels (*elevate/depress*). Myocardial O_2 consumption increases. Arrhythmias may occur because of the effects of the chemicals _____ and _____. If the pain is severe, nausea, vomiting, and diaphoresis may occur. Therefore one of the highest priorities in the care of the patient who has acute MI is the immediate relief of _____ _____.

> sympathetic
> glucose; elevate
>
> epinephrine
> norepinephrine
>
>
> chest pain

An elevated blood pressure in the presence of chest pain is most likely caused by (*hypertension/response to stress*). Any physical or emotional stimulus that elicits a cardiovascular response may be considered a stress for the patient with coronary artery disease.

> response to stress

159 Physiological stress is usually accompanied by psychological stress. The opposite is also true. In addition to the physiological response, psychological stress may produce a syndrome of nonspecific subjective, and objective reactions and defense mechanisms. Denial, anxiety, hostility, anger, and depression are all reactions commonly seen in the patient with an acute MI. Although the physiological and psychological responses to stress involve patterned responses, the perception of stress and the specific psychological reactions manifested are highly individual. Previous experiences with stress or illness as well as available personal resources, cultural conditioning, and commonly used coping mechanisms influence an individual's perception of and response to stress.

RISK FACTORS: ASSESSMENT AND PATIENT TEACHING/DISCHARGE PLANNING IMPLICATIONS

160 The coronary artery disease syndromes—angina and acute MI—occur secondary to coronary artery narrowing or stenosis. Although the exact cause of coronary artery narrowing is unknown, contributing mechanisms have been identified.
  REMEMBER: The three major mechanisms contributing to coronary artery stenosis are the following:
  1. Lipid infiltration, or _____
  2. Thrombus formation initially related to _____ aggregation

> atherosclerosis
> platelet

3. _____ of the smooth muscle wall spasm

    Factors that precipitate or aggravate any of these processes are thought to trigger or accelerate the development of coronary artery disease. They may thus be said to place the patient at high risk for the development of coronary heart disease and are referred to as _____ _____. risk factors

161 Risk factors are most typically grouped into modifiable versus non-modifiable, or alterable versus unalterable. The nonmodifiable risk factors include age, sex, race, and family history.

    Realistic assessment and intervention should focus on the many more modifiable risk factors. Four of these modifiable risk factors are consistently referred to as the major, or most highly significant, risk factors. These are hypertension, diabetes, smoking, and hyperlipidemia. The relative importance of these top four factors is controversial and of little significance, since in any single individual the coronary disease is probably caused by multiple factors.

162 Hypertension contributes to coronary artery disease primarily by triggering or facilitating atherosclerosis or _____ lipid infiltration into the vessel lining. Hypertension is associated with increased arterial wall tension, which causes vascular wall changes and increased permeability to even normal levels of circulating lipids, especially cholesterol. This effect is magnified in the presence of hyperlipidemia or high blood lipoprotein levels (see Frame 167). The damaged vessel lining may also attract _____ ag- platelet gregation. Hypertension also increases the cardiac workload and can thus precipitate and/or aggravate chest pain or heart failure, complicating coronary artery disease (see Unit 10).

    The risk of a cardiovascular event increases the greater the systolic or diastolic pressure, whether the blood pressure elevation is fixed or labile. Hypertension is more common in *(men/women)* and men *(blacks/whites)*. blacks

163 Diabetes aggravates both platelet aggregation and atherosclerosis. Atherosclerosis is probably aggravated by multiple interacting factors, since control of the blood glucose level alone does not prevent it. Patients with diabetes also typically have hypertension and disturbances in serum lipoproteins (increased LDL, VLDL and decreased HDL levels). Many are also obese. The atherosclerotic effects of diabetes are particularly significant in younger women. The incidence of both heart failure and coronary artery disease is increased in the diabetic patient.

164 Smoking is a particular significant risk factor because it is avoidable and can be linked to all three mechanisms of coronary stenosis. Nicotine can alter the blood lipoproteins, decreasing the HDL/LDL ratio (see Frame 167) and increasing the vascular _____ to them. Smoking can also increase heart rate and blood pressure.

permeability

Moderate smoking doubles the risk of the other risk factors. Quitting smoking results in an immediate risk reduction: 2 years later, the risk is only slightly higher than that of nonsmokers. Hyperlipidemia is a syndrome associated with increased blood _____. These lipoprotein levels are affected by heredity, diet, and exercise. They are also altered by each of the other three major risk factors: _____, _____, and _____ (see Frames 168 to 175 for a more extensive discussion).

lipoproteins

hypertension
diabetes; smoking

165 Other identified risk factors include stress, weight, and lack of exercise. Stress has been closely linked to the popular Type A and Type B personality types. The stress-prone personality is the Type A, who is typically competitive, impatient, ambitious and desirous of squeezing the most amount of tasks into the least amount of time. However, even patients with Type B personalities may become susceptible to the ill effects of multiple, severe, or prolonged stressors.

REMEMBER: Stress triggers a *(sympathetic/parasympathetic)* response, which results in the release of _____ and _____. These chemicals are also referred to as _____.

sympathetic
epinephrine
norepinephrine
catecholamines

Catecholamines can affect all three mechanisms of coronary stenosis.

REMEMBER: Like smoking, these chemicals can increase _____ _____ and trigger _____ _____. Coronary spasm is most typically associated with *(rest/effort)* angina. Patients with this type of angina can particularly benefit from psychological counseling and stress reduction technique. Catecholamines can also *(increase/decrease)* heart rate and *(increase/decrease)* blood pressure and predispose to high lipid levels.

platelet aggregation
coronary spasm
rest

increase
increase

Stress reduction techniques include exercise, adequate rest and diet, relaxation techniques, biofeedback, hobbies, and pesonality analysis and modifications.

166 Risk factor control is thought to be effective in preventing or limiting existing coronary disease. Prevention before clinical symptoms appear is referred to as "primary prevention." Prevention after clinical symptoms already exist is referred to as "secondary prevention." Risk factor control in this setting is probably more effective in _____ the disease and maximizing the remaining cardiovascular function.

limiting

Role of lipoproteins

167 LET US REVIEW: Fats (lipids) are carried witin the plasma in two forms: _____ _____ _____ and _____. The free fatty acids act as immediate energy sources, whereas the lipoproteins act as backup energy sources and are stored within _____ and _____ cells. The linings of the coronary arteries as well as the wall of the heart contain muscle. Lipoproteins are absorbed into the coronary vessel walls and initiate the process of atherosclerosis, which contributes to the thickening and narrowing of the vessel lumen.

free fatty acids
lipoproteins

fat; muscle

The major fats implicated in coronary artery disease—cholesterol and triglycerides—are carried in these large fat compounds in varying proportions. Routine serum cholesterol levels are a reflection of the *total cholesterol* carried in all these lipoproteins. The total serum cholesterol level is an effective initial screening tool for the risk of coronary artery disease. Serum levels of less than 200 mg/dl are considered optimal.

168 Different types of serum lipoproteins can be separated, identified, and measured by electrophoresis. This procedure is also referred to as "cholesterol fractionation."

The lipoproteins are divided into two major categories: (1) alpha (α) lipoproteins, commonly referred to as high-density lipoproteins, or HDL-cholesterol; and (2) beta (β) lipoproteins, commonly referred to as low-density lipoproteins, or LDL-cholesterol.

It is the cholesterol carried primarily within LDL which is absorbed into the vessel wall. Cholesterol is also contained within HDL. The HDL compound absorbs cholesterol and helps to transport it away from the vessel wall and other tissue cells to the liver for excretion.

169 Thus some fats in the form of lipoproteins protect against coronary artery disease, whereas others produce the disease. Increased HDL cholsterol levels can help *(raise/lower)* serum LDL cholesterol levels, thus *(producing/protecting against)* coronary artery disease.

lower
protecting against

Assessment of the serum HDL/LDL ratio is a more accurate reflection of the associated risk of atherosclerotic disease than assessment of the total serum _____ or LDL level alone. HDL/LDL level and ratios are clearly indicated when the total serum cholesterol level exceeds 239 mg/dl. Serum cholesterol levels between 200-239 are typically handled by dietary control. Decreased HDL levels alone may be a significant risk factor even in the presence of normal serum cholesterol levels. The decreased HDL levels found in women after menopause appears to coincide with the increased risk of coronary artery disease at that time.

cholesterol

LIPIDS AND CORONARY ARTERY DISEASE

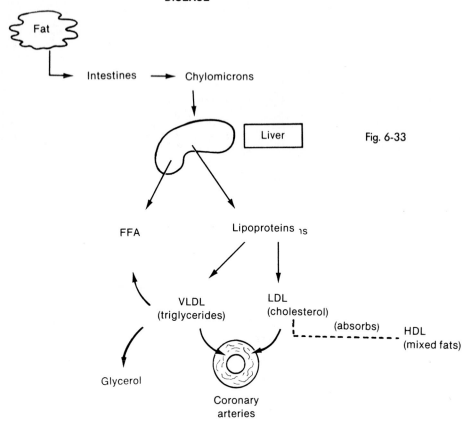

Fig. 6-33

170 Exercise has been shown to raise HDL levels. This is one of the reasons a carefully monitored exercise program is beneficial for the patient with known coronary artery disease and may prevent coronary artery disease in the normal individual. All the major risk factors for coronary artery disease have been either directly or indirectly linked to lipoprotein abnormalities (see Frames 162 to 164).

Mild alcohol consumption can also raise HDL levels, thus *(protecting/harming)* the heart. However, this concept should be approached cautiously, since excessive alcohol consumption can reverse the effect and also product direct damage to the cardiac muscle cell (cardiomyopathy). Excessive alcohol consumption can also contribute to arrhythmias and hypertension.

protecting

171 The two major fats linked to coronary artery disease are LDL-cholesterol and _____. The serum triglycerides are primarily contained within the very-low-density lipoproteins (VLDL). However, the VLDL contain small amounts of cholesterol

triglycerides

244

as well, which can be released when these fats are broken down for energy.

REMEMBER: Triglycerides may be broken down into _____ and _____, which can be used as energy sources.

FFA (free fatty acids); glycerol

The role of the triglycerides or *(LDL/VLDL)* in the production of atherosclerotic disease is not well established, since increased serum triglycerides alone have not been shown to be a significant risk factor. These lipoproteins are thought to contribute to coronary risk primarily when found in combination with other risk factors. However, it is interesting that significantly elevated serum triglycerides are more often found in middle-aged men than in middle-aged women. The role of these lipoproteins may be closely related either to the small amounts of cholesterol carried within them or to their role in fat storage and obesity, which further contribute to hypertension.

VLDL

REMEMBER: Triglycerides are the major fat _____ form. About 95% of the body's fatty tissue is composed of this lipoprotein. Weight reduction alone can effectively lower serum triglyceride levels.

storage

172 Serum triglyceride levels fluctuate throughout the day and are significantly affected by alcohol, glucose consumption, exercise, and stresses, such as pregnancy. Accurate levels require fasting for at least 12 hours and abstention from alcohol for at least 24 hours. Levels also should be drawn before any major exercise. Excessive alcohol intake *(raises/lowers)* triglyceride levels and for this reason *(should/should not)* be avoided in the patient with coronary artery disease.

raises; should

173 Five types of familial elevated blood lipid patterns (hyperlipidemias) have been identified and are thought to be major risk factors for coronary artery disease. They are classified according to the type of blood lipid elevated: LDL (cholesterol), VLDL (triglycerides), or chylomicrons. *Chylomicrons* are the form in which fat is transported from the intestines to the liver, where the lipoproteins are formed (Fig. 6-34).

Types II and IV are the most common forms of hyperlipidemias. Type II is associated with high cholesterol levels. Type IV is associated with high triglyceride levels. These patterns are typically associated with familial disorders such as diabetes and hypothyroidism. Diabetes may be associated with either Type II or Type IV hyperlipidemia or both. Hypothyroidism is predominantly associated with Type II hyperlipidemia or high *(cholesterol/triglyceride)* levels.

cholesterol

174 Therapy for Type II hyperlipidemia consists of diet cholesterol control and/or administration of cholesterol antagonists, such as colestipol (Colestid), cholestyramine (Questran), probucol (Lorelco), or niacin (vitamin B_3). A diet low in total fat content as well as saturated fats and cholesterol is recommended for diet control. Therapy in Type IV hyperlipidemia consists of diet, calorie, fat, and alcohol restriction, weight reduction, exercise and/or administering a _____ antagonist, such as clofibrate (Atromid-S). The effects of therapy on controlling the severity of coronary artery disease are still controversial. Diet control is usually preferred over drug therapy, since it is effective and associated with less risks.

triglyceride

The serum cholesterol of most individuals, with the exception of those with severe familial hyperlipidemia, can be maintained at the optimal level by diet modification alone.

EXERCISE STRESS (TOLERANCE) TESTING: DIAGNOSTIC AND PATIENT TEACHING/DISCHARGE PLANNING IMPLICATIONS

175 Exercise stress testing is a noninvasive procedure that involves the monitoring of the cardiac electrical and mechanical response to continuous, progressively strenuous, dynamic exercise. The exercise acts as a "stress" or *work load challenge* to the heart to determine normal versus abnormal function and work load capacity. The use of the word "stress" in stress testing can be misleading and disturbing, since it is easily confused with the stress response, which is potentially harmful to the heart and is regarded as a risk factory (see Frame 146). The alternate use of the term exercise *tolerance* testing (ETT) has been suggested and is gaining popularity.

Stress testing is used primarily to detect and evaluate the *functional impact* of coronary artery disease.

176 Although stress testing is primarily a diagnostic procedure, it is also commonly used to guide and evaluate intervention, rehabilitation, and physical conditioning. When compared to the invasive procedure, cardiac catheterization, it is more effective in evaluating coronary function and predicting prognosis and less effective in evaluating coronary structure.

REMEMBER: Noninvasive procedures are also generally associated with *(more/less)* risk and expense.

less

177 Stress testing is often adequate to allow for initiation of appropriate medical therapy. However, before any surgical intervention, visualization of the exact coronary anatomy or _____ is critical and can only be done during _____ _____.

structure

cardiac
catheterization

178 Two major modes of exercise are used for stress testing in the United States: treadmill and bicycle ergometry. The treadmill is used most commonly in routine stress testing or in combination with thallium radionuclide imaging. Bicycle ergometry is most commonly used in combination with gated pool radionuclide angiography because of the patient _____ required (see Frame 113).

positioning

The major diagnostic use of stress testing is to unmask an impaired coronary artery system. It may be used to screen those at high risk for having coronary artery disease (CAD) as well as apparently healthy individuals in the coronary age group who want to pursue cardiovascular conditioning programs.

179 Pursuit of a CV exercise program by the healthy person can potentially reduce or prevent many risk factors that are associated with the development of CAD.

REMEMBER: Regular exercise has been shown to raise *(high-density/ low-density)* lipoproteins, which protect against the effects of _____. Hypertension, obesity, and psychological _____ may also be reduced by a cardiovascular fitness program.

high-density

cholesterol

stress

180 In the patient with known coronary artery disease, individualized exercise prescriptions determined from stress testing results can also provide _____ _____ control, limiting existing disease. Unnecessary myocardial strain and related complications may be prevented by not exceeding the _____ _____ capacity. Psychological confidence and responsibility for self-care is promoted when the patient's exercise tolerance is determined and discussed with the patient before discharge.

risk factor

work load

As a prognostic tool stress testing has been shown to predict both mortality and morbidity, especially in patients recovering from acute MI. The immediate and long-term effects of drug therapy, coronary artery bypass surgery, and exercise, as well as the progress of the disease, can be evaluated.

Normal physiological responses to exercise

181 Let us now consider the normal cardiovascular response to exercise as a background for understanding parameters monitored during stress testing.

The normal response to dynamic exercise is an *(increase/decrease)* in oxygen demand by the body. The cardiovascular system is designed to respond to this increased demand for oxygen.

increase

REMEMBER: The heart serves as a pump to deliver _____ blood to meet the metabolic demands of the tissue (see Unit 1). The amount of blood put out by the heart per minute is known as the _____ _____. Cardiac output is a product of

oxygenated

cardiac output

_____ _____ and   heart rate

_____ _____. The heart rate is   stroke volume

primarily determined by the integrity of the _____   electrical

system. The stroke volume is primarily determined by the pumping

efficiency of the _____ _____.   cardiac muscle

   Thus the ability of the heart to respond to the body's increased

demands for oxygen is both an _____ and a   electrical

_____ phenomenon.   mechanical

182 Neural influences also play a role in the body's ability to meet the
increased oxygen demands imposed by exercise. The sympathetic
nervous system is the compensatory mediator that provides for this
increase in cardiac output. Sympathetic stimulation occurs even with
the anticipation of exercise. As the sympathetic chemicals are released from cardiovascular nerve endings, there is an increase in _both_
the heart rate and stroke volume. The stroke volume is increased because of an increased force of myocardial contraction and a mild
vasoconstriction with an increase in venous return. The net effect is

an increase in _____ _____ and   cardiac output

blood pressure.

   REMEMBER: BP = _____ _____   cardiac output

   × _____   _____   peripheral vascular

   _____.   resistance

183 As the duration and intensity of the exercise increases, local metabolic alterations occur in working muscles. These metabolic changes
result in the release of local chemicals, which produce vasodilation in
an attempt to maximize tissue O_2 delivery. The systemic vasoconstriction is balanced by the local vasodilation, and as a result the _di-
astolic pressure_ remains close to baseline as the exercise progresses.

   The cardiac output, however, continues to increase as the body
responds to increased oxygen demands. This rise in cardiac output
is proportionately greater than the changes in PVR, so the systolic

arterial pressure continues to _(rise/fall)_. This results in a widening of   rise

the pulse pressure.

184 The greater these compensatory increases in cardiac output and
blood pressure, the greater the work load on the heart. This work
load is commonly expressed as the product of the heart rate and
mean arterial pressure; it is known as the _rate pressure product (RPP),_
or _double product_. This product reflects the myocardial O_2 consumption at any given exercise work load.

   Double product calculation reflects the influence of both _heart rate_
and _arterial blood pressure_ increases on the work load of the left ventricle. These are considered the major determinants of myocardial

_____ _____ during exercise. O_2 consumption

248

The conditioned person will have a *(lower/higher)* pressure product at a given work load than the unconditioned person and *(more/less)* myocardial O_2 consumption.

lower
less

185 LET US REVIEW: Normally, as the intensity and duration of exercise increase, both heart rate and arterial pressure *(increase/decrease)*.

increase

Heart rate and arterial pressure responses in exercise can be used to evaluate cardiovascular fitness as well as serve as markers of myocardial _____ _____.

oxygen demand

The conditioned person will perform a given work load at a *(lower/higher)* heart rate and double product than will the unconditioned person.

lower

The ability of the cardiovascular system to respond in these normal physiological ways is modulated by the intensity and duration of the effort, degree of physical fitness, emotion, and presence or absence of cardiac disease—especially coronary artery disease.

186 This cardiovascular response to exercise also has normal physiological limits. The ability of the heart rate to increase in response to increased demands for cardiac output is characteristically limited by an unique age-related ceiling on rate. Normal compensatory increases in heart rate do not occur beyond this maximal point, logically referred to as the _____ heart rate. Curiously, the stroke volume reaches its normal compensatory limits at about the same time the peak heart rate is reached. Thus further increases in cardiac output *(are/are not)* possible.

maximal

are not

REMEMBER: Cardiac output = _____ × _____ .

rate
stroke volume

187 When these physiological limits are reached, oxygen demands can no longer be effectively met, and myocardial and systemic hypoxia occur. Extended periods of hypoxia are potentially harmful and life threatening and are best prevented by cessation of the exercise at this point. Continued, sustained exercise beyond this point can be said to act as a true stressor, although the heart rate can no longer typically respond.

REMEMBER: The stress response typically refers to a *(specific/nonspecific)* local and multisystem response to _____ psychological or physiological work loads or injury. Harmful stress responses are triggered when normal compensatory mechanisms have been exceeded or _____ .

nonspecific
excessive

exhausted

In unconditioned individuals or patients with coronary artery disease, a true stress response can be triggered before reaching maximal heart rate (see Frames 146 to 160).

188 Although the *normal* individual typically tolerates exercise *up to* maximal heart rate without significant systemic or myocardial hypoxia, *sustained* exercise *beyond* this point is potentially harmful and is best avoided. For this reason, suggested target heart rates for conditioning programs are usually 70% to 80% of the maximum predicted heart rate.

Maximum heart rate is commonly estimated by subtracting the patient's age from 220—theoretically, at least, the maximal achievable heart rate of a newborn. A mean deviation of 10 points is then allowed.

For example, a 50-year-old man would have a maximal predicted heart rate of 170 ± 10, or a range of 160 to 180 beats per minute. This method is used in a variety of cardiovascular conditioning programs and during diagnostic stress testing as a normal end point.

189 Patients with coronary artery disease are more prone to *(myocardial/peripheral)* hypoxia than is the normal individual. In these patients signs of significant myocardial hypoxia typically occur *before* achieving maximal heart rate. These signs are probably caused by the increased myocardial work load associated with even the normal compensatory response to exercise and/or a stress response.

REMEMBER: Both heart _____ and blood _____ increase in response to exercise placing a greater work load on the heart. This work load is estimated by multiplying the heart rate by the _____ arterial pressure to obtain the _____ _____ product, or double product. The double product is considered a measure of myocardial work load or _____ _____. Because of the importance of more subtle heart rate changes in coronary artery disease, careful monitoring of heart rate is emphasized during diagnostic stress testing and as part of rehabilitative prescriptions after MI or bypass surgery.

myocardial

rate
pressure

mean
rate pressure

O_2 consumption

190 Patients with coronary artery disease should also be watched during stress testing and/or exercise for other early signs of myocardial hypoxia. Myocardial hypoxia may be reflected as *electrical* abnormalities detected on the _____, as *mechanical*, or as hemodynamic abnormalities detected by decreases in cardiac output, or _____ _____, or as hypoxic *metabolic* changes reflected by symptoms such as _____ _____.

These manifestations are all a direct or indirect result of _____ _____ and hypoxia.

REMEMBER: Oxygen is necessary for cells to metabolize *(aerobically/anaerobically)* and produce adequate amounts of the high-energy phosphate _____. Failure of the cells to produce adequate

ECG

blood pressure
chest pain

myocardial ischemia
aerobically

ATP

amounts of ATP results in inactivation of critical ion pumps, which are responsible for electrical and mechanical stability in cardiac cells.

191 The electrical instability results primarily from the effects of K^+ shifts on the resting cell charge and automaticity and is manifested as ST segment shifts and ventricular arrhythmias. Hypoxia may produce arrhythmias related to conduction abnormalities as well as instability or _____.

automaticity

The mechanical abnormalities probably result from Ca^{++} sequestration in cardiac cells and compliance changes and is manifested by decreases in _____ _____ and/or a _____ in arterial pressure.

cardiac output
fall

These are the signs typically associated with a positive stress test and cessation of the procedure regardless of the heart rate achieved.

192 LET US REVIEW: If an individual's usual physiological limits are exceeded and compensatory mechanisms are exhausted, significant _____ and _____ hypoxia can occur.

systemic; myocardial

Exercise should be stopped before the stage of severe exhaustion and hypoxia is reached, even in the normal individual. In this way, serious _____, _____, and _____ cardiac complications can be avoided. One measure of these physiological limits in the normal individual is the _____ heart rate. It signals the onset of the exhaustion stage. In the patient with coronary artery disease symptoms of electrical, mechanical, and/or metabolic compromise typically occur *(before/after)* reaching this maximal heart rate.

electrical; mechanical
metabolic

maximal

before

The appearance of these symptoms can be used to detect or unmask latent coronary disease or to predict and prevent further coronary events.

Treadmill exercise stress (tolerance) testing

193 With this background let us now consider the exercise stress (tolerance) test in more detail. Currently the most popular method for evaluating the cardiovascular septum through exercise is the treadmill protocol with progressive increases in work load.

REMEMBER: The two major modes of exercise used for stress testing in the United States are _____ and _____ ergometry. The method most commonly used during routine stress testing or in combination with thallium imaging is the _____.

treadmill
bicycle

treadmill

194 The Bruce Multistage Test is the most popular treadmill protocol. Work loads are increased by changes in the treadmill speed and/or grade independently or simultaneously. The response of the patient at different work loads or stages is then evaluated.

In this particular protocol the speed and grade (or elevation) of the treadmill are increased at 3-minute intervals until significant symptoms appear or the patient complains of fatigue. This protocol allows the patient to judge his maximal ability to a greater extent than other protocols. Other protocols may also differ with regard to factors such as the method of exercise used, the initial speed or grade of the treadmill, or the increments of increase in speed or grade.

195 Before stress testing patients must be examined by a physician to exclude those for whom the test could be dangerous. There is absolute contraindication for those with severe acute cardiovascular disease, including recent (usually less than 2 weeks), acute MI, unstable angina, pericarditis, myocarditis, heart failure, life-threatening arrhythmias, recent systemic embolus or thrombophlebitis, and dissecting or enlarging aneurysm. Patients with severe disease associated with limited mobility or work capacity would obviously not be candidates for stress testing. These include patients with severe pulmonary or renal failure, orthopedic or neurological impairment, or systemic infection. These patients may be referred instead for radionuclide studies.

REMEMBER: Radionuclide studies can be performed either at _____ or during exercise and may also serve as diagnostic   rest
tests for _____ _____ disease.   coronary artery

196 Once the screening is accomplished, the patient may be scheduled and receive instructions to prepare for the test (see Nursing Orders, p. 273).

Patient medications are continued unless specified otherwise by the physician. The nurse should be aware that certain medications may alter test results. Included are such medications as digitalis, which alters the ST segment; beta blockers, which reduce the ability to achieve maximum heart rates; and others, such as valium, antihistamines, tricyclic antidepressants, and lithium, all of which have been cited as altering the ST segment, T wave, or heart rate.

REMEMBER: The electrical changes associated with a positive stress test are typically _____ changes. To avoid exhaustion and   ST
myocardial compromise, _____ heart rates are   maximal
used as limiting end points.

197 Immediately before beginning the test a resting ECG is obtained to verify the absence of acute disese and provide a baseline for evaluation of abnormalities.

REMEMBER: Stress testing is contraindicated in acute states
such as _____ MI or _____   acute; unstable angina
_____.

Some practitioners record a resting ECG in both the recumbent (or sitting) and standing positions to determine if there are orthostatic ST-T shifts. The patient may be also asked to hyperventilate to document any ST shifts associated with increased respiratory rate and depth. A multilead monitoring system is now used by most stress testing laboratories during testing to afford maximal views of the heart wall as well as to aid in arrhythmia interpretation.

198 Multistage exercise stress tests are usually symptom-limited or heart-rate limited. They are classified as maximal or submaximal, depending on whether the patient reaches his or her physiological limits or stops at some arbitrarily predetermined end point.

The patient may be allowed to determine his or her own physiological limits subjectively, based on feelings of fatigue or exhaustion or some symptoms of cardiovascular decompensation, such as chest pain. More commonly, the more objective determination of maximal heart rate is correlated with subjective symtomatology in determining the end points of a maximal test.

A submaximal test, with regard to an objective parameter such as heart rate, might have to be terminated when the patient reaches 70% to 80% of the age-predicted maximum heart rate.

199 Some investigators feel that maximal tests provide more accurate information of physical performance capacity. However, submaximal tests are clearly indicated for selected subsets of patients, such as those tested early (2 to 3 weeks) after MI or after bypass surgery or those known to have significant CAD.

In a negative exercise stress test the patient is able to achieve a maximum heart rate without signs of _____ decompensation. A negative test does not exclude the presence of CAD, but it does mean that if the disease is present, the risk of complications are low.

cardiovascular

200 A positive exercise stress test is one which must be terminated before the predicted maximal or submaximal limits are achieved through signs or symptoms of _____ decompensation.

cardiovascular

Generally the earlier the signs and symptoms of cardiovascular decompensation become manifested, the more serious is the extent of the disease.

The major clinical parameters monitored during stress testing are those that signal cardiac decompensation.

REMEMBER: These signals may be manifested electrically as _____ changes or _____, hemodynamically as changes in _____ _____ or _____ _____, or symptomatically by the occurrence of _____ _____.

ECG; arrhythmias
heart rate
blood pressure
chest pain

Assessment of the ECG during stress testing

201 Let us consider in more detail the electrocardographic changes that signal cardiac decompensation. The most common electrical sign of cardiovascular decompensation with stress testing is ST segment depression on the ECG. Although it is not a specific change seen only in CAD, it is well established that when it occurs in this setting, it is usually evidence of compromised subendocardial blood flow.

REMEMBER: The first layer of the heart wall to be compromised in the face of myocardial ischemia is the _____. This is because the subendocardium has a *(richer/poorer)* blood supply than the epicardium has. Significantly compromised subendocardial flow is a predictor of future transmural compromise and potential myocardial infarction.

subendocardium

poorer

202 Compromised subendocardial blood flow can result in either ST segment changes (injury) or T wave changes (ischemia) caused by myocardial _____ and related *(electrical/mechanical)* changes.

hypoxia; electrical

REMEMBER: On the majority of the standard epicardial leads subendocardial injury is reflected as ST segment *(elevation/depression)* (see Frames 59 to 65).

depression

203 Decreased subendocardial blood flow may be described physiologically as _____. However, this physiological ischemia *(is/is not)* synonymous with the electrical ischemia that specifically refers to a *(QRS/ST/T wave)* change.

ischemia

is not

T wave

ST depression serves as a sign of physiological subendocardial ischemia or decreased _____ _____ and electrical *(injury/ischemia/necrosis)*. This change thus becomes an important ECG manifestation of cardiac decompensation.

blood flow

injury

204 Other factors that may contribute to acute or preexisting ST shifts and/or ST-T abnormalities must be compensated for during a stress test. Examples of such factors include drugs, electrolyte imbalances, hypertrophy, hyperventilation, and orthostatic phenomena. J point depression may precede ST depression on the ECG.

REMEMBER: The J point is the junction between the _____ _____ and the _____ _____.

QRS complex

ST segment

Pain may be experienced while the pattern of ST segment depression is recorded and would provide additional support for terminating the test.

205 The stress test is considered positive for myocardial ischemia when the magnitude and configuration of the ST segment fulfills any of the following criteria:
1. 1 millimeter (mm) *flat* (horizontal) ST segment depression lasting for 0.08 second or

2. 1 mm *downsloping* ST segment depression lasting for 0.08 second
or
3. 1.5 to 2.0 mm *upsloping* ST segment depression lasting for 0.08
second.

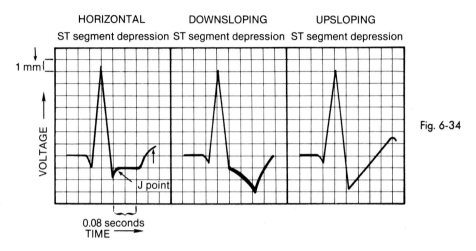

Fig. 6-34

NOTE: ST upsloping is the least predictive of the three criteria.
Some feel that ST upsloping *alone* should not constitute a positive response and should be interpreted as equivocal. In contrast, ST depression with a downsloping ST segment has the *highest* predictive
value for coronary artery disease.

Generally the earlier the ST shift occurs within the test protocol
and the greater its magnitude, the greater is the extent of the coronary artery disease. Although less commonly seen, ST segment elevation of 1 mm for at least .08 second has the same significance as
ST segment depression.

REMEMBER: ST segment elevation typically indicates
_____ injury. Some investigators have documented   epicardial
that ST elevation occurring with stress testing is caused by LV aneurysm and/or wall motion abnormalities.

206 The occurrence of life-threatening arrhythmias may also serve as a
marker of cardiac decompensation. Most investigators feel that severe exercise-induced arrhythmias are strongly suggestive of coronary artery disease. The presence of PVCs alone in apparently
healthy individuals being routinely tested is of little prognostic significance. Arrhythmias present before testing even in those with
known CAD may be abolished as the heart rate *(increases/decreases)*   increases
with exercising.

Generally arrhythmias that would require treatment in a CCU
necessitate termination of the stress test. Of particular concern are
the life-threatening ventricular arrhythmias.

Emergency cardiac drugs and intravenous supplies as well as a defibrillator and other resuscitative equipment should be available for immediate use in the stress testing laboratory in case the need arises.

Assessment of hemodynamic parameters—heart rate and BP

207 Heart rate and blood pressure responses to stress testing not only serve as parameters to assess cardiovascular conditioning but also serve as markers of physical limitation and cardiovascular _____.

> decompensation

Originally, exercise testing protocols emphasized only ECG changes. The use of BP and heart rate responses have been found to increase the predictive value of the test significantly.

Impairment of heart rate response has been shown to correlate with impaired left ventricular function. Maximum BP achieved with exercise has been shown to be one of the best predictors of mortality. Generally the lower the heart rate and blood pressure at which a test becomes positive, the more likely that it is a _true positive._

REMEMBER: The product of the heart rate and mean BP is a reflection of the myocardial work load and is also referred to as the _____ _____. Individuals with-

> double product

out coronary artery disease are usually able to tolerate work loads up to their _____ heart rate. However, patients with

> maximal

coronary artery disease typically develop symptoms earlier, depending on their specific work load tolerance. This tolerance or intolerance is usually a reflection of the _____ extent of

> functional

the disease and _____ of future complications.

> risk

The double product is calculated by multiplying the mean arterial pressure (MAP) by the _____

> heart rate

_____ and dividing by _____.

> 100

Achievement of a double product of 250 with a normal ECG is said to exclude critical coronary artery disease necessitating surgery.

208 Failure to achieve target or maximal heart rates before termination of the stress test, in the absence of drugs that negate the chronotropic response (that is, beta blockers) has been shown to prognosticate the high likelihood of a future coronary event.

REMEMBER: The maximal, or _____, heart rate

> target

to be achieved with stress testing can be roughly estimated by subtracting the patient's age from _____ and allowing for a

> 220

mean deviation of 10 points. Submaximal stress tests (with reference to heart rate) would use a target heart rate that is approximately 70% to 85% of the predicted maximum.

209 The occurrence of bradycardia with stress testing is also a sign of CV decompensation and an indication for test termination. The arterial

BP response to exercise is also indicative of cardiovascular conditioning and is an important marker of cardiovascular decompensation.

REMEMBER: The normal response to progressively intense dynamic exercise is a rise in the arterial pressure. This rise in pressure is primarily *(systolic/diastolic)* and occurs as a result of the increase in *(cardiac output/peripheral vascular resistance)*.

systolic; cardiac output

Most investigators terminate the exercise test when the systolic BP approaches 250 mm Hg.

210 Failure to raise the BP or a sudden drop in BP with dynamic exercise is a sign of cardiovascular _____.

decompensation

Hypotension manifested during exercise, especially at low work loads, is a *poor* pronostic sign indicative of severe cardiac disease. Dizziness, sudden pallor, or gait disturbances may precede a drop in blood pressure.

NOTE: The cardiac disease may be obstructive or valvular or cardiomyopathic, as well as CAD.

211 LET US REVIEW: The normal hemodynamic response to increased tissue oxygen demands with exercise is to increase the _____ _____ and the _____ _____. Failure to raise the BP or a sudden drop in BP during stress testing is a *(poor/good)* prognostic sign indicative of *(moderate/severe)* cardiac disease.

heart rate
blood pressure
poor
severe

Assessment of chest pain and other symptoms

212 Another sign of cardiovascular decompensation with stress testing is the development of chest pain.

REMEMBER: Chest pain is a manifestation of myocardial ischemia and results from the accumulation of excessive metabolic end products causing irritation of nerve endings.

Chest pain by itself may not necessitate exercise termination unless it is part of a typical anginal syndrome (see Frames 10 to 12) or is accompanied by ST segment _____.

depression

Anginal chest pain occurring during stress testing has been shown to be useful in predicting the likelihood of subsequent coronary events. Generally the lower the work load at which the pain occurs, the higher is the likelihood of a coronary event.

Anginal pain accompanied by ST segment _____ prognosticates the likelihood of a coronary event even more.

depression

213 Other indications for termination of a stress test include complaints of general fatigue or exhaustion, feelings of breathlessness or dizziness, the development of AV block or branch bundle block, or failure of the ECG monitoring system. Some practitioners use an exertion scale visible to the patient during stress testing so that the patient may numerically indicate his perceived level of exertion or fatigue during the test.

False positive and false negative results

214 There are many reasons for false positive and false negative test results. ST segment depression is not specific for coronary disease and may be caused by a myocardial abnormality unrelated to coronary artery disease. For example, such factors as hyperventilation, vasomotor instability associated with postural changes and drugs, and electrolyte abnormalities may alter the ST segment and/or T wave. ECG abnormalities such as LBBB and LV hypertrophy may also render test interpretation difficult.

False negative tests may occur because of the effects of drugs, such as beta blockers and nitrates, that obscure the ischemic response, as well as by other factors.

Thallium imaging with stress testing

215 Supplementing the exercise stress test with thallium imaging has been shown to improve the diagnostic accuracy up to 95% and also aids in localizing the area of ischemia. However, thallium should only be used in problem cases in which definitive results are uncertain as an alternative to angiography.

REMEMBER: Thallium is a radioactive analog of _____. Thallium, like potassium, is actively absorbed by *(healthy/ischemic)* tissue.

potassium
healthy

Thallium thus can serve as a tracer for _____ tissue and *(would/would not)* be taken up by ischemic or infarcted tissue. At rest the proportion or ratio of blood flow to normally perfused and potentially ischemic myocardium is such that thallium uptake in both areas is *uniform*. Rest thallium scans thus provide a baseline for evaluation of what happens with exercise.

healthy
would not

A rest scan *(would/would not)* show a defect of thallium uptake, or _____ spot, in a previously infarcted area.

would
cold

216 With exercise the blood flow ratio to normally perfused and ischemic myocardium changes dramatically. Thallium is then taken up only by the nonischemic, or _____, tissue.

healthy

The ischemic zone shows up as a *(cold spot/hot spot)*, or filling defect.

cold spot

With exercise testing, thallium is injected at peak exercise, and the test is continued for 1 minute to allow the chemical to distribute within the heart muscle. The patient is then rapidly transferred to the nuclear department for imaging. Within 4 hours the tracer has redistributed, so that a repeat scan at this time is almost identical to a resting scan; this prevents the need for two injections.

Comparison of the exercise and rest thallium scan allows for evaluation of potentially _____ areas.

ischemic

217 After stress testing the patient is asked to sit or lie down until the heart rate and ECG have returned to baseline levels.

A 12-lead ECG and series of rhythm strips are recorded every few minutes. During this time, it is also important to auscultate the heart carefully, assessing the patient for other signs of cardiac compromise, such as gallops and murmurs.

Implications for discharge exercise prescriptions

218 The results of the exercise stress test may be used as the basis for individualized discharge instructions after MI or after bypass surgery. It may also be used to guide the individual without known coronary artery disease who is starting out in a cardiovascular conditioning program.

The stages of the exercise stress testing protocols are commonly correlated with various levels of oxygen demands known as MET. *MET* is an abbreviation for *met*abolic equivalent. A MET corresponds to the equivalent of the usual metabolic, or amount of O_2 used per minute, at rest. The concept of MET is supported by the American Heart Association. MET can also be correlated to calories, especially for diet and weight control.

219 The usual MET requirements of the first stage in the Bruce protocol is about 5 MET. For this reason, stress tests taken after myocardial infarction are not usually performed until immediately before discharge.

REMEMBER: Stress testing is usually _____ less than 2 weeks after acute MI.

contraindicated

Predischarge activities should generally be kept below this level of _____ METs. These activities can include flexion and extension of the limbs, lateral trunk bending, partial squatting, and walking down the corridor at progressively further distances and at a gradually increasing pace. The effects of these activities are cautiously monitored according to increases above the resting heart rate. For example, in one protocol, activity is stopped when the heart rate exceeds 20 beats above the patient's resting level.

5

REMEMBER: Heart rate is one of the major components of the _____-pressure product or _____ _____, which in turn is a reflection of the individual patient's myocardial work load tolerance.

rate; double product

220 Energy expenditures of routine household, occupational, and recreational activities have also been classified according to METs and can be discussed with the patient before discharge. Activities immediately following discharge should also generally not exceed _____ METs.

5

Most routine household activities, such as cooking, making beds, and washing clothes and mild recreational activities, such as horseback riding, bowling, and playing golf fall below the 5-MET level.

Examples of activities requiring greater than 5 METS include mowing the lawn, climbing more than two flights of stairs, and lifting items weighing more than 20 lbs. Patients recovering from an acute MI should be instructed to *(participate in/avoid)* such activities immediately after discharge.

avoid

221 True conditioning programs usually require some form of regular aerobic or sustained activity of at least moderate intensity and are not usually begun until 6 to 8 weeks after discharge. The major form of aerobic activity used before discharge is _____. Sustained activity is considered aerobic because it allows time for cardiovascular O_2 compensation to develop fully as the major skeletal muscle metabolic source. Conditioning exercise sessions involve a warm-up phase, aerobic phase, and cool-down phase. The frequency and duration of the activity can be extended to compensate for intensity and maintain the same aerobic benefit with a lesser cardiac work load. High energy-expenditure exercises, such as jogging (at 10 METS for 1 mile in 10 minutes) are initially best avoided by the patient with documented coronary disease. However, after about 6 months of regular exercise, activities similar to those individuals with normal health may be safely tolerated. Activity programs such as these for patients with coronary artery disease are best guided by regular treadmill studies and individualized, regularly updated exercise prescriptions. Programs for patients having had coronary bypass surgery have similar principles but may be initiated earlier and progress more rapidly. Major benefits in this group include decreased postsurgical stiffness and guarding, prevention of atelectasis, and decreased postoperative depression.

walking

222 Certain principles regarding cardiovascular conditioning should be emphasized to the patient when an exercise prescription is given. They include the following five points:

1. Instruct the patient always to begin an exercise session with a warm-up period and end it with a _____ period.

cool-down

The warm-up period may be as long as 5 to 15 minutes. It allows the cardiovascular system to adapt gradually rather than abruptly to *(increased/decreased)* oxygen demands associated with exercise. A warm-up also may prevent musculoskeletal pulls and injuries.

increased

The cool-down period after exercise should also be *(gradual/abrupt)* so that the body can adapt to any oxygen debt incurred with exercise.

gradual

A gradual tapering-off of exercise, especially when the patient is upright, also prevents the pooling of blood in the extremities and the possible development of symptomatic hypotension.

Relaxation techniques following the cool-down may also be used to reduce the heart rate and blood pressure further.

2. Instruct the patient to avoid exercising in bad weather, after heavy meals, or during mild illnesses or injuries.

REMEMBER: Ingestion of heavy meals diverts blood to the _____ tract, thus reducing blood flow to the heart and working muscles.

GI

3. With the patient, appropriate exercises with regard to MET level, preference, and cardiovascular conditioning considerations.

REMEMBER: Exercises that involve continuous rhythmic muscle movement (isotonic muscle movement) are those best suited for cardiovascular conditioning. This type of exercise improves the ability of the body to take in and utilize oxygen and is known as _____ exercise. Examples of such exercise include walking, swimming, jogging, rowing, and cycling. Arm training should receive equal emphasis.

aerobic

4. Instruct the patient to avoid exercises that require (1) tensing of muscle against muscle or muscle against extreme resistance, such as lifting weights and pushing furniture, and (2) sudden bursts of activity and competition, such as tennis and racquet ball.

The muscle tensing, or isometric, type of exercise promotes the use of the Valsalva maneuver and exaggerated blood pressure responses. It is especially hazardous for the sedentary adult or cardiovascular patient. Exercises requiring sudden bursts of activities also may impose excessive oxygen demands on the myocardium.

5. Teach the patient to take his or her own pulse so that a target heart rate can be used to gauge exercise limits.

223 NURSING ORDERS: Exercise stress testing

1. Explain the procedure to the patient and obtain his or her signed consent.
2. Assess the patient with special attention to risk factors, exercise patterns, and presence of abnormal heart or lung sounds.
3. Instruct the patient to fast and avoid stimulants, such as smoking or caffeine, before stress testing.
4. Have the patient wear nonrestrictive, comfortable clothing and rubber-soled, supportive shoes. Women should wear bras, unless special supportive shirts are available.

5. Instruct the patient to continue all usual medications, unless specified otherwise by the physician.
6. Do not schedule stress testing on the same day as a glucose tolerance test or barium enema. A glucose load may produce ST shifts and thus alter test results. The laxative preparation used with barium enemas may induce hypokalemia, which also produces ST-T abnormalities.
7. Validate the presence and operation of all emergency equipment.
8. Record a baseline ECG BP and heart rate immediately before testing.
   REMEMBER: Hyperventilation and postural changes may alter the _____ segment and _____ wave.   ST; T
9. Demonstrate the correct stance and gait for the patient, and allow for practice on the treadmill before beginning the test.
10. Emphasize with the patient the importance of reporting even subtle symptoms that could indicate myocardial ischemia.
11. Assess the patient's heart rate, blood pressure, and ST segment carefully during stress testing, recording rhythm strips at intervals specified by the physician. Correlate the responses with the level of work load and other symptomatology.
12. Observe the patient for subtle signs of exercise intolerance, such as changes in facial expression, gait, respiratory rate, skin temperature and color; correlate them with the work load.
13. Encourage the patient to continue with the test if there is no adverse symptomatology or if the target heart rate has not been attained.
14. When the test is terminated, allow the patient to sit; record the heart rate and blood pressure every 1 to 3 minutes, until it has returned to baseline.
15. Instruct the patient not to shower for 1 hour after stress testing to prevent vasomotor alterations that could occur with extremely cold or hot water temperatures.

SUGGESTED READINGS
Pathophysiology of coronary artery disease risk factors

Ackerman AM and others: The multiple risk factor intervention trail (MRMT): implications for nurses, Progress Cardiovasc Nurs 2(3):92, 1987.

Barret-Connor FL: Obesity, atherosclerosis, and coronary artery disease, Part 2, Ann Intern Med 103(6):1010, 1985.

Brown, WV and others: Treatment of common lipoprotein disorders, Progress Cardiovasc Dis 27(1):1, 1984.

Cohn PF: Total ischemic burdern: pathophysiology and prognosis, Am J Cardiol 59(7):7C, 1987.

Cohn PF: Prognostic significance of asymptomatic coronary disease, Am J Cardiol 58(4):51B, 1986.

Conti CR: Unstable angina before and after infarction: thoughts on pathogenesis and therapeutic strategies, Heart Lung 15(4):361, 1986.

Deanfield JE and others: Clinical evaluation of transient myocardial ischemia during daily life, Am J Med 79(3A):18, 1985.

Deutscher S et al: Determinants of lipid and lipoprotein levels in elderly men, Atherosclerosis 60(3):221, 1986.

Dunn FG: Arteriosclerotic heart disease in the elderly, Cardiol Clin 4(2):253, 1986.

Gould KL: Assessing coronary stenosis severity a recurrent clinical need, J Am Coll Cardiol 8(1):91, 1986.

Hallfrisch J and others: Modification of the United States' diet to effect changes in blood lipids and lipoprotein distribution, Atherosclerosis 57(2):179, 1985.

Hanby RI and others: Symptomatic coronary disease for 20 or more years: clinical aspects, angiographic findings, and therapeutics implications, Am Heart J 112(11):65, 1986.

Kannel WB: Metabolic risk factors for coronary heart disease in women: perspective from the Framingham study, Am Heart J 114(2):413, 1987.

Kennel WB and Schatzkin A: Risk factor analysis, Progress Cardiovasc Dis 26(4):309, 1984.

Kannel WB: Lipids, diabetes, and coronary heart disease: insights from the Framingham Study, Am Heart J 110(5):1100, 1985.

Klein DM: Angina: physiology, signs, and symptoms, Nursing 14(2):44, 1984.

Lewis B and others: The hyperacute phase of right ventricular infarction, Heart Lung 13(6):682, 1984.

Maseri A and others: Mechanisms of ischemic cardiac pain and silent myocardial ischemia, Am J Med 79(3A):7, 1985.

Maseri A: A symposium: the concept of the total ischemic burden, Am J Cardiol 59(7):1C, 1987.

McGill HC Jr: The cardiovascular pathology of smoking, Part 2, Am Heart J 115(1):250, 1988.

Paoletti R and others: Pharmacological control of serum lipid levels: currently available drugs, Eur Heart J (Suppl)8(E):87, 1987.

Pepper GA: Preventing myocardial infarction: cholestyramine (Questran) and other hypolipidemics, Nurse Pract 11(3):84, 1986.

Pepine CJ and Hill JA: Management of the total ischemic burden in angina pectoris, Am J Cardiol 59(7):7C, 1987.

Raichler JS and others: Importance of risk factors in the angiographic progression of coronary artery disease, Am J Cardiol 57(2):66, 1986.

Roberts R: Stable angina as a manifestation of ischemic heart disease: medical management, Part 2, Circulation 72(6):145, 1985.

Schneider JR: Effects of caffeine ingestion on heart rate, blood pressure, myocardial oxygen consumption, and cardiac rhythm in acute myocardial infarction patients, Heart Lung 16(2):167, 1987.

Singh BN and others: Newer concepts in the pathogenesis of myocardial ischemia: implications for the evaluation of antianginal therapy, Drugs 32(1):1, 1986.

Silinsky J: Your patient's lipid profile, RN 47(9):102, 1984.

Valladares BK: Platelet aggregation and atherosclerosis, Heart Lung 15(2):211, 1986.

Serum enzymes

Gibler W: Myoglobin as an early indicator of acute myocardial infarction, Ann Int Med 16(8):851, 1987.

Ingwall JS and others: The creatine kinase system in normal and diseased human myocardium, N Engl J Med 313(17):1050, 1985.

Pauletto P and others: Changes in myoglobin, creatine kinase and creatine kinase-MB after percutaneous translumial coronary angioplasty for stable angina pectoris, Am J Cardiol 59(9):999, 1987.

Roberts R: Enzymatic diagnosis of acute myocardial infarction, Chest (Suppl):35, 93(1) 1988.

Yusuf S: Significance of elevated MB isoenzyme with normal creatine kinase in acute myocardial infarction, Am J Cardiol 59(4):245, 1987.

ECG changes

Aldrich HR: Identification of the optimal electrocardiographic leads for detecting acute epicardial injury in acute myocardial infarction, Am J Cardiol 59(1):20, 1987.

Ambutas S: A teaching module: EKG interpretation in acute myocardial infarction, Crit Care Update 10(4):48, 1983.

Barold SS and others: Significance of transient electrocardiographic Q waves in coronary artery disease, Cardiol Clin 5(3):367, 1987.

Conner RP: The electrocardiographic diagnosis of posterior myocardial infarction, Crit Care Nurse 5(2):20, 1985.

Conover MB: Understanding electrocardiography: arrhythmias and the 12 lead ECG, ed 5, St. Louis, 1988, The C.V. Mosby Co.

Diamond T: The ST segment axis: a distinguishing feature between acute pericarditis and acute myocardial infarction, Heart Lung 14(6):629, 1985.

Funk M: Diagnosis of right ventricular infarction with right precordial ECG leads, Heart Lung 15(6):562, 1986.

Goldberger AL: Normal and noninfarct Q waves, Cardiol Clin 5(3):357, 1987.

Hoagland P: Right ventricular infarction, CCQ 7(4):19, 1985.

Hoffman JR: Influence of electrocardographic findings on admission decision in patients with acute chest pain, Am J Med 79(6):699, 1985.

Lewis BS: The hyperacute phase of right ventricular infarction, Heart and Lung 13(6):682, 1984.

Pina IL et al: Lead systems: sensitivity and specificity, Cardiol Clin 2(3):329, 1984.

Reddy GV and Schamroth L: The electrocardiography of right ventricular myocardial infarction, Chest 90:756, 1986.

Roberts R: Recognition, pathogenesis, and management of non-Q-wave infarction, Mod Concepts of Cardiovasc Dis 56(4):17, 1987.

Rossignol M and others: Assessment and treatment of right ventricular infarction, Focus Crit Care 12(6):20, 1985.

Severi S and others: Electrocardiographic manifestations and in-hospital prognosis of transient acute myocardial ischemia at rest, Am J Cardiol 61(1):31, 1988.

Singh BN: Hemodynamic and electrocardiographic correlates of symptomatic and silent myocardial ischemia: pathophysiologic and therapeutic implications, Am J Cardiol 58(4):3B, 1986.

Schamroth L: An introduction to electrocardiography, ed 6, Edinburgh, 1982, Blackwell Scientific Publications.

Sweetwood H: Clinical Electrocardiography for Nurses, Rockville, Maryland, 1983, Aspen Publishers Inc.

Tzivoni D and others: The significance of ST abnormalities in myocardial infarction, Cardiol Clin 5(3):419, 1987.

Trasover T: A conceptual approach to the electrocardiogram, Crit Care Nurse 66:76, 1982.

Villaneuva K:; A closer look at inferior wall myocardial infarction, Heart and Lung 14(3):255, 1985.

Warner RA and others: Recent advances in the diagnosis of myocardial infarction, Cardiol Clin 5(3):381, 1987.

Cardiac catheterization/PTCA

Armstrong R and Finisiwer C: Cardiac catheterization, Crit Care Update pgs. 7-15, 1983.

Berger E et al: Sustained efficacy of percutaneous transluminal coronary angioplasty, Am Heart J 111(2):233, 1986.

Disler L: Cardiogenic shock in evolving myocardial infarction: treatment by angioplasty and streptokinase, Heart Lung 16(6):649, 1987.

Galan K and Hollman J: Recurrence of stenoses after coronary angioplasty, Heart Lung 15(6):585, 1986.

Loan T: Nursing interaction with patients undergoing coronary angioplasty, Heart Lung 15(4):368, 1986.

Melchoir JP; Percutaneous transluminal coronary angioplasty for chronic total coronary arterial occlusion, Am J Cardiol 59(6):535, 1987.

Valladares B and Lemberg L: Percutaneous transluminal coronary angioplasty: An update, Heart Lung 14(1):102, 1985.

Watkins L: Preparation for cardiac catheterization: tailoring the content of instruction to coping style, Heart Lung 15(4):382, 1986.

Willerson JT: Selection of patients for coronary arteriography, Part 2, Circulation 72(6):V3, 1985.

Radionuclide studies

Altschule MD: Thallium 201 myocardial imaging: seeing is believing—believing what ?, Chest 89(6):880, 1986.

Bentley LJ: Radionuclide imaging techniques in the diagnosis and treatment of coronary heart disease, Focus Crit Care 14(6):27, 1987.

Beller G: Role of nuclear cardiology in evaluating the total ischemic burden in coronary artery disease, Am J Cardiol 59(7):31C, 1987.

Corbitt J and others: Prognostic value of submaximal exercise radionuclide ventriculography after myocardial infarction, Am J Cardiol 52:82A, 1983.

Gibbons RJ and others: Non-invasive identification of severe coronary artery disease using exercise radionuclide angiography, J Am Coll Cardiol 11(1):28, 1988.

Iskandrian AS and others: Radionuclide evaluation of exercise left ventricular performance in patients with coronary artery disease, Am Heart J 110(4):851, 1985.

Steinberg EP and others: Exercise thallium scans: patterns of use and impact on management of patients with known or suspected coronary artery disease, Am J Cardiol 59(1):50, 1987.

Winters W and Cashion R: Imaging techniques in patients with acute myocardial infarction, Heart Lung 14(3):259, 1985.

Stress and psychological aspects

Boykoff SL: Visitation needs reported by patient with cardiac disease and their families, Heart Lung 15(6):573, 1986.

Bramwell L: Wives' experiences in the support role after husbands' first myocardial infarction, Heart Lung 15(6)578, 1986.

Burgess AW and others: Patient's perception of the ecardiac crisis: key to recovery, Am J Nurs 86(5):568, 1986.

Costa PT Jr: Influence of the normal personality dimension of neuroticism on chest pain symptoms and coronary artery disease, Am J Card 60(18):20J, 1987.

Fournet K and others: What about spouses? S-O-S !, Foc Crit Care 13(1):14, 1986.

Jones JG and others: Goal setting; a method to help patients escape the negative effects of stress, Postgrad Med 83(1):237, 1988.

Moreno CK: Concepts of stress management in cardiac rehabilitation, Focus Crit Care 14(5):13, 1987.

Nyamathi AM: The coping responses of female spouses of patients with myocardial infarction, Heart Lung 16(1):86, 1987.

Pollock SE: The stress response, CCQ 6(4):1, 1984.

Ramsey PW: Bringing a patient through ICU psychosis, RN 49(9):42, 1986.

Rowe MA and others: The CCU experience: stressful or reassuring ?, Dimens Crit Care Nurs 6(6):341, 1987.

Runion J: A program for psychological and social enhancement during rehabilitation after myocardial infarction, Heart Lung 14(2):117, 1985.

Talbert R: Pharmacotherapeutic modification of the stress response by anxiolytics, CCQ 6(4):58, 1984.

Tzivoni D and others: Myocardial ischemia dur-

ing daily activities and stress, Am J Cardiol 58(4):47B, 1986.

Weiss S: Psychophysiologic effects of care giver touch on incidence of cardiac dysrhythmia, Heart Lung 15(5):495, 1986.

Woods JH and others: The relationship of stress management training to the experience of pain in clients with intractable angina, J Holistic Nurs 5(1):11, 1987.

Williams RB: Refining the type A hypothesis: emergence of the hostility complex, Am J Cardiol 60(18):27J, 1987.

Patient teaching, rehabilitation, and exercise stress testing

Blumenthal JA and others: Comparison of high and low intensity exercise training early after acute myocardial infarction, Am J Cardiol 61(1):26, 1988.

Boogard MA: Rehabilitation of the female patient after myocardial infarction, Nurs Clin North Am 19(3):433, 1984.

Burke L and others: Nursing diagnoses, indicators, and interventions in an outpatient cardiac rehabilitation program, Heart Lung 15(1):70, 1986.

Caplin M: Early mobilization of uncomplicated myocardial infarct patients, Focus Crit Care 13(2):36, 1986.

Chavez CW and Faber L: Effect of an education-orientation program on family members who visit their significant other in the intensive care unit, Heart Lung 16(1):92, 1987.

Clark PI: Arrhythmias and conduction disturbances: impact on exercise testing, Cardiol Clin 2(3):359, 1984.

Clark PI: Physiologic signs and symptoms: contribution to the interpretation of the exercise test, Cardiol Clin 2(3):355, 1984.

Coplan NL: Principles of exercise prescription for patients with coronary artery disease, Am Heart J 112(1):145, 1986.

Crean P and others: Exercise electrocardiography in coronary heart disease, QJ Med 62(237):7, 1987.

Crowther M: Sex questions a cardiac patient may be too scared to ask, RN 49(10):44, 1986.

Ehsani AA: Cardiac rehabilitation, Cardiol Clin 2(1):63, 1984.

Fletcher G: Exercise and exercise testing: current state of the art, Heart Lung 13(1):5, 1984.

Glasser SP: Exercise-induced S-T segment alterations, Cardiol Clin 2(3):311, 1984.

Jesson A: Planning patient care: rehabilitation after myocardial infarction, Nurs Times 82(42): 44, 1986.

Mickus D: Activities of daily living in women after myocardial infarction, Heart Lung 15(4):376, 1986.

Mills G and others: An evaluation of an inpatient cardiac patient/family education program, Heart Lung 14(4):400, 1985.

Moynihan M: Assessing the educational needs of post-myocardial infarction patients, Nurs Clin North Am 19(3):441, 1984.

Swahn E and others: Predictive importance of clinical findings and a predischarge exercise test in patients with suspected unstable coronary artery disease, Am J Cardiol 59(4):208, 1987.

VanCamp SP and others: Cardiovascular complications of outpatient cardiac rehabilitation programs, JAMA 256(9):1160, 1986.

Wenger N: Early ambulation physical activity: myocardial infarction and coronary artery bypass surgery, Heart Lung 13(1):14, 1984.

Wenger NK: Cardiovascular drugs: effects on exercise testing and exercise training of the coronary patient, Cardiovasc Clin 15(2):133, 1985.

Miscellaneous

Ahnve S and others: Limitations and advantages of the ejection fraction for defining high risk after acute myocardial infarction, Am J Cardiol 58:872, 1986.

Andreoli KG and others: Comprehensive cardiac care, ed 6, St. Louis, The CV Mosby Co.

Armstrong WF: Echocardiography in coronary artery disease, Progr Cardiovasc Dis 30(4):267, 1988.

Boylan A and others: Myocardial infarction, Nurs Times 81(46):35, 1985.

Braunwald E, editor: Heart disease: a textbook of cardiovascular medicine, ed 3, Philadelphia, 1988, WB Saunders Co.

Boone S and others: Nursing management of the patient with acute myocardial infarction, Cardiovasc Clinics 16(3):73, 1986.

Bondestam E and others: Pain assessment by patients and nurses in the early phase of myocardial infarction, J Adv Nurs 12(6):677, 1987.

DeBusk RF and others: Identification and treatment of low-risk patients after acute myocardial infarction and coronary bypass surgery, N Engl J Med 314:161, 1986.

Doenges ME and Moorhouse MF: Nursing diagnoses with interventions, ed 2, Philadelphia, 1986, FA Davis Co.

Goldstein JA and others: Evaluation of left ventricular thrombi by contrast-enhanced computed tomography and two-dimensional echocardiography, Am J Cardiol 57(10):757, 1986.

Gordon M: Nursing diagnosis: process and application, ed 2, New York, 1987, McGraw-Hill Inc.

Goldberg RJ and others: Outcome after cardiac arrest during acute myocardial infarction, Am J Cardiol 59:251, 1987.

Hurst WJ and Logue RB, editors: The heart, arteries, and veins, ed 6, New York, 1986, McGraw-Hill Inc.

Jaffe AS: Complications of acute myocardial infarction, Cardiol Clin 2:79, 1984.

Klein DM: Angina: physiology, signs, and symptoms, Nursing 14(2):44, 1984.

Meador B: Warning signs to watch for in your post-MI patient, RN 44(7):25, 1981.

Moorhouse MF and others: Critical care plans: guidelines for patient care, Philadelphia, 1987, FA Davis Co.

Moore CA and others: Post-infarction ventricular septal rupture: the importance of location of infarction and right ventricular function in determining survival, Circulation 74:45, 1986.

Riegal BJ: The role of nursing in limiting myocardial infarct size, Heart Lung 14(3):247, 1985.

Schneider AC: Unreported chest pain in a coronary care unit, Focus Crit Care 14(5):21, 1987.

Turi ZG and others: Electrocardiographic, enzymatic, and scintigraphic criteria of acute myocardial infarction as determined from study of 726 patients (A MILIS study), Am J Cardiol 55:1463, 1985.

Valladares BK and others: Coronary and esophageal diseases: symptoms overlap, Heart Lung 14(3):310, 1985.

White RD and others: Segmental evaluation of left ventricular wall motion after myocardial infarction: magnetic resonance imaging versus echocardiography, Part 1, Am Heart J 115(1):166, 1988.

Yacone L: Acute MI: the first crucial hours, RN, pp. 20-27, 1986.

Yacone L: Acute MI: the road to recovery, RN 49(2):45, 1986.

Electrical Complications in Coronary Artery Disease: Arrhythmias

---

1 The heart has been described as having both electrical and mechanical properties. The *three* electrical properties of the heart are: (1) _____, (2) _____, and (3) _____.   automaticity; excitability conductivity

    REMEMBER: The ability of the heart to *initiate electrical* impulses is known as _____. The ability of the heart to *respond* to electrical impulses is known as _____. The ability of the heart to *transmit* electrical impulses is known as _____.   automaticity

excitability

conductivity

2 When there are disturbances in the electrical activity of the heart, arrhythmias occur.

    Arrhythmias, then, are manifestations of abnormal _____ _____. They may also be referred to as *dysrhythmias*. Generally arrhythmias may be considered to be a result of disturbances in *automaticity, conduction,* or *both*.   electrical; activity

    NOTE: Arrhythmias are considered to be *ectopic* when they originate outside the SA node.

    Before discussing the pathophysiology of arrhythmias, let us again consider the innervation of the heart and its relationship to *automaticity* and *conduction*.

3 The heart is richly innervated by both sympathetic and parasympathetic nerves.

    REMEMBER: The sympathetic nervous system supplies the _____ node, the _____ muscle, the _____ _____ tissue, and the _____ muscle.   SA; atrial

AV junctional

ventricular

    Sympathetic stimulation: (1) (*increases/decreases*) automaticity in the SA node and (2) (*accelerates/slows*) AV conduction.   increases

accelerates

    Parasympathetic (vagal) fibers supply the _____ node, the _____ muscle, and the _____ _____ tissue.   SA

atrial; AV junctional

Parasympathetic stimulation: (1) (*increases/decreases*) automaticity in the SA node and (2) *(accelerates/slows)* AV conduction.

    Thus the sympathetic and parasympathetic nervous systems strongly influence the properties of _____ and _____.

decreases
slows

automaticity
conduction

PATHOPHYSIOLOGY OF ARRHYTHMIAS: OVERVIEW

4 Arrhythmias may be *generally* considered as resulting from disturbances in _____ or _____ or both.

automaticity; conduction

5 *Automaticity* is the ability of certain areas of the heart to _____ electrical impulses. The areas of the heart that normally have the property of automaticity are the _____ node, the AV _____ tissue, and the _____ _____ system of the ventricles. In the presence of certain pathologies, the *atria* can also have the property of automaticity. Disturbances in automaticity may result in arrhythmias that arise from the normal pacemaker area, the _____ node, or in *ectopic* sites.

    REMEMBER: Arrhythmias are considered to be ectopic when they originate *(within/outside)* the SA node. Ectopic arrhythmias typically result in tachyarrhythmias and may be either ventricular or supraventricular in origin. Ectopic supraventricular arrhythmias originate above the ventricles in the _____ or AV _____.

initiate
SA
junctional; bundle
  branch-Purkinje

SA

outside

atria
junction

6 Conduction is the ability of an impulse to be _____.

    Transmission of a cardiac impulse normally occurs in a *uniform* and *synchronous* manner. Disturbances in conduction may result in either *blocks* in conduction and bradyarrhythmias or in the *generation* of *ectopic impulses* and tachyarrhythmias.

transmitted

Tachyarrhythmias

7 Tachycardias are defined as rhythms with ventricular rates exceeding 100 beats per minute. Therefore tachyarrhythmias are arrhythmias with rates exceeding _____ beats per minute. Tachyarrhythmias are potentially clinically significant because they may cause a symptomatic *fall in cardiac output,* increase the O_2 demands of the myocardium, and decrease coronary blood supply. Tachyarrhythmias originating in the ventricles are particularly clinically significant because they may degenerate into *ventricular fibrillation.*

100

8 Tachyarrhythmias may result from either enhanced automaticity or altered conduction.

9 The clinical factors that have been identified as *enhancing automaticity* in a patient with acute MI may be grouped into three categories: (1) lack of oxygen, (2) chemical toxicity, and (3) stretch. A more complete list of factors can be incorporated under these three major headings:

  I. Lack of oxygen
    A. Local myocardial ischemia
    B. Respiratory dysfunction with hypoxemia
    C. Systemic hypoxia (shock)
    D. Metabolic demands (fever, sepsis, hyperthyroidism)
    E. Anemia
  II. Chemical toxicity
    A. Drug toxicity (digitalis, isoproterenol (Isuprel), epinephrine)
    B. Electrolyte imbalances (decreased K^+, Ca^{++}, Mg^{++})
    C. Acid-base imbalances
    D. Stress
 III. Stretch
    A. Heart failure
    B. Aneurysm

10 Tachyarrhythmias may also be produced by _____ conduction.   **altered**

The clinical factors that *alter conduction* and result in tachyarrhythmias are very similar to those that enhance automaticity. They include:

1. Hypoxia
2. Electrolyte imbalances
3. Acid-base imbalances
4. Drugs
5. Surgical incisions (areas of edema)
6. Scar tissue

ARRHYTHMOGENIC FACTORS

(Automaticity and reentry)

1. **Hypoxia**
    A. Local ischemia
    B. Systemic (O_2/blood supply)
    C. Metabolic needs (O_2 demands)

Fig. 7-1.

2. **Toxicity**
    A. Drugs/stress/hormones
    B. Lytes
    C. Acid/base

3. **Stretch**
    A. CHF
    B. Aneurysms

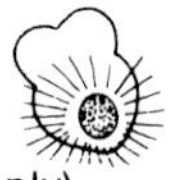

Disturbances in conduction produce ectopic impulses and tachyarrhythmias by the process known as *reentry* (see Frames 39 to 51). The related clinical factors are similar to those enhancing automaticity.

Bradyarrhythmias

11 Bradycardias, or bradyarrhythmias, are usually associated with ventricular rates of less than 60 beats per minute. When automaticity, conduction, or both are *depressed,* bradyarrhythmias, or *(fast/slow)* rates, occur.   slow

In the presence of *depressed automaticity,* the rate of impulse discharge from automatic centers *(decreases/increases).* When *conduction* is   decreases
depressed, the transmission of an impulse may be *delayed* or *blocked* in any structure of the conduction system. Depressed automaticity and depressed conduction often occur together and thus in conjunction cause bradyarrhythmias, or _____ rates.   slow

12 Bradyarrhythmias are clinically significant *when:* (1) they cause a symptomatic fall in cardiac output, and (2) they allow for the breakthrough of dangerous tachyarrhythmias. Clinical factors that have been identified as *depressing automaticity* and *conduction* include:
1. Ischemia or infarction of the conduction structures
2. Electrolyte imbalances (increased K^+, Ca^{++}, Mg^{++})
3. Drug toxicity (digitalis, propranolol [Inderal])
4. Parasympathetic stimulation such as that associated with Valsalva maneuvers (rectal stimulation, carotid sinus pressure)

CLINICAL SIGNIFICANCE OF ARRHYTHMIAS

13 Arrhythmias may be grouped according to clinical significance into either *acutely* life threatening or *potentially* life threatening. The acutely life-threatening arrhythmias are those indicating actual cardiac arrest and are therefore associated with absence of
_____. They include standstill or asystole; ventricular fi-   pulse
brillation (VF) and ventricular tachycardia (VT). VT may or may not indicate a cardiac arrest, depending on the individual response. Initial therapy for this arrhythmia varies accordingly. Ventricular fibrillation may be further divided into coarse and fine (see Figs. 7-2, 7-29, and 7-30 and Frames 84 to 87).

14 Cardiac arrest may also be associated with electromechanical dissociation (EMD). EMD refers to the absence of a pulse in the presence of normal electrical activity.
REMEMBER: Electrical activity prepares the heart for
_____ activity. Although abnormal electrical activity is eas-   mechanical
ier to correct, mechanical activity is more important because it is the
ensurance of actual _____ action. For every beat on the   pump

CARDIAC ARREST

• Electrical

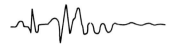

(Acutely life-threatening arrhythmias)

Fig. 7-2

Asystole   VT   VF

• Mechanical

(EMD)

ECG, there should be a corresponding _____. When there are normal beats on the ECG without a corresponding pulse, the phenomenon is referred to as _____ dissociation; it can occur in severe _____, cardiac _____, or tension pneumothorax (see Unit 1, Frame 32).

pulse

electrical-mechanical

CHF; tamponade

15 The *potentially* life-threatening arrhythmias are those that are either associated with significant symptoms or signify impending cardiac arrest. Arrhythmias become potentially life threatening under three conditions: (1) when they originate in the *ventricles*, (2) when they result in a critically *slow ventricular rate*, and (3) when they result in a critically *fast ventricular rate*. Therefore, the three most significant types of arrhythmias are (1) the _____ tachyarrhythmias, (2) the _____ arrhythmias, and (3) the supraventricular tachyarrhythmias.

ventricular

brady-

POTENTIALLY LIFE-THREATENING
ARRHYTHMIAS

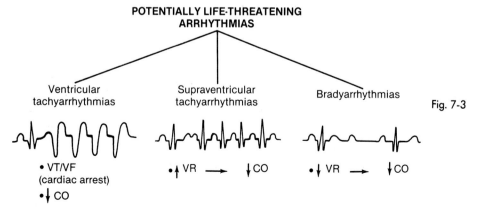

Ventricular
tachyarrhythmias

Supraventricular
tachyarrhythmias

Bradyarrhythmias

Fig. 7-3

• VT/VF
(cardiac arrest)
• ↓ CO

• ↑ VR → ↓ CO

• ↓ VR → ↓ CO

16 Ventricular arrhythmias are clinically significant because they may result in ventricular tachycardia (VT) or _____ _____. VT is clinically significant because it may result in a symptomatic fall in _____ _____ or cardiac arrest, or it may lead to _____, another form of _____ _____.

    VF is clinically significant because it is essentially a state of no _____ _____, or clinical _____. Ventricular arrhythmias potentially leading to VF are the most _____ significant. The ventricular arrhythmias commonly leading to VF in the setting of acute MI are the following:
1. PVC on T wave (R on T phenomenon)
2. Frequent PVCs (> 6/min)
3. Multifocal PVCs
4. Consecutive PVCs with a ventricular rate > 100 (see Frames 77 to 79).

ventricular
fibrillation (VF)
cardiac output
VF
cardiac arrest

cardiac output; death

clinically

17 Bradyarrhythmias are clinically significant when (1) they result in a symptomatic fall in cardiac output, or (2) they allow for the breakthrough of dangerous tachyarrhythmias. Bradyarrhythmias may cause a fall in cardiac output because

    Cardiac output = stroke volume × _____ _____

heart rate

The following symptoms reflect a significant fall in cardiac output:
1. Hypotension (cold, clammy skin)
2. Sensorium changes
3. Left ventricular failure
4. Fall in urinary output

18 Supraventricular tachyarrhythmias are clinically significant when they result in a fall in cardiac output and compromise cardiac function. Tachyarrhythmias may decrease cardiac output by shortening ventricular filling time in *(systole/diastole)*. The coronary arteries receive their blood supply during *diastole*. In the presence of tachyarrhythmias, therefore, coronary blood flow may be reduced.

diastole

    Fast supraventricular arrhythmias may decrease cardiac output by (1) *(decreasing/increasing)* ventricular filling time, and (2) *(decreasing/increasing)* coronary blood flow.

decreasing; decreasing

19 Initial therapy in the management of ventricular arrhythmias is directed toward depressing _____ _____ in the ventricles. Subsequent therapy would be directed toward correcting the _____ cause. In the setting of acute MI, ventricular arrhythmias are most commonly a manifestation of (1) electrical _____ caused by ischemic areas, (2) electrolyte imbalance (hypo _____), and (3) drug _____.

ectopic activity

underlying

instability
kalemia; toxicity

Initial therapy in the management of bradyarrhythmias is directed toward accelerating the _____ _____.   ventricular rate

REMEMBER: The most common cause of bradyarrhythmias in the setting of a CCU is probably *IWMI.*

Initial therapy in the management of fast supraventricular arrhythmias in directed toward decreasing the _____   ventricular rate
_____. Subsequent therapy may be directed toward depressing _____ automaticity and correcting the   atrial
_____ cause.   underlying

REMEMBER: The most common cause of fast supraventricular arrhythmias in the setting of acute MI is _____   heart
_____.   failure

20 NURSING ORDERS: The patient with an arrhythmia
1. Anticipate and be prepared for *bradyarrhythmias* and *ventricular* arrhythmias in the first 48 hours.
   —In anticipation of bradyarrhythmia, have atropine, isoproterenol (Isuprel), an external transthoracic pacemaker and equipment for pacemaker insertion available.
   —In anticipation of ventricular arrhythmias, have lidocaine (Xylocaine), procainamide (Pronestyl), bretylium, and equipment for countershock available.
2. If life-threatening arrhythmias should occur, immediate IV therapy is required. Therefore make certain the patient has a patent IV at all times.
3. Monitor for the effects of drugs, electrolyte imbalances, hypoxic states, and any changes in the QRS morphology with a standard 12-lead ECG.
   REMEMBER: Consider low Mg^{++} as well as low K^+ levels in repetitive VF.
4. When an arrhythmia occurs, observe how the patient is tolerating the arrhythmia. Report:
   —Changes in sensorium.
   —Changes in skin color and temperature.
   —Change in the rate or character of respirations.
   —Hypotension.
   —Left ventricular failure (rales, gallops).
   —Decrease in urinary output.
5. Record on ECG strip an example of any arrhythmia. If possible, record the initiating factor.
6. Have resuscitation equipment and emergency drugs immediately available as per American Heart Association standards. (For more specific information refer to the Nursing Orders for ventricular and supraventricular arrhythmias and bradyarrhythmias and the related drug therapy in Unit 10.)

DISTURBANCES IN AUTOMATICITY: ROLE OF NA⁺/CA⁺⁺

21 Cells which normally demonstrate the property of automaticity are characteristically unstable cells.

REMEMBER: Automaticity is a normal property of conduction structures such as the _____ node, the _____ node (or AV junction) and ventricular _____ fibers. Tachyarrhythmias or bradyarrhythmias may be caused by these normally automatic areas when their automaticity or *(stability/instability)* is suppressed or enhanced by clinical factors (Fig. 7-1). Arrhythmias may also be caused by normally stable cells that have become unstable or _____ secondary to pathological changes.

SA; AV
Purkinje

instability

automatic

22 The electrical characteristics of stable atrial and ventricular muscle cells are described in Unit 4.

REMEMBER: The cell membranes of electrically *stable* cells allow them to maintain an *(electronegative/electropositive)* resting charge until a *stimulus* arrives. Depolarization in these stable cells is typically *(Na⁺ dependent/Ca⁺ dependent)*. The resting cell charge or _____ _____ potential is typically _____ mV in these stable cells.

electronegative
Na⁺ dependent
resting membrane
−90

23 Cells with *unstable* cell membranes are not able to sustain this electronegative resting state until a stimulus arrives. Instead, they spontaneously start to lose their electronegativity and begin to depolarize. These cells *(do/do not)* require a stimulus to alter their resting state and initiate depolarization.

do not

REMEMBER: The ability of areas of the heart to spontaneously generate an impulse is known as _____. Automatic cells are electrically *(stable/unstable)* cells that can *(depolarize/repolarize)* spontaneously.

automaticity
unstable; depolarize

24 The resting cell charge of automatic cells is typically lower or less negative than that of nonautomatic cells.

REMEMBER: A lower resting membrane potential favors the opening of *(Na⁺/Ca⁺⁺)* gates or channels. Thus spontaneous depolarization in highly automatic cells such as the SA node or AV junction is predominantly *(Na⁺/Ca⁺⁺)* dependent. Spontaneous depolarization within the ventricular Purkinje fibers remains predominantly *(Na⁺/Ca⁺⁺)* dependent but may also be influenced by Ca⁺⁺ (see Fig. 7-4).

Ca⁺⁺

Ca⁺⁺
Na⁺

Pharmacological Ca⁺⁺ calcium channel blockade results in *(increased/decreased)* automaticity of both the _____ node and _____ junction, especially in the presence of preexisting SA or AV node disease. The effect on the AV junction is the major therapeutic effect of these drugs in arrhythmia control. However, ventricular automaticity *(should/should not)* be significantly affected by Ca⁺⁺ calcium blockade. Enhanced ventricular automaticity is most

decreased
SA
AV

should not

effectively treated by (Na^+/Ca^{++}) channel blockade. (See Unit 10, Antiarrhythmic agents.)

25 Both the resting cell charge and spontaneous depolarization are also influenced by K^+.

REMEMBER: The electronegative resting state or _____ _____ _____ depends on the integrity of the _____ _____ and its resting permeability to _____.

Stable polarized cell membranes are normally permeable to K^+ but not to _____ at rest. Depolarization does not occur until an external stimulus increases _____ permeability.

However, the cell membranes of automatic cells are characteristically (stable/unstable). They lose their selective permeability to K^+ spontaneously while at the same time increasing their permeability to Na^+ or Ca^{++}. Depolarization is thus _____ triggered. Low serum K^+ levels enhance this early shift in permeability, especially in Na^+-dependent cells. Thus a low serum K^+ (increases/decreases) automaticity, especially in the (SA node/ventricles). This effect is magnified in the presence of ischemia, which further alters the integrity and stability of the cell membrane.

26 The electrical changes occurring in automatic cells can be recorded graphically for further consideration and understanding.

REMEMBER: When a single cell is activated by a stimulus, local electrical changes occur, producing an *action current,* or _____ _____ (see Unit 4).

This action potential from one cell can be recorded on graph paper, producing a pattern (see Unit 4, Frames 86 to 94). Phases 0, 1, 2, and 3 of the action potential graph collectively represent phases of electrical action, or electrical (systole/diastole). Phase 4 represents the reestablishment of the resting _____ _____, or electrical (systole/diastole).

27 Automatic cells *depolarize spontaneously* during electrical diastole, or phase _____.

Therefore the property of automaticity is also referred to as phase-4 depolarization, or spontaneous _____ depolarization (SDD). This spontaneous depolarization is associated with the influx of Na^+ and/or Ca^{++} depending on the _____ cell charge (see Fig. 7-4).

28 The ability of an automatic cell to spontaneously depolarize is determined by three interrelated factors: (1) the slope of phase 4, (2) the level of membrane potential at the time of activation (threshold),

Na^+

resting membrane potential

cell membrane
K^+

Na^+
Na^+

unstable

spontaneously

increases
ventricles

action potential

systole
membrane potential
diastole

4

diastolic

resting

and (3) the *maximal* resting membrane potential (RMP) or diastolic potential.

NOTE: For simplification we will use the term "resting membrane potential" (RMP) for maximal diastolic potential.

AUTOMATICITY
Pacemaker cell (SA node)

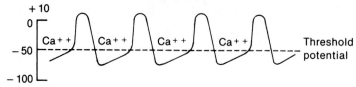

Latent pacemaker (His-Purkinje fiber)

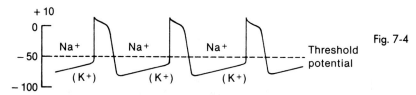

Fig. 7-4

Nonpacemaking cell (contractile muscle fiber)

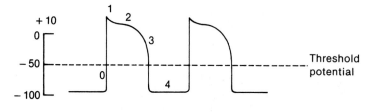

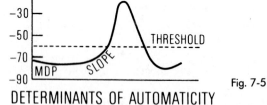

Fig. 7-5

DETERMINANTS OF AUTOMATICITY

1. MAXIMUM DIASTOLIC POTENTIAL
2. THRESHOLD
3. SLOPE

29 The slope or incline of phase 4 reflects the *rate* of diastolic depolarization. The more gradual the slope, or incline, the *(slower/faster)* the rate of automatic discharge. The steeper the slope, or incline, the

slower

(slower/faster) the rate of automatic discharge. Ectopic impulses fire more rapidly when there is an *(increase/decrease)* in the slope of phase 4.

faster
increase

THRESHOLDS

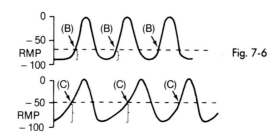

Fig. 7-6

30 Automatic cells must reach a certain level of membrane potential before an action potential is generated. This critical level of membrane potential is known as *threshold.* The automatic cell in Fig. 7-6 begins to depolarize spontaneously during the period indicated below the dotted line. However, an action potential is not generated until the time denoted by the letters *B* and *C.*

Threshold is that critical level of membrane potential at which a cell generates an _____ _____.

action potential

31 The higher the threshold, the *harder* it is for the automatic cell to generate an action potential. *Lowering* the threshold allows the cell to generate an impulse (action potential) more easily because it takes *(more/less)* time for the threshold to be reached. In Fig. 7-6, the threshold at level C is *(higher/lower)*, or less negative, than the former level designated by the letter *B.* Thus it is *(harder/easier)* for the cell to reach the threshold *(C)* for activation and to _____ an impulse. Ectopic impulses are more easily generated when the threshold is *(elevated/lowered).*

less
higher
harder
generate

lowered

32 A third factor relating to automaticity is the level of resting membrane potential at which a cell *starts* to depolarize spontaneously. The greatest resting potential achieved in diastole (phase 4) is called the *resting membrane potential, (RMP).* The more electronegative the cell in phase 4, or the *greater* the RMP, the slower is the rate of automatic firing. That is because the cell will take *(less time/more time)* to reach the threshold.

more time

33 LET US REVIEW: Automaticity is a property of *(stable/unstable)* cells. Disturbances in automaticity can occur in normally automatic cells or in pathologically altered, typically stable cells. The disturbances in automaticity can result in either tachyarrhythmias or _____, which may be either Na^+ dependent or

unstable

bradyarrhythmias

_____ dependent. Automaticity within Na⁺-dependent cells is enhanced in the presence of a *(high/low)* serum K⁺ and _____.

AV junctional arrhythmias are more typically _____-dependent, whereas ventricular arrhythmias are more typically _____ dependent. Supraventricular arrhythmias are most effectively treated by *(Na⁺/Ca⁺⁺)* blocking agents. Ventricular arrhythmias are usually most effectively treated by *(Na⁺/Ca⁺⁺)* blocking agents and by monitoring the serum _____ level, especially in the presence of _____.

Enhanced automaticity can occur in clinical states that either (1) *(increase/decrease)* the slope of phase 4, (2) *(elevate/lower)* the threshold, or (3) *(elevate/lower)* the RMP.

Ca^{++}
low
ischemia
Ca^{++}
Na^+
Ca^{++}
Na^+
K^+
ischemia
increase; lower
lower

DISTURBANCES IN CONDUCTION

34 Conduction is the ability of the heart to _____ electrical impulses. Electrical impulses are transmitted in the heart by the specialized conduction system through the muscle tissue.

transmit

REMEMBER: Transmission of a cardiac impulse normally occurs in a _____ and _____ manner. Disturbances in conduction may result in either conduction _____ or _____ impulses. Disturbances in conduction may produce ectopic impulses by the process of reentry (see Frames 39 to 51). Na⁺ and Ca⁺⁺ play a major role in conduction as well as automaticity and may contribute to the development of reentry circuits.

uniform; synchronous
blocks
ectopic

Role of Na⁺/Ca⁺⁺

35 Depolarization via Na⁺ channels occurs more rapidly than depolarization via Ca⁺⁺ channels. The term "fast cell" is used to describe areas of the heart that depolarize _____ using *(Na⁺/Ca⁺⁺)* channels. The term "slow cell" is used to describe areas of the heart that depolarize _____ using *(Na⁺/Ca⁺⁺)* channels.

rapidly; Na^+

slowly; Ca^{++}

Transmission of the depolarization signal from cell to cell is known as _____. The rate of depolarization and conduction is closely related to the resting cell charge or _____ _____ _____.

conduction

resting membrane potential (RMP)

REMEMBER: Generally, the *more* electronegative the cell, or the greater the RMP, the *(slower/faster)* is the rate of depolarization (activated or spontaneous) and conduction. Na⁺-dependent, fast cells typically have a *(high/low)* RMP of _____ mV. Ca⁺-dependent, slow cells typically have a *(higher/lower)* RMP.

faster

high; −90
lower

NOTE: Initial treatment in the management of supraventricular arrhythmias is directed toward the control of the ventricular rate via the AV node (slow cell) transmission. Complete abolishment of the arrhythmia may require the addition of an Na^+-channel blocking to stabilize the atrial (fast cell) Purkinje fibers.

36 Factors such as drugs, electrolyte imbalance, and ischemia may lower the resting membrane potential and *(hypopolarize/hyperpolarize)* the myocardial muscle and/or conduction structures. This effect may depress the conduction of the normally fast ventricular cells or facilitate their conversion to slow cells. Depressed and/or nonuniform conduction within ventricular Purkinje fibers can facilitate the development of ventricular reentry circuits and contribute to ventricular arrhythmias. Ventricular arrhythmias caused by either automaticity or reentry (altered conduction) are most effectively treated—at least initially—by *(Na^+/Ca^{++})*-channel blocking agents.

hypopolarize

Na^+

NOTE: Ventricular arrhythmias unresponsive to Na^+-channel blockade may respond to subsequent Ca^{++}-channel blockade, since these arhythmias may be associated with pathologically converted slow cells. However, the greater sensitivity of the AV node to Ca^{++} blockade must be carefully considered, since AV block usually occurs before the effects on ventricular arrhythmias are seen.

37 Cells that have a low RMP are *(more/less)* electronegative in the resting state than other cardiac cells. For this reason slow cells may also be described as *(hyperpolarized/hypopolarized)*. Hypopolarization favors a *(Ca^{++}/Na^+)* channel or *(fast/slow)* cell activity.

less

hypopolarized
Ca^{++}; slow

Slow cells depolarize and conduct *(rapidly/slowly)*. Fast cells depolarize and conduct *(rapidly/slowly)*. Slow cells depolarize slowly because of the low RMP and slow *influx* of Ca^{++}. They also repolarize slowly because of an extended refractory period that is closely related to the extended action of Ca^{++} into early repolarization.

slowly
rapidly

REMEMBER: Unlike Na^+, the effects of Ca^{++} extend into _____ as the Ca^{++} gates remain open and then _____ close (see Unit 4, Frames 81, 87, and 94).

repolarization
slowly

38 This effect on repolarization as well as depolarization may further contribute to the development of reentry circuits.

Slow-channel activity contributes to the normal delay in AV node conduction and recovery and facilitates AV node reentry. This type of reentry plays a major role in *(ventricular/supraventricular)* arrhythmias and is highly susceptible to Ca^{++}-channel blockade. Thus ectopic supraventricular arrhythmias caused by either automaticity or reentry (altered conduction) are most effectively treated—at least initially—by *(Na^+/Ca^{++})*-channel blocking agents.

supraventricular

Ca^{++}

Concept of reentry

39 Let us now consider how alterations in conduction and refractoriness occurring in either slow or fast cells may contribute to the formation of ectopic impulses and ventricular or supraventricular tachyarrhythmias.

Local disturbances in conduction may produce ectopic impulses by the process known as *reentry*. Reentry is defined as the ability of an impulse to reexcite some region of the heart through which it has already passed. Reentry usually occurs when an impulse deviates around a circular conduction pathway, forming a loop.

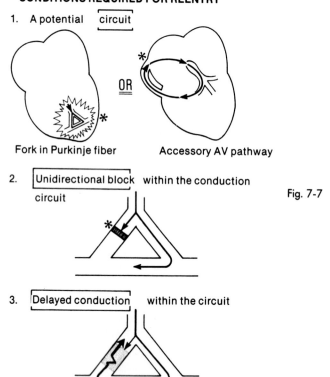

CONDITIONS REQUIRED FOR REENTRY

1. A potential   circuit

OR

Fork in Purkinje fiber   Accessory AV pathway

2. Unidirectional block within the conduction

circuit   Fig. 7-7

3. Delayed conduction   within the circuit

40 Three conditions are necessary for reentry to occur. They include (1) a potential conduction circuit, or _____ conduction _____; (2) block within part of the circuit; and (3) delayed conduction within the remainder of the circuit.

circular
pathway

41 Many small potential circuits (microcircuits) normally exist within the conduction system. These circuits are classically noted within the AV node and in atrial and ventricular conduction tissue where terminal Purkinje fibers attach to cardiac muscle (Fig. 7-8).

REENTRY CIRCUIT (MICRO)

AV node   **Purkinje fibers**

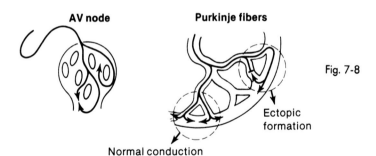

Fig. 7-8

Ectopic
formation

Normal conduction

42 Macrocircuits, or larger _____ paths, may also form. These circuits are at least partially composed of cardiac conduction tissue. Examples include circuits formed by congenital accessory pathways or by the AV node microcircuits *functionally* grouped together into two major pathways (Fig. 7-9).

circular

REENTRY CIRCUIT (MACRO)

AV node   **Kent pathway** (WPW)

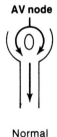 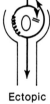 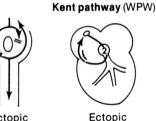

Fig. 7-9

Normal   Ectopic   Ectopic
                formation   formation

43 The macrocircuits are thought to play a major role in potentially life-threatening arrhythmias that are not necessarily associated with acute MI. These include the supraventricular tachyarrhythmias. Microcircuits within the ventricle probably play a more significant role in the setting of acute MI. Although currently a popular theory, their confirmed existence is still questioned by certain authorities in the field of cardiology.

44 Normally the impulse travels through the conduction fibers in an *even* and *synchronous* manner and collides with itself in the potential circuits (see Figs 7-4 and 7-5). However, ischemia can affect selected portions of these conduction fibers, depressing conduction or converting fast cells to slow or *(hypopolarized/hyperpolarized)* cells. Slow cells also recover slowly from previous impulses. Thus they may not conduct new approaching impulses.

hypopolarized

REMEMBER: Slow cells have extended _____ periods.

refractory

45 An impulse entering a circuit that is altered in this way may be *blocked* anterogradely in one arm of the circular path (see Fig. 7-7).

  When an impulse is blocked in *one direction* through a pathway, *unidirectional block* is said to exist. When unidirectional block occurs, the electrical impulse detours away from the blocked area. The impulse subsequently deviates around the circular conduction pathway, forming a _____. Impulse transmission is thus *nonuniform,*   loop
or *asynchronous.*

46 The impulse enters the ischemic area in a *retrograde* direction and is conducted through this tissue *slowly.*

  REMEMBER: These ischemic (slow) cells have *(prolonged/shortened)*   prolonged
refractory periods. If tissue surrounding the previously blocked area has recovered excitability, the emerging impulse will reenter this adjacent tissue. As a result, the *original impulse* will reexcite or depolarize an area through which it has previously passed. A normal impulse, in this way, may result in the generation of an _____   ectopic
impulse (Fig. 7-10).

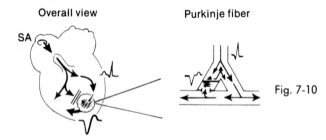

Overall view   Purkinje fiber

SA

Fig. 7-10

REENTRY

47 If the reentrant impulse exits early in repolarization, when the disparity in recovery is still pronounced, the impulse may recycle within the circuit, producing a *chain reaction response.* This response may disintegrate further into chaotic electrical activity and corresponds with the _____period of the heart (see Unit 2, Frames   vulnerable
20 to 23).

48 Ectopic impulses generated as a result of reentry are usually precipitated by *fast rates,* which limit recovery time. Ectopic impulses caused by enhanced automaticity are typically abolished in the presence of fast rates and facilitated in the presence of slow rates. Reentrant tachycardias are characteristically *interrupted* by delivery of single electrical stimuli that break the circuit. They are also typically *triggered* by single electrical stimuli.

49 The formation of a reentrant ectopic impulse is closely related to the conduction of the preceding impulse. Thus the ectopic impulse occurs at a fixed distance from the original impulse. This fixed interval is known as the *coupling interval*.

ECG SUPPORT

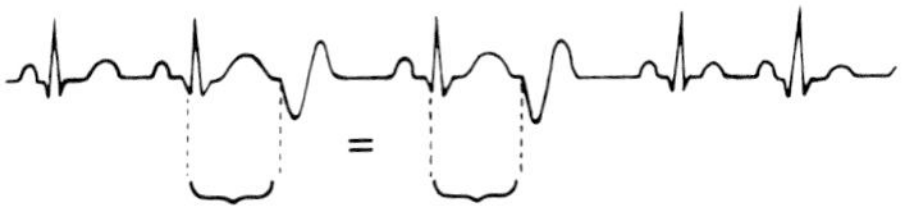

Fig. 7-11

Coupling intervals

When ectopic beats of the same focus occur at fixed coupling intervals, their mechanism of origin is *more likely (automaticity/reentry)*.

reentry

The existence of a reentrant phenomenon is also assumed when tachyarrhythmias are precipitated by *(fast/slow)* rates and are initiated and/or terminated by single _____ _____.

fast
electrical stimuli

50 LET US REVIEW: Reentry occurs because of alterations in _____ of an impulse. Reentry is defined as the ability of an impulse to _____ some region through which it has previously passed. Conditions necessary for reentry to occur include (1) a potential _____, (2) unidirectional _____, and (3) slow _____. A circuit is a circular _____, or _____, through which impulses that exit at a critical time during recovery may pass again, producing a _____ _____ response. Reentrant ectopic beats from the same focus typically exhibit fixed _____ intervals.

conduction
reexcite

circuit
block; conduction
pathway; loop

chain reaction

coupling

51 The clinical factors that may enhance reentry are very similar to those that enhance automaticity. They include the following:
1. Hypoxia
2. _____ imbalances
3. Acid-base imbalances
4. _____
5. Surgical incisions (areas of edema)

electrolyte

drugs

In acute MI, peak occurrences of reentry have been reported in immediate (first 24 hours) and delayed (after 3 days) phases.

IDENTIFICATION OF ARRHYTHMIAS ON THE ECG

52 When identifying arrhythmias, nurses are encouraged to use the following systematic approach:
1. Analyze the _____ complex.
2. Analyze the _____ wave.
3. Analyze the relationship between the P wave and the QRS _____: the _____ interval.

QRS
P

complex; PR

The first part of the ECG to be considered is the _____ complex.

QRS

REMEMBER: The QRS complex represents depolarization of the _____.

ventricles

53 Analysis of the QRS complex provides information about the origin of the ventricular impulse. The origin of the impulse may be *ventricular* or *supraventricular*.

If the impulse originates *in the ventricles*, the rhythm is described as _____. If the impulse originates *above the ventricles*, the rhythm is described as _____.

ventricular
supraventricular

REMEMBER: The structures above the ventricles that have the ability to initiate impulses are: the _____ node, the _____, and the _____ _____ tissue.

SA
atria; AV junctional

Therefore, sinus, atrial, and nodal or junctional arrhythmias are classified as _____ arrhythmias.

supraventricular

Supraventricular impulses are usually transmitted through the *normal* AV conduction pathways to the ventricles. When an impulse reaches the ventricles through these normal AV pathways, the ventricular musculature is depolarized *rapidly* and the resulting QRS complex is *narrow*, that is, less than 0.12 second.

Thus supraventricular impulses will *usually* produce *(narrow/wide)* QRS complexes.

narrow

If we considered one patient, we would expect that *all* impulses arising *above* the ventricles should be conducted similarly through the AV node, His bundle, and the bundle branches to reach the ventricles. Therefore all supraventricular impulses in a particular patient should produce QRS complexes having the *same* configuration.

Supraventricular impulses may therefore be described as producing QRS complexes that are *(narrow/wide)* and unchanging.

narrow

54 Impulses arising in the ventricles *(are/are not)* transmitted through the normal conduction pathways. As a result, depolarization of the ventricular musculature occurs *slowly* or with *delay*. Thus ventricular impulses *usually* produce a QRS complex that is *(narrow/wide)*. Another characteristic of ventricular impulses is that they *always* produce QRS complexes *different* from the patient's normal complexes.

are not

wide

Ventricular impulses may therefore be described as producing QRS complexes are *usually (narrow/wide)* and *always* _____ from the patient's normal complexes.

wide
different

Thus analysis of the QRS complexes enables us to ascertain whether the origin of an impulse is _____ or _____.

ventricular
supraventricular

55 Analysis of the P wave and calculation of the atrial rate aid in the differential diagnosis of supraventricular arrhythmias. Analysis of the PR interval provides information about the relationship between the atria and the ventricles and aids in the diagnosis of atrioventricular (AV) blocks.

NOTE: The origin of the rhythm is determined first. Next the discharge sequence—rate or timing of the impulse—is determined; and finally the conduction sequence is noted.

DISTURBANCES IN A SA NODE FUNCTION

56 REMEMBER: The SA node normally has the property of *automaticity*. Normally, electrical impulses arise from the SA node and drive the heart at a rate of _____ to _____ beats per minute.   60; 100

NOTE: The sinus rate may be calculated on the ECG by measuring the _____ wave rate (see Unit 2).   P

Sinus tachycardia

57 When automaticity in the SA node is enhanced, impulse discharge will *(increase/decrease)*.   increase

Increased automaticity in the SA node may result in an arrhythmia known as _____ tachycardia.   sinus

Sinus tachycardia generally falls in the range of 101 to 150 beats per minute.

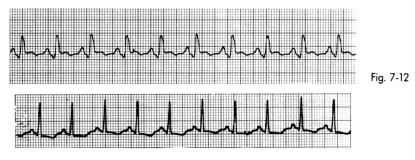

Fig. 7-12

58 Some factors have been identified as enhancing automaticity in the SA node. In the setting of acute MI, the most significant factors are (1) sympathetic stimulation (fever, pain, anxiety); (2) heart failure; (3) hypoxia; and (4) drugs (atropine, isoproterenol, aminophylline). Initial therapy in the management of sinus tachycardia is directed toward correcting the *underlying cause* rather than depressing automaticity. For example, if the sinus tachycardia is associated with heart failure, initial therapy would be directed toward improving cardiac function and decreasing cardiac work load.

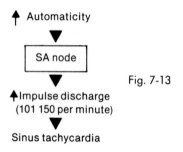

Fig. 7-13

Sinus tachycardia

59 NURSING ORDERS: The patient with sinus tachycardia
1. Is patient symptomatic from the fast rate?
   —Check blood pressure, sensorium, skin color, and temperature.
2. Is the tachycardia associated with heart failure?
   —Auscultate lungs for rales.
   —Check CVP readings, fluid balance, wedge pressure.
3. Assess adequacy of oxygenation.
   —Check skin color and temperature.
   —Observe character and rate of respirations.
   —Assess arterial blood gas values, especially pH, P_{CO_2}, and P_{O_2}.
4. Is the tachycardia associated with drug therapy?
   —Isoproterenol (Isuprel), atropine, aminophylline, epinephrine, or dopamine.
5. Are there any stressors that may elicit a sympathetic response and thus increase the heart rate?
   —Fever
   —Pain
   —Anxiety

Sinus bradycardia

60 When automaticity is depressed in the SA node, the rate of impulse discharge from this area will *(increase/decrease)*. Slowing of the sinus rate to less than 60 beats per minute results in an arrhythmias known as *sinus bradycardia*.

decrease

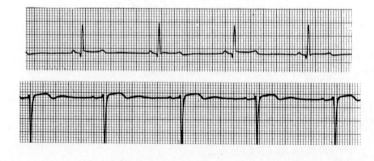

Fig. 7-14

286

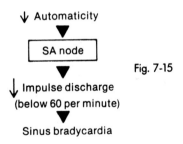

Fig. 7-15

62 Some factors have been identified as depressing automaticity and conduction in the SA node. In the setting of acute MI, the most significant factors are (1) ischemia (to the SA node); (2) parasympathetic or vagal stimulation (ischemia to the vagal fibers, carotid sinus pressure, Valsalva maneuver); (3) drugs (digitalis, propranolol); and (4) electrolyte imbalances (hyperkalemia). Sinus bradycardia is clinically significant *when* it causes a symptomatic fall in cardiac _____.

output

REMEMBER: Cardiac output = _____ _____ × stroke volume.

heart rate

Sinus bradycardias are also significant because *slow rates* may precipitate the development of dangerous tachyarrhythmias. Initial therapy in the management of sinus bradycardia is directed toward *(accelerating/slowing)* the ventricular rate.

accelerating

63 NURSING ORDERS: The patient with sinus bradycardia
1. Is the patient symptomatic from the slow rates?
   —Watch for the development of hypotension and sensorium changes.
   —Check for changes in skin color and temperature and for diaphoresis.
   —Check for ventricular arrhythmias associated with the slow rate.
2. Is the bradycardia associated with infarction of the inferior wall?
   NOTE: Slow rates classically accompany IWMI.
3. Is the sinus bradycardia associated with any drug therapy?
   —Is the patient receiving digitalis or propranolol therapy?
4. Is the patient hypoxic?
5. Have serum K^+ levels increased?
   REMEMBER: Increased K^+ acts as a cardiac depressant.
6. Have atropine at the bedside.
7. Is bradycardia associated with Valsalva maneuvers or other vagal stimulation?

Sinus arrhythmias

64 The SA node and the lungs are both innervated by the parasympathetic nervous system via the vagus nerve. The SA node therefore *(may/may not)* be affected by respirations. The rate of the SA may *gradually* increase with inspiration and *gradually* decrease with expiration. If these effects are marked, the overall rhythm will appear *(regular/irregular)*. This irregularity is considered a *normal* physiological process and is especially marked in young people.

may

irregular

    This physiological variation in heart rate has been attributed to the *Bainbridge reflex*, which is activated by volume receptors located in *both atria.* Distention of these receptors by a sudden *increase* in atrial volume increases impulse transmission to the vasomotor center via *vagal* (parasympathetic) *sensory pathways.* The motor response is via sympathetic pathways and results in an *(increase/decrease)* in the heart rate. This sympathetic response appears to be selective in that other sympathetic effects, such as increased contractility and vasoconstriction, are not associated with it. This increase in heart rate that occurs in response to *increased atrial volume* promotes emptying of the atria and prevents "damming up" of blood.

increase

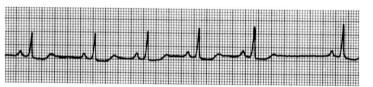

Fig. 7-16

Wandering pacemaker

65 The term *wandering pacemaker* is used to refer to a change of the pacemaker of the heart to another supraventricular focus. It usually occurs as a result of sinus rate slowing.

    REMEMBER: The lower portions of the atria and the AV junctional tissue have the property of automaticity. Therefore they *(are/are not)* potential pacemakers of the heart.

are

    If the lower portion of the atria gains control of the heart's rhythm, there will be a *change* in P wave morphology. This *may* be accompanied by a slight change in the P and QRS rates or PR interval and is of minimal clinical significance.

    If the AV *junctional* tissue gains control of the heart's rhythm, the P wave may disappear or become inverted on lead II. There may be a significant decrease in ventricular rate. The clinical significance is identical to that of a junctional rhythm.

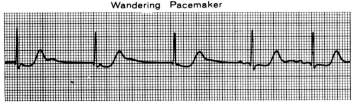

Wandering Pacemaker

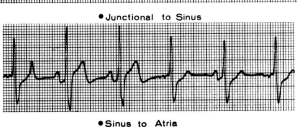

• Junctional to Sinus

Fig. 7-17

• Sinus to Atria

VENTRICULAR ARRHYTHMIAS

66 REMEMBER: A ventricular arrhythmia is a manifestation of abnormal electrical activity in the _____.

ventricles

   Some factors have been identified as contributing to the development of ventricular arrhythmias. In the setting of acute MI, the most significant factors are (1) electrical instability caused by infarction, (2) hypokalemia, (3) hypoxia, (4) slow rates, (5) CHF, and (6) drugs (digitalis, isoproterenol, aminophylline, dopamine, epinephrine). Ventricular arrhythmias produce a QRS complex that is *different* from the patient's normal complex and usually appears *(narrow/wide)*.

wide

Premature ventricular beats

67 An early sign of abnormal electrical activity in the ventricles is the appearance of *premature ventricular beats*. Premature beats are beats that occur before the next expected natural impulse has occurred. Premature ventricular beats occur before the next expected *(P wave/ QRS complex)*.

QRS complex

   The early, or premature, beats arise in the _____. Therefore it can be expected that the QRS complexes of the premature beats will appear _____ from the patient's supraventricular beats and usually wide.

ventricles

different

   One early ventricular impulse is known as a *premature ventricular contraction* (PVC). PVCs are also known as ventricular extrasystoles or ventricular ectopic beats.

68 PVCs that arise from the same foci in the ventricles will have the same shape or morphology and are known as *unifocal PVCs*.

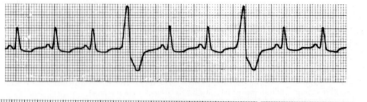

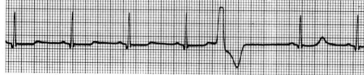

Fig. 7-18

When a single PVC falls on the T wave of a previous beat, this timing should be noted.

REMEMBER: The T wave is referred to as the _____ period of the heart. One stimulus during this period may produce multiple responses known as _____ _____ responses.

vulnerable

chain reaction

PVC ON T WAVE

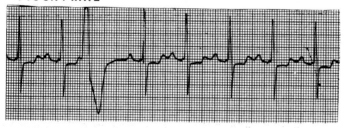

Fig. 7-19

PVCs that arise from different areas in the ventricles have different shapes and are known as *multifocal PVCs*.

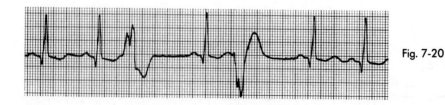

Fig. 7-20

69 PVCs may increase in frequency and appear every other beat. When a discharge sequence appears that consists of a sinus beat, a PVC, a sinus beat, a PVC, and so on, forming groups of two, the arrhythmia is known as *ventricular bigeminy*.

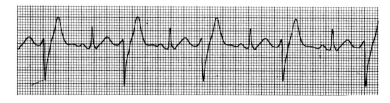

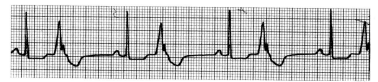

Fig. 7-21

The term *ventricular trigeminy* may be used to describe any ventricular arrhythmias that, together with the sinus beat, form groups of *three*. The term therefore can refer to *either* two sinus beats followed by one PVC *or* to one sinus beat followed by two *consecutive* PVCs. The term is best avoided unless its intended meaning is carefully defined, because the clinical significance of the two rhythms differs greatly.

70 The following are characteristics of PVCs, or ventricular extrasystoles:
1. They are *early,* or *premature.*
2. The QRS complexes of the premature beats are *different* from the patient's normal complexes and are usually *wide.*
3. They are *usually* but *not always* followed by a full compensatory pause.
4. They may be preceded by *nonpremature* P waves.

    When the pause following a premature beat is fully compensatory, the distance between the sinus beat that precedes the premature beat and the sinus beat that follows the premature beat is equal to the sum of two consecutive sinus intervals (Fig. 7-22).

71 An *incomplete* compensatory pause typically occurs with a premature atrial contraction (PAC) because premature atrial beats are able to penetrate and reset the sinus (P wave) rate. A *full* compensatory pause typically occurs with PVCs because ventricular beats *usually* do not conduct retrogradely into the atria. For this reason, PVCs *(are/ are not)* able to penetrate and reset the SA node. The sinus cycle is thus uninterrupted.

are not

72 The QRS complex of a PVC is often superimposed on the sinus P wave, masking its appearance on the surface ECG. However, when PVCs are only slightly premature, the P wave is not obscured by the ectopic QRS complex and may be seen immediately preceding the PVC. This P wave indicates *(sinus/ectopic)* discharge and thus remains

sinus

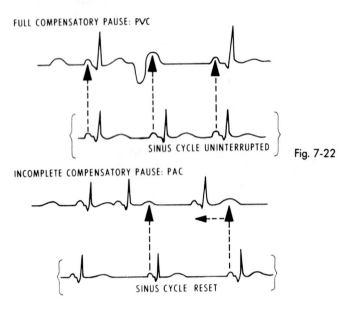

FULL COMPENSATORY PAUSE: PVC

SINUS CYCLE UNINTERRUPTED

Fig. 7-22

INCOMPLETE COMPENSATORY PAUSE: PAC

SINUS CYCLE RESET

consistent with the underlying sinus (P wave) cycle, that is, nonpremature. PVCs can be preceded by nonpremature P waves but *(should/should not)* be preceded by premature P waves (see Frames 102, 103, 115 to 132, and 137 to 138).

should not

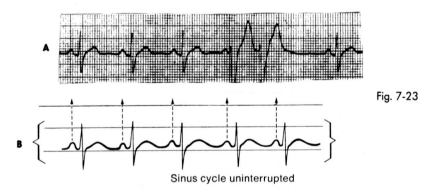

A

B

Sinus cycle uninterrupted

Fig. 7-23

73 PVCs may be described as either *early* or *late* according to their exact timing with reference to the underlying RR cycle. Early PVCs are distinctly premature, that is, close to the T wave of the preceding impulse. The term *late* PVC is used to describe those PVCs that occur late in diastole—that is only slightly early. They are also commonly referred to as *end-diastolic PVCs* (see Fig. 7-19). End-diastolic PVCs are only slightly premature and are thus typically preceded by the sinus P wave on the ECG. They may be difficult to distinguish from fusion beats because the timing is similar (see Frames 76 to 85 and 90 to 98).

74 In the presence of significantly premature, early, PVCs, the sinus P wave may follow the ectopic QRS complex at a sufficient distance to allow the ventricles to recover and immediately conduct this sinus P wave. Thus these PVCs *(will/will not)* be followed by a pause. Because   will not
the PVC appears between two normal beats without a pause, this beat is referred to as an *interpolated* PVC. The presence of slow sinus rates further facilitates the occurrence of interpolated PVCs. Interpolated PVCs have the same clinical significance significance as non-interpolated PVCs. They appear differently on the ECG only because of the timing of the ectopic beat relative to the underlying
_____ cycle.   QRS

Interpolated PVC

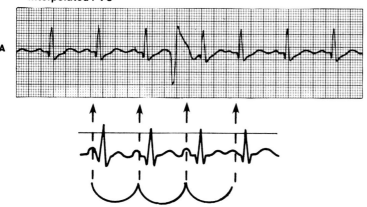

A

Noninterpolated PVC (same focus)

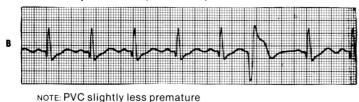

B

Fig. 7-24

NOTE: PVC slightly less premature

Interpolated PVC (slow sinus rate)

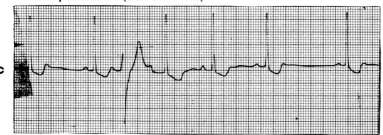

C

75 NOTE: This P wave following an interpolated PVC is typically conducted with a prolonged PR interval (Fig. 7-24). This altered conduction occurs as a result of AV node refractoriness caused by retrograde penetration by the PVC. The presence of retrograde AV node penetration following PVCs is usually not seen on an ECG. Its presence is inferred because of its effect on the subsequent sinus beat. This phenomenon is referred to as *concealed conduction*. Prolongation of the PR interval may help differentiate an interpolated PVC from artifact.

76 PVCs are clinically significant because they are (1) a manifestation of an underlying problem, and (2) often the precursors to more serious and life-threatening arrhythmias.

LET US REVIEW: PVCs produce QRS complexes that are characteristically *(wide/narrow)* and _____ from the patient's   **wide; different**
normal beats. Other characteristics of PVCs include: (1) they are
early, or _____; (2) they may be followed by a full   **premature**
compensatory pause; and (3) they may be preceded by a
_____ P wave. PVCs that arise from different foci   **nonpremature**
in the ventricles are known as _____ PVCs. When   **multifocal**
a PVC occurs in a discharge sequence after every sinus beat, the arrhythmia is known as ventricular _____. PVCs are   **bigeminy**
significant because they are often the precursors to ventricular fibrillation.

Ventricular tachycardia

77 PVCs may increase in frequency until they begin to occur consecutively in groups of two or three. When *three* or more PVCs occur in a row and their rate exceeds 100 beats per minute, the arrhythmia is

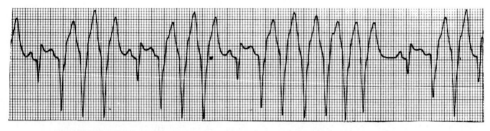

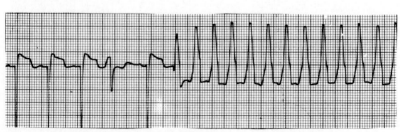

Fig. 7-25

labeled *ventricular tachycardia* (VT). However, because two consecutive PVCs with a ventricular rate greater than 100 beats per minute may rapidly lead to VT, their significance is equally ominous.

When the rate of a ventricular arrhythmia exceeds 100 beats per minute, it is known as ventricular _____.

REMEMBER: A rhythm is currently not classified as a tachycardia until the rate exceeds _____ beats per minute.

tachycardia

100

78 The ventricles normally initiate impulses at a rate of _____ to _____ per minute. Thus a ventricular arrhythmia with a rate greater than 40 but less than 100 beats per minute is still normally fast. Ventricular rhythms with rates greater than 40 but less than 100 beats per minute are referred to as *accelerated idioventricular rhythms*. These rhythms are considered separately following this section.

20
40

VT has ectopic ventricular rate greater than _____ beats per minute. It may break through in spite of an adequate sinus rate and often appears *suddenly*. VT has also been called *paroxysmal VT*. It is *usually* initiated by an early PVC, one that is distinctly premature, occurring close to or on the T wave of the previous beat.

100

REMEMBER: A stimulus that falls on the T wave may cause _____ _____.

repetitive firing

79 VT is a malignant arrhythmia and frequently deteriorates into VF. It therefore requires *immediate* therapy. Pulseless VT is treated like VF. When a pulse is present, VT is initially treated pharmacologically or with synchronized countershock (i.e., cardioversion) depending upon the accompanying symptoms. Therapy is usually directed toward *depressing* the ectopic focus in the ventricles.

NOTE: If VT appears in the setting of a slow rate, initial or subsequent therapy may be directed toward accelerating the underlying bradycardia.

LET US REVIEW: VT has a ventricular rate greater than _____ beats per minute. It is usually initiated by an _____ PVC. VT may appear in the presence of *fast* or _____ rates. It is clinically significant because it frequently deteriorates into _____. Initial therapy in the management of VT is *usually* directed toward depressing the ectopic focus in the _____.

100
early
slow
VF

ventricles

Ventricular fibrillation

80 VF represents the most disintegrated electrical activity that can occur in the _____. It is usually initiated by a single PVC on the T wave or a run of VT. In VF the electrical activity is so chaotic that the complexes have no distinct QRS-T wave morphology and are uneven in height. Thus in the presence of VF no distinct

ventricles

_____ complexes will be seen on the ECG. The electrical QRS
activity is so disintegrated in this arrhythmia that the heart cannot
receive a signal to pump and quivers ineffectually. As a result there
is no pulse, no cardiac output, and clinical death occurs. VF is a
form of cardiac arrest.

81 VF is divided into two types according to the size of the fibrillatory
waves: *fine* (Fig. 7-27) and *coarse* (Fig. 7-26, *A* and *B*).

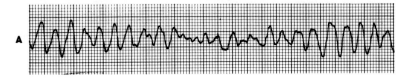

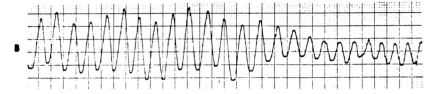

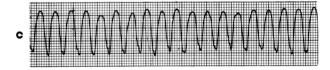

Fig. 7-26

In coarse VF the waves are of large amplitude. Coarse VF implies
that the fibrillation is of recent onset in a stronger heart and that
electrical intervention will usually abolish the arrhythmia.

Ventricular flutter (Fig. 7-26, *C*) differs from coarse ventricular
fibrillation in that the complexes remain regular or equal in height
and have thus not fully disintegrated. However, the QRS-T complexes have lost the more distinct shape still seen in VT. Thus this
arrhythmia gives the appearance of a regular, wavy baseline. The
ventricular rate of ventricular flutter is usually 300 beats per minute.
Its clinical significance is identical with that of coarse VF. In fact, this
intermediate stage between VT and VF is not commonly seen. If
coarse VF is not terminated immediately, the heart will become an-
oxic and depressed. The fibrillatory waves will then become fine.
Pharmacological and mechanical intervention is then necessary before this arrhythmia will respond to electrical therapy.

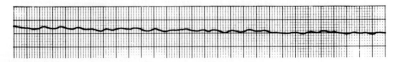

Fig. 7-27

82 LET US REVIEW: The most chaotic electrical activity that can occur in the ventricles is known as _____.

VF is usually initiated by a single _____ or a run of _____. In the presence of VF distinct QRS complexes *(will/will not)* be seen on the ECG. The electrical activity is so disintegrated in this arrhythmia that the heart _____ ineffectually. As a result there is no _____ _____, and _____ death occurs. Coarse VF can usually be terminated by _____ intervention. Fine VF, however, usually requires _____ and _____ intervention before it will respond to electrical therapy.

VF

PVC

VT; will not

quivers

cardiac output

clinical

electrical

mechanical; pharmacological

83 NURSING ORDERS: The patient with a ventricular arrhythmia
1. Have lidocaine at the bedside.
2. Medicate patient as necessary (according to institutional policy).
3. Evaluate the underlying causes.
   —In first 48 hours following infarction, ventricular arrhythmias are usually a result of electrical instability.
   —Check for hypokalemia.
   —Is patient hypoxic?
   —Is arrhythmia arising in the presence of slow rates?
   —Is patient receiving drugs such as isoproterenol (Isuprel), digoxin, aminophylline, dopamine?
   —Is there evidence of heart failure?
4. Make sure a cardioverter defibrillator is immediately available and in good working order.

Idioventricular rhythm

84 Let us now discuss another ventricular arrhythmia that usually appears in the presence of depressed conduction. When conduction is depressed, the ventricles may assume control of the rhythm.

REMEMBER: Depressed conduction results in *(slow/fast)* rates. The ventricles normally have the ability to initiate impulses at a rate of _____ to _____ per minute.

slow

20; 40

When the ventricles assume control of the rhythm at this rate, the arrhythmia is known as *idioventricular rhythm*. The QRS complex in the presence of idioventricular rhythm is usually *(wide/narrow)* because it is originating in the ventricles.

wide

Idioventricular rhythm is clinically significant because (1) it is slow and may cause a symptomatic fall in cardiac output, and (2) it may allow for the break-through of dangerous tachyarrhythmias. Initial therapy in the management of idioventricular rhythm is usually directed toward *accelerating* the ventricular rate. This rhythm should *never* be suppressed.

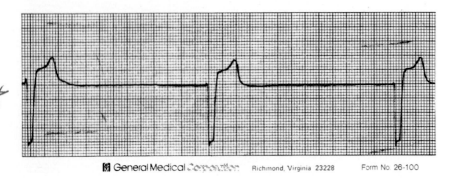

Fig. 7-28

85 LET US REVIEW: When the ventricular rate of a ventricular rhythm is between 20 and 40 beats per minute, the arrhythmia is known as
_____ _____.   idioventricular rhythm

Idioventricular rhythm characteristically appears in the presence of depressed _____. An idioventricular rhythm is   conduction
clinically significant because (1) it is slow and may result in a _____ fall in _____ _____, and   symptomatic; cardiac output
(2) it may allow for the breakthrough of life-threatening _____.   tachyarrhythmias

Accelerated idioventricular rhythm

86 A ventricular rhythm with a rate greater than 40 but less than 100 beats per minute is known as an *accelerated idioventricular rhythm* (AIVR). AIVR has been divided into two types. This classification was recently developed because the pathophysiology, clinical significance, and management of the two types differ.

Type I AIVR characteristically is initiated by a *ventricular escape beat, fushion beat,* or end-diastolic PVC (*late PVC*) and appears when the sinus rate slows.

REMEMBER: The term *late PVC* is used to describe those PVCs that occur _____ in electrical *diastole*. An escape beat is   late
one that occurs because the next supraventricular impulse fails to appear. Ventricular fusion beats are discussed in Frames 90 to 98.

Type I AIVR is usually a *regular rhythm,* the mechanism of which is most likely *enhanced automaticity.* It represents the activity of a "protective" ventricular focus and therefore is usually considered *benign.* Termination occurs with a *fusion beat,* prompt return to sinus rhythm, or both (Fig. 7-29).

A fall in cardiac output may occur with Type I AIVR because of loss of the atrial contribution to cardiac output. In this case therapy is usually directed toward accelerating the underlying ventricular _____.   rate

298

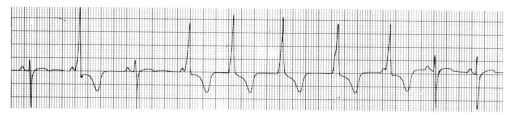

Fig. 7-29

87 *Type II AIVR* characteristically is initiated by a *distinctly premature ventricular beat*. It is usually an *irregular rhythm*, the mechanism of which is most likely depressed conduction. The presence of irregularity is the most useful clue in distinguishing Type II from Type I AIVR. Type II AIVR is considered *more dangerous* than Type I because it usually masks a *VT*. Termination follows a *compensatory pause* like that often seen following a *PVC* (Fig 7-30).

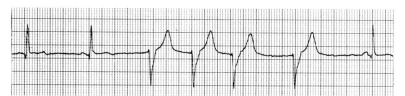

Fig. 7-30

Let us consider the pathophysiology of Type II AIVR in more detail. Ventricular ectopic beats may fail to *exit* from their site of origin when their conduction pathway is *temporarily* blocked. This temporary block referred to as an *exit block*. Exit block is a manifestation of *(depressed/enhanced)* conduction and may result from such factors as ischemia, electrolyte imbalance, and drug toxicity. When impulses are intermittently or consecutively blocked, the true inherent rate of a ventricular focus may be *masked* on the ECG. Thus the rhythm may appear *deceptively benign*.

depressed

88 The irregularity of Type II AIVR is probably a result of intermittent, random exiting of the *ventricular focus*. Type II AIVR should be considered clinically significant because it probably represents an underlying _____. It has the potential for acceleration, and thus therapy is usually directed toward *depressing* the *ectopic focus*. If the underlying rhythm is a bradycardia, therapy should be directed toward *(accelerating/slowing)* the underlying rhythm. The figure below illustrates a true VT (VR > 100), which initially appeared to be a benign focus.

VT

accelerating

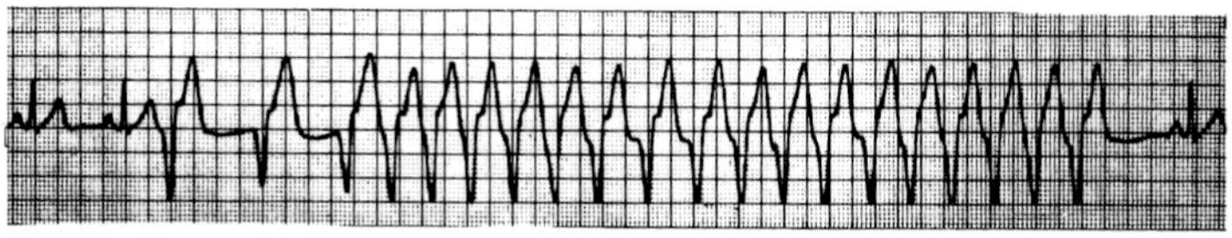

Fig. 7-31

The acceleration occurs by a *(Type I/Type II)* mechanism.

Type II

89 LET US REVIEW: AIVRs have ventricular rates greater than
_____ but less than _____ beats per minute.
Type I AIVR is usually initiated by an *(early/late)* PVC and is terminated by a *(fusion beat/compensatory pause)*. It is considered a *(benign/
dangerous)* arrhythmia and therefore usually *(does/does not)* require intervention. Type II AIVR is characteristically a(n) *(regular/irregular)*
rhythm and in most cases *masks* a _____.

40; 100
late
fusion beat; benign
does not
irregular
VT

The irregularity of Type II AIVR probably represents an intermittent _____ _____ of a ventricular focus. Type
II AIVR should be considered clinically significant and has the potential for acceleration. Therapy should be directed toward depressing the ectopic focus in the _____.

exit block

ventricles

Fusion beats

90 Depolarization of the same chamber of the heart by two or more simultaneous impulses may result in a blending or a *fusing* of these
impulses within a single chamber. The resulting beat is known as a
_____ beat.

fusion

When a ventricular focus discharges an impulse at the same time
or slightly before a supraventricular impulse has entered the ventricles, a fusion beat can occur. The ventricles will be partially depolarized by the supraventricular impulse and partially depolarized by the
ectopic _____ impulse. The resulting QRS com-
plex will appear as a blend, or fusion, of the two contributing impulses in both contour and duration. This discussion is limited to
ventricular fusion beats—by far the most common form.

ventricular

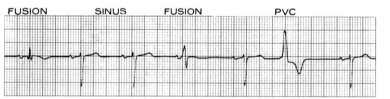

Fig. 7-32

91 The first step in the identification of fusion beats is to establish the
probability that fusion could occur. This probability is determined
by evaluating the timing of the ectopic QRS complex relative to the
underlying RR cycle.

REMEMBER: Fusion beats occur when two impulses are attempting
to control the ventricles *at the same time.*

The presence of a sinus P wave preceding the ectopic QRS complex can also indicate the probability that fusion could occur.

REMEMBER: PVCs can be preceded by _____ P
waves that are consistent with the PP intervals of the underlying sinus rhythm.

nonpremature

The presence of a sinus P wave with a short PR interval indicates the probability of a sinus impulse's attempt to enter the ventricles together with the ventricular ectopic beat. However, neither the presence of a sinus P wave nor a short PR interval *confirms the existence* of fusion.

REMEMBER: Sinus P waves also precede _____   end-diastolic
PVCs.

92   A diagnosis of fusion beats can be made only when there is ECG evidence that at least two distinct foci are attempting to control the ventricles and have blended together. Therefore the second step in the identification of fusion beats is to identify the QRS complex of each distinct focus in its naturally occurring form and then determine if the ectopic QRS configuration is a blend of these in _____ and _____.   contour; duration

Fusion beats occur when two or more impulses _____   blend
in _____ and _____. Therefore,   contour; duration
when fusion beats occur, there *(will/will not)* be a change in the QRS   will
configuration. The QRS complex of a fusion beat is partially formed by the patient's supraventricular impulse. Therefore the QRS complex of a fusion beat may be partially *(narrow/wide)*. However, the fu-   narrow
sion complex will appear *(the same as/different from)* the normal QRS   different from
complex of the supraventricular impulse. That is because of the presence of a concurrent *(ventricular/supraventricular)* impulse.   ventricular

93   The clinical significance of a fusion beat is that there is an ectopic ventricular focus attempting to control the ventricles. Therefore fusion beats are significant not for their supraventricular component but for their _____ component. These beats may   ventricular
appear multifocal when initially compared with the nonfused form of the same ectopic focus (Fig. 7-32). However, multifocal beats are more typically *both* early PVCs and do not demonstrate blending characteristics when compared with the normal QRS complexes.

94   Common examples of ventricular fusion beats are the following:
    1. Sinus beat with a late (end-diastolic) PVC (Fig. 7-33).

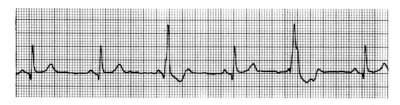

Fig. 7-33

2. Sinus beat with a pacemaker beat (Fig. 7-34)

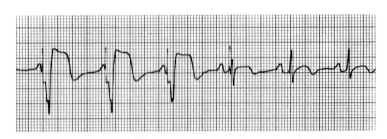

Fig. 7-34

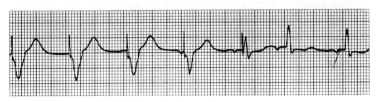

NOTE: Fusion beats may also occur, less commonly, when two ventricular ectopic impulses fuse and appear as a third focus.

REMEMBER: Fusion beats are not significant for their _____ component but for their _____ component.

supraventricular;
ventricular

95 The purpose of a pacemaker is to induce a ventricular focus. Therefore fusion beats are expected in the presence of normal pacemaker function and *(are/are not)* clinically significant. When fusion beats result from spontaneous ectopic ventricular impulses, however, they may be clinically significant. A sequence of three or more consecutive fusion beats may indicate the presence of either VT or *(Type I/ Type II)* AIVR. Occasionally fusion beats are followed by a distinctly premature form of the same focus, indicating an irregular ectopic rate, or AIVR-Type II phenomenon. Consecutive fusion beats therefore *(may be/may never be)* clinically significant. For this reason, single fusion beats are treated like PVCs until their consecutive rate is established and confirmed to the benign.

are not

Type I

may be

96 In the setting of tachycardias, the appearance of fusion beats may help confirm the presence of a *(ventricular/supraventricular)* ectopic focus. They may thus aid in distinguishing VT from supraventricular tachycardia with aberrant conduction (see Frames 115 to 132, 140, and 142).

ventricular

97 LET US REVIEW: Fusion beats are usually regarded clinically as *(ventricular/supraventricular)* and are produced by *(early/late)* or _____ diastolic ventricular beats. Most commonly they result from the _____ of a _____ and

ventricular
late
end-
fusion; supraventricular

302

_____ impulse in the _____.
The resulting QRS complex appears as a _____ of these
two impulses in _____ and
_____.

ventricular; ventricles

blend

contour

duration

98 NURSING ORDERS:

1. When identifying fusion beats, look for end-diastolic beats
preceded by a nonpremature P wave and short PR interval.
This finding is evidence of a possible supraventricular as well
as ventricular component. Then identifying each contributing
focus in its pure form and document blending.
2. Report fusion beats:
—When they are isolated but occur more frequently than 5
per minute.
—When they are consecutive, which may indicate the presence
of VT or AIVR.
—When they are associated with a bradyarrhythmia.
3. If fusion beats are occurring consecutively in the presence of
an adequate supraventricular rate, have lidocaine (Xylocaine)
at the bedside.
4. When fusion beats occur in the presence of a bradyarrhythmia, have atropine at the bedside.

REMEMBER: Fusion beats that occur in the presence of normal
pacemaker function are benign.

ECTOPIC SUPRAVENTRICULAR ARRHYTHMIAS

99 Analysis of the QRS complex provides information about the origin
of the impulse: ventricular or _____. The term *su-*
praventricular implies that the origin of the impulse is *(above/below)*
the ventricles.

supraventricular

above

REMEMBER: Supraventricular impulses may arise in the
_____ node, the _____, or the _____
_____ tissue. Supraventricular impulses *(are/are*
not) usually transmitted through the normal conduction pathways to
the ventricles. Therefore supraventricular impulses will usually produce a *(narrow/wide)* unchanging QRS complex.

SA; atria; AV junctional

are

narrow

Thus the presence of a narrow, unchanging QRS complex can be
used as a guide when one is diagnosing a *(supraventrciular/ventricular)*
arrhythmia. Analysis of the P wave and calculation of the atrial rate
provides the information for the differential diagnosis of supraventricular arrhythmias.

supraventricular

Atrial arrhythmias

100 Atrial arrhythmias are a manifestation of abnormal electrical activity
in the _____. Some factors have been identified as contrib-

atria

uting to the development of atrial arrhythmias. In the setting of acute MI, the most significant factors are (1) atrial distention, as in heart failure; (2) ischemia resulting from hypoxia or IWMI; (3) drugs (digitalis toxicity); (4) pericarditis; and (5) chronic disease of the SA node.

101 REMEMBER: When diagnosing supraventricular arrhythmias, one must analyze the _____ wave and calculate the _____ rate.   P; atrial
When assessing supraventricular arrhythmias, one must locate the P waves. We suggest the following points be utilized when locating P waves:
1. P waves are usually best visualized on either lead II or V_1 (MCL_1).
2. P waves are small forces and may be best seen when the amplitude, or gain, is increased.
3. Premature P waves are often hidden on the T wave of the previous beat. The T wave configuration of that beat should be compared with that of the patient's usual T waves.

Premature atrial beats

102 An early sign of abnormal electrical activity in the atria is the appearance of premature atrial beats. Premature atrial impulses will appear on the ECG as *early P waves.*
REMEMBER: Atrial depolarization is represented on the ECG by the _____ wave.   P
Premature beats are beats that occur before the next expected impulse has occurred. Premature atrial beats occur before the next expected P wave as compared with the underlying *(PP/PR)* cycle.   PP
They disrupt the regularity of the PP interval. A single early atrial impulse is known as a premature atrial contraction (PAC).
NOTE: PACs are also known as *atrial extrasystoles* and *atrial ectopic beats.* Throughout this discussion, these terms will be used interchangeably.

103 PACs have these characteristic features: (1) the P wave is early, or _____; and (2) the P wave appears different from   premature
the normal sinus P wave on at least one lead. The P wave appears different from the normal sinus impulse because it is originating in the atria and not in the _____ node. However, this differ-   SA
ence is often slight and may be difficult to detect on single monitoring leads.

104 Premature atrial impulses are usually transmitted through the normal conduction pathways to the ventricles. Therefore the premature P wave of a PAC *(is/is not)* usually followed by a QRS complex. The   is
QRS complex produced is usually *(narrow/wide)*, or *(the same as/different from)* that of the basic rhythm, or both.   narrow; the same as

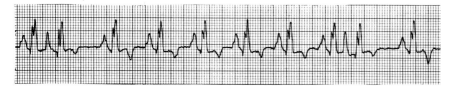

Fig. 7-35

105 If a premature atrial impulse finds the ventricles completely *refractory*, it *(will/will not)* be conducted through to the ventricles. Therefore the P wave *(will/will not)* be conducted. The impulse is known as ture/late) _____ wave that is not followed by a _____ complex.

will not

will not

P

QRS

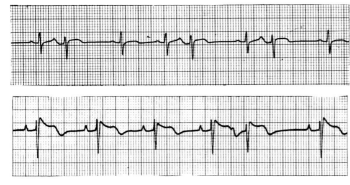

Fig. 7-36

106 If the premature atrial impulse finds the ventricles *partially* refractory, the impulse will be conducted with delay. A wider QRS complex conducted differently, or *aberrantly,* may follow the premature P wave. A PAC conducted in this manner is referred to as an aberrantly conducted PAC (see Frames 115 to 132). It is not unusual to see PACs conducted in all of these three ways in a given patient (Fig. 7-37).

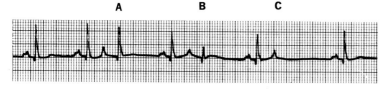

Fig. 7-37

The criteria common to all of the above PACs is the premature
_____ wave.   P

NOTE: PACs may be conducted with normal, short, or long PR intervals. They are most commonly conducted with a PR interval that
is longer than normal because the ectopic atrial impulse finds the
AV node partially refractory. Following a PAC, there is an incomplete compensatory pause because the ectopic atrial impulse prematurely discharges the SA node and resets the sinus cycle. (See Frames
70 to 72 for definition of a complete compensatory pause.)

107 PACs are clinically significant because (1) they may indicate an underlying problem (for example, in the setting of acute MI, they frequently indicate the presence of CHF), and (2) they may be precursors to more serious atrial arrhythmias.

NOTE: Just one PAC that falls during the vulnerable period of the
atria may produce atrial flutter of fibrillation. PACs may increase in
frequency and, in this way, also be precursors of atrial tachycardia,   premature
flutter, or fibrillation.

Atrial bigeminy

108 PACs may increase in frequenty until they begin to occur consecutively. As they increase in frequency, they may occur every other
beat in a bigeminal pattern.

NOTE: In atrial bigeminy, the second beat is usually the ectopic
impulse. That can be more clearly demonstrated by obtaining the
underlying rhythm.

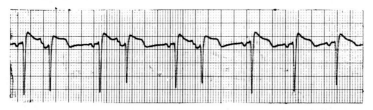

Fig. 7-38

Atrial trigeminy

109 The term *atrial trigeminy* may be used to describe any
_____ arrhythmias that, together with the sinus beat, form   atrial
groups of _____ (Fig. 7-39). The term therefore can refer   three
to *either* two sinus beats followed by one _____ or to   PAC
_____ sinus beats followed by two _____   one; consecutive
PACs.

Fig. 7-39 illustrates the more benign form of atrial trigeminy and
may be interpreted as sinus rhythm with atrial trigeminy (PAC every
third beat). In this form the PACs are *(more/less)* frequent than in   less
atrial bigeminy. However, in the setting of an acute MI, frequent
PACs—even less frequent than atrial bigeminy— *(are/are not)* clini-   are
cally significant and should be immediately reported.

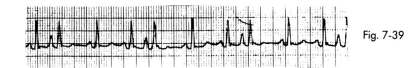

Fig. 7-39

Atrial tachycardia

110 When three or more PACs occur in a row, the arrhythmia is known as atrial tachycardia.

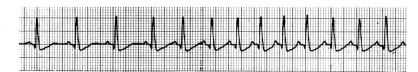

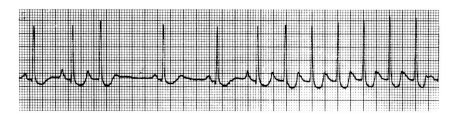

Fig. 7-40

Since this arrhythmia appears and disappears suddenly, it is frequently known as a *paroxysmal tachycardia* (PAT). In atrial tachycardia the atrial rate may range between 150 and 250 beats per minute. Characteristically, the atrial rate is in the lower range—150 beats per minute.

REMEMBER: The atrial rate may be calculated by measuring the _____ wave rate.

P

If the AV node is functioning normally, every atrial impulse should be conducted through to the _____. Therefore in atrial tachycardia the ventricular rate will usually be the same as the _____ rate.

ventricles

atrial

111 If some of the atrial impulses are not conducted through to the ventricles, the arrhythmia is then known as *atrial tachycardia with block,* or PAT with block.

NOTE: This arrhythmia is classically associated with digitalis toxicity (Fig. 7-41).

Atrial flutter

112 An increase in the atrial rate leads to an arrhythmia known as *atrial flutter.* In atrial flutter the atrial rate usually falls between 250 and 350 beats per minute. Characteristically, the atrial rate is in the middle of this range—300 beats per minute. In atrial flutter, the atria

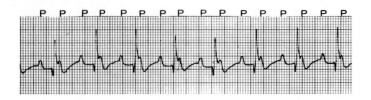

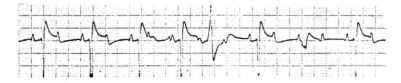

Fig. 7-41

are initiating impulses so rapidly that this arrhythmia may assume a sawtooth appearance.

NOTE: This characteristic sawtooth pattern should not be relied on when one is diagnosing atrial flutter; the atrial rate should first be measured. The ventricular response may be either regular or irregular.

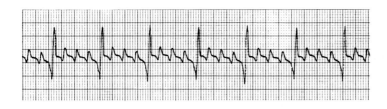

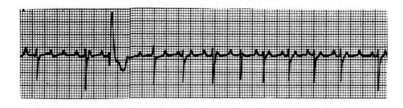

Fig. 7-42

113 In atrial flutter, *not* every atrial impulse is usually conducted through to the _____. The atria are discharging impulses so rapidly that even the healthy AV node is not able to transmit all of the impulses.

ventricles

REMEMBER: The physiological function of the AV node is to protect the ventricles from rapid atrial rhythms.

Characteristically, the atrial rate in atrial flutter is approximately 300 beats per minute. Most commonly there is a two-to-one conduction ratio: every other impulse is conducted to the ventricles. Thus there would be two P waves for every _____ complex. The ventricular rate would be half of the atrial rate, or approximately _____ beats per minute. This arrhythmia is described as atrial flutter with two-to-one conduction.

QRS

150

Lead I

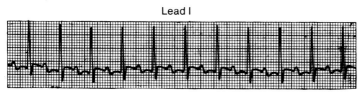

A

Lead aV_F

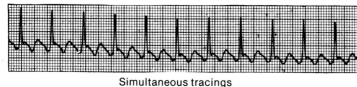

Fig. 7-43

Simultaneous tracings

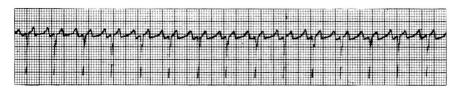

NOTE: Detection of this arrhytmia is difficult because P waves may be hidden in the T waves or QRS complexes. It is suggested that in the presence of a supraventricular arrhythmia with a ventricular rate of approximately 150 beats per minute, the possibility of atrial flutter with two-to-one conduction should always be considered. An extra P wave may be found halfways in-between the more clearly visible P waves if one searches for it carefully (Fig 7-43, B). The conduction ratio may vary, depending on the adequacy of AV conduction.

NOTE: It is important to record the rate of the ventricular response when one is diagnosing this arrhythmia.

Atrial fibrillation

114 The rate of impulse discharge from the atria may become faster and may result in an arrhythmia known as *atrial fibrillation*. In the presence of this rapid atrial rate, the shape or morphology of the _____ waves will begin to deteriorate. At this point the atria are initiating impulses so rapidly that a distinct, regular P wave rate can no longer be identified. The ventricular response is typically *(rapid/slow)*.

P

rapid

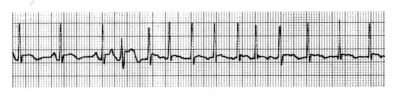

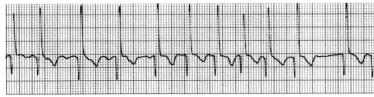

Fig. 7-44

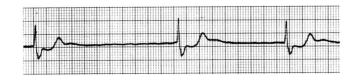

115 In the presence of atrial fibrillation, the AV node is being bombarded with impulses. The AV node selects and conducts impulses randomly. Therefore in atrial fibrillation the ventricular response will always be *(regular/irregular)*. We suggest, when a consistent P wave rate cannot be measured in the presence of a supraventricular arrhythmia and there is an irregular ventricular response, that the arrhythmias be diagnosed *atrial fibrillation*.

    NOTE: It is important to note the rate of the ventricular response when one is labeling this arrhythmia—for example, atrial fibrillation with a rapid ventricular response of 180.

116 In summary:

    Atrial arrhythmias are clinically significant because:

1. They may result in a fast ventricular response, which will compromise cardiac output and thus decrease coronary blood flow. These arrhythmias may also increase O_2 consumption of the myocardium and cause patient symptoms.
2. The atrial contribution to cardiac output may be lost.
3. They usually indicate an underlying problem, such as CHF with hypoxemia or hypoxia or both, pericarditis, drug toxicity or stress, and SA node dysfunction.

    Initial therapy in the management of persistent atrial tachycardia, atrial flutter, or atrial fibrillation is usually directed toward decreasing the _____ rate. Subsequent therapy is directed toward correcting the underlying cause, depressing ectopic activity in the _____, or both.

irregular

ventricular

atria

NOTE: Atrial arrhythmias are diagnosed by the P wave rate but are treated initially by the _____ rate. If the ventricular rate is slow, therapy is directed towards (*increasing/decreasing*) the ventricular rate.

ventricular

increasing

117 NURSING ORDERS: The patient with an atrial arrhythmia
1. Evaluate the ventricular response.
   —Is the rate fast?
   —Is the patient tolerating the fast rate?
   —Check blood pressure, sensorium, skin color, and temperature.
   —Does the patient have coronary artery disease?
   —Notify physician of frequent PACs or any atrial arrhythmias.
   —Have patient perform Valsalva maneuver or cough
   —Obtain and elevate wedge or PA pressure if Swan/Ganz in place (see Unit 9).
2. Assess patient for evidence of heart failure.
   —Auscultate lungs for cracker (rales).
   —Auscultate heart for gallop rhythms.
   —Check to see if the patient was in sinus tachycardia before the arrhythmia began.
   —Check fluid balance, serum Na^+, and hematocrit values.
   —Check urine output.
3. Could the patient be hypoxemic?
   —Check for signs of respiratory distress.
   —Position for optimal chest expansion.
   —Have the O_2 mask and prongs been removed by the patient or family?
   —Check ABG.
   —Increase O_2 supply if indicated or substitute with other mode of O_2 therapy if the respiratory pattern is variable.
4. Could the arrhythmias be stress related?
   —Watch for nonverbal as well as verbal expressions of anxiety.
   —Is any event (for example, family or staff visits) associated with the arrhythmias?
5. Does the patient have evidence of pericarditis?
6. Could drug therapy (isoproterenol, dopamine) be associated with the arrhythimas?
7. If the rhythm is PAT with block, it is probably digitalis toxicity.
   —Check serum K^+ level and serum Mg^{++} level.
   —Watch patient for anorexia, nausea, and vomiting.
8. Have verapamil (Isoptin) and esmolol (Brevibloc) on hand. Discuss the possible need for these as well as possible cardio-

version or the need for carotid sinus pressure, digitalis, or quinidine therapy with the physician.

Nodal or junctional arrhytmias

118 Nodal, or junctional, arrhythmias originate in the AV junctional tissue. Junctional arrhythmias are therefore *(ventricular/supraventricular)*.

supraventricular

REMEMBER: The differential diagnosis of supraventricular arrhythmia is dependent on the analysis of the _____ wave.

P

When a nodal, or junctional, arrhythmia occurs, the atria are depolarized in a reverse direction. This is known as retrograde atrial depolarization. Retrograde depolariation of the atria results in inversion of the _____ wave.

P

As a result of the P wave in lead II appears *(negative/positive)*.

negative

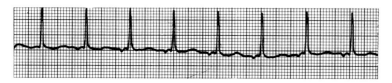

Fig. 7-45

In this type of arrhythmia, the P wave may be seen either *before* or *after* the QRS complex. If the P wave appears in front of the QRS complex, the PR interval will be *short* (less than 0.12 second) because activation of the atria only *slightly* precedes activation of the ventricles.

119 If the atria are depolarized at the same time as the ventricles, the P wave may become hidden within the QRS complex. The ventricular response will remain regular, thus distinguishing this rhythm from _____ _____ in which P waves are also not clearly visible.

atrial fibrillation

Junctional arrhythmia

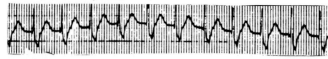

Atrial fibrillation

Fig. 7-46

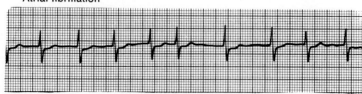

120 Junctional arrhythmias can result from anything that (1) depresses automaticity and conduction in the SA node (for example, sinus bradycardia, digitalis) or (2) increases automaticity in the AV junctional tissue (for example, digitalis intoxication, isoproterenol).

121 Just as single premature beats may originate in the atria, they may also originate in the AV junctional tissue. Premature beats that originate in the AV junctional tissue are known as *premature junctional contractions* (PJCs). The following are characteristics of PJCs: (1) they are early, or premature; and (2) if a P wave is associated with the premature beat, it will be inverted or hidden.

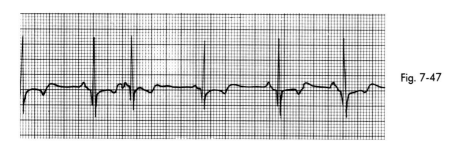

Fig. 7-47

NOTE: PJCs occur less frequently than do PACs and are usually not clinically significant.

122 When the normal pacemaker in the SA node is *depressed,* the AV junctional tissue may assume control of the rhythm at a rate usually between 40 and 70 beats per minute. That is known as *idiojunctional* rhythm.

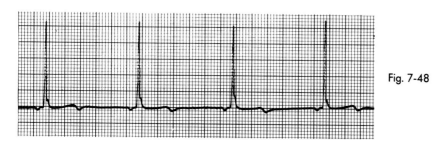

Fig. 7-48

123 When automaticity is *enhanced* in the AV junctional tissue, the rhythm may again be controlled by the _____ node.　　AV

　　When that occurs and the ventricular rate is greater than 100 beats per minute, the arrhythmia is known as *junctional,* or *nodal, tachycardia.*

　　REMEMBER: Tachycardias are defined as those rhythms with ventricular rates exceeding _____ beats per minute. A junc-　　100

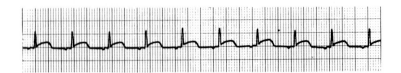

Fig. 7-49

tional rhythm with a rate greater than 70 but less than 100 beats per minute *(is/is not)* abnormally fast for the junctional site.

is

A junctional rhythm with a ventricular rate exceeding 70 but less than 100 beats per minute may be referred to as _____ *junctional rhythm.*

accelerated

Accelerated junctional rhythm is a manifestation of enhanced _____ but is often facilitated by depressed automaticity in the _____ node, as in idiojunctional rhythm.

automaticity
SA

124 Occasionally, the AV junction will be unable to penetrate the atria in a _____ fashion. That most commonly occurs when the sinus and junctional rates are almost the same. Both atria and ventricles will beat independently, and the P wave, when seen, will be upright in lead II (see Frames 178 to 184). However, the focus controlling the *ventricular* response is still the _____ _____. Thus AV dissociation with a junctional pacemaker has the same clinical significance as _____ rhythm. AV dissociation may occur in the presence of either idiojunctional rhythm, accelerated junctional rhythm, or junctional tachycardia.

retrograde

AV junction

idiojunctional

125 Junctional arrhythmias are clinically significant when (1) they indicate an underlying problem; (2) they are fast and compromise cardiac output and thus cardiac function; (3) they are slow and result in a symptomatic fall in cardiac output.

NOTE: Cardiac output may be compromised because the atrial contribution may be lost. Initial therapy in the management of junctional arrhythmias is usually directed toward: (1) correcting the underlying cause, (2) increasing the rate of the SA node, and (3) depressing automaticity in the AV junctional tissue in an attempt to decrease the ventricular rate.

126 NURSING ORDERS: The patient with a junctional arrhythmia
    1. Evaluate the ventricular response.
        —Is the rate too fast or too slow?
        —Check blood pressure, sensorium, skin color, and temperature.
        —If the patient is symptomatic because of a slow ventricular rate, have atropine at bedside.

—If the patient is symptomatic because of junctional tachycardia with a fast ventricular response, have diphenylhydantoin (Dilantin) available.

2. Rule out digitalis toxicity.

NOTE: Digitalis intoxication is the most common cause of junctional tachycardia.

Aberration

127 Aberrantly conducted beats produce *changing QRS complexes* and thus appear to be ventricular in origin. However, these beats are most commonly premature *supraventricular* impulses (usually PACs) that have *deviated* from their normal ventricular conduction pathways.

REMEMBER: Normally, when a premature supraventricular impulse (PAC) reaches the ventricles, it is uniformly conducted through the bundle branch system. The premature P wave of a PAC is therefore usually followed by a *(normal/abnormal)* QRS complex.

normal

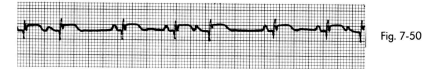

Fig. 7-50

If the supraventricular impulse (PAC) is significantly premature, the bundle branches of the ventricles may still be completely refractory. The premature atrial impulse is *not* conducted at all and is referred to as a _____ PAC. The premature P wave *(is/is not)* followed by a QRS complex.

nonconducted

is not

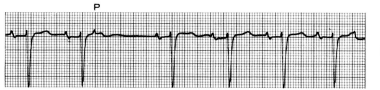

Fig. 7-51

128 If a premature atrial impulse finds the bundle branch system partially refractory, the impulse will be conducted with *delay, deviation,* or both. This deviation from the normal conduction pathway is referred to as _____ conduction. It is associated with *variations* in *bundle branch refractory periods.*

aberrant

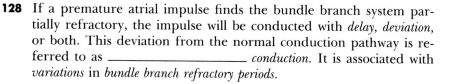

Fig. 7-52

In most patients the right bundle branch has the longest refractory period. Therefore aberrantly conducted PACs usually find the _____ bundle branch refractory and are conducted with a *_____ bundle branch block* (RBBB) pattern.

right
right

NOTE: Although most aberrant beats are PACs, PJCs are also supraventricular impulses and may be conducted aberrantly. However, these beats are particularly difficult to distinguish from PVCs. Therefore, unless distinctly characteristic QRS patterns are present, QRS complexes different from normal and *not* preceded by a *premature* P wave should first be considered *ventricular ectopic in origin*.

129 RBBB patterns are best detected in leads V_1 and V_6. An upright QRS configuration (rsR^1 or qR) occurs typically in lead V_1. Lead V_6 may assume either a qRs or Rs configuration (see Unit 8).

The *most* characteristic configuration is a *triphasic pattern* in both leads V_1 and V_6 (rsR^1 in V_1 and qRs in V_6).

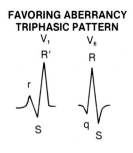

FAVORING ABERRANCY
TRIPHASIC PATTERN

Fig. 7-53

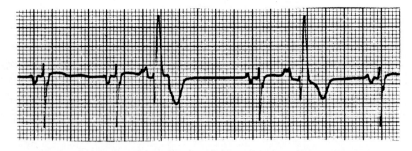

Fig. 7-54

NOTE: These PACs are conducted aberrantly with RBBB pattern or rsR^1 in lead V_1.

130 The deflections of the QRS complex produced by ectopic impulses on lead V_1 mimic the ears of a rabbit. The peaks of these deflections were recognized and initially described by a few CCU nurses as the "rabbit ear" phenomenon. When the *right peak* (ear) of the ectopic beat is taller than the left, aberrant conduction may be involved. However, when the *left* peak (ear) is taller, aberrant conduction is *highly unlikely,* and the pattern is therefore considered ventricular ectopy (PVC).

REMEMBER: RBBB pattern characteristically produces a terminal right peak referred to as the *R′ wave* and is compatible with the "rabbit ear" phenomenon.

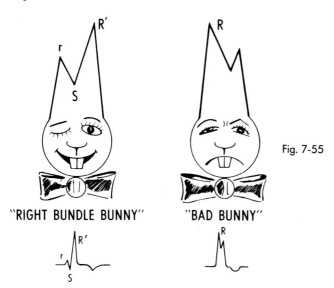

Fig. 7-55

"RIGHT BUNDLE BUNNY"   "BAD BUNNY"

131 LET US REVIEW: The best criteria supporting a diagnosis of an aberrant supraventricular beat is the presence of a _____ p wave.

The most characteristic QRS configuration in aberrantly conducted beats is a *(right/left)* bundle branch pattern.

The leads most helpful in the diagnosis of aberrantly conducted beats are _____ and _____.

The most characteristic QRS configuration in these leads is a *(monophasic/triphasic)* pattern, most typically _____ in lead V_1 and _____ in lead V_6.

premature	
right	
V_1; V_6	
triphasic; rsR′	
qRs	

132 The initial deflection of an RBBB pattern is the same as the patient's normal beat.

REMEMBER: The initial deflection seen in lead V_1 represents _____ depolarization. This electrical force originates in the left bundle branch and is thus unchanged by RBBB. Because aberrantly conducted beats are most commonly associated with RBBB patterns, the *initial* deflection of an aberrantly conducted beat is often *(the same as/different from)* the patient's normal beat.

septal

the same as

133 Bundle branch refractory periods vary according to the length of the preceding RR cycle. A *long* RR cycle prolongs the refractory period of the *second beat* in the next cycle. Thus the refractory period of an impulse is determined by the *timing of the preceding impulse.* Long RR cycles or *slow rates* are associated with *(long/short)* refractory periods. When preceded by long RR cycles, premature beats are *(more likely/less likely)* to find the bundle branches of the previous beat *still refractory.* Thus aberrant conduction is more likely to occur.

long

more likely

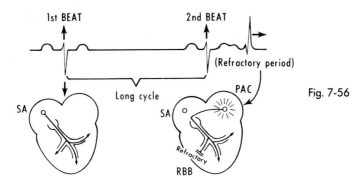

Fig. 7-56

NOTE: The PAC in Fig. 5-56, because of its prematurity, ends or forms a *short* cycle. This short cycle is preceded by the *long* cycle, promoting _____ conduction.

aberrant

Ventricular ectopic impulses also commonly end short cycles preceded by long cycles in settings such as ventricular bigeminy. Thus the presence of a different QRS complex ending a short cycle in the absence of other strong evidence favoring aberration (that is, premature p wave, triphasic pattern in leads V_1 and V_6) is *not* strong support for aberration.

134 PACs may increase in frequency until they begin to occur consecutively, thus producing a tachycardia. Aberrantly conducted PACs may also initiate runs of supraventricular tachycardia. When the first PACs is aberrantly conducted, consecutive impulses *may or may not* be aberrantly conducted. If only the first PAC is preceded by a *long cycle,* it may be the only impulse conducted aberrantly.

NOTE: In the above traces, only the first atrial impulse is aberrantly conducted. This PAC triggers a run of atrial flutter. Aberrant PACs end or form short cycles preceded by _____ cycles. The second and third beats in the burst of tachycardia end or form *short* RR cycles but *(are/are not)* preceded by long cycles. They therefore *(are/are not)* aberrantly conducted. Each aberrant beat in the example above appears *second* in a *group* of beats. However, it is actually the *first* ectopic beat in a run of ectopic beats.

long

are not

are not

This phenomenon, depicted in Fig. 7-57, is sometimes referred to as the *second-in-a-group rule.* When *only* the second in a group of rapid supraventricular beats is conducted differently, _____ conduction should be suspected.

aberrant

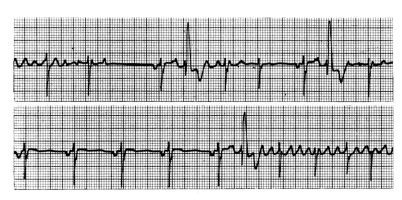

Fig. 7-57

135 The long-short cycle sequence promoting aberration is known as *Ashman's phenomenon.* It is depicted in the *second-in-a-group rule* mentioned above and in other rules related to aberration. In the presence of atrial fibrillation, RR cycle lengths vary. The length of the bundle branch refractory periods therefore also varies predisposing the patient to the occurrence of Ashman's phenomenon in which a long RR cycle is followed by a short cycle. In the presence of atrial fibrillation the impulse ending or forming the cycle *(is/is not)* likely to be conducted aberrantly. This long-short cycle sequence producing aberrant conduction is another illustration of _____ phenomenon.

is

Ashman's

Lead V₁

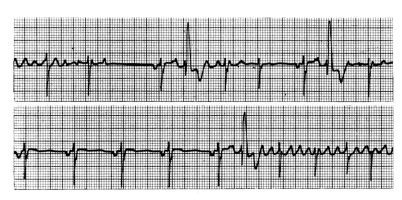

Fig. 7-58

The third beat in Fig. 7-58 ends a short cycle preceded by a long cycle. It has an _____ configuration on lead V₁. Therefore it is likely to be an _____ conducted beat. In the setting of atrial fibrillation, aberrantly conducted beats are a *common* occurrence. Unfortunately, in atrial fibrillation the best indicator of an aberrantly conducted PAC—the premature P wave—is lost. The diagnosis must be based on the resulting QRS patterns.

rsR'

aberrantly

REMEMBER: Ventricular ectopic beats may also occur in a cycling pattern. Therefore in the setting of atrial fibrillation—unless characteristic QRS patterns favoring aberration are also seen—a diagnosis of ventricular ectopy should be made. This is especially important in the setting of acute MI, in which ventricular ectopy *(is/is not)* likely to occur.

is

136 Aberrant conduction may produce less characteristic QRS patterns. When this variation occurs, it may be more difficult to differentiate between aberrantly conducted supraventricular beats and ventricular ectopy. *Anteroseptal MI* produces electrical distortions that prevent the QRS complex from assuming the typical aberrant patterns (see Unit 8).

REMEMBER: The initial small r wave in lead V_1 represents septal depolarization.

In patients with anteroseptal MI, septal depolarization is altered. Therefore in lead V_1 the initial r wave *(will/will not)* be seen. In these patients the normal QRS in lead V_1 has a QS configuration instead of the classic rS. Thus the RBBB pattern *(will/will not)* have an initial r wave. Instead, the QRS complex assumes a qR configuration. Aberrantly conducted beats in anteroseptal MI produce a qR pattern that may identically mimic *left* ventricular PVCs in *lead* V_1. In this setting, aberrant beats *cannot* assume the typical rsR' configuration and become difficult to differentiate from PVCs or VT, especially at rapid rates (see Fig. 7-59).

will not

will not

Lead V_1

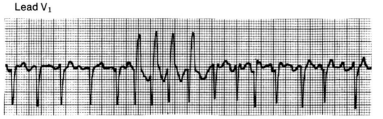

Fig. 7-59

NOTE: The occasional appearance of an initial r wave is artifactual in this case.

137 The analysis of leads V_1 and lead V_6 in patients with atrial fibrillation may be helpful in distinguishing supraventricular beats that are conducted from ventricular ectopy.

LET US REVIEW: The best criteria supporting a diagnosis of an aberrant SV beat is a preceding _____ p wave. However, in atrial fibrillation the p wave *(is/is not)* normally visible. Therefore other criteria for aberration must be used.

premature

is not

A _____ QRS pattern in leads V_1 and V_6 also strongly supports a diagnosis of aberration. Lead V_1 typically assumes a _____ pattern, and lead V_6 assumes a _____ pattern with *aberrant* beats.

triphasic

rsR'

qRs

Less typically the QRS complex of an aberrant impulse may produce a _____ pattern in lead V_1. This may occur if the patient has had an _____ infarction. When these less typical QRS patterns occur, it becomes more difficult to differentiate aberrant beats from ventricular ectopy. In the setting of acute MI, the diagnosis of *(aberration/ventricular ectopy)* should take priority.

qR
anterior

ventricular ectopy

138 Let us now consider the morphology of typical ventricular ectopy in more detail.

REMEMBER: Like aberrant beats, PVCs produce QRS patterns different from the patient's _____ beats.

normal

PVCs may also be preceded by a p wave as aberrant beats are; however, the p wave *(will/will not)* be premature (see Frames 70 to 72).

will not

The most characteristic QRS patterns produced by PVCs are either *monophasic* or *biphasic*.

PCVs originating in the *left ventricle* typically produce a monophasic R or biphasic qR pattern in lead V_1, resulting in a predominantly positive complex that may at first glance mimic the RBBB (aberrant) complex. A biphasic rS or QS pattern is most typically seen in lead V_6. This predominantly *negative* pattern in lead V_6 is a major clue helpful in differentiating left ventricular ectopic beats from aberrant SV beats. It *(does/does not)* mimic the RBBB (aberrant) complex in V_6, since it typically remains *(negative/positive)*.

does not
positive

FAVORING VENTRICULAR ECTOPY

MONOPHASIC PATTERNS

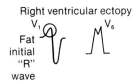

Left ventricular ectopy   Right ventricular ectopy

Fig. 7-60

139 In the setting of acute MI, most PVCs are *(left/right)* ventricular in origin. However, right ventricular ectopic beats and/or rhythms may also occur. These are usually easier to differentiate from aberrant supraventricular beats. Unlike LV PVCs, the QRS complexes are negative in V_1 and *(do/do not)* mimic the typical RBBB pattern.

left

do not

PVCs originating in the right ventricle typically produce a predominately _____, biphasic, rS pattern in lead V_1 and a monophasic R wave in lead V_6.

negative

The pattern of *right* PVCs is very similar to that produced by an LBBB pattern (see Unit 8, Frame 88).

140 The single most characteristic sign favoring ventricular ectopy is the presence of *fusion beats.*

REMEMBER: Fusion beats represent simultaneous depolarization of the same chamber of the heart by both _____ and   supraventricular
_____ impulses. Fusion beats are thus evidence that a   ventricular
_____ focus is firing.   ventricular

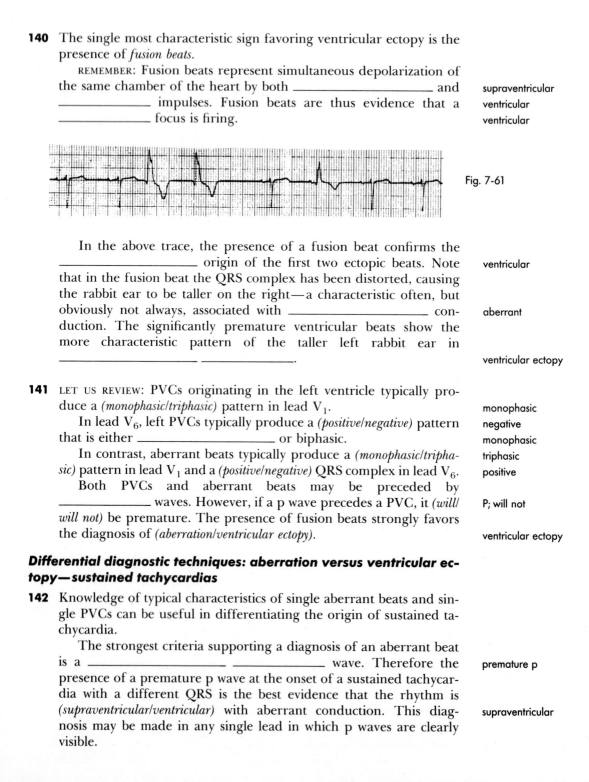

Fig. 7-61

In the above trace, the presence of a fusion beat confirms the _____ origin of the first two ectopic beats. Note   ventricular
that in the fusion beat the QRS complex has been distorted, causing
the rabbit ear to be taller on the right—a characteristic often, but
obviously not always, associated with _____ con-   aberrant
duction. The significantly premature ventricular beats show the
more characteristic pattern of the taller left rabbit ear in
_____ _____.   ventricular ectopy

141 LET US REVIEW: PVCs originating in the left ventricle typically produce a *(monophasic/triphasic)* pattern in lead V$_1$.   monophasic
In lead V$_6$, left PVCs typically produce a *(positive/negative)* pattern   negative
that is either _____ or biphasic.   monophasic
In contrast, aberrant beats typically produce a *(monophasic/triphasic)* pattern in lead V$_1$ and a *(positive/negative)* QRS complex in lead V$_6$.   triphasic
positive
Both PVCs and aberrant beats may be preceded by
_____ waves. However, if a p wave precedes a PVC, it *(will/*   P; will not
will not) be premature. The presence of fusion beats strongly favors
the diagnosis of *(aberration/ventricular ectopy).*   ventricular ectopy

Differential diagnostic techniques: aberration versus ventricular ectopy—sustained tachycardias

142 Knowledge of typical characteristics of single aberrant beats and single PVCs can be useful in differentiating the origin of sustained tachycardia.
The strongest criteria supporting a diagnosis of an aberrant beat
is a _____ _____ wave. Therefore the   premature p
presence of a premature p wave at the onset of a sustained tachycardia with a different QRS is the best evidence that the rhythm is
(supraventricular/ventricular) with aberrant conduction. This diag-   supraventricular
nosis may be made in any single lead in which p waves are clearly
visible.

The strongest criteria supporting a diagnosis of ventricular ectopy is the presence of ventricular _____ beats.

fusion

REMEMBER: Fusion beats typically represent simultaneous depolarization of the same chamber of the heart by both a _____ and a _____ impulse. Therefore ECG documentation of fusion beats in the presence of a sustained tachycardia with a different QRS strongly supports that the idea that the rhythm is ventricular tachycardia. The diagnosis of fusion beats may also be made on single leads.

supraventricular; ventrciular

When either fusion beats or captured beats interrupt a sustained tachycardia with wide QRS complexes, these beats are referred to as Dressler's beats. Dressler's beats confirm the presence of _____ _____.

ventricular ectopy

143 After single-lead assessment, if doubt exists as to the origin of the tachycardia, clinical trials of antidysrhythmic agents such as lidocaine (Xylocaine) or procainamide (Pronestyl) should be considered. If the arrhythmia is abolished after the administration of Xylocaine or Pronestyl, then the diagnosis of VT is supported. (See Unit 10 for a discussion of potential hazards with this approach.)

Clinical signs of AV dissociation may be helpful in differentiating between ventricular taachycardia and SV tachycardia with aberrant conduction.

REMEMBER: Ventricular tachycardia usually results in a form of a dissociated rhythm (see Frame 179).

When clinical signs of AV dissociation such as intermittent _____ waves and varying intensity of _____, are present, a diagnosis of _____ _____ is strongly supported.

cannon
S_1; ventricular ectopy

NOTE: Junctional tachycardia with aberrant conduction may result in AV dissociation and mimic VT but is highly unusual.

144 When a premature p wave cannot be verified or fusion beats identified at the onset of a tachycardia, and clinical signs are not helpful, analysis of the QRS patterns in both leads V_1 and V_6 will provide further information.

REMEMBER: Aberrant SV impulses usually conduct with a(n) _____ bundle branch block pattern.

right

The most characteristic QRS morphology favoring an aberration is a(n) _____ pattern in both leads V_1 and V_6.

triphasic

The lead V_6 morphology remains predominantly (*positive/negative*).

positive

Left ventricular rhythms, in contrast, would characteristically produce a monophasic or biphasic pattern in leads V_1 and V_6. Lead V_6 in this setting is predominantly (*positive/negative*) and is especially

negative

helpful in this situation because of the sharp differences in morphology seen with the two rhythms.

145 Multilead assessment may also be beneficial in the presence of a sustained tachycardia. Multilead assessment allows for simultaneous observation of the limb leads and chest leads and calculation of the electrical axis.

The presence of an abnormal left axis or indeterminate axis (see Unit 8), particularly if the QRS morphology is QS in the inferior leads, favors a ventricular origin.

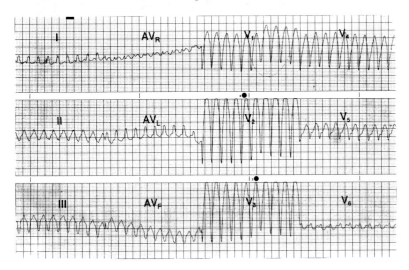

Fig. 7-62

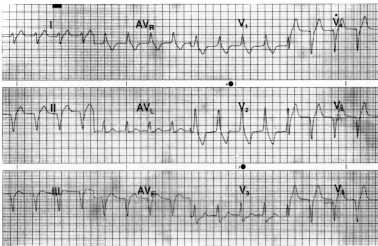

NOTE: This is an example of a ventricular ectopic rhythm showing characteristic features of ventricular ectopy, although the ventricular rate is not consistently greater than 100 (see accelerated idioventricular rhythm, or AIVR).

146 The presence of all upright QRS patterns or all negative QRS patterns throughout the precordial leads to (V₁ to V₆) also favors a diagnosis of VT. This phenomenon is referred to as precordial concordance and is *not* commonly seen.

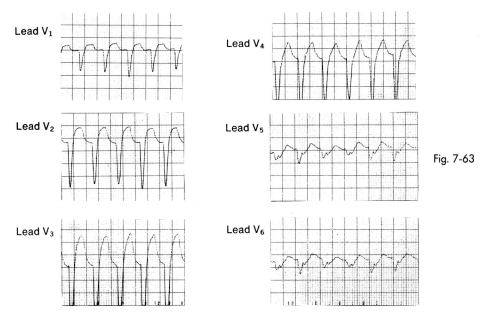

Fig. 7-63

The "rabbit ear" phenomenon has also been used to support a diagnosis of ventricular rhythms (see Frame 130). When the left rabbit ear in lead V₁ is taller than the right, a diagnosis of *(ventricular/supraventricular)* ectopy is supported.

ventricular

Table 8. Differential diagnosis of ventricular arrhythmias and supraventricular aberrations

Ventricular arrhythmias favoring ventricular ectopy	Supraventricular aberration favoring aberrantly conducted supraventricular beats
A. Single beats	
1. If preceded by p wave, should *not* be premature	1. Premature p wave (indicates PAC)
2. QRS: biphasic or monophasic pattern: qR or R on lead V₁; QS or rS on lead V₆	2. QRS; triphasic pattern (RBBB); rsR¹ on lead V₁; qRs on lead V₆
3. Presence of fusion beats; "rabbit ear" higher on left in lead V₁*	3. Long-short cycle sequence: second in-a-group rule; long-short sequence in atrial fibrillation*

*Weak criteria.   *Continued.*

Table 8. Differential diagnosis of ventricular arrhythmias and supraventricular abberations—cont'd

Criteria favoring VT	Criteria favoring SVT with aberrations
B. Sustained tachycardias	
1. Captured beats or fusion beats during tachycardia (Dressler's beats)	1. Premature p wave at onset of paroxysm
2. Disappears with lidocaine (Xylocaine) or procainamide	2. Triphasic pattern in leads V_1 and V_6; rsR^1 in lead V_1 and qRS in lead V_6
3. Clinical signs of AV dissociation: intermittent cannon "a" waves, varying intensity of S_1-independent p waves	3. Grossly irregular; responds to vagal manuever
4. Monophasic or biphasic QRS in leads V_1 and V_6; lead V_1—upright; lead V_6—negative	
5. Extreme axis deviation with QS patterns in leads, II, III, and aV_F	
6. Concordant negativity or positivity*	

*Weak criteria.

147 NURSING ORDERS: The patient with aberration
1. When analyzing premature beats that have a different or wide QRS morphology:
   —Look for preceding *premature P waves.*
   —Monitor on lead V_1 or MCL_1 and also check lead with best P waves if not lead V_1.
   —If no P waves are clearly visible, analyze the QRS configuration on leads V_1 and V_6 on their monitoring equivalents, MCL_1 and MCL_6.
   —Look for an rSR' pattern on lead V_1.
   —Check lead V_6 for triphasic (qRS) configuration.
   —Look for fusion beats.
   —Consider the clinical setting in which the abnormal beats occur. Is the patient in atrial fibrillation? Does the patient have an acute MI, especially anteroseptal MI?
   —Has the patient been having PACs?
   —Consider an antiarrhythmic trial.
2. In the presence of atrial fibrillation
   —Monitor on lead V_1 or its equivalent, MCL_1.
   —Look for cycling (Ashman's phenomenon).*
   —Check to see if the patient was previously in RSR with ectopic beats.
   NOTE: The presence of a triphasic configuration on both leads V_1 and V_6, together with cycling, is the strongest evidence favoring aberration in this setting.

3. Rule out aberration:
   —If the premature impulses are end-diastolic and, especially, preceded by nonpremature P waves.
   —If there are fusion beats present.
   —If less characteristic QRS patterns are present on the chest leads.
   —If the premature or ectopic impulses are preceded by a short rather than long RR cycle.*
   —When the "rabbit ear" of the ectopic beat is taller on the left in lead V_1.*
4. In the presence of a sustained tachyarrhythmia with changing or wide QRS complexes
   —When central pulses are absent, thus confirming the diagnosis of ventricular ectopy, administer electrical intervention.
   —Note the presence or absence of patient symptoms. VT is less likely to be asymptomatically tolerated, although asymptomatic VT does occur.
   —If the patient loses consciousness or develops any of the typical sensorium changes accompanying hypoxia (see Unit 3), always treat the arrhythmia initially as ventricular.
   —Note the presence of cannon waves and/or the varying intensity of S_1, which favor VT.
   —Consider an antiarrhythmic trial.
   —Note the presence of the second-in-a-group phenomenon.*
   —Obtain recordings on multiple monitoring leads; then document by obtaining a 12-lead ECG.
   —Look for Dressler's beats.
   —Rule out aberration if Dressler's beats are present, if concordance appears on the chest leads, if there is indeterminate axis deviation on the limb leads, or if the ectopic rhythm disappears following lidocaine (Xylocaine) therapy.
   —Suggest carotid sinus pressure.
5. When in doubt, in the setting of an acute MI, consider the ectopic beat ventricular in origin and attempt a therapeutic antiarrhythmic trial with lidocaine (Xylocaine) or procainamide (Pronestyl).

HEART BLOCKS

148 Let us now consider a group of arrhythmias that occur as a result of depressed conduction—the *heart blocks*.

REMEMBER: The heart's conduction system allows for the rapid transmission of electrical impulses from the _____ node, through the _____ _____ tissue, to the _____.

SA
AV junctional
ventricles

An electrical impulse can be *delayed* or *blocked* at any point in this

---

*Weak criteria

conduction system. The group of arrhythmias that occur as a result of depressed conduction are known as heart _____.

blocks

Blocks may occur in any structure of the conduction system: the _____ node, the _____ _____ tissue, or the bundle _____ system.

SA; AV junctional
branch

SA block

149 SA block occurs because conduction is depressed between the SA node and the _____.

atria

When SA block occurs, the normal sinus impulse is formed but fails to reach the atria. As a result the atria and the ventricles *(will/ will not)* be depolarized.

will not

REMEMBER: Atrial depolarization is represented on the ECG by the _____ wave. Ventricular depolarization is represented on the ECG by the _____ complex.

P
QRS

Therefore at the onset of an SA block, a _____ wave and a _____ complex will suddenly be dropped.

P
QRS

150 When the *onset* of SA block is not recorded, it is difficult to differentiate between this arrhythmia and *sinus bradycardia*. When a sinus rate of 80 *suddenly* drops to 40 beats per minute, the arrhythmia is most likely *SA block*. The pause in the rhythm associated with an SA block is usually equal to a multiple of original p wave cycles.

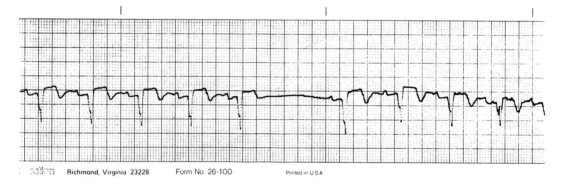

Richmond, Virginia 23228   Form No. 26-100   Printed in U.S.A.

Fig. 7-64

REMEMBER: SA *block* is a manifestation of depressed *conduction* between the _____ node and the _____. *Sinus bradycardia* is a manifestation of depressed _____ in the SA node.

SA; atria
automaticity

Another arrhythmia that may appear similar on the ECG is *sinus arrest,* which occurs when the sinus node is depressed so that the impulses are not formed. Unlike an SA block, the pause in the rhythm associated with a sinus arrest is of no predictable length.

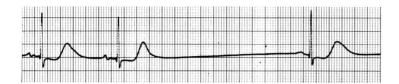

Fig. 7-65

151 SA block and sinus arrest are potentially clinically significant because they may result in a *slow rate* and cause a symptomatic fall in cardiac output.

Therapy in the management of SA block is directed toward accelerating conduction between the SA *node* and the *atria*. Therapy in the management of sinus arrest is directed toward enhancing the _____ of the SA node. Both therapeutic goals can usually be achieved with a single drug.

automaticity

152 LET US REVIEW: SA block is a manifestation of depressed conduction between the _____ _____ and the _____. When the SA block occurs, the normal *sinus* impulse fails to reach the _____.

SA node
atria
atria

SA block is diagnosed on the ECG by the sudden absence of a _____ wave and a _____ _____. If the onset of SA block is not recorded, it may be difficult to distinguish between this arrhythmia and sinus _____ on the ECG.

P; QRS complex

bradycardia

Another arrhythmia that may appear as SA block on the ECG is sinus _____.

arrest

Both sinus arrest and SA block are clinically significant when they result in a sustained slow rate and thus cause a symptomatic fall in _____ _____.

cardiac output

Therapy in the management of SA block is directed toward accelerating conduction between the _____ node and the _____.

SA
atria

AV blocks

153 AV blocks are a manifestation of depressed conduction between the *atria* and the *ventricles.* Therefore, to detect AV blocks on the ECG, the _____ interval must be analyzed.

PR

Analysis of the *p wave rate* should precede assessment of the pr interval because an accelerated atrial rate may indicate the presence of an atrial arrhythmia or predispose the patient to more severe forms of AV blocks.

AV blocks are classified (1) according to their location in relation to the His bundle and (2) by degrees according to ECG criteria.

AV blocks are classified as occurring either *above* or *below* the His bundle. AV blocks that occur *above* the His bundle at the AV node are known as "supra-Hisian" blocks.

AV blocks occurring below the His bundle in the bundle branch system are known as *(supra/infra)*-Hisian blocks.

infra

154 The classification of AV blocks according to degrees (first, second, and third) is based on analysis of the ECG. Although it is generally true that second-degree and third-degree AV blocks are more severe disturbances than is first-degree AV block, it is not always the case. The most important clinical parameters to assess when the patient develops an AV block are the following:

1. The ventricular rate
2. The patient's tolerance of this ventricular rate (that is, is he or she exhibiting signs of a symptomatic fall in cardiac output?)
3. The setting in which the block is occurring (that is, is it more likely that the block is above or below the His bundle?)

REMEMBER: The atrial rate should also be identified when the patient develops an AV block, since an _____ atrial rate may predispose the patient to AV block.

accelerated

First-degree AV block

155 First-degree AV block is a manifestation of *delayed conduction* time between the SA node and the ventricles. Although there is a delay in conduction time, *all* impulses are conducted to the ventricles.

REMEMBER: On the ECG, the conduction time between the SA node and the ventricles is represented by the _____ interval.

PR

In first-degree AV block, the only abnormality on the ECG is a prolonged _____ interval.

PR

REMEMBER: The normal PR interval is from _____ to _____ second.

0.12
0.20

Therefore a diagnosis of *first-degree AV block* is made when the PR interval is greater than _____ second. First-degree AV block may occur as a result of pathology either *above* or *below* the His bundle. To determine the location of the block, the rhythm must be analyzed within the clinical setting in which it occurs.

0.20

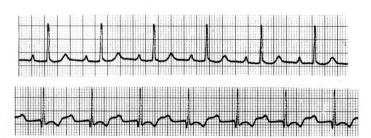

Fig. 7-66

NOTE: Complete analysis of the strips on page 330 require assessment of the atrial rate. For example, in Fig. 7-66, regular sinus rhythm with first-degree AV block would be the complete diagnosis.

The clinical significance of first-degree AV block is related to (1) the _____ _____ and symptoms indicating a fall in _____ _____ and (2) the location of the AV block in relation to the His bundle. The location of the AV block in relation to the His bundle is determined from the _____ _____ in which it occurs (see Frame 177).

ventricular rate
cardiac output

clinical setting

156 LET US REVIEW: In first-degree AV block, the sinus impulse is delayed in reaching the _____. First-degree AV block is diagnosed on the ECG by the presence of a *(prolonged/shortened)* PR interval. In first-degree AV block, each P wave *(will/will not)* be followed by a QRS complex.

ventricles
prolonged
will

157 **In summary:**
In first-degree AV block:
1. Sinus impulses are delayed in reaching the ventricles.
2. The block may be as a result of pathology *above* or *below* the His bundle.
3. PR intervals are greater than 0.20 second.
4. Each P wave is followed by a QRS complex.

Second-degree AV block

158 When second-degree AV block occurs, *one* or *more* sinus impulses fail to activate the ventricles. Atrial depolarization occurs normally, but ventricular depolarization *does not always* follow. Therefore, in the presence of second-degree AV block, P waves *(will/will not)* be present. Every P wave, however, will not be followed by a _____ complex. ECG diagnosis of second-degree AV block requires that there be at *least* one *nonconducted* P wave or *dropped* QRS complex.

will

QRS

REMEMBER: AV blocks are classified according to their location in relation to the _____ _____.

His bundle

159 Generally, *Type I,* or *Wenckebach,* second-degree AV blocks occur *above* the His bundle at the AV *node.*
NOTE: These blocks are also known as *Mobitz I.*
Blocks of the *Wenckebach* type occur *(above/below)* the His bundle at the AV node.
REMEMBER: The AV node is primarily supplied by the *(right/left)* coronary artery.
Blocks that occur at the AV *node* are *usually* associated with *right*

above

right

coronary artery pathology. Right coronary artery occlusion produces _____ wall MI.

inferior

Thus second-degree AV blocks of the Wenckebach type are associated with _____ wall MI.

inferior

NOTE: Wenckebach-type second-degree AV blocks may also occur as a result of *digitalis toxicity* or chronic lesions of the conduction system.

Wenckebach blocks occur in the presence of IWMI as a result of (1) ischemia to the _____ node or (2) ischemia to the parasympathetic (vagal) fibers that supply the AV node. In IWMI the ischemia at the AV node is *reversible*. Thus the AV blocks that occur as a result of this ischemia are (*transient/permanent*).

AV

transient

Second-degree AV blocks of the Wenckebach type are thus described as being *ischemic* and *transient* in *nature*.

160 Type I (Wenckebach) block is diagnosed when a dropped QRS complex is preceded by progressive *prolongation* of the PR interval. The progressive prolongation of the PR interval eventually causes the P wave to fall *in the refractory period* of the ventricles, and thus a P wave eventually becomes blocked.

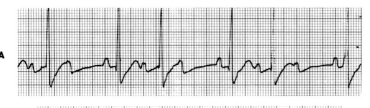

A

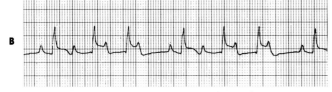

B

Fig. 7-67

NOTE: In Fig. 7-67, *A*, the rhythm could be described as *RSR* with 2° AV block—Wenckebach—because the P wave rate is _____ beats per minute. In Fig. 7-67, *B*, the rhythm could be described as *sinus tachycardia* because the P wave is _____ beats per minute. In this case slowing of the atrial rate may have resulted in resolution of the AV block. Other characteristics of Type I, or Wenckebach, block are (1) constant PP intervals and (2) irregular and decreasing RR intervals.

100

120

161 Wenckebach block is clinically significant because (1) it may result in a slow rate and cause a symptomatic fall in cardiac output, and (2) it may be the precursor of third-degree AV block.

Initial therapy in the management of second-degree AV block of the Wenckebach type is directed toward *accelerating (SA/AV)* conduction and thus increasing the ventricular rate.

NOTE: Because of its ischemic nature, Wenckebach block usually responds well to pharmacological intervention. Temporary pacing may be required in some patients.

162 LET US REVIEW: Wenckebach block is classified as a *(first-degree/second-degree)* AV block and occurs *(above/below)* the His bundle at the _____ node. Type I, or Wenckebach, blocks are associated with _____ wall MI. They may also be a manifestation of _____ toxicity. Wenckebach blocks classically occur as a result of _____ to the AV node and are *(transient/permanent)*.

ECG diagnosis of Type I block requires the presence of: (1) progressive _____ interval prolongation preceding the dropped QRS complex, (2) regular intervals between _____ waves, and (3) irregular intervals between _____ waves.

Initial therapy, in the management of Wenckebach block is directed toward accelerating _____ conduction.

Wenckebach second-degree AV block requires therapy when it results in a slow ventricular rate and causes a _____ fall in cardiac output.

163 Generally, Type II (Mobitz II) second-degree AV blocks occur *below* the His bundle in the *bundle branch system.*

REMEMBER: The left coronary artery supplies most of the right bundle branch and the anteriorsuperior division of the _____ branch. The posteroinferior division of the left branch is also partially supplied by the _____ coronary artery.

Blocks that occur *below the His bundle* are usually associated with *left* coronary artery pathology. Left coronary artery occlusion produces _____ wall MI. Thus Type II, or Mobitz II, blocks may be associated with _____ wall MI.

NOTE: Type II blocks may also occur as a result of *chronic lesions* of the conduction system.

Type II (Mobitz II) blocks occur in AWMI as a result of the *necrotic* process. In AWMI the blocks that occur in the bundle branch system may thus be described as being *necrotic* in *nature.*

164 Mobitz II block is diagnosed when a dropout QRS complex that is *not* preceded by a progressive prolongation of the PR interval is seen. When this type of block occurs, the PR interval remains fixed, and the dropped beat occurs without warning. Another characteris-

AV

second-degree
above
AV
inferior
digitalis
ischemia
transient

PR

P

R

AV

symptomatic

left
left

anterior
anterior

tic of Type II second-degree AV block is a regular interval between
P waves.

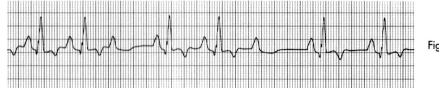

Fig. 7-68

NOTE: Complete diagnosis of Fig. 7-68 is RSR with second-degree
AV block, Type II (Mobitz II).

165 Let us now consider the pathophysiology of Type II Mobitz block in
more detail.

    REMEMBER: Type II block occurs as a result of pathology in the
_____ _____ system.

    The bundle branch system is composed of *three fascicles:* the right
bundle branch, the anterosuperior division of the _____
branch, and the _____ division of the
_____ branch (see Unit 8).

    A block in *one* of these fascicles is known as a *monofascicular* block.

    A block in *two* of these fascicles is known as a *bifascicular* block.

    A block in *all three* of these fascicles is known as a *trifascicular*
block.

    Type II second-degree AV block usually occurs as a result of an
intermittent trifascicular block.

bundle branch

left

posterior
left

166 When Type II block occurs, a sinus impulse fails to activate the ventricles because *all conduction pathways* between the His bundle and the
ventricles are _____.

blocked

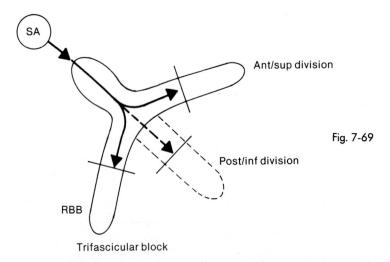

Fig. 7-69

334

REMEMBER: ECG diagnosis of Mobitz II block requires that there be a dropped *(P wave/QRS complex)* that is *not* preceded by progressive prolongation of the _____ interval.

QRS complex
PR

To diagnose Type II, or Mobitz II, block, there must also be *evidence* of *preexisting bundle branch pathology*. The probability that trifascicular block is likely to occur must be demonstrated. There must be pathology in at least two of the three fascicles for it to be probable that the trifascicular, or _____, block will occur. Therefore a bifascicular block in the presence of AWMI *(would/would not)* be evidence that trifascicular block could occur. The presence of a monofascicular block *(is/is not)* evidence that trifascicular block is *likely* to occur.

Mobitz
would

is not

167 Mobitz II block is clinically significant because (1) it may be associated with a symptomatic fall in cardiac output, and (2) it is the precursor of third-degree, or complete, AV block.

Initial therapy in the management of Type II second-degree AV block is directed toward accelerating *(SA/AV)* conduction thus the ventricular rate.

AV

NOTE: Because the pathology in the bundle is necrotic in nature, Type II second-degree AV block usually responds poorly to pharmacological intervention. Electrical intervention is usually necessary to manage the arrhythmia.

168 LET US REVIEW: Type II, or Mobitz II, block occurs as a result of pathology in the _____ _____ system. Type II second-degree AV blocks are associated with _____ wall MI. They may also occur as a result of chronic lesions of the _____ _____. Type II second-degree AV blocks usually occur as a result of intermittent _____ fascicular block.

bundle branch

anterior
conduction system

tri-

To diagnose Type II, or Mobitz II, block on the ECG the following must exist:
1. A fixed PR interval preceding the dropped _____ complex

QRS

2. Regular intervals between _____ waves

P

3. Evidence that the patient has preexisting _____ _____ pathology

bundle branch

Mobitz II block is clinically significant when it is associated with a symptomatic fall in _____ _____.

cardiac output

Fixed ratio second-degree AV block

169 Fixed ratio second-degree AV block (for example, two to one, three to one, or four to one) may be an end result of either a Wenckebach or a Mobitz II block. Unless the onset of the fixed ratio block is recorded, it is difficult to conclude whether it results from a Wenckebach to a Mobitz II block. Fixed ratio blocks should thus be analyzed in the clinical setting in which they occur.

In fixed ratio blocks that occur as an end result of a Wenckebach block, the QRS complexes are generally *narrow*.

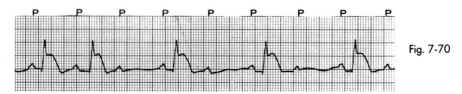

Fig. 7-70

In fixed ratio blocks that occur as an end result of a Mobitz block, the QRS complexes are generally *wide*.

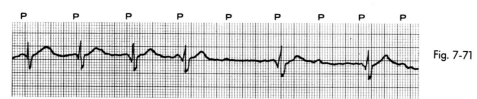

Fig. 7-71

170 In summary:

Table 9. Second-degree AV blocks

Wenckebach (Type I)	Mobitz (Type II)
AV lesion: supra-Hisian	Lesion in bundle branch system: infra-Hisian
Associated with IWMI, digitalis toxicity, chronic lesion of conduction system	Associated with AWMI, chronic lesions of the conduction system
Described as ischemic, reversible, and transient in nature	Described as necrotic in nature
Dropped QRS complex preceded by progressive prolongation of the PR interval	Dropped QRS complex preceded by a fixed PR interval
Regular PP intervals	Regular PP intervals
Usually responds well to pharmacological intervention	Usually not responsive to pharmacological intervention
May require temporary pacing in symptomatic patients	Requires electrical intervention

171 LET US REVIEW: In *first-degree* AV block, all sinus impulses are conducted to the ventricles, but the conduction occurs with _____. In *second-degree* AV block, *some* of the sinus impulses fail to activate the ventricles and some are _____.

delay

conducted

336

The pathology involved in AV block can progress in severity *until all sinus impulses are blocked.* When this occurs, the AV block is known as *third-degree,* or complete, *AV block.*

REMEMBER: As with all AV blocks it is important to identify the atrial rate together with the degree of the block.

Third-degree AV block

172 In third-degree AV block, all of the sinus impulses fail to activate the

_____.   ventricles

There is no relationship between the *atria* and the *ventricles.* Therefore it can be expected that there will be no *fixed* relationship between the _____ wave and the _____ complex.   P; QRS

REMEMBER: The interval that denotes the relationship between the atria and the ventricles is the _____   PR interval

_____.

One of the characteristics of third-degree AV block is a *highly* ✳ *variable* PR interval.

173 Third-degree AV block may occur as an end result of Type I (Wenckebach) second-degree AV block.

REMEMBER: Wenckebach block occurs *(above/below)* the His bundle   above
at the _____ node.   AV

When third-degree AV block occurs following a Wenckebach block, the ventricles will usually be under control of the AV node, and the controlling rhythm will be *idiojunctional.*

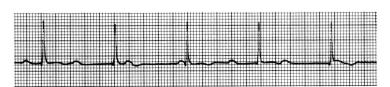

Fig. 7-72

NOTE: The complete ECG diagnosis of Fig. 7-72 is RSR rhythm with third-degree complete AV block and idiojunctional rhythm. Longer tracing of this rhythm often reveals occasional captured beats, suggesting that this AV block is actually not complete—especially when the ventricular rate remains about 40.

REMEMBER: The ventricular rate of an *idiojunctional* rhythm is *usu-   70
ally* between 40 and _____ beats per minute, and the QRS   narrow
complexes are *(narrow/wide)* unless bundle branch block is present.

174 Third-degree Av block may also occur as an end result of Type II Mobitz second-degree AV block.

REMEMBER: Mobitz blocks occur *(above/below)* the His bundle in the   below
_____ _____ system.   bundle branch

When the third-degree AV block occurs following Type II block, the ventricles will usually control the rhythm and the controlling rhythm will be *idioventricular*.

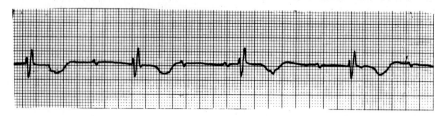

Fig. 7-73

NOTE: Complete diagnosis of Fig. 7-73 is RSR rhythm with complete AV block and idioventricular rhythm.

REMEMBER: The ventricular rate of an *idioventricular rhythm* is usually between _____ and _____ beats per minute, and the QRS complexes are (narrow/wide).

20; 40
wide

175 Third-degree, or complete, AV block is clinically significant *when* it is associated with a symptomatic fall in cardiac output.

Third-degree AV block that follows a Wenckebach Type I second-degree AV block may *not* require therapy because the controlling rhythm is commonly idiojunctional at a VR between _____ and _____ per minute.

40; 70

Third-degree AV block that occurs as an end result of a Mobitz Type II second-degree AV block usually results in a symptomatic fall in cardiac output because the ventricular rate is between _____ and _____ per minute.

20; 40

Initial therapy in the management of third-degree AV block is directed toward accelerating AV conduction and thus the _____ rate.

ventricular

LET US REVIEW: When third-degree AV block occurs, there is *no* relationship between the _____ wave and the _____ complex. As a result there will be a highly variable _____ interval.

P
QRS
PR

176 In summary:

In third-degree AV block:

1. Highly variable PR intervals occur, since no relationship exists between P waves and QRS complexes.
2. There are regular PP intervals.
3. There are regular RR intervals.
4. Following Wenckebach the controlling rhythm will usually be *idiojunctional*.
5. Following Mobitz II the controlling rhythm will usually be *idioventricular*.

338

177 NURSING ORDERS: The patient with an AV block
   1. Is the *AV block* resulting in symptomatic bradycardia?
   2. Identify the type of MI associated with the AV block.
   3. If AV block is associatd with IWMI:
      —Have atropine at the bedside.
   REMEMBER: AV blocks associated with IWMI are *ischemic* in nature and usually respond well to pharmacological intervention.
      —Watch for the development of Type I (Wenckebach) second-degree AV block.
      —Watch for the development of third-degree AV block with idiojunctional rhythm.
   4. If AV block is associated with AWMI:
      —Monitor the patient with first-degree AV block for the development of intraventricular conduction disturbances (see Unit 8), and observe for the development of Mobitz II block.
      —In anticipation of Type II (Mobitz) block, have a transthoracic pacemaker at the bedside or an (Isuprel) drip if a tranthoracic pacemaker is not available.
      —Watch for the development of third-degree AV block with idioventricular rhythm.

AV DISSOCIATION

178 In various cardiac arrhythmias, the atria beat independently of the ventricles. Examples of such arrhythmias include the following:
   1. VT without retrograde conduction.
   2. Junctional tachycardia without retrograde conduction
   3. Complete heart block (CHB)
   The term *AV dissociation* is therefore a general term and might apply to any of the entire group of arrhythmias, with varying clinical significance.

179 AV dissociation is a general term that may be used to describe any cardiac arrhythmia in which the _____ and the _____ beat independently. The best indication of a constant relationship, or occasion, between the atria and the ventricles is the presence of a fixed _____ interval. Therefore, in the presence of AV dissociation, the PR inverval *(does/does not)* remain the same.

atria
ventricles

PR
does not

180 AV dissociation is a *(specific/general)* term. It is a description, not a diagnosis. If the term *AV dissociation* is used to describe an arrhythmia, a more complete interpretation is required, such as:
   1. AV dissociation resulting from VT
   2. AV dissociation resulting from junctional rhythm, or tachycardia

general

3. AV dissociation resulting from CHB
4. AV dissociation resulting from ventricular pacing
   When AV dissociation occurs as a result of VT, the ventricles generally beat *(faster/slower)* than the atria.

faster

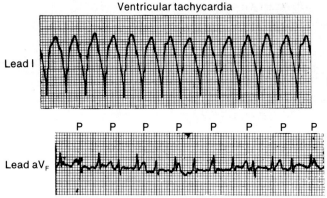

Ventricular tachycardia

Lead I

Lead aV$_F$

Fig. 7-74

(Simultaneous tracings) NOTE: Observe the dissociation between the P waves and QRS complexes in lead aV$_F$.

181 Let us now consider another example of AV dissociation. When the SA node slows, the _____ _____ tissue may assume control of the ventricles. If that occurs and the atria remain under the control of the SA node, the atria and the ventricles will become *(associated/dissociated)*.

AV junctional

dissociated

   This rhythm is best identified as AV dissociation with a(n) _____ _____ pacemaker. When this arrhythmia occurs, the ventricular rate is usually only slightly greater that the atria rate. Thus the P waves appear to march into the QRS complex, forming a characteristic pattern.

AV junctional

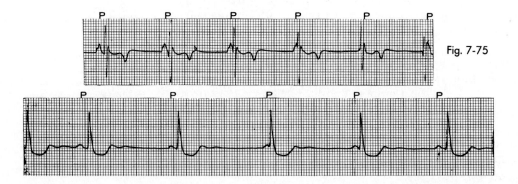

Fig. 7-75

NOTE: When the atrial and ventricular rates remain almost the same, this arrhythmia may be referred to as *isorhythmic AV dissociation.*

340

182 AV dissociation with a junctional pacemaker has the same clinical significance as a(n) _____ rhythm. This arrhythmia is terminated when the SA node accelerates and again controls the heart. If therapy is indicated in the management of this arrhythmia, the drug of choice is _____.

junctional

atropine

When AV dissociation occurs as a result of CHB, the ventricles beat *(faster/slower)* than the atria (Fig. 7-76).

slower

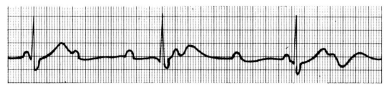

Fig. 7-76

NOTE: AV dissociation caused by normal ventricular pacing mimics this pattern. The major difference is the appearance of the pacing spike preceding each QRS complex. The ventricular rate is also faster.

183 Clinical signs may aid in the diagnosis of AV dissociation. When the atria and ventricles beat independently, atrial and ventricular depolarization and contraction may randomly *coincide*.

REMEMBER: During ventricular systole, the AV valves are closed. *Reflux* of *blood* occurs when the atria attempt to empty their contents against these closed valves. This reflux is seen as an accentuation of normal neck vein pulsations. These accentuated atrial waves are known as *cannon waves*. These large intermittent pulsations are easily visible if one inspects the neck.

184 LET US REVIEW: When AV dissociation occurs, atrial and ventricular contractions will randomly _____. When that occurs, the atria will contract against *(closed/open)* AV valves. Reflux of atrial contents into the venous system results in accentuation of neck vein _____. These accentuated waves are a clinical sign of a dissociated rhythm and are known as _____ _____.

coincide
closed

pulses

cannon waves

Another clinical sign indicative of a dissociated rhythm is varying intensity of the first heart sound.

REMEMBER: The first heart sound is known as _____ and represents closure of the *(AV/SL)* valves. It marks the onset of ventricular *(systole/diastole)*.

S_1
AV
systole

The intensity of S_1 is related to the *timing* of ventricular systole. If ventricular systole occurs when the valves are widely opened, a *loud* sound will be produced. Short PR intervals are associated with widely opened AV valves and *loud* first heart sounds.

A short PR interval implies that the atria and ventricles contract in *rapid* sequence. The AV valve is widely reopened when atrial systole occurs and then rapidly slammed shut as ventricular systole immediately follows.

In the presence of a *long* PR *interval,* the atria and ventricles contract in *(fast/slow)* sequence, producing a less intense or *(louder/softer)* S_1.

slow; softer

When AV dissociation occurs, *the PR interval (does/does not)* remain the same. Thus the intensity of S_1 constantly varies. Intermittent cannon waves and varying intensity of S_1 are clinical signs of a _____ rhythm.

does not

dissociated

MULTILEAD ASSESSMENT OF ARRHYTHMIAS

185 Multiple ECG views facilitate the accurate interpretation of rhythm disturbances. This concept is particularly critical in the following arrhythmias: (1) *narrow PVCs,* (2) isolated *ventricular ectopy* as opposed to *aberrant conduction,* (3) *atrial arrhythmias* (PAC, atrial flutter, and atrial fibrillation), and (4) *ventricular tachycardia* as opposed to *supraventricular tachycardia with aberrant conduction.*

186 PVCs may appear somewhat narrow or less characteristic when analyzed on a single lead. Selection of another lead may provide a more characteristic pattern (Fig. 7-77).

Lead I

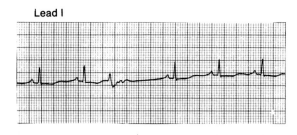

Lead II

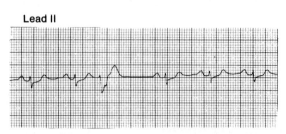

Lead V$_1$

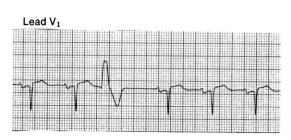

Fig. 7-77

Recording of leads V_1 and V_6 may be unnecessary unless aberrant conduction is suspected.

Example A: Selected monitoring lead ⬛ Lead I ⬛

Lead I

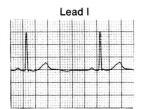

Lead II

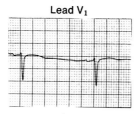

Lead III

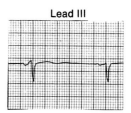

Lead V₁

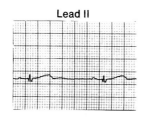

Example B: Selected monitoring lead ⬛ Lead V₁ (MCL₁) ⬛

Lead I

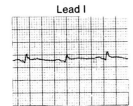

Lead II

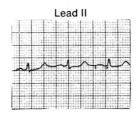

Lead III

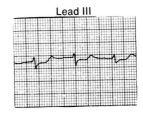

Fig. 7-78

Lead V₁

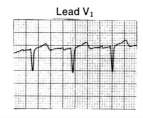

Lead V₂

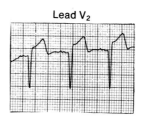

Example C: Selected monitoring lead ⬛ Lead I ⬛

Lead I

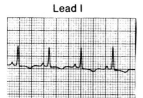

Lead II

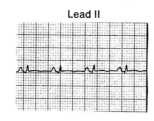

Lead III

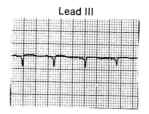

Lead V₁

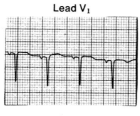

187 There is no ideal monitoring lead for every patient. A critical consideration when selecting an ideal monitoring lead for a given patient is determining which lead has the most clearly visible P waves. Selection of a lead providing the clearest P waves facilitates the interpretation of atrial arrhythmias, junctional arrhythmias, and AV block, as demonstrated by the examples in Fig. 7-78.

NOTE: In example C, the P waves are clearly visible on lead II but not the QRS complexes, making concurrent ventricular arrhythmias or AV blocks difficult to diagnose. Lead _____ would be preferred.

II

188 In atrial flutter, the characteristic sawtooth appearance is most clearly seen on leads II, III, and aV$_F$. However, the P waves may also be clearly identified in lead V$_1$ in the absence of a sawtooth appearance (Fig. 7-79).

Lead I

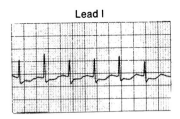

Lead II

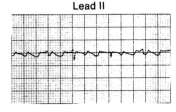

Fig. 7-79

Lead III

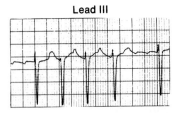

Lead V$_1$

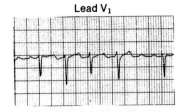

As previously mentioned, assessment of leads V_1 and V_6 as well as the full 12-lead ECG during a sustained tachycardia is invaluable in the differentiation of aberration from ventricular ectopy (see Frames 127 to 147).

ATRIAL ELECTROGRAMS

189 Recording of intracardiac electrical signals known as *electrograms* is helpful in detecting the exact origin and/or mechanism of an arrhythmia. *Atrial electrograms* or AEGs are recordings taken directly from or near the atria and are the type most commonly recorded in the coronary care unit. They may be displayed on a monitor and or recorded on a standard ECG machine.

Recording directly from the atria allows for clearer visualization of *P waves* known as *a waves* on the AEG. This allows for a more accurate diagnosis of a supraventricular rhythm as well as clearer differentiation between *supraventricular* and *ventricular arrhythmias.*

190 The atrial deflection on the AEG, known as an _____ a wave, appears as a spike similar to a pacemaker impulse. The atrial impulse is easily seen because the electrodes are sensing directly from or near the atria. The ventricular deflection on the AEG is known as the *V wave* and may or may not be visible depending on the mode in which it is recorded (see Figure 7-80).

Unipolar AEG

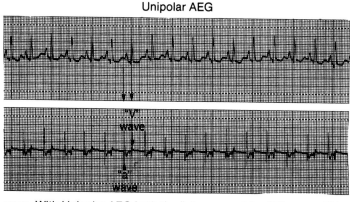

Fig. 7-80

NOTE: With Unipolar AEG both the "a" wave and the "V" wave will be visible.

Atrial electrograms may be sensed (1) from *endocardial electrodes* within the atria, such as those on an ordinary pacing catheter, or the multipolar catheters used in electrophysiologic labs; (2) from *esophageal electrodes* positioned in the esophagus near the atria, or *most commonly;* (3) from temporary *epicardial wire electrodes* attached directly to the atria during cardiac surgery (see Unit 11). Esophageal electrodes are attached to a wire and are then surrounded with a dissoluable capsule, which is swallowed to allow the electrode to pass into the esophagus.

191 It is best to record the AEG simultaneously with the ECG to compare the waveforms directly on a one to one basis. If this is not possible then sequential recording of the ECG followed by the AEG will be useful in making a differential diagnosis. Some monitoring systems have a special module that can be plugged into the monitor to detect and display the AEG. The monitoring cable, which attaches to this module, contains three terminals—RA, LA, and LL. The *atrial electrodes* are connected to the *right arm* and *left arm* terminals. The left leg terminal is attached to a skin surface electrode. A lead selector on the module enables the operator to switch from one lead to another. With the monitor on *lead I* a *bipolar* recording is displayed because both the _____ _____ and _____ _____ are connected with the atrial electrodes.

right arm
left arm

REMEMBER: A *bipolar* recording utilizes _____ electrodes in contact with the atria or near the atria. The ventricular event will not be seen or will be very small when the AEG is in the bipolar mode (Figure 7-81).

two

Bipolar AEG

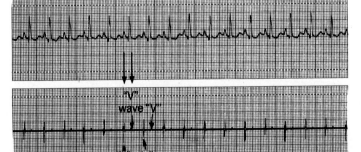

Fig. 7-81

NOTE: P wave on ECG correlates with "a" wave on AEG. QRS complex on ECG correlates with "V" wave on AEG. With bipolar AEG "V" wave will be very small or not visible.

192 Switching to *lead II,* or lead *III* will allow for a *unipolar* recording to be obtained because only the RA (in Lead II) or the LA (in Lead III) will be sensing atrial activity.

REMEMBER: with a *unipolar system* only *(one/two)* electrode(s) is in contact with the heart. The indifferent electrode is some distance from the body, and thus a large area of electrical activity is recorded and *both atrial* and *ventricular* events will be visible. The unipolar recording is useful to see the exact sequence of atrial and ventricular

one

activation and thus confirm the relationship between atrial and ventricular events (see Figure 7-81).

193 LET US REVIEW: the bipolar AEG primarily records _____ activity. The unipolar AEG records both _____ and _____ activity. If a regular ECG machine is used to record the AEG, then the atrial wires or electrodes can be connected with a special adapter or alligator clamps to the RA and LA electrodes on the ECG machine. With the machine on lead I, a bipolar AEG will be recorded. With machine on lead II or III a _____ recording will be obtained.

    The AEG allows for clearer detection of _____ waves. This allows for clearer differentiation of supraventricular arrhythmias and _____ and _____ arrhythmias.

    The atrial signal is easily seen on the AEG because electrodes are sensing directly from or near the _____.

    A bipolar AEG is recorded with the atrial electrodes connected to the _____ and _____ electrodes and the monitor or ECG machine selected on lead _____.

    A unipolar ECG is recorded when the monitor or ECG is on lead _____ or _____ because only *(one/two)* electrode(s) is near or in contact with the heart.

	atrial
	atrial
	ventricular
	unipolar
	P
	supraventricular; ventricular
	atria
	RA; LA
	I
	II; III; one

194 In Figure 7-82 the ECG shows a *(supraventricular/ventricular)* tachycardia at a ventricular and apparent atrial rate of approximately 130 BPM. The AEG taken simultaneously reveals a regular, actual atrial rate of approximately _____ per minute. The arrhythmia can be diagnosed definitively from the AEG as _____ _____ with a 2:1 conduction ratio.

	supraventricular
	270
	atrial flutter

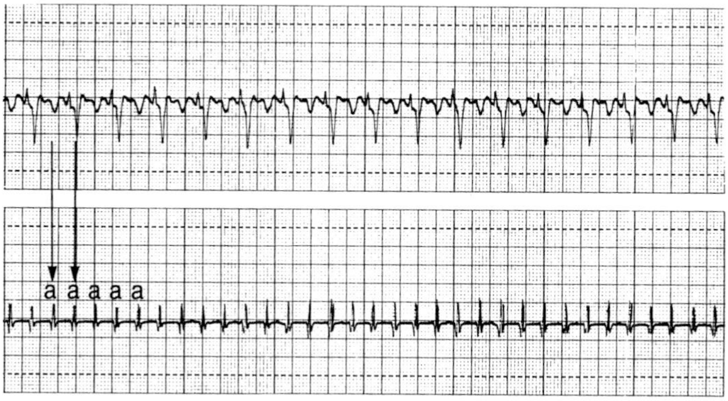

Fig. 7-82

NOTE: Bipolar AEG reveals regular "a" waves at a rate of approximately 270 per minute, consistent with a diagnosis of atrial flutter—the ECG shows a regular ventricular rate of approximately 130 per minute. Thus the rhythm is definitely diagnosed as atrial flutter = 2:1 conduction.

195 In Figure 7-83 the rhythm appears to be a *(ventricular/supraventricular)* tachycardia. The unipolar AEG shows *a waves* wandering throughout the rhythm and *V waves* corresponding with the ventricular complexes of the tachycardia. The AEG showing A-V dissociation confirms the diagnosis of *(supraventricular/ventricular)* tachycardia.

ventricular

ventricular

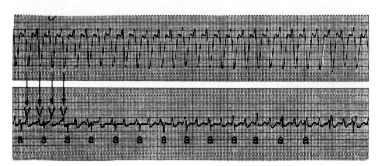

Fig. 7-83

NOTE: ECG shows what appears to be ventricular tachycardia—AEG confirms this diagnosis showing "a" waves marching through the tachycardia—AV dissociation. "V" waves at a rate of 180 correlate with QRS complexes.

OVERVIEW: ARRHYTHMIAS IN ACUTE MI

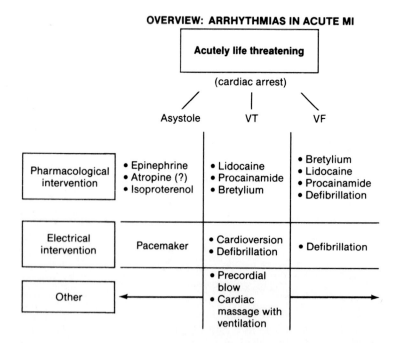

	Asystole	VT	VF
Pharmacological intervention	• Epinephrine • Atropine (?) • Isoproterenol	• Lidocaine • Procainamide • Bretylium	• Bretylium • Lidocaine • Procainamide • Defibrillation
Electrical intervention	Pacemaker	• Cardioversion • Defibrillation	• Defibrillation
Other		• Precordial blow • Cardiac massage with ventilation	

Fig. 7-84

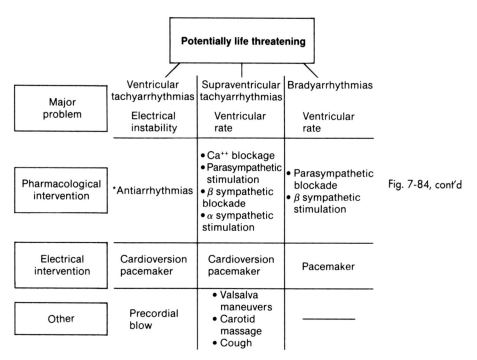

	Ventricular tachyarrhythmias	Supraventricular tachyarrhythmias	Bradyarrhythmias
Major problem	Electrical instability	Ventricular rate	Ventricular rate
Pharmacological intervention	*Antiarrhythmias	• Ca⁺⁺ blockage • Parasympathetic stimulation • β sympathetic blockade • α sympathetic stimulation	• Parasympathetic blockade • β sympathetic stimulation
Electrical intervention	Cardioversion pacemaker	Cardioversion pacemaker	Pacemaker
Other	Precordial blow	• Valsalva maneuvers • Carotid massage • Cough	————

Fig. 7-84, cont'd

*See Unit 10 for specific drugs

Table 10. Summary of arrhythmia categories (ECG criteria/clinical significance)

Rhythm	Significance	ECG	Treatment
Tachyarrhythmias: ventricular			
Ventricular premature contractions (PVCs)	May lead to: —Ventricular tachycardia (see VT), or —Ventricular fibrillation (cardiac arrest)	QRS: "different" (i.e., changing) and premature —May be preceded by nonpremature p wave —May or may not have a pause —May or may not be obviously wide	Acute:—Lidocaine (Xylocaine) —Procainamide (Pronestyl) —> 6/min —On T wave ("close coupled") —Multifocal —2 or more consecutive (VR > 100* unless written exceptions ordered by physician) Long-term: —Quinidine —Procainamide (Pronestyl) —Disopyramide (Norpace) —Propranolol (Inderal) (PO)

Continued.

Table 10. Summary of arrhythmia categories (ECG criteria/clinical significance)—cont'd

Rhythm	Significance	ECG	Treatment
Tachyarrhythmias: ventricular—cont'd			
Ventricular tachycardia (VT)	May ↓ CO or indicate a form of cardiac arrest, or lead to ventricular fibrillation (cardiac arrest)	QRS: "different" (i.e., changing) —3 or more consecutive beats —VR > 100	Acute: —Lidocaine (Xylocaine) —Procainamide (Pronestyl) —Bretylium —Cardioversion NOTE: without pulse treat as VF Long-term: (see PVCs) Also pacemakers (bursting, scanning, dual demand)
Ventricular fibrillation (VF)	Cardiac arrest	QRS: "disintegrated" —No distinct QRS/T complexes —Wave of uneven height (coarse) —May appear as wavy baseline only mimicking asystole (fine)	Acute: —Check pulse —Precordial blow —Defibrillation —Lidocaine (Xylocaine) —Bretylium Long-term: (see PVCs/VT)
Tachyarrhythmias: supraventricular (ectopic)			
Atrial Premature atrial contractions (PACs)	May lead to: —Other sustained atrial arrhythmias with rapid VR and ↓ CO —Often indicate CHF or hypoxemia	p wave: premature (irregular pp)	Acute: None Long-term: —Digitalis —Verapamil (PO) —Propranolol (Inderal) (PO) —Quinidine —Procainamide (Pronestyl) —treat cause
Atrial tachycardia (PAT)	↑ VR (↓ CO)	p wave rate: 150-250 (typically: 150)	Acute: —Verapamil (IV) or Esmolol (IV) —Cardioversion —Digitalis —Valsalva maneuver —Carotid sinus pressure Long-term: (see PACs)
Atrial flutter	↑ VR (↓ CO)	p wave rate: 250-350 (average: 300)	Acute: (see PAT) Long-term: (see PACs)
Atrial fibrillation	↑ VR (↓ CO)	p wave: "disintegrated" —No distinct visible p waves —QRS complexes: irregular	Acute: (see PAT) Long-term: (see PACs)
Junctional premature contractions (PJCs)	Usually of no clinical significance	p wave: not visible, or if visible, inverted on lead II with short PR	Acute: None Long-term: None

Table 10. Summary of arrhythmia categories (ECG criteria/clinical significance)—cont'd

Rhythm	Significance	ECG	Treatment
Tachyarrhythmias: supraventricular (ectopic)—cont'd			
Junctional tachycardia (JT)	↑ VR (↓ CO) R/O digitalis toxicity	p wave: not visible, or if visible, inverted on lead II with short PR —QRS complexes (regular) —VR > 100	Acute: —Diphenylhydantoin (Dilantin) —Propranolol (Inderal) (avoid digitalis and verapamil, unless diagnosis unclear, i.e., "SVT")
Bradyarrhythymias: AV blocks			
First-degree AV block	↓ VR (↑ CO) —Block in AV node or bundle branches	PR interval: prolonged (> 0.20 sec)	Acute (if symptomatic only): —Atropine —pacemaker (transthoracic) —Isoproterenol (Isuprel) —Pacemaker (transvenous)
Second-degree AV block	↓ VR (↓ CO)	PR interval: Some p waves not followed by QRSs	Acute (if symptomatic only): —Atropine —pacemaker (transthoracic) —Isoproterenol (Isuprel) —pacemaker (transvenous)
—Fixed ratio (example: "2 to 1")	Block in AV node or bundle branches	—RR regular —constant PR in those p's followed by QRS complex	Long-term: Pacemaker (permanent)
—Wenkebach (Mobitz I)	Block in AV node (usually)	—RR irregular —"4 p's": previous, progressive, pR, prolongation	
—Mobitz II	—Block in bundle branches (usually) —May result in sudden asystole	—RR irregular —No previous progressive PR change	
Third-degree AV block	—↓ VR (↓ CO), or —asystole (especially if in bundle branches)	PR interval: —Some p waves not followed by QRS —RR regular —Varying PR in those p's followed by QRS complexes	Acute: (see second-degree AV block) Long-term: (see second-degree AV block)
Bradyarrhythmias: other			
SA block	↓ VR (↓ CO)	p wave: absent (pause = multiples of original p wave cycles)	Acute (if symptomatic only): —Atropine —pacemaker (transthoracic) —Isoproterenol (Isuprel) —Pacemaker (transvenous) Long-term: Pacemaker (permanent)

Continued.

Table 10. Summary of arrhythmia categories (ECG criteria/clinical significance)—cont'd

Rhythm	Significance	ECG	Treatment
Bradyarrhythmias: other—cont'd			
Escape beats (ventricular)	Compensatory, prevent ↓ VR (↓ CO)	QRS: "different" (i.e., changing) timing: after the next expected natural QRS has not appeared	Acute: None, or support with atropine DO NOT SUPPRESS
Idioventricular rhythm	↓ VR (↓ CO)	QRS: "different" (i.e., changing) —3 or more consecutive beats —VR < 40	Acute: —Atropine —pacemaker (transthoracic) —Isoproterenol (Isuprel) —Pacemaker (transvenous) Long-term: Pacemaker (permanent) DO NOT SUPPRESS
Accelerated idioventricular rhythm (AIVR)	↓ VR (↓ CO)	QRS: "different" (i.e., changing) —3 or more consecutive beats —VR > 40 < 100	Acute: None or support with atropine
Junctional rhythm	↓ VR (↓ CO)	QRS: normal p wave: not visible, or if visible, inverted on lead II with short PR —VR < 100	Acute (if symptomatic only): —Atropine —pacemaker (transthoracic) —Isoproterenol (Isuprel) —Pacemaker (transvenous)

Table 11. Arrhythmia recognition matrix

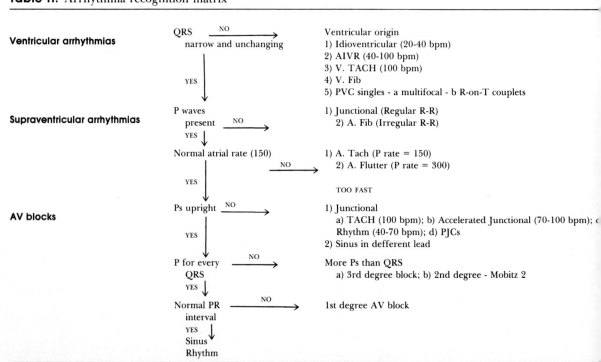

Ventricular arrhythmias

QRS —NO→ Ventricular origin
narrow and unchanging
1) Idioventricular (20-40 bpm)
2) AIVR (40-100 bpm)
3) V. TACH (100 bpm)
YES
4) V. Fib
5) PVC singles - a multifocal - b R-on-T couplets

Supraventricular arrhythmias

P waves present —NO→ 1) Junctional (Regular R-R)
YES 2) A. Fib (Irregular R-R)

Normal atrial rate (150)
—NO→ 1) A. Tach (P rate = 150)
2) A. Flutter (P rate = 300)
YES
TOO FAST

AV blocks

Ps upright —NO→ 1) Junctional
YES a) TACH (100 bpm); b) Accelerated Junctional (70-100 bpm); c Rhythm (40-70 bpm); d) PJCs
2) Sinus in defferent lead

P for every QRS —NO→ More Ps than QRS
YES a) 3rd degree block; b) 2nd degree - Mobitz 2

Normal PR interval —NO→ 1st degree AV block
YES
Sinus Rhythm

(Courtesy Linda Kisner, R.N.)

SUGGESTED READINGS

Boag F and others: Cardiac arrhythmias and myocardial ischemia related to cocaine and alcohol consumption, Postgrad Med J 61(721:997, 1985.

Braunwald E, editor: Heart disease: a textbook of cardiovascular medicine, ed 3, Philadelphia, 1988, WB Saunders Co.

Bryant M: Abnormalities in cardiac rhythm: sinus and atrial dysrhythmias, J Nephrol Nurs 3(3):112, 1986.

Brugada P and Wellens H: To beat or not to beat: arguments for use of the term ventricular premature depolarization, Am J Card 55:1113, 1985.

Castellanos A, editor: Cardiac arrhythmias: mechanisms and management, Cardiovascular Clinic Series, Philadelphia, 1980, FA Davis Co.

Catalano JT: PVC quiz, Crit Care Nurse 7(2):121, 1987.

Chapman PD and others: Pseudo P waves: a cause of diagnostic confusion in wide QRS tachycardia, Clin Cardiol 9(1):30, 1986.

Cudworth K: Is that funny looking beat dangerous? RN 49(5):32, 1986.

Conover MB: Understanding electrocardiography, ed. 5, St. Louis, 1988, The CV Mosby Co.

Dongas J and others: Value of preexisting bundle branch block in the electrocardiographic differentiation of supraventricular from ventricular origin of wide QRS tachycardia, Am J Card 55:717, 1985.

Euler D and Moore EN: Continuous fractioned electrical activity after stimulation of the ventricles during the vulnerable period: evidence for local reentry, Am J Card 46:783, 1980.

Edwards JD and others: Significance and management of intractable supraventricular arrhythmias in critically ill patients, Crit Care Med 14(4):280, 1986.

Francis GS: Development of arrhythmias in the patient with congestive heart failure: pathophysiology, prevalence, and prognosis, Am J Card 57(3):3B, 1986.

Geddes LE: Monitoring the patient with conduction disturbances and blocks, Nurs Clin North Am 22(1):33, 1987.

Gilmour R and Zipes D: Slow inward current and cardiac arrhythmias, Am J Card 55:89B, 1985.

Grogan EW: Management of SVT, Cardiovasc Clin 16:215, 1985.

Hancock EW: Wide complex tachycardia in acute myocardial infarction, Hosp Pract (Off) 23(1):109, 1988.

Hodd and others: Early atrial fibrillation during evolving myocardial infarction: a consequence of impaired left atrial perfusion, Circulation 75:146, 1987.

Huang S and others: Coronary care nursing, Philadelphia, 1983, WB Saunders Co.

Julian DG: Nomenclature in cardiology: more on 'extrasystole', Heart Lung 16(2):121, 1987.

Keefe DL and others: Supraventricular tachyarrhythmias: their evaluation and therapy, Am Heart J 111(6):1150, 1986.

Lange HW: Prevalence and clinical correlates of non-Wenckebach, narrow-complex second-degree atrioventricular block detected by ambulatory ECG, Part 1, Am Heart J 115(1):114, 1988.

Lazzara R and Scherlag B: Electrophysiologic basis for arrhythmias in ischemic heart disease, Am J Card 53:1B, 1984.

Loeb J: Cardiac electrophysiology: basic concepts and arrhythmogenesis, CCQ 7(2):21, 1984.

Looks like SVT, Lancet 2:8507, 1986.

Lundermann JP and others: Potential biochemical mechanism for regulation of the slow inward current: theoretical basis for drug action, Am Heart J 103:746, 1982.

Morady F and Scheinman N: Paroxysmal supraventricular tachycardia, Part I—Diagnosis, Mod Concepts Cardiovasc Dis 51(8):107, 1982.

Morady F and Scheinman N: Paroxysmal supraventricular tachycardia, Part II—Treatment, Mod Concepts Cardiovasc Dis 51(9):113, 1982.

Marriott HJL and Conover MH: Advanced concepts in arrhythmias. St. Louis, 1983, The CV Mosby Co.

Nieminski K and others: Current concepts and management of the sick sinus syndrome, Heart Lung 13(6):675, 1984.

Nordrehaug JE and others: Serum potassium concentration as a risk factor of ventricular arrhythmias in early acute myocardial infarction, Circulation 71:645, 1985.

Norsen L and others: Detecting dysrhythmias, Nursing 16(11):34, 1986.

Ordonez RV: Monitoring the patient with supraventricular dysrhythmias, Nurs Clin North Am 22(1):49, 1987.

Parmley WW and others: congestive heart failure and arrhythmias: an overview, Am J Card 57(3):34B, 1986.

Porth C and others: The Valsalva maneuver: mechanisms and clinical implications, Heart Lung 13(5):507, 1984.

Quaal S and others: Aberrant ventricular conduction during atrial fibrillation, Heart Lung 14(1):101, 1985.

Rapeport N and others: A study of ventricular ectopy during atrial fibrillation, Heart Lung 14(2):191, 1985.

Reyes AV: Monitoring and treating life-threatening ventricular dysrhythmias, Nurs Clin North Am 22(1):61, 1987.

Roberts WC: Ventricular premature complex, Am J Card 55:1117, 1985.

Rosequist CC: Current Standards and guidelines for cardiopulmonary resuscitation and emergency cardiac care, Heart Lung 16(4):408, 1987.

Schamroth L: The disorders of cardiac rhythm, ed. 2, Edinburgh, 1980, Blackwell Scientific Publications, Inc.

Sugiura T and others: Atrial fibrillation in acute myocardial infarction, Am J Card 56:57, 1985.

Ten Eick RE and others: Ventricular dysrythmia: membrane basis of currents, channels, gates, and cables, Prog Cardiovasc Dis 24:157, 1981.

Sweetwood H: Clinical electrocardiography for nurses, Rockville, Md, 1983, Aspen Publications.

Valladares BJ: Ventricular arrhythmias: a perspective on management, Heart Lung 14(4):417, 1985.

Walsh RA: Emergency treatment of tachyarrhythmias, Med Clin N Am 70(4):791, 1986.

Ward JW: EKG of the month (myocardial infarction with complete heart block), Crit Care Nurse 5(1):14, 1985.

Waxman MB and others: Interaction between the autonomic nervous system and tachycardias in man, Cardiovasc Clin 15(3):115, 1985.

Wellens HJ: Diagnosis of ventricular tachycardia from the 12-lead electrocardiogram, Cardiol Clin 5(3):511, 1987.

Wessman JP: Preventing ventricular dysrhythmia following myocardial infarction, DCCN 4(1):24, 1985.

Willoughby M: The treatment of atrial fibrillation and flutter: a review, Heart Lung 13(5):578, 1984.

Witt AL and Rosen MR: Cellular electrophysiology of cardiac arrhythmias, Mod Concepts Cardiovasc Dis 50:1, 1981.

Atrial electrograms

Conover MB: Understanding electrocardiography, ed. 5, St. Louis, 1988, The CV Mosby Co.

Hammill SC and Pritchett ELC: Simplified esophageal electrocardiography using bipolar recording leads. Ann Intern Med 98:14-18, 1981.

Sulzbach LM: The use of temporary atrial wire electrodes to record atrial electrograms in patients who had cardiac surgery. Heart Lung, 14(16):540-547, 1985.

Waldo AL and Maclean WAH: Diagnosis and treatment of cardiac arrhythmias following open heart surgery, emphasis on the use of atrial and ventricular epicardial wire electrodes. Mount Kisco, NY, 1980, Futura Publishing Co Inc.

UNIT 8

Intraventricular Conduction Disturbances

---

1 The intraventricular conduction system has three main components: the *His bundle,* the *right bundle branch,* and the *main left branch.* The main left branch subdivides into two fascicles: the *anterosuperior* and the *posteroinferior.*

    The components of the intraventricular conduction system are best visualized in the *horizontal plane.*

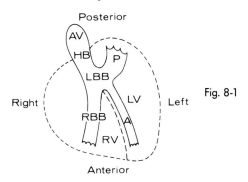

Fig. 8-1

2 REMEMBER: The borders of the horizontal plane are _____, _____, _____, and _____.

    NOTE: In this plane the anterosuperior division of the left bundle lies _____. The posteroinferior division of the left bundle lies _____.

anterior

posterior; right; left

anteriorly

posteriorly

DEFINITIONS

Let us now define some terms commonly used when discussing blocks in the intraventricular conduction system. The term *bundle branch* will be used when referring to the major branches of the intraventricular conduction system. The major branches of the intraventricular conduction system are the _____ _____ _____ and the _____ _____ _____. Blocks

right bundle branch

main left branch

355

that occur in the major branches are known as
_____ _____ blocks.

bundle branch

Examples of bundle branch block are right bundle branch block (RBBB) and left bundle branch block (LBBB).

4 Blocks that occur in half of the left branch are known as *hemiblocks*. The term *hemiblocks* therefore refers to a block in either the _____ or _____ division of the left bundle.

anterosuperior; posteroinferior

A block in the anterosuperior division is known as *left anterior hemiblock (LAH)*.

A block in the posteroinferior division is known as *left posterior hemiblock (LPH)*.

5 In this discussion the term *fascicle* will be used when referring to any branch of the intraventricular conduction system. The fascicles of the intraventricular conduction system are the _____

right bundle branch

_____ _____ and the _____ and _____ divisions of the main left branch.

anterosuperior; posteroinferior

6 Blocks that occur in the fascicles are known as _____ *blocks.*

fascicular

Fascicular blocks can further be described according to the number of fascicles involved.

7 A block in *one* fascicle is called a *monofascicular block.* Examples of monofascicular blocks are LAH, LPH, and RBBB. A block in *two* fascicles is called a *bifascicular block.* Examples of bifascicular blocks are RBBB and LAH or RBBB and LPH. A block of *three* fascicles is called a _____ *fascicular block.* An example of trifascicular block is RBBB, LAH, and LPH occurring together.

tri-

NORMAL VENTRICULAR ACTIVATION AND BLOCKS

8 Before discussing blocks that occur in the intraventricular conduction system, let us first review *normal ventricular activation.* The first part of the ventricles to be depolarized is the _____.

septum

The septum is normally activated from *left* to *right* and _____ to _____. Depolarization of the septum produces the small *(q/r)* wave seen in lead V_1 and the small *(q/r)* seen in lead V_6. The waves of depolarization then spread through both the *right* and *left* ventricles.

posteriorly; anteriorly
4
q

9 REMEMBER: The left ventricle lies posteriorly. Therefore the sum of all electrical forces traveling through the ventricles is a force shifted slightly to the _____ and _____.

left; posteriorly

Main left branch and complete left bundle branch block

10 Each branch of the intraventricular conduction system and its associated conduction disturbance will not be considered. The main left branch emerges from the bundle of His and lies against the septum. *Septal* depolarization is normally initiated in this area. Two fascicles are emitted from the main left branch. The main left bundle may be compared to the trunk of a tree. The anterosuperior and posteroinferior fascicles are analogous to the branches of this tree.

The main left bundle is supplied by both the *right* and *left* coronary arteries. Although the main left bundle can be blocked as a result of acute MI, a more common cause of complete left bundle branch block (CLBBB) is *sclerosis*, or calcification, of this area.

11

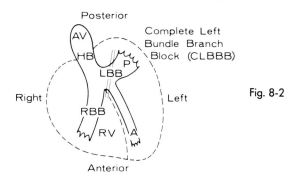

Fig. 8-2

12 In the presence of CLBBB there is *abnormal* septal depolarization.

REMEMBER: Normal septal depolarization occurs from _____ to _____ from the main _____ bundle branch.

left; right; left

In CLBBB, the septum is depolarized from _____ to _____. This reversal results in a loss of the *small r wave* in lead _____ and of the *small q wave* in lead _____.

right
left
V₁; V₆

13 In the presence of CLBBB the only fascicle still conducting impulses to the ventricles is the _____ bundle branch. Therefore the ventricles are activated through this branch.

right

14 When ventricular activation occurs in this way, the impulse is *delayed* in reaching the left ventricle. It can then be expected that in the presence of CLBBB the QRS will be *(narrow/wide)*. This delay is seen on the ECG as a *medial* change in the QRS complex. *Medial* means the delay is seen in the *(middle/last)* portion of the QRS complex.

wide

middle

15 Bundle branch blocks are best visualized in the *horizontal* plane.

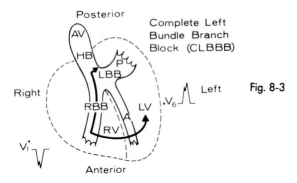

Posterior

Complete Left
Bundle Branch
Block (CLBBB)

Fig. 8-3

Right

Left

Anterior

16 *Leads V_1 and V_6 are used in the ECG diagnosis of bundle branch blocks.*

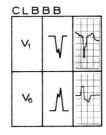

Fig. 8-4

Right bundle branch and right bundle branch block

17 The right bundle branch and the anterosuperior division of the left bundle exist in a common portion of the septum for a short segment. Then the right bundle emerges as a thin, single fascicle.

18 The right bundle branch is primarily supplied by the left coronary artery.

REMEMBER: The left coronary artery supplies the *(inferior/anterior)* surface of the left ventricle. It can then be anticipated that RBBB will be seen most frequently in the presence of *(anterior/inferior)* wall MI.

anterior

anterior

19

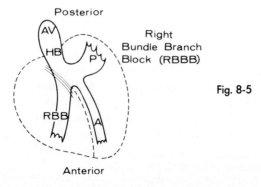

Posterior

Right
Bundle Branch
Block (RBBB)

Fig. 8-5

Anterior

20 When RBBB occurs, septal depolarization is usually not altered. Septal depolarization occurs normally from _____ to _____. Therefore the small r wave in lead V_1 and the small q in lead V_6 *(will/will not)* be seen.

left

right

will

21 In the presence of RBBB the only fascicle still conducting impulses to the ventricles is the _____ bundle branch. Therefore ventricular activation occurs *through* the *left bundle branch*. In RBBB the left ventricle is activated normally, but the *right ventricle* is activated with *delay*. This delay is seen on the ECG as a *terminal* change in the QRS. Terminal delays occur in the *(middle/last)* portion of the QRS complex.

left

last

22 REMEMBER: Bundle branch blocks are best visualized in the horizontal plane. Therefore leads V_1 and V_6 are also used to diagnose RBBB on the ECG.

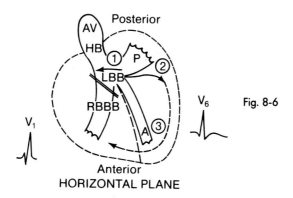

Fig. 8-6

HORIZONTAL PLANE

23 NOTE: If the septal forces are lost, as in anteroseptal MI, the small r in lead V_1 and small q in lead V_6 will not be present. The QRS will then assume a qR configuration in lead V_1 rather than the classic rSR′ pattern shown in the example below. However, it will still be a predominantly upright complex in lead V_1, exhibiting terminal delay.

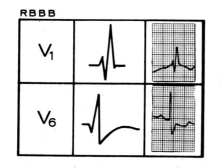

Fig. 8-7

24 SUMMARY: The right bundle branch

    I. Singular blood supply is from the left coronary artery.

    II. RBBB commonly occurs in the presence of *anterior* wall MI.

    III. Characteristics of RBBB:

        A. Septal depolarization is usually not altered.

        B. Terminal delay is indicated by slurring and widening of S wave in lead V_6.

        C. A sR′ or aR configuration occurs in lead V_1 (predominantly upright complex).

Left branch and hemiblocks

25 The main left subdivides into two fascicles: the _____ division and the _____ division.

      It is possible that a conduction block may occur in only *half* of the left bundle. The term used to describe these half blocks is _____.

                                           anterosuperior; posteroinferior

                                           hemiblock

26 When a hemiblock occurs, there are still normal conduction pathways to the ventricles. Therefore, in the presence of hemiblocks, only minimal changes in the QRS duration are seen on the ECG. However, hemiblocks do cause shifts in the *electrical axis of the heart;* therefore, before considering the identification of hemiblocks on the ECG, we will discuss a method for calculating the electrical axis.

Calculating the electrical axis

27 LET US REVIEW: Axis is defined as the summation force, or summation _____.

                                           vector

      REMEMBER: The left ventricle has *(more/less)* electrical forces than does the right ventricle. Therefore in the normal adult the axis is shifted toward the *(right/left)*.

                                           more

                                         left

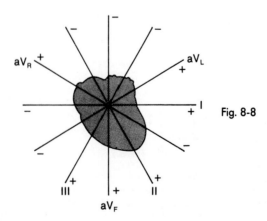

Fig. 8-8

28 The electrical axis is usually considered and calculated in the *frontal plane*.

REMEMBER: The limb leads are derived in the _____ plane.

frontal

29 This reference system can be divided into four quadrants, with leads I and aV_F serving as coordinates.

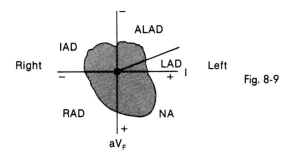

Fig. 8-9

30 If the electrical axis lies within the lower left quadrant, the axis is _____ *(NA)*. If the axis deviates toward the lower *right* quadrant, it is considered to be _____ axis deviation *(RAD)*. If the axis deviates toward the upper *left* quadrant, it is considered to be _____ axis deviation *(LAD)*.

normal

right

left

Left axis deviation is further subdivided into *left axis* and *abnormal left axis*. Abnormal left axis deviation *(ALAD)* occurs when the axis is shifted far to the left. If the heart's electrical forces deviate toward the *upper right* quadrant, the axis is considered to be *indeterminate* axis deviation *(IAD)*.

31 The coordinates may be joined by a circle, and degrees assigned to them as reference points.

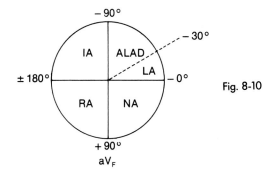

Fig. 8-10

32 Normal axis lies between ± 0° and + _____.

90°

Right axis lies between +90° and + _____.

180°

Left axis lies between ±0° and − _____.   90°

Abnormal left axis lies between −30° and − _____.   90°

Indeterminate axis lies between + _____ and +   180°
_____.   240°

33 For the purposes of this discussion, it is not necessary to learn the degrees presented in each quadrant. It is more important to assess the QRS *morphology* in the presence of normal and abnormal axes and determine why the axis shifts in different clinical settings.

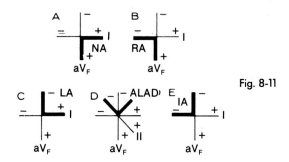

Fig. 8-11

34 When the axis is within *normal* limits, the net ventricular forces travel toward both the *(positive/negative)* pole of lead I and toward the *(positive/negative)* pole of lead aV$_F$. The QRS complex therefore should be *(positive/negative)* in lead I and *(positive/negative)* in lead aV$_F$ when the axis is normal.

positive; positive

positive; positive

35 When the axis is shifted to the right, the QRS complex is *(positive/negative)* in lead I and *(positive/negative)* in lead aV$_F$.

negative
positive

36 When the axis is shifted to the left, the QRS complex is *(positive/negative)* in lead I and *(positive/negative)* in lead aV$_F$.

positive
negative

37 When diagnosing *abnormal left axis,* we must consider the QRS morphology in lead II as well as in leads I and aV$_F$. When the axis is *abnormal left,* the QRS complex is *(positive/negative)* in lead I and *(positive/negative)* in leads II and aV$_F$.

positive; negative

38 When the axis is indeterminate, the QRS complex is *(positive/negative)* in lead I and *(positive/negative)* in lead aV$_F$.

negative
negative

39 The clinical causes of axis deviation in the setting of acute MI are presented in the remainder of this chapter. We give special emphasis to axis deviation and hemiblocks here.

40 In summary:

	I	aV_F	II
NA			
RA			
LA			
ALAD			
IA			

Fig. 8-12

Left anterior hemiblock

41 The anterosuperior division of the left bundle branch has a common anatomical origin with the _____ bundle branch. Thus these two fascicles are often injured simultaneously.

right

42 The anterosuperior division is supplied by the *(left/right)* coronary artery. Thus the anterosuperior division will commonly be involved in infarctions of the *(anterior/inferior)* wall of the heart.

left

anterior

43 The anterosuperior division of the left bundle is thought to be the *most* vulnerable structure of the intraventricular conduction system. This vulnerability is caused by (1) anatomical location in the hemo-dynamically turbulent aortic area, (2) its thinness and length, and (3) its single blood supply—the _____ coronary artery.

left

44 A block of the anterosuperior division of the left bundle is known as _____ _____ _____ _____.

left anterior hemiblock
(LAH)

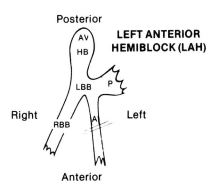

LEFT ANTERIOR HEMIBLOCK (LAH)

Posterior

AV
HB

LBB   P

Right   Left

RBB

Anterior

Fig. 8-13

45 ECG diagnosis of *hemiblocks* is made on the basis of *axis* shifts. In the presence of LAH the axis shifts to abnormal left.

REMEMBER: When ALAD occurs, the QRS complex is *(positive/neg-ative)* in lead I and *(positive/negative)* in leads II and aV_F.

positive
negative

46 Let us now consider *the reasons why* the a xis shifts to abnormal left in the presence of LAH. We will also derive the specific QRS patterns associated with this conduction disturbance.

47 The electrical axis is calculated by examining leads I, _____, and _____.
REMEMBER: These leads are derived in the *frontal plane*. Therefore, to understand the axis shifts associated with hemiblocks, we must visualize the intraventricular conduction system in the frontal plane.

II; aV_F

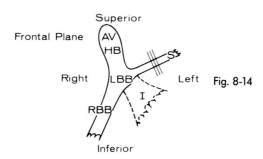

Fig. 8-14

48 As seen in the frontal plane, the anterosuperior division of the left bundle lies *(inferiorly/superiorly)*. The posteroinferior division lies *(inferiorly/superiorly)*.
When the *anterosuperior* division of the left bundle is blocked (LAH), activation of the left ventricle occurs through the *posteroinferior* division of the left bundle.

superiorly; inferiorly

49 Because activation occurs through the posteroinferior division, the initial forces in LAH are shifted *inferiorly* and to the right. This *initial* force produces small r waves in leads II and aV_F and a small q in lead I.

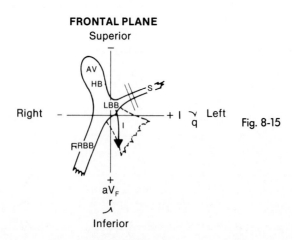

Fig. 8-15

364

REMEMBER: Leads II and aV$_F$ relfect the electrical activity of the *inferior* wall of the left ventricle.

50 The *main* forces then shift *superiorly* and to the *left*. These forces produce deep S waves in leads II and aV$_F$ and a large R wave in lead I.

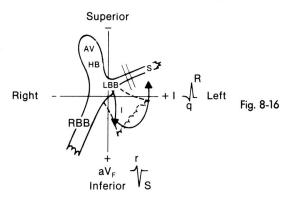

Fig. 8-16

51 Because the *main* forces are shifted superiorly and to the left, in LAH the axis shifts to *abnormal* left.

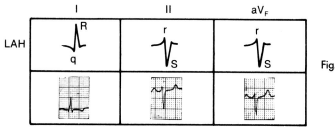

Fig. 8-17

52 Another cause of ALAD is *inferior* wall MI.

It is important to differentiate between the QRS patterns seen in IWMI and LAH. In both IWMI and LAH, lead I is *(positive/negative)* and leads II and aV$_F$ are *(positive/negative)*. However, the morphology of the QRS complexes in these two settings differ.

positive

negative

53 In IWMI, leads II and aV$_F$ are negative and assume a *large Q, small r* configuration (Qr). Lead I is positive and has a *small q, large R* configuration (qR).

NOTE: The large Q waves in leads II and aV$_F$ represent necrosis of tissue in the *(anterior/inferior)* wall.

inferior

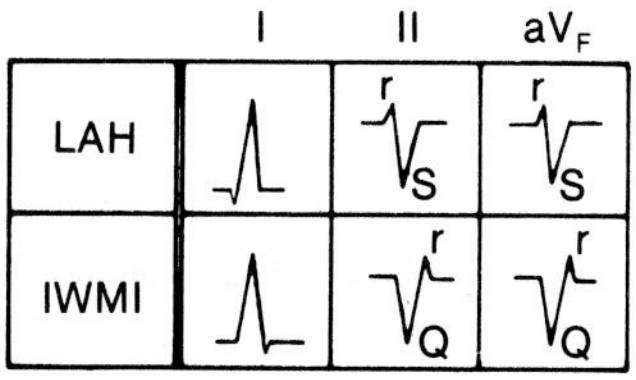

	I	II	aV$_F$
LAH			
IWMI			

Fig. 8-18

NOTE: In LAH leads II and aV$_F$ are *(positive/negative)* and the QRS pattern has a(n) _____ configuration. In IWMI leads II and aV$_F$ are again *(positive/negative)*, but the QRS pattern has a(n) _____ configuration. In both settings lead I is *(positive/negative)*.

negative
rS

negative
Qr

positive

54 Other causes of ALAD include right apical pacing; left ventricular pacing via the middle cardiac vein; Wolff-Parkinson-White syndrome, Type B; hyperkalemia; severe COPD; and left coronary arteriography.

55 LET US REVIEW: LAH most commonly occurs in combination with *(RBBB/LAH)*.

RBBB

LAH plus RBBB are known as a _____ block. LAH and RBBB are most frequently seen in the presence of _____ wall MI.

bifascicular

anterior

To diagnose LAH on the ECG, there must be *(LAD/ALAD)*. When LAH occurs, the QRS complex is *(positive/negative)* in led I and *(positive/negative)* in leads II and aV$_F$. There are also specific QRS patterns in LAH. In leads II and aV$_F$, the QRS pattern assumes a(n) *(rS/Qr)* configuration.

ALAD
positive
negative

rS

56 SUMMARY: Left anterior hemiblock
  I. Anterior division supplied by left coronary artery.
 II. LAH seen in setting of *anterior* wall MI.
III. LAH often accompanies RBBB.
IV. ECG diagnosis of LAH:
   A. There must be ALAD.
   B. Lead I is positive; leads II and aV$_F$ are negative.
   C. Lead I has a qR configuration.
   D. Leads II and aV$_F$ have an rS configuration.

Left posterior hemiblock

57 The posteroinferior division of the left bundle branch is the first fascicle emitted from the His bundle. It appears as the true continuation of the main left branch because of its thickness.

58 The posteroinferior division of the left bundle is supplied by both the _____ and _____ coronary arteries.

right; left

59 The posteroinferior division of the left bundle is the *least* vulnerable structure of the intraventricular system. This fact is attributed to its (1) anatomical location in a hemodynamically nonturbulent area, (2) thickness and length, and (3) dual blood supply—the _____ and _____ coronary arteries.

right; left

60 A block of the posterior division of the left bundle is known as
_____ _____ _____
_____.

left posterior hemiblock (LPH)

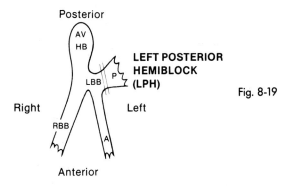

Fig. 8-19

61 ECG diagnosis of hemiblocks is made on the basis of _____ shifts. In the presence of LPH the axis shifts to the *right*.

REMEMBER: When RAD occurs, the QRS complex is *(positive/negative)* in lead I and *(positive/negative)* in lead aV$_F$.

axis

negative
positive

62 Let us now consider the *reasons why* the axis shifts to the right in the presence of LPH. We will also derive the specific QRS pattern associated with this conduction disturbance.

63 The electrical axis is calculated by examining leads I, _____, and _____.

REMEMBER: These leads were derived in the _____ plane. Therefore, to understand the axis shifts associated with hemiblocks, we must visualize the intraventricular conduction system in the _____ plane.

II; aV$_F$

frontal

frontal

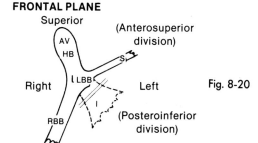

Fig. 8-20

64 In the frontal plane the *posteroinferior* division of the left bundle lies *(inferiorly/superiorly)*. The anterosuperior division lies _____. When the *posteroinferior* division of the left

inferiorly
superiorly

367

bundle is blocked (LPH), activation of the left ventricle occurs through the _____ division of the left bundle.

anterosuperior

65 Because activation occurs through the *anterosuperior* division, the *initial* forces in LPH are shifted, superiorly and to the left. This initial force produces a *small q wave* in lead aV$_F$ and a *small r wave* in lead I.

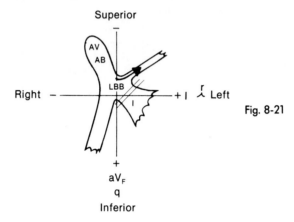

Fig. 8-21

66 The *main* forces, then, shift *inferiorly* and to the *right*. These forces produce large R waves in leads II and aV$_F$.

   REMEMBER: Leads II and aV$_F$ reflect the electrical activity of the _____ wall of the left ventricle.

inferior

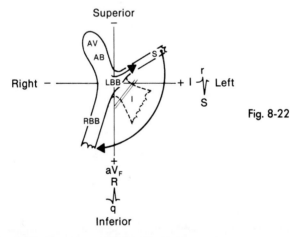

Fig. 8-22

67 Because the main forces are shifted inferiorly and to the right, in the presence of LPH the axis shifts to the *right*.

   NOTE: LPH is the *exact* mirror image of LAH.

68 Another cause of RAD is *lateral* wall MI. It is important to differentiate between the QRS patterns seen in lateral wall MI and LPH.

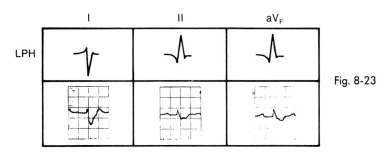

LPH | I | II | aV_F

Fig. 8-23

In both AWMI and LPH lead I is *(positive/negative)*, and leads II and aV_F are *(positive/negative)*. However, the morphologies of the QRS complexes in these two settings *differ*.

negative
positive

69 In lateral wall MI, lead I is negative and assumes a *large Q, small r* configuration (Qr). Leads II and aV_F are positive and have a small q, large R configuration (qR).

NOTE: The large Q wave in lead I represents necrosis of tissue in the *(lateral/inferior)* wall.

lateral

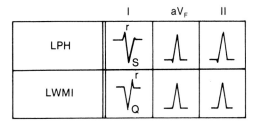

	I	aV_F	II
LPH			
LWMI			

Fig. 8-24

NOTE: In LPH lead I is negative and the QRS pattern has a(n) _____ configuration. In LWMI lead I is also negative, but the QRS has a(n) _____ configuration. In both settings leads II and aV_F are *(positive/negative)*.

rS
Qr
positive

70 LPH cannot be diagnosed on the ECG unless other causes of RAD are excluded: right ventricular hypertrophy; chronic lung disease; pulmonary emboli; Wolff-Parkinson-White syndrome, Type A; right ventricular pacing via the outflow tract; left ventricular pacing via the great cardiac vein; dextrocardia; and right coronary arteriography.

71 LET US REVIEW: LPH is often seen in combination with *(RBBB/LAH)*. When LPH occurs, it indicates *(mild/severe)* coronary artery disease. The ECG diagnosis of LPH is dependent on the presence of *(RAD/ ALAD)*. In the presence of LPH the QRS complex is *(positive/negative)* in led I and *(positive/negative)* in leads II and aV_F.

The QRS pattern in lead I assumes a(n) *(rS/Qr)* configuration. In leads II and aV_F the QRS pattern assumes a(n) *(rS/qR)* configuration.

RBBB
severe
RAD
negative
positive
rS
qR

72 SUMMARY: Left posterior hemiblock

    I. Posterior division is supplied by both the _____ and _____ coronary arteries. LPH indicates severe coronary artery disease.

    II. LPH is usually seen in combination with _____.

    III. ECG diagnosis of LPH:

        A. There must be RAD.

        B. Lead I is negative; leads II and aV_F are positive.

        C. Lead I has a rS configuration.

        D. Leads II and aV_F have a qR configuration.

right
left

RBBB

73

Summary:	I	aV_F	II	V_1
Normal	(waveform)	(waveform)	(waveform)	(waveform)
LAD	(waveform)	(waveform)	(waveform)	(waveform)
ALAD caused by IWMI	(waveform)	(waveform)	(waveform)	(waveform)
ALAD caused by LAH	(waveform)	(waveform)	(waveform)	(waveform)
RBBB	(waveform)	(waveform)	(waveform)	(waveform)
RBBB + LAH	(waveform)	(waveform)	(waveform)	(waveform)
RAD caused by LWMI	(waveform)	(waveform)	(waveform)	(waveform)
RAD caused by LPH	(waveform)	(waveform)	(waveform)	(waveform)
RBBB + LPH	(waveform)	(waveform)	(waveform)	(waveform)

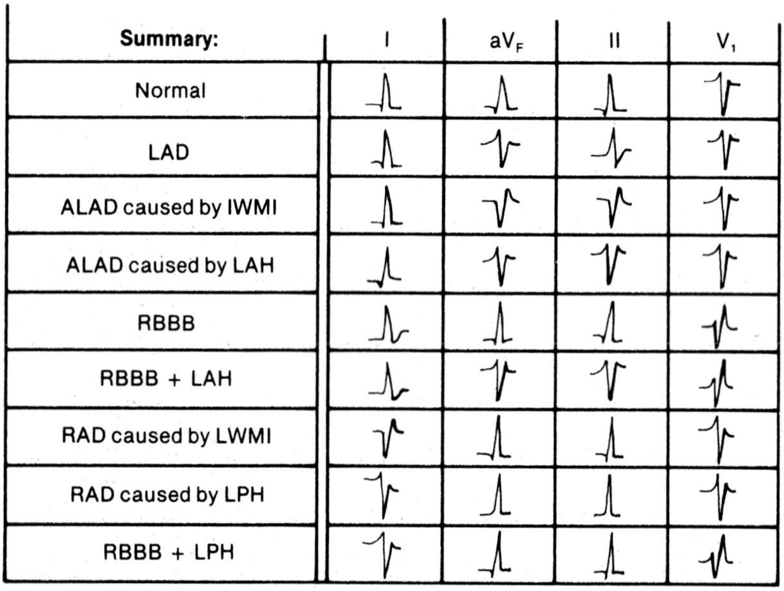

Fig. 8-25

IMPLICATIONS OF BLOCKS FOR NURSES

74 Bundle branch blocks and hemiblocks are clinically significant because they are the precursors of symptomatic Type II, or Mobitz II, AV blocks (see Unit 7).

    REMEMBER: Type II blocks usually occur as a result of *(right/left)* coronary artery pathology and are associated with infarctions of the _____ wall.

left

anterior

75 LET US REVIEW: A block that occurs in *one* fascicle is known as a _____ fascicular block.

    Examples of monofascicular blocks are _____, _____, and _____.

mono-
RBBB;
LAH; LPH

A block that occurs in *two* fascicles is known as _____ bifascicular block.

bi-

Examples of bifascicular blocks are _____ plus
_____ and _____ plus _____.

RBBB;
LAH; RBBB; LPH

A block that occurs in *three* fascicles is known as _____
fascicular block.

tri-

A trifascicular block occurs when the RBBB and the
_____ and _____ divisions of the
left bundle are blocked simultaneously.

anterior; posterior

76 Trifascicular block may occur transiently or may be permanent.
Type II (Mobitz) second-degree AV block occurs as a result of a
transient, or intermittent, _____ fascicular block.

tri-

Complete heart block may be a manifestation of *sustained* trifascicular block

77 Symptomatic AV block is usually preceded by the development of
bundle branch blocks and hemiblocks. Nurses who can diagnose
bundle branch blocks and hemiblocks can anticipate the development of symptomatic AV block.

78 Evidence of pathology in *two* of the three fascicles demonstrates that
there is probability that trifascicular block may occur.

NOTE: In bifascicular block, there is only *one fascicle* still conducting impulses to the _____. Therefore a bifascicular
block in the presence of AWMI *(is/is not)* evidence that trifascicular
block could occur.

ventricles
is

79 In the setting of AWMI bifascicular block is usually a result of *RBBB
and LAH.*

REMEMBER: AWMI is associated with *(right/left)* coronary pathology. Both the right bundle branch and the anterior division of the
left bundle branch are supplied by the _____ coronary artery.

left
left

NOTE: LPH may also occur in the presence of extensive AWMI
and diffuse coronary artery disease.

80 Therefore, in the presence of AWMI, the nurse should monitor the
patient for the development of _____ and _____
because these blocks frequently occur together. Bifascicular blocks
(may/may not) be precursors of symptomatic AV block. RBBB is
diagnosed by a change in the QRS morphology in lead
_____ or _____. LAH is diagnosed by the
development of _____ and changes in the QRS morphology.

RBBB; LAH

may

V₁; V₆
ALAD

81 If no fascicular blocks are present in the setting of AWMI, the patient should be monitored on either lead II or V_1. If LAH occurs, the develoment of an ALAD can best be observed on lead _____. If RBBB develops it can be best observed on lead _____.

II
V_1

82 In the presence of RBBB the patient should be observed for the development of _____. Therefore this patient should be monitored on lead _____.

LAH
II

83 In the presence of either LPH or LAH the patient should be observed for the development of _____. Therefore the patient should be monitored on lead _____.

RBBB
V_1

84 In the presence of a bifascicular block the patient should be monitored closely for any further conduction abnormalities.

REMEMBER: In bifascicular block there is (are) only _____ fascicle(s) still conducting impulses to the ventricles.

one

When a bifascicular block occurs suddenly, the nurse should notify the physician, prepare an isoproterenol (Isuprel) drip, and prepare for prophylactic pacemaker insertion.

85 LET US REVIEW: Bifascicular blocks may be precursors of the development of _____ fascicular block. In the setting of AWMI the most common type of bifascicular block is _____ plus _____.

tri-
RBBB
LAH

Transient trifascicular block became apparent as TypeII, or _____, AV block. Sustained trifascicular block may also appear as _____ or _____ AV block.

Mobitz
third-degree; complete

The development of symptomatic AV block may be observed by monitoring the patient for _____ fascicular blocks.

bi-

86 NURSING ORDERS: The patient with bundle branch block
1. Place chest electrodes in the same position or as near the same position as possible each day. If electrodes are changed, note on hourly rhythm strips.
2. If gain (size of complex) is changed for any reason, note on hourly rhythm strips.
3. If no fascicular blocks are present, monitor the patient on lead II or V_1.
4. In the presence of RBBB monitor the patient on lead II to observe for the development of LAH.
5. In the presence of LPH or LAH monitor the patient on lead V_1 to observe for the development of RBBB.

6. In the presence of bifascicular block (such as RBBB plus LAH or RBBB plus LPH) monitor the patient closely for conduction abnormalities (such as first-degree AV block, second-degree AV block [Mobitz II], or complete AV block). Monitor on whatever lead shows both clear P waves and QRS complexes so that AV block may be more easily detected.

7. When a bifascicular block occurs suddenly in the setting of AWMI:
   —Notify the physician immediately.
   —Prepare an isoproterenol (Isuprel) drip on stand-by.
   —Prepare for pacemaker insertion.

8. If no fascicular blocks are present in the setting of AWMI, monitor the patient on lead II or V_1. If LAH occurs, observe for the development of ALAD on lead _____. If RBBB develops, observe it on lead _____.

II

V_1

9. In addition to continuous monitoring, document leads I, II, aV_F and V_1 every 4 hours to make a more comprehensive analysis of the intraventricular conduction system.

ECTOPY ASSOCIATED WITH BUNDLE BRANCH BLOCK AND FASCICULAR BLOCK PATTERNS

87 The QRS patterns associated with bundle branch blocks and hemiblocks are important not only in predicting the onset of AV blocks, but also in determining the origin of ventricular ectopy. The V leads are used to diagnose conditions in which there are differences in the time between right and left ventricular activation.

REMEMBER: The V leads were used in the diagnosis of bundle branch blocks.

The V leads may also be used to determine the origin of ventricular ectopy.

Right ventricular ectopy

88 LET US REVIEW: When an impulse is blocked in the left bundle branch (LBB), the QRS comlex in lead V_1 is *(positive/negative)* and *(narrow/wide)*. Depolarization of the left ventricle occurs across the ventricular *(conduction tissue/muscle tissue)*, and this pathway accounts for the width of the QRS complex.

negative; wide

muscle tissue

89 When a ventricular ectopic beat originates in the *right ventricular* His-Purkinje tissue, the impulse activates the left ventricular muscle without first activating the LBB. The LBB is not physiologically blocked, but activation occurs in such a way that this pathway is not used. Thus the resulting QRS pattern associated with right ventricular ectopy is similar to that occurring in _____.

LBBB

The predominant forces travel from right to left, *(away from/toward)* lead V_1 and across the ventricular muscle tissue, resulting in a *(positive/negative)* and *(wide/narrow)* QRS complex in this lead.

away from

negative; wide

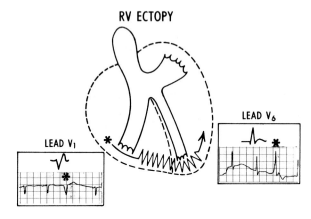

Fig. 8-26

Left ventricular ectopy

90 LET US REVIEW: When an impulse is blocked in the right bundle branch (RBB), the QRS complex in lead V_1 is *(positive/negative)* and *(narrow/wide)*. Depolarization of the right ventricle occurs across the ventricular *(conduction tissue/muscle tissue)*, and this pathway accounts for the width of the QRS complex.

postive

wide

muscle tissue

91 When a ventricular ectopic beat originates in the *left ventricular* His-Purkinje tissue, the impulse activates the right ventricular muscle without first activating the RBB. The RBB is not physiologically blocked, but activation occurs in such a way that this pathway is not used. The resulting QRS pattern associated with left ventricular ectopy is thus similar to that occurring in _____.

RBBB

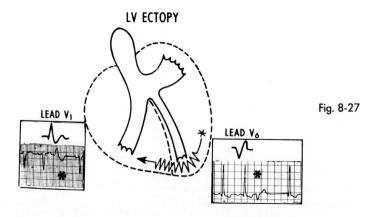

Fig. 8-27

The predominant forces travel from left to right, *(away from/to-*   **toward**
ward) led to V_1 and across the ventricular muscle tissue, resulting in
a *(positive/negative)* and *(wide/narrow)* complex in this lead.   **positive; wide**

92 We suggest monitoring on lead V_1 to determine the origin of ventricular ectopy. In the setting of acute MI most ventricular ectopic
beats originate from the left ventricle because this is the ventricle
most commonly injured. Ventricular ectopic beats that originate in
the right ventricle may also be the result of injury, but more likely
they result from another mechanism, such as catheter irritation of
the ventricular wall.

Fascicular ectopy

93 Recent studies have proved that at times ventricular ectopic beats may
result in QRS complexes with only minimal widening. These studies
have shown that these narrow PVCs may originate in the fascicles.
    REMEMBER: The LBB has two fascicles—the
_____ fascicle and the _____   **anterosuperior; posteroinferior**
fascicle.

94 When ectopy originates in the divisions or fascicles, the QRS configuration will resemble the patterns associated with a *hemiblock*.
    REMEMBER: Hemiblocks are diagnosed by shifts in the electrical
_____, and they produce changes in the QRS morphology   **axis**
in leads _____, _____, and aV_F.   **I; II**
    Thus leads I, II, and AV_F are also used in the diagnosis of fascic-
ular ectopy.

Anterosuperior fascicular ectopy

95 LET US REVIEW: When an impulse is blocked in the posteroinferior
fascicle (LPH), there is *(RAD/ALAD)*. Lead I becomes *(negative/posi-*   **RAD; negative**
tive) with an rS morphology, and lead aV_F becomes positive with a
qR pattern.

96 When a ventricular ectopic beat originates in the anterosuperior fascicle, the impulse activates the left ventricular muscle without first
activating the posterior fascicle. The posterior fascicle is not physiologically blocked, but activation occurs in such a way that this pathway is not used. Thus the pattern associated with anterior fascicular
ectopy is the same as that occurring in _____.   **LPH**
    There is RAD associated with the ectopy because the forces travel
inferiorly and to the right, *(away from/toward)* lead I and *(away from/*   **away from; toward**
toward) lead aV_F.
    NOTE: The anatomical relationship of the anterior fascicle to the
RBB is such that ectopic beats that arise in the anterior fascicle may
not be delayed in their activation of the right ventricle.

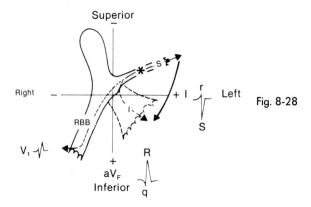

Fig. 8-28

Posterior fascicular ectopy

98 LET US REVIEW: When an impulse is blocked in the anterosuperior fascicle (LAH), there is *(RAD/ALAD)*. Lead I is predominantly *(positive/negative)* with a qR pttern, and leads II and aV$_F$ become *(positive/negative)* with an rS pattern.

ALAD; positive
negative

99 When a ventricular ectopic beat originates in the posteroinferior fascicle, the impulse activates the left ventricular muscle without first activating the anterior fascicle. The anterior fascicle is not physiologically blocked, but activation occurs in such a way that this pathway is not used. Thus the pattern associated with posterior fascicular ectopy is the same as that occurring in _____.

LAH

There is ALAD associated with the ectopy because the forces travel superiorly and to the left *(away from/toward)* lead I and *(away from/toward)* lead aV$_F$.

toward; away from

100

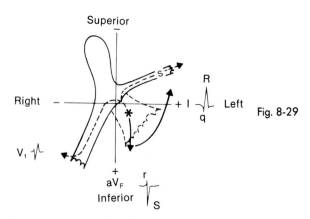

Fig. 8-29

NOTE: The anatomical relationship of the posterior fascicle to the RBB is such that impulses arising in this fascicle usually have some associated degree of RBBB.

101 PVCs with narrow QRS complexes have the same potential for producing repetitive ventricular firing or cardiac arrest when falling during the vulnerable period of a preceding beat as has the usual PVC with a wide QRS complex.

SUGGESTED READINGS

Braunwald E, editor: Heart disease: a textbook of cardiovascular medicine, ed. 3, Philadelphia, 1988, WB Saunders Co

Castellanos A, editor: Cardiac arrhythmias: mechanisms and management, Cardiovascular Clinic Series, Philadelphia, 1980, FA Davis Co.

Castellanos A: Recent advances in the diagnosis of fascicular blocks, Cardiol Clin 5(3):469, 1987.

Castellanos A: Unstable intraventricular conductiondisorders, Cardiol Clin 5(3):489, 1987.

Conover MB: Understanding electrocardiography, ed. 5, St. Louis, 1988, The CV Mosby Co.

Fisch G and others: Bundle branch block and sudden death, Prog Cardiovasc Dis 23:187, 1980.

Hammond C: Bundle branch blocks: when to sound the alarm, RN 44(1):55, 1981.

Hollander G and others: Bundle branch block in acute myocardial infarction, Am Heart J 105:738, 1983.

Kernicke J and Weiler KM: Electrocardiography for nurses: physiological corrleates, New York, 1981, John Wiley and Sons, Inc.

Klein RC and others: Intraventricular conduction defects in acute myocardial infarction: incidence, prognosis, and therapy, Am Heart J 108:1007, 1984.

Levy D and others: Electrocardiographic changes with advancing age: A cross-sectional study of the association of age with QRS axis, duration, and voltage, J Electrocardiography (suppl) 20:53, 1987.

Marriott HJL: Practical electrocardiography, ed. 7, Baltimore, 1983, Williams & Wilkins.

McAnulty JH and Rahimtoola S: Bundle branch block, Prog Cardiovasc Dis 26(4):333, 1984.

Narula OS: Intraventricular conduction defects: current concepts and clinical significance. In Castellanos A, editor: Cardiac arrhythmias: electrophysiology, diagnosis, and management, Philadelphia, 1980, William & Wilkins.

Sweetwood H: Clinical electrocardiography for nurses, Rockville, Md, 1983, Aspen Publications.

Mechanical Complications in Coronary Artery Disease: Heart Failure and Shock

HEART FAILURE

1 In previous units we discuss normal and abnormal electrical activity in the heart. Let us now consider the mechanical activity of the heart, or its role as a _____.

    pump

        The function of the heart is to provide an adequate *supply of* _____ *blood* to meet the metabolic *demands* of the body's tissues.

    oxygenated

        REMEMBER: In an attempt to meet the demands of the tissues, the heart pumps out a certain amount of oxygenated blood per minute. This amount of blood is known as the _____ _____.

    cardiac output

2 When the cardiac output falls as a result of mechanical (muscle) dysfunction and the demands of the tissues are no longer effectively met, the heart has failed to perform as an effective pump. This state is referred to as *heart failure*. Thus, heart failure may be defined as cardiac output not adequate to meet the demands of the tissues in which the *pump* is the *direct* cause of the imbalance.

3 If the fall in cardiac output is severe, resulting in tissue symptoms of hypoxia, the patient experiences and exhibits a _____ fall in cardiac output. The clinical state of *hypoxia* caused by inadequate cardiac output is known as _____ (see Unit 3, Frames 3 to 8).

    symptomatic

    shock

        In the presence of heart failure resulting from acute MI there *(is/is not)* a fall in cardiac output. Therefore heart failure caused by acute MI has the potential—if the patient's condition deteriorates—of leading to a symptomatic fall in cardiac output, or _____.

    is

    shock

        Shock occurring as a consequence of heart failure is known as _____ _____.

    cardiogenic shock

4 LET US REVIEW: Hypoxia caused by inadequate cardiac output is manifested by cellular _____ changes and _____ symptoms (see Unit 3). Heart failure is distinguished from cardiogenic shock by the *absence* of _____ _____.

metabolic

tissue

tissue symptoms

The symptoms of heart failure are initially an indirect rather than a direct manifestation of the fall in _____ _____ (see Frame 8). In contrast, the symptoms of shock are a(n) *(direct/indirect)* manifestation of the fall in cardiac output. Heart failure *(may/may not)* later evolve into the shock state.

cardiac output

direct

may

5 Let us now focus on the problem of heart failure.

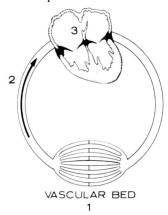

VASCULAR BED
1

Fig. 9-1

The function of the heart as a pump depends on three main factors: (1) resistance to ejection of blood *(systemic vascular _____)*; (2) venous return to the heart, which is related to venous tone and total *blood _____*; and (3) contractility of the heart *_____*.

resistance

volume

muscle

The systemic vascular resistance is also known as the heart's *afterload*. The venous return is also known as the heart's *preload*. Disturbances in any of these variables may either cause or enhance mechanical dysfunction of the heart and result in a discrepancy between the _____ of blood and the _____ of the body's tissue. The heart then may *fail* in its function as a pump. This condition is known as heart _____.

supply; demands

failure

6 If the heart must pump blood against an increased systemic vascular resistance or _____ load, heart _____ may occur.

after; failure

REMEMBMER: Systemic vascular resistance is a major determinant of blood _____. Systemic hypertension, then, is an example of a *(volume/pressure)* load.

pressure

pressure

If the heart is presented with excessive volume or a _____ load that it is unable to pump, _____ _____ may occur. Administration of large amounts of intravenous fluid is an example of a *(volume/pressure)* load.

pre-; heart failure

volume

Fluid overload is thus a potential source of heart failure in patients with borderline cardiac reserve. Mitral insufficiency and VSD are examples of internal volume loads that can occur in acute MI and can further overload the heart.

7 If the heart *muscle*, or *myocardium*, is damaged, _____ _____ may occur. In acute MI, the myocardium *(is/is not)* damaged. It can then be expected that in acute MI some manifestations of _____ _____ will be seen.

heart failure

is

heart failure

REMEMBER: Most MIs predominantly involve the *(right/left)* ventricle. Therefore, heart failure in the setting of MI is usually *(right/left)*-sided heart failure.

left

left

8 When the heart fails to pump enough blood forward, the cardiac output falls, and there is ineffective emptying of the left ventricle. As a result, blood becomes dammed up within the left ventricle. This result produces congestion in the heart and in the blood vessels that drain into the heart. The patients will exhibit symptoms that are caused by this congestion. Heart failure is thus frequently referred to as _____ *heart failure*, or CHF.

congestive

The symptoms of CHF are a consequence of either pulmonary or systemic congestion. These symptoms reflect an *indirect* rather than a direct manifestation of the fall in cardiac output. The major direct manifestations of the fall in cardiac output are less specific and include sinus tachycardia, decreased urine output, and changes in serum and urine electrolytes (see Unit 3), which promote fluid retention and further compromise borderline cardiac reserve.

9 The right and left sides of the heart may fail together or *separately*. We therefore speak of *right* ventricular failure or _____ ventricular failure. Heart failure in the setting of acute MI is usually *(right/left)* ventricular failure.

left

left

Left ventricular failure

10 When the left ventricle is damaged, the heart cannot function efficiently as a(n) _____. As a result, blood is dammed up within the _____ _____.

pump

left ventricle

This effect produces congestion and increased *pressure* within the left ventricle. The increase in ventricular contents and pressure interferes with effective filling. Thus the filling, or *(systolic/diastolic)*, pressure rises (see Frames 44 to 57). This pressure is transmitted retrogradely to the communicating left atrium and to the

diastolic

_____ _____ draining into the left side   **pulmonary veins**
of the heart. The atrial distention commonly produces atrial
arrhythmias.

11   Failure of the left ventricle, then, results in an *(increase/decrease)* in   **increase**
pressure, which is transmitted retrogradely to the communicating
left _____, the pulmonary _____, and the pul-   **atrium; veins**
monary capillaries. This increase in pulmonary capillary pressure
and pulmonary congestion causes fluid to escape from the alveolar
capillaries into the interstitial spaces of the _____.   **lungs**

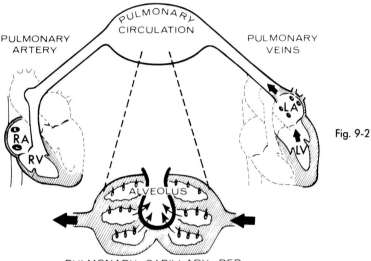

Fig. 9-2

12   Left ventricular failure may result in congestion of blood in the
_____ vascular bed. This congestion could result   **pulmonary**
in transudation of fluid into the lungs. Initially fluid transudates into
the *interstitial* spaces of the lungs. When fluid is in the interstitial
spaces, this state is known as *interstitial pulmonary edema.* Fluid may
then move into the *alveoli.* The presence of fluid in the alveoli may
interfere with gas exchange and thus produce significant patient
symptoms.

13   The *pulmonary congestion* may be manifested by certain symptoms: (1)
dyspnea and cough, (2) orothopnea, (3) rales or wheezes, and (4)
frothy, bloody sputum (hemoptysis).

14   *Dyspnea* is a subjective sensation of difficulty in breathing. In the setting of congestive heart failure this symptom is directly related to an
(increase/decrease) in pulmonary pressure secondary to *(left/right)* ven-   **increase; left**
tricular failure. The resulting pulmonary congestion causes the
lungs to become stiff and less compliant. The effect is a(n) *(increase/*   **increase**

decrease) in the work of breathing, manifested symptomatically as
_____. *Cough* is another symptom of *(right/left)* ven-
tricular failure and frequently accompanies dyspnea.

dyspnea; left

15 The symptoms of dyspnea are related to position. *Orthopnea* implies that a patient with stiff, congested lungs has greater dyspnea
when in the recumbent position and less dyspnea when in the
_____ position.

upright

In the upright position, venous return is decreased, hydrostatic
pressure is decreased, and lung capacity is increased.

16 Auscultation of the lungs in the patient with heart failure may reveal
abnormal breath sounds. The movement of air through abnormal *fluid*
in the terminal air passages or alveoli produces a noise known as a
crackle *(rale).* The *quality* of the rales is dependent on their *origin.*
The movement of air into fluid-filled *alveoli* produces fine crackling
sounds. These crackles (rales) are heard best at the *end of inspiration*
and do not disappear with coughing. Fine and inspiratory crackles
(rales) indicate fluid in the _____ or mild _____
ventricular heart failure.

alveoli; left

17 The rales of heart failure may be heard bilaterally or unilaterally on
the *right side.*

NOTE: Early left ventricular failure may be detected on chest x-ray
films as pulmonary venous engorgement *before* _____ may
be heart at the bedside.

rales

Refer to Unit 3 for a more complete discussion of pulmonary
assessment.

18 LET US REVIEW: When the left ventricle fails, blood is
_____ _____ within the _____
ventricle. This increase in ventricular content interferes with left
ventricular _____.

dammed up; left
filling

As a result the left ventricular filling pressure *(rises/falls).*

rises

The increased left ventricular pressure is transmitted retrogradely to the _____ _____ and the
_____ _____ draining into the
left side of the heart. The rise of pressure in the pulmonary veins
and capillaries results in _____ congestion.

left atrium
blood vessels
pulmonary

Severe (acute) pulmonary edema

19 Let us now briefly consider the problem of severe pulmonary
edema. Severe pulmonary edema is a result of *(right/left)* ventricular
failure.

left

REMEMBER: Pulmonary congestion and edema may be manifested
by the symptoms listed on page 383.

1. _____ or _____   dyspnea; cough
2. _____   orthopnea
3. _____ and _____   rales; wheezes
4. _____   hemoptysis

NOTE: Pulmonary congestion in *acute* pulmonary edema is severe, and its symptoms are dramatic. All of the symptoms just noted are present.

20 Pulmonary congestion and edema may be rapidly corrected by decreasing the *venous return* to the heart and lungs, decreasing the *circulating blood volume,* or *both.*

Rapid reduction of venous return (preload) may be accomplished by such measures as supporting the patient in high Fowler's position with legs dangling, sitting the patient in a chair with legs dependent; or applying rotating tourniquets. These measures facilitate trapping of blood in the extremities.

21 Morphine, an agent commonly used in the management of chest pain, also has a beneficial effect on venous return. Thus it may be useful for treating the patient with pulmonary edema. Morphine acts by dilating peripheral veins and decreasing the respiratory rate, thus causing a(n) *(increase/decrease)* in venous return.   decrease

REMEMBER: Inspiration *(raises/lowers)* intrathoracic pressure and   lowers
(increases/decreases) venous return. Thus the rapid respiratory rates   increases
occurring in response to acute pulmonary edema *(increase/decrease)*   increase
venous return, further congesting the lungs. Suppression of these
rapid respiratory rates stabilizes the venous return, thus decreasing
the _____ congestion.   pulmonary

22 The administration of *intermittent positive pressure ventilation* can also serve to decrease venous return to the heart *mechanically.* However, complete positive pressure with measures such as *continuous positive airway pressure* (CPAP) or positive end expiratory pressure (PEEP) may have a more sustained effect and, in addition, improve gas exchange. Alcohol may be administered in conjunction with positive pressure or in a separate nebulizer as a defoaming agent.

Vasodilator drugs may also be used to decrease the venous return and thus *(increase/decrease)* the pulmonary   decrease
_____. Although vasodilators are generally consid-   congestion
ered as afterload-reducing agents, many also dilate the venous bed
and thus effectively reduce the *(preload/afterload).*   preload

23 REMEMBER: Pulmonary congestion may also be decreased by agents
that decrease _____ blood volume.   circulating

Phlebotomy, also referred to as *plasmapheresis* when the red blood cells are returned, is a rapid way of decreasing circulating blood volume by directly withdrawing it from the circulation. This blood may then be discarded or may be returned without the plasma to the patient. Sterile technique in withdrawing the blood is critical.

Diuretics also decrease circulating blood volume. Selective diuretics may exert a venodilating effect and thereby also decrease venous return of _____.

preload

24 Myocardial O_2 demands (MV_{O_2}) may also be reduced by measures directed toward promoting patient comfort and relieving anxiety (see Frame 43).

REMEMBER: Left ventricular failure in the setting of acute MI represents a severe discrepancy between mycardial O_2 supply and demand. Much of the therapy is directed toward decreasing O_2 demands. However, therapy may also be directed toward improving blood or O_2 supply.

Supplementary oxygen may be given to patients to increase arterial O_2 supply temporarily and compensate for the interference in pulmonary O_2 transport. In addition, tachycardias compromising coronary blood flow are controlled.

25 Aminophylline acts to reverse the bronchospasm accompanying bronchiolar congestion. Aminophylline is a peripheral vasodilator and may also be given to decrease pulmonary congestion by decreasing _____ _____. Common side effects associated with the use of aminophylline include tachyarrhythmias and nausea or vomiting. Hypotension may also occur because of the ability of aminophylline to relax smooth muscle.

venous return

Aminophylline should be administered with caution to patients with acute MI because of its ability to increase the heart rate, increase automaticity, and stimulate contractility, thereby *(increasing/decreasing)* MV_{O_2}.

increasing

Right ventricular failure

26 The most common cause of *right* ventricular failure is left ventricular failure. Left ventricular failure increases the pressure of the _____ circulation. This pressure can eventually overload the right ventricle. The earliest sign of right ventricular pressure is an increased right atrial pressure. Right atrial pressure is also called *central venous pressure* (CVP). A catheter may be placed in the right atrium and the pressure measured against a column of water. This measurement is called the _____ _____ _____ measurement, or CVP.

pulmonary

central venous pressure

27 An increase in CVP indicates an increase of pressure in the *(right/left)* side of the heart. An increased CVP therefore reflects *(right/left)* ven-

right
right

tricular failure. An increased CVP *may indirectly* reflect left ventricular failure; however, an increased CVP *(does/does not)* *always* reflect left ventricular failure.

does not

REMEMBER: The most common cause of right-sided heart failure is _____ heart failure. Therefore an increased CVP may indirectly reflect _____ _____ _____.

left-sided

left ventricular failure

28 An increase in CVP can be observed clinically as distention of the *neck veins,* which feed into the superior vena cava and the _____ atrium.

right

Congestion in the right side of the heart may progress beyond the right atrium into the *(venous/aterial)* side of the systemic circulation. Just as pulmonary edema is a symptom of left ventricular failure, *systemic edema* is a manifestation of _____ ventricular failure.

venous

right

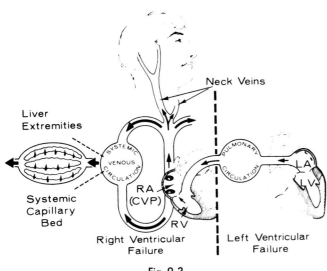

Fig. 9-3

29 The problem of systemic congestion may be manifested by certain symptoms: (1) liver enlargement and (2) peripheral edema. The *liver* may become enlarged as a result of chronic, passive congestion related to _____ _____. The development of *peripheral edema,* a late sign of _____ _____, is best seen in the dependent parts of the body, usually the feet and ankles.

heart failure
heart failure

NOTE: Patients with chronic left ventricular failure may develop right ventricular failure over a period of time. However, in acute MI, it is *uncommon* to see the symptoms of *(left/right)* ventricular failure.

right

30 LET US REVIEW: The most common cause of right ventricular failure is
_____ _____ failure. One of the earliest   left ventricular
signs of right ventricular failure is an increase in *(left atrial/right*   right atrial
atrial) pressure.

Changes in the right atrial pressure may be demonstrated by
changes in the measurement of the _____. The failure of   CVP
the right side of the heart may result in _____   systemic
congestion.

Right ventricular infarction as a form of right ventricular failure

31 Another potential cause of right ventricular failure in the setting of
coronary artery disease is right ventricular infarction.

REMEMBER: Most myocardial infarctions involve the *(right/left)* ven-   left
tricle.

Right ventricular infarctions are rarely isolated from left ventricular infarctions and occur mostly commonly in combination with
_____ wall MI.   inferoposterior

REMEMBER: The *(right/left)* coronary artery supplies the inferior   right
posterior wall of the left ventricle. The right coronary artery also
supplies the right ventricle.

Thus right coronary artery occlusion could result in infarction of
the inferior posterior wall of the _____ ventricle as well as   left
infarction of the _____ ventricle.   right

Extremely high cardiac enzymes in the setting of inferoposterior
MI with minimal signs of left ventricular dysfunction are an early
suggestion of right ventricular infarction.

32 Right ventricular infarction may not be clinically significant in terms
of overall cardiac function unless the right ventricle fails to perform
its function as a pump.

REMEMBER: The function of the right ventricle is to deliver
_____ blood from the body to the _____   unoxygenated; lungs
and subsequently to the _____ ventricle.   left

Right ventricular failure could thus result in failure to fill the
lungs, and subsequently the _____ ventricle, adequately.   left

If the right ventricle fails to fill the left ventricle, the patient may
appear to be in a shocklike state, with hypotension and signs and
symptoms of decreased tissue perfusion.

REMEMBER: A shocklike state occurring as a consequence of heart
failure is known as _____ shock.   cardiogenic

33 Right ventricular infarction is not easily recognizable on a standard
ECG. An ECG with "reversed" chest leads should be obtained (see
Unit 6, Frame 49). Hemodynamic and radionuclide techniques cor-

related with clinical signs and symptoms have made recognition of right ventricular infarction at the bedside possible.

34 Right ventricular failure and decreased tissue perfusion are signs and symptoms of a clinically significant right ventricular infarction.

REMEMBER: Signs and symptoms of right ventricular failure include distended _____ veins (reflecting the increase in right _____ pressure), liver enlargement (reflecting systemic venous congestion), and—less commonly in this setting—peripheral _____. The patient may also have a systolic murmur caused by *(mitral/tricuspid)* insufficiency manifested as large V waves in the neck veins. The lung fields would be *(congested/clear)* with right ventricular infarction, since the right ventricle rather than the left ventricle is failing. If the right ventricular failure is extremely severe, the patient may present with shocklike symptoms caused by the right ventricle's inability to fill the _____ ventricle.

neck
atrial

edema
tricuspid

clear

left

These signs and symptoms might include hypotension, cool, clammy skin, decreased urinary output, and mental confusion (see Frames 122 to 140).

35 Classic hemodynamic findings in right ventricular infarction include an elevated right atrial pressure or _____ with a normal, low, or only minimally elevated left atrial pressure (wedge pressure, LVEDP) and normal right ventricular (RV), systolic and pulmonary artery (PA) pressure (see Frames 44 to 70).

CVP

This hemodynamic pattern gives the impression of equalization of right-sided and left-sided pressures.

The clinical and hemodynamic findings with right ventricular infarction are thus similar to those seen with cardiac tamponade and require different action in acute settings.

36 Noninvasive tests such as echocardiography and radionuclide studies are useful in establishing a differential diagnosis. The clinical presentation of RV infarction is also similar to that seen with pulmonary embolism. However, with pulmonary embolism the RV and PA systolic pressures are elevated.

The major clinical significance of RV infarction is the potential shocklike state that may result if the RV fails to fill the _____ ventricle.

left

Therapy in the management of RV infarction is thus directed toward supporting the filling of the right and left ventricles by the administration of fluids. Inotropic support may also be required in the setting of severe hypotension.

37 LET US REVIEW: Right ventricular infarction occurs most commonly in conjunction with *(inferoposterior/anterior)* wall MI.

    Right ventricular infarction becomes clinically significant when it results in right _____ _____.

    Right ventricular infarction *(is/is not)* easily recognizable on the ECG but should be suspected when cardiac enzymes are extremely *(increased/decreased)* and the ECG show signs of _____ wall MI.

    The clinical picture is similar to that seen with cardiac _____ and requires differentiation in acute settings. Signs and symptoms of a clinically significant right ventricular infarction include _____ neck veins, _____ lungs, *(increased/decreased)* right atrial pressure or CVP, normal left _____ or wedge pressure, and *(hypotension/hypertension)*.

    Therapy in the management of right ventricular infarction is directed toward supporting the filling of the *(right/left)* ventricle through the administration of intravenous _____.

inferoposterior

ventricular failure
is not

increased
inferoposterior

tamponade

distended; clear
increased
atrial; hypotension

left
fluids

38 In summary:

    The patient with heart failure exhibits symptoms caused by either _____ or _____ congestion or both. In right ventricular failure the patient exhibits symptoms caused by _____ congestion. In left ventricular failure, the patient exhibits symptoms caused by _____ congestion.

    REMEMBER: These symptoms reflect an _____, rather than a direct, manifestation of the fall in cardiac output. When symptoms appear as a direct consequence of a fall in cardiac output, the heart failure has evolved into the _____ state.

pulmonary; systemic

systemic

pulmonary

indirect

shock

39 In most settings the *decreased cardiac output* and *congestion* have a *common* underlying mechanism: *decreased myocardial contractility*. Therefore initial therapy in the management of heart failure in acute MI is directed toward *decreasing* the *work load* of, or the demand on, the weakened myocardium.

    This management may be accomplished by any of the following:
1. Reduction of preload (ventricular filling) with diuretic therapy, or sodium and fluid restriction (see Unit 10)
2. Reduction of preload (ventricular _____) by measures directly decreasing venous return (see Frames 43 and 91)
3. Reduction of both afterload and preload by vasodilating drugs (see Unit 10)
4. Promoting physical and psychological comfort
5. Providing supplementary oxygen

filling

NOTE: Measures used to decrease preload rapidly by decreasing _____ _____ may take prece-   *venous return*
dence in the setting of *severe* pulmonary congestion, known as *acute pulmonary edema.*

Further information on the determinants of myocardial O_2 demand (consumption) is presented in Frame 57.

40 Following a reduction of cardiac work load, therapy may be directed toward stimulating *contractility.* The drug most commonly used for this purpose is digitalis. Digitalis increases myocardial _____ and thus *(increases/decreases)* the pulmonary   *Contractility; decreases*
and systemic congestion.

Digitalis is no longer considered the drug of choice in the setting of heart failure caused by acute MI because of its effect of increasing O_2 demands. Dopamine is an alternate drug that can be used in severe heart failure and has less harmful effects on O_2 demands.

41 In the setting of left ventricular failure with severe pulmonary edema, initial therapy is directed toward decreasing _____ _____. Measures used to   *pulmonary congestion*
decrease pulmonary congestion act either by directly decreasing venous return or by decreasing circulating blood volume. Subsequent therapy is directed toward first improving cardiac output and then reducing systemic congestion. Improvement of cardiac output may be accomplished by measures that decrease the _____ _____ _____ or stimulate   *cardiac work load*
_____. Reduction of systemic congestion may be ac-   *contractility*
complished by measures that decrease circulating blood volume.

42 The fall in cardiac output associated with CHF may produce functional limitation due to the associated decrease in *(O_2 supply/O_2 demands)* and energy levels. Patients may be classified into subsets which   *O_2 supply*
describe the severity of these limitations or other symptoms of CHF.

The popular New York Heart Association Classification system is based on functional limitations and is as follows:

Class I: No limitations (i.e., no symptoms of dypsnea, fatigue, or palpitation with ordinary physical activity)

Class II: Slight limitation (i.e., occurrence of the above symptoms with ordinary physical activity)

Class III: Marked limitation (i.e., occurrence of symptoms with less than ordinary activity)

Class IV: Symptoms present even at rest

The popular Killip classification system is based on the presence and severity of congestive symptomatology in patients with acute myocardial infarction and is described on page 390.

Class I: absence of crackles (rales) and S_3—i.e., absence of CHF

Class II: crackles (rales) in the lower half of the lung fields and S_3—i.e., mild to moderate CHF

Class III: acute pulmonary edema—i.e., severe CHF

Class IV: systolic BP less than 90 mm Hg with oliguria and decreased level of consciousness—i.e., cardiogenic shock

43 In summary, the goals in the management of heart failure are to decrease pulmonary and systemic congestion and to improve cardiac output. Five main principles are employed in the management of these three problems.

To decrease pulmonary congestion by:

1. Decreasing _____ _____   venous return
2. Decreasing   _____   _____   circulating blood volume
_____

To increase cardiac output and tissue oxygenation/energy levels promote more complete ventricular emptying by:

3. Decreasing cardiac _____ _____   work load
4. Strengthening the _____   myocardium
   To decrease chronic systemic congestion by:
5. Decreasing   circulating   _____   blood volume
_____

44 NURSING ORDERS: The patient with heart failure
1. Provide cardiac rest.
   —Place patient in semi-Fowler's or Fowler's position.
   —Encourage chair rest.
   —Allow use of commode chair.
   —To relieve psychological stress:
     Explain all procedures in simple terms.
     Allow patient contact with familiar objects.
     Encourage independence and self-care.
     Allow visitors, with limitations as needed.
   —Administer sedation as required.
2. Observe patient for overt signs of dyspnea:
   —Shortness of breath
   —Cough
   —Increase in respiratory rale
   —Valsalva respirations
3. Auscultate the heart and lungs when checking vital signs, check for:
   —Gallops
   —Murmurs see Frames 90 to 116
   —Variations in the normal heart sounds
   —Rales
   Alterations in the quality of the normal breath sounds

4. Check the CVP when checking vital signs.
   —If no CVP catheter is inserted, observe for the development of neck vein distention.
   —Always correlate CVP findings with lung sounds.
5. Watch for the development of tissue symptoms indicating that heart failure is evolving into the shock state.
6. In the presence of severe pulmonary edema:
   —Support the patient in high Fowler's position with legs dependent.
   —Start O_2 therapy.
   —Ensure patent IV route or limit IV fluids to keep it open.
   —Obtain vital signs
   ——Have available:
      Rotating tourniquets
      IPPB (or PEEP or CPAP, if preferred) equipment
      Resuscitation equipment
      Morphine sulfate
      Aminophylline
      Diuretics
      Digitalis
      Vasodilators (nitroglycerine, isosorbide, nitroprusside)
7. When tourniquets are required:
   —Place tourniquets in a position high in groin and axilla.
   —Check blood pressure before and during use of the tourniquets; rotating tourniquets are contraindicated if the patient is *(hypotensive/hypertensive)*.
   —Check for the presence and adequacy of arterial pulses—only the venous flow should be occluded.
   —Occlude only three extremities at one time, rotate at least every 10 to 15 minutes.
   —When discontinuing tourniquets, do *not* release all at one time.

hypotensive

HEMODYNAMIC MONITORING

45 In acute coronary artery disease (angina or acute MI), the myocardial changes and resulting mechanical dysfunction alter the movement of blood through the heart and blood vessels. The study of the movement of blood is known as *hemodynamics*. The monitoring of hemodynamic changes is logically referred to as _____ monitoring.

hemodynamic

Since the movement of blood occurs within the cardiovascular system, hemodynamics simply refers to the assessment of the function or physiology of the _____ system.

cardiovascular

46 Cardiovascular function (i.e., hemodynamics) can be assessed both invasively and non-invasively. Non-invasive evaluation includes monitoring of heart sounds and detection of clinical signs of pulmonary congestion and decreased cardiac output mentioned earlier in this unit (see Frame 8-18).

Another currently used noninvasive method of evaluating left ventricular function (both systolic and diastolic) is *echocardiography*. A beam of sound is directed through the chest wall from the anterior to the posterior wall. The beam bounces back vibrating, or echoing, when it makes contact with any dense structure, such as the ventricular wall or valves. The pattern of these vibrations is recorded and provides information about the function of the mechanical structures.

47 Noninvasive techniques of hemodynamic monitoring have not provided as practical, accurate, or early information about LV function as the invasive modes to date. The advent of the flow-directed, balloon-tipped pulmonary artery catheter (first known as the Swan-Ganz catheter) popularized the use of invasive techniques at the bedside. The term hemodynamics is currently used more clinically to describe the invasive monitoring of cardiovascular function.

48 The focus of hemodynamic monitoring is assessment of function or dysfunction of *mechanical* structures of the cardiovascular system.

REMEMBER: The mechanical structures of the heart are the _____, blood vessels, and _____. The mechanical activity of the heart refers to its role as a _____. The state where the heart fails to perform as an effective pump is known as _____ _____ and is associated with a fall in _____ _____. If the cardiac output falls significantly enough to produce tissue symptoms of hypoxia, this state may evolve into _____.

muscle; valves

pump

heart failure

cardiac output

shock

The assessment of hemodynamic changes, therefore, allows us to detect or anticipate the presence of _____ _____ or _____.

heart failure

shock

Flow/Pressure/Resistance Relationships

49 The three major physiologic parameters reflecting the mechanical function or dysfunction of the cardiovascular system are *flow, pressure,* and resistance. The heart as a pump creates the driving force that initiates the *flow* of blood. This flow of blood put out by the heart is more commonly referred to as the _____ _____.

cardiac output

The blood vessels direct the flow to the individual tissues and/or back to the heart by vasoconstriction and/or vasodilation of their smooth muscle lining.

50 *Pressure* is generated *within the blood vessels* as the force of the blood flow from the heart (i.e., the Cardiac Output) meets resistance or "interference" in the vessel tubes. Resistance is determined primarily

by the _____ and/or _____ of the
smooth muscle lining.

Pressure is also generated *within the heart itself* as the blood is forced against the chamber walls during systole and/or diastole. The *compliance* of the chamber wall determines the amount of "interference" to flow during ventricular filling or *(systole/diastole)*.

Compliance may be defined as the opposition to ventricular _____ due to the natural distensibility or stiffness of the muscle wall. It is more accurately reflected by changes in pressure for a given volume. ($\Delta V/\Delta P$)

vasoconstriction; vasodilation

diastole

filling

51 Systemic Blood Pressure is the measurement of the pressure within the *(blood vessel/heart)*. Therefore, the major determinants of systemic BP are the _____ _____ and peripheral vascular _____. More specifically, BP reflects the force of the blood against the walls of the *arteries* during cardiac systole and diastole.

blood vessels
cardiac output
resistance

IN SUMMARY: The movement of blood within the cardiovascular system is affected by the amount of *flow* within the blood vessels or within the cardiac chambers (and the corresponding _____ or compliance changes). The pressure generated within the blood vessels or heart itself is a reflection of these parameters. Therefore, complete hemodynamic monitoring involves monitoring of all of these parameters by information obtained from both within the _____ _____ and within the _____ itself. Systemic BP reflects only the changes occurring within the _____ _____, specifically the peripheral *(arteries/veins)*.

resistance

blood vessels
heart
blood vessels
arteries

52 The *Cardiac Ouptut* is the amount of blood _____ put out by the heart *per minute*. Cardiac output is determined by heart _____ and *stroke volume* (blood flow *per beat*). Stroke volume is in turn determined by the *preload, contractility,* and *afterload*.

flow

rate

REMEMBER: The preload is the stretch on the ventricle with filling prior to contraction and is equivalent to the blood volume and/or venous tone (i.e., _____ _____). The afterload is the resistance to ejection and is equivalent to the systemic _____ _____ or mean arterial pressure.

venous return

vascular resistance

Hemodynamic changes in acute myocardial infarction

53 The first clinically perceptible change in acute myocardial infarction occurs in *diastole* due to a decrease in compliance of the left ventricle. This decrease in compliance is the result of an immediate inflammatory response to decreased coronary blood supply and thus occurs during episodes of angina as well as during myocardial infarction.

393

REMEMBER: Compliance is the opposition to ventricular _____ due to the distensibility or _____ of the muscle wall. Compliance is more accurately defined as a change in _____ for a given change in volume. As the left ventricle becomes less compliant, it has difficulty accepting the entering blood volume, and the diastolic _____ rises.

filling

stiffness

pressure

pressure

The first sign of left ventricular dysfunction in acute MI is a rise in _____ ventricular _____ _____, caused by alterations in _____.

left; diastolic pressure

compliance

54 Left ventricular filling occurs in two major phases. The first phase occurs as the AV valves open and is known as the *rapid filling phase.* The second phase occurs at the end of diastole as atrial contraction completes diastolic filling.

A slightly damaged left ventricle can accommodate the blood that enters during the *initial* filling phase. However, because of alterations in compliance, the left ventricle cannot efficiently accommodate the *added* volume that enters with atrial contraction at the end of filling.

REMEMBER: Atrial contraction occurs at the *(beginning/end)* of ventricular diastole. Thus left ventricular pressure first rises at the *end* of the diastole.

end

The first hemodynamic change seen as a result of acute MI is—more accurately—a rise in left ventricular _____ diastolic pressure (LVEDP).

end-

This change results in only slight increases in LVEDP, which are usually tolerated asymptomatically and are detected clinically only with invasive monitoring (See Frames 63-72) or by the presence of an S_4 gallop (See Frames 95-97).

55 The LVEDP reflects the stretch or *load* on the left ventricle *prior to* systole. This filling load is also known as the *left ventricular preload.* Left ventricular filling is directly affected by pulmonary venous return, which is a function of the systemic venous return (i.e., blood volume), and right ventricular filling. Thus the venous return is often clinically referred to as the *heart's preload.*

A significant increase in preload (blood volume, venous return) may increase LVEDP, while a significant decrease in preload (blood volume, _____ _____) may compromise cardiac output. Both of these changes can result in patient symptomatology (See Frames 71 and 72).

venous return

56 The second clinically perceptible change in mechanical function affects ventricular *systole,* resulting in a fall in cardiac output. This early fall in cardiac output may be clinically detected by invasive techniques only or by its secondary effects on ventricular diastole (see Frame 57).

NOTE: In the initial stages of myocardial damage, the *unaffected* fibers may increase their contractility and overcompensate for the loss of effective contractile structures. Thus there is no initial net loss in contractility, and the cardiac output is maintained.

Subsequent loss of myocardial function results in the inability of intact fibers to compensate for this loss. The cardiac output therefore falls. When the cardiac output falls as a result of mechanical dysfunction, this state is known as *heart failure.*

57 In heart failure, as the cardiac output falls, the fraction of the blood ejected by the left ventricle during systole (left ventricular ejection fraction) decreases.

NOTE: The fraction of the left ventricular diastolic volume ejected during systole is known as the *left ventricular ejection fraction.*

As a result the residual volume remaining in the left ventricle at the end of systole rises. Thus at the onset of diastole the left ventricle is already partially full and has difficulty accepting even the initial amounts of entering blood. As a result, the diastolic pressure rises further.

58 REMEMBER: During *ventricular diastole,* the valves separating the left atrium from the left ventricle are *(open/closed).*　　　　　　　　　　open

The left atrial and left ventricular pressure is transmitted to the left atrium. This increase in pressure is further transmitted retrogradely to the communicating pulmonary _____ and pulmonary _____, resulting in *pulmonary congestion* (see Fig. 9-2, Frames 10 to 17).　　veins capillaries

The pulmonary congestion corresponds with the decrease in the LV _____ fraction and a further increase in LVEDP. In this hemodynamic phase, the *(systolic/diastolic)* changes are more clinically significant. However, they occur secondary to systolic changes.　　ejection diastolic

59 In response to the fall in cardiac output, there is a compensatory rise in systemic vascular resistance. This rise in systemic resistance is the body's attempt to maintain the *mean* arterial pressure in the presence of a fall in cardiac output.

However, this reflexive rise in SVR may further impede and actually *decrease* the cardiac output.

REMEMBER: Blood pressure = cardiac output × systemic vascular resistance.

The rise in systemic vascular resistance is not accompanied initially by any significant change in cuff pressure other than a narrowing pulse pressure and thus may not be detected noninvasively.

60 With more extensive damage, the cardiac output may continue to fall to the point that tissue perfusion becomes compromised in spite of compensatory efforts. When tissue symptoms result from this significant fall in cardiac output, the state is known as *shock*.

Tissue O_2 demands may be estimated by determining the body surface area. The comparison of cardiac output to this body surface area is referred to as the *cardiac index* (CI) and is a reflection of tissue _____ _____.

O_2 demands

$$CI = \frac{cardiac\ output}{BSA\ (M_2)}$$

The determination of cardiac index requires an exact and, therefore, invasive measurement of cardiac output (see Frames 82-83). Body surface area (BSA) is determined by obtaining the patient's height and weight and plotting them on a Dubois BSA chart.

If the cardiac index falls significantly, a state of _____ is imminent. When this state occurs as a consequence of heart failure it is associated with a high LV *(systolic/diastolic)* pressure and is known as _____ _____.

shock

diastolic
cardiogenic shock

61 In summary:

The three progressive hemodynamic phases that may occur as a result of acute MI are:
1. A rise in left ventricular _____ diastolic pressure (LVEDP) caused by altered _____.

end
compliance

2. An initial fall in cardiac output and decreased ejection LV fraction accompanied by a further rise in LVEDP with _____ _____ and a reflexive rise in _____. This state is referred to clinically as congestive _____ _____.

pulmonary congestion
SVR
heart failure

3. A significant fall in cardiac output resulting in a low cardiac _____ and _____ symptoms. This state is referred to clinically as _____.

index; tissue
shock

The major hemodynamic alterations in acute MI involve changes in left ventricular *pressure*, cardiac _____ and/or _____ and _____. Therefore, the monitoring of hemodynamic changes in these patients should include attempts at monitoring at least these major parameters.

output
index; SVR

62 When considering the disturbances in myocardial function that occur in the setting of acute MI, one must also evaluate the factors affecting myocardial O_2 consumption. The determinants of myocardial O_2 consumption (MV_{O2}) are:
1. *Heart rate*
2. *Preload,* which influences wall tension in diastole
3. *Afterload,* which influences wall tension with systole

4. Contractile state

NOTE: Both preload and afterload influence wall tension. Thus some authors consider intramyocardial wall tension as a link between preload and afterload.

Ironically, these are also the major determinants of an adequate cardiac output. While a significant increase in any of these parameters can increase the myocardial O_2 demands, a significant decrease in any of these may compromise the cardiac output. Thus both extremes are to be avoided.

Monitoring pressures (invasive techniques)

63 LET US REVIEW: The first mechanical changes occuring in acute MI affect *left ventricular (systolic/diastolic)* pressure.

Maximum diastolic pressures are reached at the *(beginning/end)* of diastole. Thus minor increases in filling pressures can be first detected at the _____ of diastole. The goal of monitoring pressure changes in acute MI is to detect, as accurately as possible, early changes in _____.

diastolic

end

end

LVEDP

64 The most accurate measure of LVEDP is obtained directly by a left ventricular catheter. However, since the right side of the heart is more easily accessible via the venous system, indirect monitoring of left ventricular change is done with catheters introduced into the right side of the heart.

65 *Early* attempts to monitor left ventricular function were done through catheters introduced into the right atrium to record the _____ _____ pressure. However, the right atrium communicates with the *(right ventricle/left ventricle)* only during ventricular diastole and thus reflects changes only in *(RVEDP/LVEDP)*.

central venous

right ventricle

RVEDP

66 Pressures recorded from the pulmonary artery were found to correlate more closely with left ventricular function because the pulmonary artery is obviously anatomically closer to the left ventricular cavity than are the right atrium and right ventricle.

In addition, the catheter is situated beyond the pulmonary valve. Closure of the pulmonary valve during ventricular diastole interrupts communication with the *(right/left)* side of the heart. However, direct communication is maintained with the pulmonary circulation and the *(right/left)* atrium (Fig. 9-4).

Because the left atrium, in turn, communicates with the left ventricle during diastole, communication is established between the pulmonary artery and left ventricle. Thus pulmonary artery *end-*diastolic pressure (PAEDP) closely approximates the pressure in the _____ circulation, and, in the absence of pulmo-

right

left

pulmonary

nary disease, _____ atrial pressure, and _____. left; LVEDP
Continuous monitoring of pulmonary artery pressure is made possible with a balloon-tipped flow-directed pulmonary artery catheter (first known as the Swan/Ganz catheter). Once the tip is positioned in the pulmonary artery, the balloon is deflated and should remain deflated to prevent inadvertent movement into the wedge position (See Frame 69).

MONITORING OF VENTRICULAR DIASTOLIC PRESSURES

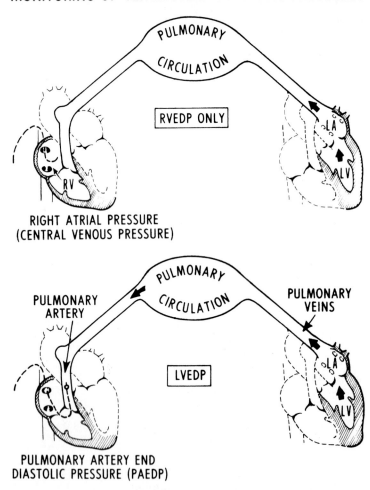

Fig 9-4

67 Pulmonary artery (PA) catheters are typically provided with another lumen, which is positioned in the RA when the distal tip is positioned in the pulmonary artery. This lumen is labeled on the connecting port/outlet as the proximal opening and allows for concurrent monitoring of RA pressure and/or the administration of RA pressure and/or the administration of fluids or medications. This port is also used in conjunction with a thermistor port for the measurement of cardiac output (See Frames 82 and 83).

Additional optional features currently available include an outlet for concurrent monitoring of venous O_2 saturation (SvO2) and five electrodes for concurrent dual chamber pacing (three atrial and two ventricular (Fig 9-5) (See Unit 3: frames for discussion of Sv_{O_2} monitoring and Unit 11 for discussion of dual chamber pacing).

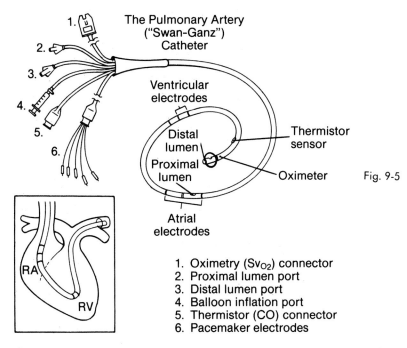

The Pulmonary Artery ("Swan-Ganz") Catheter

Ventricular electrodes

Distal lumen

Proximal lumen

Thermistor sensor

Oximeter

Fig. 9-5

Atrial electrodes

1. Oximetry (Sv_{O_2}) connector
2. Proximal lumen port
3. Distal lumen port
4. Balloon inflation port
5. Thermistor (CO) connector
6. Pacemaker electrodes

In the presence of pulmonary disease, the pulmonary artery vascular resistance and systolic as well as diastolic pressure are typically elevated. Severe CHF may also elevate these pressures. Thus, the PA systolic pressure *(is/is not)* helpful in differentiating pulmonary disease from CHF. In the absence of pulmonary disease, the PA *(systolic/diastolic)* pressure correlate best with LV dysfunction.

is not

diastolic

68 Although the monitoring of pulmonary artery *(systolic/diastolic)* pressure in acute MI is a useful index of left ventricular function, a still more accurate measurement may be obtained. The balloon of the pulmonary artery (PA) catheter can be re-inflated so that the catheter may be advanced farther into one of the branches of the pulmonary artery. When the catheter is in position within this branch, it is said to be *wedged* in the vessel. The pressure obtained after the catheter is wedged is known as the _____ pressure.

diastolic

wedge

PULMONARY CAPILLARY WEDGE PRESSURE

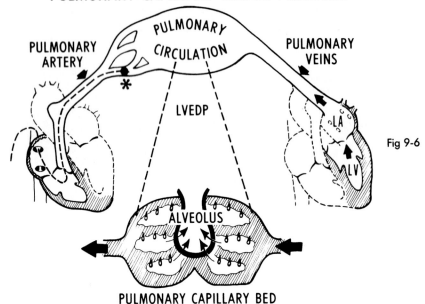

Fig 9-6

PULMONARY CAPILLARY BED

69 Because the catheter is closer in this position to the pulmonary capillary bed than it is to the main pulmonary artery, the pressure recording obtained at this site is known more completely as *pulmonary* _____ *wedge pressure*. Since a pulmonary artery branch is temporarily occluded while obtaining this pressure reading, this pressure is also known as the *pulmonary artery occlusion pressure (PAOP)*.

    capillary

    The wedging of the catheter in the pulmonary artery branch not only interrupts communication with the *(right/left)* side of the heart but also interrupts communication with part of the pulmonary circulation. Therefore, as compared with the pulmonary artery pressure, pulmonary capillary wedge pressure is a *(more/less)* accurate index of left atrial and left ventricular end-diastolic function.

    right

    more

70 The most common potential complications associated with the use of Swan-Ganz catheters are (1) *right ventricular PVCs* and *VT* resulting from mechanical stimulation of the ventricular wall during insertion and during monitoring if the catheter slips back into the right ventricle and (2) *pulmonary infarction* caused by prolonged pulmonary ischemia if the catheter remains inflated in the wedge position or inadvertently floats into this position during PA monitoring. Pulmonary infarction is more likely to occur in susceptible individuals, such as those with pre-existing pulmonary hypertension or COPD.

    NOTE: The length of time the catheter is tolerated in the wedge position is individually determined. However, prophylactically, wedge readings should be taken as quickly as possible, and the balloon should be deflated immediately until a pulmonary artery pulse pattern is again obtained.

Other reported complications include: infection, thromboembolism, right bundle branch block, and catheter knotting. Balloon rupture, although common after the balloon has been inflated multiple times, does not produce patient complications unless large amounts of air are introduced. Failure to wedge after the introduction of 1.5 cc of air and the loss of resistance to inflation are suggestive of balloon rupture.

71 Normally, LVEDP is approximately 6 to 12 mm Hg. Some sources quote lower normal limits of 4 to 12 mm Hg. Elevations in LVEDP of up to 15 mm Hg are expected in the setting of acute MI and may be caused by altered compliance even in the absence of CHF. However, the LVEDP is not considered *critically* elevated until it exceeds 18 mm Hg.

PAEDPs, in the absence of lung disease, and pulmonary capillary wedge pressures usually *(do/do not)* reflect LVEDP. Therefore PAEDP and wedge pressure readings should not exceed _____ mm Hg in acute MI. Increases in pressure beyond this level may indicate greater *(right ventricular/left ventricular)* dysfunction and predict impending _____ congestion. Such changes indicate Pulmonary congestion typically occurs when the LVEDP and pulmonary capillary pressure 18 mm Hg. Pressures exceeding this critical level may indicate significant left ventricular _____. PAEDP is normally within 2-4 mm Hg of the LVEDP or _____ pressure.

do

18
left ventricular

pulmonary

exceeds

failure
wedge

72 A wedge pressure of 5 mm Hg would indicate a(n) *(low/high)* LVEDP although still within normal limits, if the cardiac output is compromised. The most likely explanation would be decreased left ventricular filling caused by blood volume depletion. Indicated therapy would consist of administering *(IV fluids/diuretics)*.

Even a damaged myocardium requires a certain amount of stretch during diastole to promote effective contraction and cardiac output during systole. Stretching of cardiac muscle fibers, within limits, is thus needed and actually promotes contraction. This property of cardiac muscle is described by Starling's law of the heart. Starling's law states that the greater the stretch on a muscle fiber (as in diastole), the more effective the subsequent fiber shortening (or _____). The detection of a low wedge pressure in the presence of a low cardiac output indicates that the cardiac output has been most likely compromised by inadequate _____ or stretch before contraction and the administration of _____ is indicated.

low

IV fluids

contraction

filling
volume

REMEMBER: The stretch of the left ventricle with filling, *before* contraction, is known as the left ventricular _____.   preload

Thus a low wedge pressure indicates insufficient left ventricular _____.   preload

Monitoring pressure pulse patterns

73 Continuous monitoring of the pressure pulse patterns is necessary to (1) effectively monitor catheter position and (2) record pressures accurately and thus avoid complications. Although pressure values may be recorded with a catheter-manometer system, a record of the pulse pattern can be obtained only with the use of a catheter-transducer system.

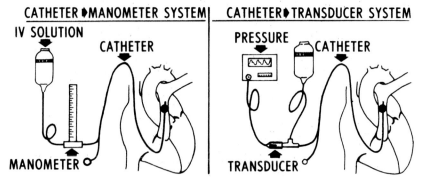

Fig. 9-7

74 With the use of a catheter-transducer system, characteristic patterns may be recorded from either *atria, ventricles,* or *arteries.* Recognition of these characteristic mechanical patterns has added a new dimension to the nursing management of critical care patients.

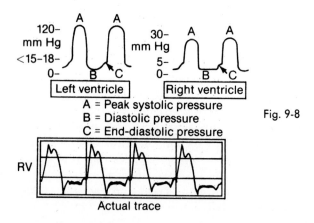

Fig. 9-8

75 Pressure within the right and left ventricles rises quickly with the onset of ventricular contraction, or *(systole/diastole)*. It rapidly reaches a peak point. This point is known as the peak _____ pressure.

systole

systolic

As systolic ejection is completed, the *(AV/semilunar)* valves close, separating the ventricles from the _____ leaving them. The pressure in the ventricles drops abruptly as ventricular filling, or _____, begins.

semilunar

vessels

diastole

The ventricular *end*-diastolic pressure is recorded just before the onset of the next systole.

Arterial patterns

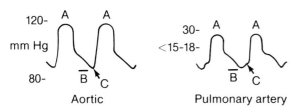

Aortic   Pulmonary artery

A = Peak systolic pressure
B = Lowest diastolic pressure
C = End-diastolic pressure

Fig. 9-9

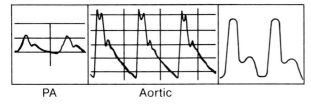

PA   Aortic

Actual trace

76 NOTE: Peripheral arteries (brachial, femoral, or radial) may mimic either of the two examples of aortic patterns above. The pulmonary artery pattern may also closely mimic the aortic or peripheral arterial pattern in a given patient (see Frame 75), but is more likely to have cyclic changes related to respirations. (See Frame 80).

The pressure within the major arteries (pulmonary artery and aorta) rises quickly as blood is ejected into them with the onset of ventricular systole. It also rapidly reaches a peak _____ pressure.

systolic

Because the valves separating the ventricles and vessels are *(open/closed)* during the ventricular systole, ventricular systolic pressures and arterial systolic pressures *(are/are not)* equivalent. Arterial systolic pressure reflects the changes occurring within the arteries during _____ systole.

open

are

ventricular

77 With the onset of ventricular diastole, the semilunar valves *(open/close)*, separating the ventricles and the blood vessels. The pressure

close

in the vessels drops *gradually* as the blood still within them is dispersed throughout the vascular bed to the tissues.

REMEMBER: Ventricular diastolic pressure drops *(gradually/ abruptly)*. Therefore ventricular and arterial *systolic* patterns are *(similar/different)* but their diastolic patterns are distinctly *(the same/different)*.

abruptly

similar

different

The record obtained from a catheter is a peripheral artery such as the *brachial* or *radial* artery may closely mimic the pulmonary artery or aortic patterns.

Mean pressures are also obtained with arterial tracings. The mean pressure equals the diastolic pressure + ⅓ of the difference between the systolic and diastolic. Thus it correlates more closely with the *(systolic/diastolic)* pressure.

diastolic

Atrial patterns (or pulmonary capillar wedge pattern)

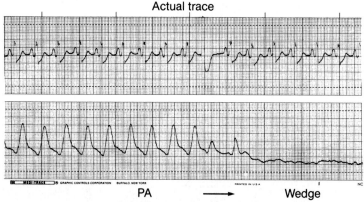

Mean

RA—0-5 mm Hg (>12 mm Hg critical)
LA—6-12 mm Hg (>18 mm Hg critical)

a = Atrial contraction
c = Bulging of AV valve into atria with early ventricular contraction
v = Ventricular contraction
x and y = Drop in pressure with atrial relaxation and filling

Actual trace

Fig. 9-10

PA   ⟶   Wedge

78 Pressures within the right and left atria rise quickly with the onset of atrial contraction, producing an atrial systolic pulse wave recorded as the *a wave*. The a wave in an atrial pulse pattern represents _____ _____.

atrial contraction

79 Because the force of atrial contraction is not as great as the force of ventricular contraction the atrial systolic pulse is not usually as distinctly noted on an oscilloscope record.

Ventricular mechanical events also directly influence atrial events, producing extra pulsations in the pressure pattern (Fig. 9-9). As a result the atrial pattern *(does/does not)* exhibit systolic and dias-

does not

tolic curves as distinct as ventricular and arterial patterns. Instead, it assumes a wavy configuration. An average, or *mean*, pressure level is usually recorded.

NOTE: Because *pulmonary capillary wedge pressure* most directly reflects left atrial pressure, the characteristic wedge pulse pattern closely resembles the atrial pattern (Fig. 9-9) (see Frames 65 to 67). Venous pulse patterns, such as those present in the neck veins, also resemble the atrial pattern because of their direct communication with the right atrium.

80 Mitral regurgitation produces a giant V wave distorting both the PA and wedge tracing, making it more difficult to distinguish between them. The V wave immediately follows the systolic peak in the PA tracing resulting in a notched appearance. As the balloon is inflated, this notch disappears, leaving only the V waves. Mitral regurgitation or insufficiency occurs in angina and/or MI due to _____ muscle ischemia or _____.   papillary; infarction
In this setting, the a wave pressure correlates the most closely with LVEDP.

The changes in intrathoracic pressure occurring with inspiration and expiration are transmitted to the RA, PA, and wedge pressure tracings as cyclic increases and decreases in pressure. The intrathoracic pressure is more *negative* on *inspiration* resulting in a _____ in pressure. Labored breathing as with se-   decrease
vere pulmonary congestion magnifies these effects. With mechanical ventilation, in contrast to spontaneous breathing, the intrathoracic pressure and corresponding pressure readings are *(increased/   increased
decreased)* in inspiration. The pressure at end-expiration is the most accurate in all these situations.

81 Other distortions in the pressure patterns, which may result in inaccurate measurements, include: damped tracing, catheter whip, and lack of leveling the transducer air-fluid interface to the phlebostatic axis (mid right atrium), especially with position changes.

Catheter whip can be minimized by preventing the connecting tubing from lying across the patients chest, by adding high frequency filters to the system, introducing an air bubble into the transducer, or by having the physician reposition the catheter to avoid looping in the right ventricle or positioning of the catheter tip near the turbulent area of the pulmonic valve.

Monitoring cardiac output (invasive techniques)

82 The most accurate methods of determining cardiac output are by the invasive *indicator-dilution* techniques. Thermal dilution using a PA catheter is the most commonly used.

Dye dilution

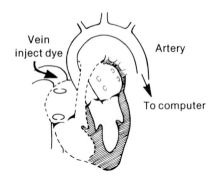

Vein inject dye

Artery

To computer

Thermal dilution

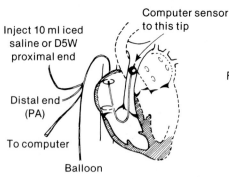

Inject 10 ml iced saline or D5W proximal end

Computer sensor to this tip

Fig. 9-11

Distal end (PA)

To computer

Balloon

NOTE: The thermistor lumen communicates with the distal tip in the pulmonary artery and is attached to a computer sensitive to temperature changes in the injected fluid, which will calculate the cardiac output.

83 LET US REVIEW: The purpose of maintaining effective cardiac output is to meet _____ O_2 demands. Tissue O_2 demands may be estimated by determining the _____ _____ _____ from the patient's height and weight using a Dubois Body Surface Area Chart. The effectiveness of cardiac output relative to these tissue O_2 demands is determined by dividing the measured cardiac output by the BSA to obtain the cardiac _____ (see Frame 60). The normal cardiac index is 2.5 - 4.2 l/min/m2. A cardiac index is considered critically low when it drops below 1.8 l/min/m2. At that point _____ is imminent.

tissue

body surface area

index

shock

Cardiac output may also be determined by estimating or calculating the A-V O_2 difference and relating this to the Fick principle. The more recent introduction of continuous Sv_{O_2} monitoring allows for the continuous evaluation of cardiac output changes relative to tissue oxygenation needs (see Unit 3).

Monitoring systemic vascular resistance and pulmonary vascular resistance

84 Systemic vascular resistance (SVR) and pulmonary vascular resistance (PVR) cannot be directly measured invasively or noninvasively. Therefore calculation of these parameters is mathematically determined from established relationships between the pressures in the arterial and venous vascular beds and the cardiac output.

$$SVR = \frac{MAP - MVP}{CO} (CVP) \times constant\ 80*$$

$$PVR = \frac{MPAP - MLAP}{CO} \text{ (wedge)} \times \text{constant } 80*$$

---

*Converts the result to resistance units or dynes/sec/cm^{-5}

85 The SVR reflects the afterload of the _____ ventricle.　　left
REMEMBER: The fall in cardiac associated with acute MI is accompanied by a rise in _____. This rise may further impede　　SVR
_____ _____.　　　　　　　　　　　　　cardiac output

The PVR reflects the afterload of the _____ ventricle.　　right
REMEMBER: In the presence of pulmonary disease. The PAEDP
cannot be used to reflect LVEDP. A wedge pressure must be
obtained.

86 NURSING ORDERS: Hemodynamic monitoring
1. While monitoring the *pulmonary arterial* pressure, note the characteristic pulmonary arterial pulse pattern on oscilloscope:
   —Watch for changes in the pulse pattern that might indicate the
   catheter has slipped back into the right ventricle.

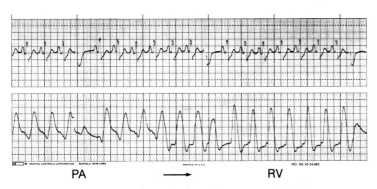

Fig. 9-12

PA　　⟶　　RV

   —Monitor on lead V_1 for right ventricular PVCs during catheter insertion and throughout monitoring period; may inflate balloon to
   cushion tip, but watch carefully for inadvertent migration back
   into the pulmonary artery and wedge position.
   —Keep lidocaine (Xylocaine) at bedside; may be given prophylactically during insertion or as per routine criteria.
   —Normal pulmonary artery pressures (systolic and diastolic) usually
   fluctuate with respirations because of the proximity of the pulmo-
   narny artery to the lungs. It is recommended that all readings be
   taken at the end of expiration. When obtaining pulmonary artery
   pressures during mechanical ventilation, take into consideration
   the mode of ventilation. With intermittent mandatory ventilation
   (IMV), differences in thoracic pressure are produced by the controlled as compared with the spontaneous ventilation. These differences are maximal during inspiration because expiration is a

passive process. Therefore record pulmonary artery pressures at the *end* of expiration, particularly in these patients. PEEP causes compression of the pulmonary vascular bed and thus elevates pulmonary capillary wedge pressures.

  —Note the presence or development of pulmonary complications that might invalidate correlations between PAEDP and LVEDP (increased pulmonary arterial systolic pressures may be a clue).

2. When obtaining pulmonary capillary *wedge* pressures:
  —Introduce only as much air as required to obtain change from pulmonary artery to wedge pulse pattern on the oscilloscope.
  —Do not introduce more air than is designated on the balloon catheter.
  —Record the mean wedge pressure quickly, deflating the balloon immediately thereafter; verify that the catheter is no longer wedged by pattern change on scope (wedge back to pulmonary artery).
  —If the wedge pattern cannot be obtained with maximum inflation, notify the physician and record PAEDP in the interim.
  —Inflate the balloon slowly to allow time for it to float into the wedge position.
  —Keep a syringe on the balloon lumen to prevent an accidental injection of liquids.

3. While monitoring pressure invasively, watch concurrently for:
  —Noninvasive signs of increased LVEDP, such as S_4 as especially S_3 gallop (see Frames 92 to 113).
  —Atrial arrhythmias.
  —Signs of *pulmonary congestion,* such as increased respiratory rate, Valsalva (forced) respiration, and end inspiratory rales not clearing with coughing.

4. Watch for spontaneous wedging detected by change in the pulmonary artery pattern to left atrium. Have the patient turn on his or her side and cough. Strike the patient's back to dislodge the catheter. If not successful immediately, notify the physician. Avoid administering continuous IV medications through the distal lumen so that any change in the pulmonary artery pressure can be noted.

5. Take initial readings and recalibrate with offgoing shift to confirm accuracy.

6. Institute nursing measure to minimize O_2 demands by preventing and/or quickly correcting factors that might increase myocardial O_2 consumption (see Frame 163).

7. Provide increased O_2 supply with supplementary oxygen; may document effectiveness on blood gas samples.

8. Watch for further mechanical complications, such as mitral insufficiency or VSD (murmurs) or aneurysm (with AWMI, palpable movement of the chest wall).

9. Watch for intermittent changes in the pulse pattern that might indicate changes in contractility and cardiac output.
   —Every other pressure pulse may be smaller in a patient with CHF because the heart cannot sustain strong pulses *(pulsus alternans)*.
   —With arrhythmias, the pulse may become irregular and/or diminished because the output with these is less.
   —The voltage of the pattern may also vary with respiration because of respiratory influences on cardiac output.
10. Give special care to catheter site for the prevention of sepsis in the form of routine prep, dressing changes, and carefully sealed dressings; monitor temperature.
11. Record serial changes in cardiac output; when evaluating the cardiac output results, relate them to the patient's BSA *(cardiac index)* and SVR.
   REMEMBER: As the cardiac output falls, the SVR rises. The rise in SVR may further impede cardiac output (see Unit 10).
12. As cardiac index begins to drop, monitor clinical signs of decreased tissue perfusion (noting a *symptomatic* fall in cardiac output) that might indicate that heart failure is evolving into the shock state.

NOTE: For nursing action in the presence of significant elevations in LVEDP and significant decreases in LVEDP and cardiac output index refer to nursing orders for CHF, Frame 43, and shock, Frame 163.

AUSCULTATION OF THE HEART

87 REMEMBER: The heart sounds serve as _____ outlining the _____ events of the heart.

parameters
mechanical

Alterations in the mechanical activity of the heart are reflected by the presence of extra (sometimes abnormal) heart sounds and variations in the normal heart sounds.

88 LET US REVIEW: The earliest mechanical alterations occurring in acute MI affect ventricular *(filling/contraction)*, which is also known as ventricular *(systolic/diastole)*.

filling
diastole

Maximum diastolic pressures are reached at the *(beginning/end)* of diastole. Thus minor changes in filling pressure can be first detected at the *end* of diastole.

end

Variations in the heart sounds are produced that correlate with these changes in *(LAEDP/LVEDP)*. The heart sounds thus provide a means for clinically evaluating the *mechanical* and *hemodynamic* changes occurring in acute MI.

LVEDP

89 The heart sounds are produced by the mechanical events that accompany valve closure. S_1 marks the onset of ventricular *(systole/diastole)*.

systole

During ventricular systole the (AV/semilunar) valves close, the ventricular muscular wall contracts, and the blood is ejected into the _____ _____.

    AV

    blood vessels

Although older theories claim that valve closure is the major factor responsible for the production of the sound, more recent theories are less definite. The sound may be produced by any of *three* factors or a combination of them:

1. *Valve closure*
2. Vibrations of the ventricular wall associated with *ventricular contraction*
3. Vibrations associated with *acceleration* and *deceleration* of blood by the force of ventricular contraction.

90 S_2 marks the onset of ventricular *(systole/diastole)*.

During ventricular diastole, the *(AV/semilunar)* valves close, the ventricular wall relaxes, and blood enters the ventricles from the _____.

    diastole

    semilunar

    atria

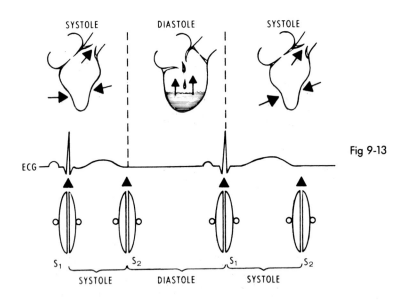

Fig 9-13

NOTE: The electrical activity is presented to emphasize its relationship to the mechanical activity.

91 The most clinically significant abnormal heart sounds occurring in the setting of acute MI are *gallops* and *murmurs*. The abnormal heart sounds that reflect left ventricular *diastolic* changes are the *gallops*.

Gallops

92 Gallops are extra sounds created by gushes of blood entering resistant, or stiffened, *ventricles*.

REMEMBER: Alterations in the resistance, or _____, of the left ventricular wall produce the first sign of mechanical dysfunction—a rise in _____. Thus gallops are manifestations of a rise in left ventricular _____ _____.

compliance

LVEDP

end-diastolic pressure

93 Gushes of blood enter the ventricles at two times during ventricular diastole: (1) during the *initial* filling phase (early to mid diastole) and (2) at the time of atrial systole (at the *end* of diastole). Gallops thus occur during early and late ventricular _____.

diastole

S_3 gallop

94 Ventricular *diastole* begins *after* the closure of the semilunar valves denoted by (S_1/S_2). The abnormal extra sound created within the ventricles at the *beginning* of ventricular diastole, immediately following the S_2, is known as S_3 *gallop*.

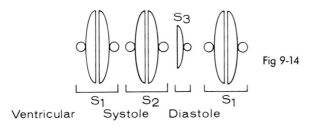

Fig 9-14

The S_3 gallop is heard immediately following _____. Another term used to describe this extra sound is *ventricular* gallop.

S_2

S_4 gallop

95 Another abnormal sound can occur as the blood enters the ventricles at the *(beginning/end)* of ventricular diastole. This sound is known as an S_4 *gallop* and is associated with _____ systole.

S_4 corresponds to _____ systole. Although all gallop sounds are created in the _____, the S_4 gallop, because it is associated with atrial systole, is frequently referred to as the *atrial gallop*. S_4 is heard at the _____ of ventricular diastole, or just *before* _____.

end

atrial

atrial

ventricles

end

S_1

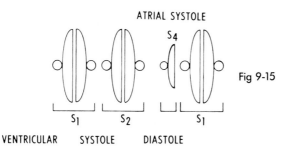

Fig 9-15

NOTE: An S_4 may occur without the presence of an S_3 because it usually represents an earlier sign of mechanical dysfunction (see Frames 102 to 107). (Conversely, an S_3 may occur without an S_4.)

96 The use of the term *gallop* with reference to an S_3 or S_4 sound implies that a pathological mechanism is responsible for its production. Either an S_3 or S_4 sound, or both, may be present in children or young adults because of normal ventricular filling. The sounds may become louder during periods of increased ventricular filling, such as with exercise or fever.

With age, however, these sounds usually become dampened and should not be heard unless ventricular filling is accentuated by the presence of pathology.

97 LET US REVIEW: An S_3 *gallop* is produced by alterations occurring at the *(beginning/end)* of ventricular diastole. An S_4 *gallop* is produced by alterations occurring at the *(beginning/end)* of ventricular diastole.

The first sign of mechanical dysfunction in acute MI occurs at the *(beginning/end)* of ventricular diastole. Therefore the earliest abnormal sound usually heard in acute MI is an _____ gallop.

Any other myocardial pathology that produces alterations in ventricular compliance (thus increasing LVEDP) may also result in the production of an S_4 gallop. Examples include left ventricular hypertrophy as occurs with hypertensive disease, the myocardiopathies, and myocardial ischemia occurring during episodes of angina.

beginning
end

end
S_4

98 REMEMBER: A *slightly* damaged left ventricle can accommodate the blood that enters through the initial filling phase, although it cannot accommodate the added volume that enters with _____ contraction.

However, when the presence of heart failure complicates acute MI, the cardiac output falls, and the injured left ventricle may not completely eject its contents. As a result, residual volume remains in the left ventricle at the end of systole and the beginning of _____.

atrial

diastole

99 When this condition is present, the left ventricle cannot fully accommodate blood that enters even during initial stages. Thus, in the presence of left ventricular failure, an abnormal sound may also be heard at the beginning of diastole. When an abnormal sound is produced at the *beginning* of diastole, it is referred to as an _____ gallop.

S_3

100 In summary:
Gallops may occur as a result of:
1. *Increased blood volume* (larger gush) producing *(increased/decreased)* ventricular filling

increased

2. *Stiffened ventricles,* which offer *(more/less)* resistance to filling   more

    The patient with left ventricular failure resulting from acute MI may have both an increased blood _____ and   volume _____ ventricles; thus the presence of ventricular gallop   stiffened sounds in this patient *(is/is not)* a common finding.   is

    Gallops reflect *(increases/decreases)* in left ventricular diastolic pressure (LVDP).   increases

    A slight rise in LVEDP *(is/is not)* an expected occurrence in acute   is MI. Early increases in LVEDP associated with initial changes in compliance are reflected by the presence of an *(S_3/S_4)* gallop. Thus the S_4 presence of an S_4 gallop *(is/is not)* an expected finding in patients   is with acute MI.

    Further increases in LVDP caused by left ventricular failure *(are/*   are *are not)* considered a *complication* of acute MI. These are reflected by the presence of an *(S_3/S_4)* gallop. S_3

101 It is not unusual to find *both* an S_3 and S_4 gallop present in a patient with left ventricular failure resulting from an acute MI. The resulting sound is a *quadruple rhythm.*

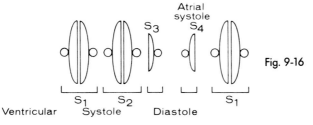

Fig. 9-16

102 REMEMBER: A manifestation of CHF is *(fast/slow)* rates. With fast rates the gallop sounds blend together, producing a summation gallop. A summation gallop sounds on auscultation like a *galloping horse—* hence its name.

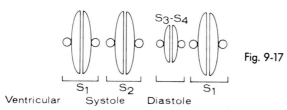

Fig. 9-17

Murmurs

103 The other major abnormal heart sound is a *murmur.* Murmurs occur because of alterations in the movement of blood—its acceleration or deceleration.

    REMEMBER: The study of alterations in the movement of blood is known as _____. Therefore murmurs *(do/do not)*   hemodynamics; do reflect hemodynamic changes.

104 The movement of blood is significantly altered when there is leakage through insufficient valves or when turbulence occurs across a narrowed outlet as with *stenotic* valves. Murmurs are labeled according to when they occur—*systolic* or *diastolic*.

Systolic murmurs

105 A *systolic* murmur is heard between the heart sounds S _____ and S _____. In *systole* the AV valves should be closed and semilunar valves should be opened. *Insufficient* _____ valves or *stenotic* _____ valves, then, may cause systolic murmurs.

1; 2

AV; semilunar

> NOTE: AV valve (mitral) insufficiency is the most likely cause of murmurs heard in acute MI. This insufficiency is usually caused by *papillary muscle dysfunction.* Another possible cause is ventricular *dilation* resulting from CHF.

> If a sudden very loud systolic murmur appears, possible causes are (1) a ruptured interventricular septum or (2) a ruptured papillary muscle.

Diastolic murmurs

106 A *diastolic* murmur is heard between the heart sound S _____ and S _____.

2; 1

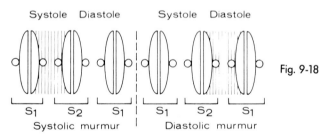

Fig. 9-18

In *diastole* the AV valves should be open and the semilunar valves should be closed. Insufficient _____ valves or *stenotic* _____ valves, then, may cause diastolic murmurs.

semilunar

AV

107 Murmurs may be further differentiated according to their quality, radiation, and graded intensity. Murmurs may be "blowing" or "honking" in quality. They may radiate to characteristic locations on the chest wall, such as the pulmonic or aortic region and sternal borders. The intensity is graded on a scale of 1 to 6, with the loudest being 6. A systolic murmur graded 3/6 would be of *(soft/average/loud)* intensity.

average

Normal variations of heart sounds

108 Because of the *dual* component to AV valve *closure,* the intensity of (S_1/S_2) may be either *loud* or *soft* (see Unit 1). The AV valves begin

S_1

closing passively because of increases in ventricular pressure occurring with ventricular filling. If the AV valves have had enough time to *start closing* passively before active closure with ventricular systole occurs, the sound of *active,* or *complete,* closure will be *soft.* If the AV valves are still wide *open* when ventricular systole begins, the valves will *slam* shut with active closure, producing a _____ sound.

loud

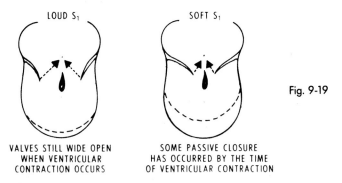

LOUD S₁

SOFT S₁

Fig. 9-19

VALVES STILL WIDE OPEN
WHEN VENTRICULAR
CONTRACTION OCCURS

SOME PASSIVE CLOSURE
HAS OCCURRED BY THE TIME
OF VENTRICULAR CONTRACTION

109 Conditions that *shorten* filling time or time for passive closure are:
1. Short PR interval (0.12 second; that is, still normal)
2. Tachycardia (supraventricular)
3. Early beats (for example, early versus late PVC)
    The above conditions *(increase/decrease)* passive closure time and therefore produce a *(loud/soft)* S₁.

decrease
loud

110 Conditions that *prolong* filling time or time for passive closure are:
1. Long _____ interval
2. *(Tachycardia/Bradycardia)*
    The above conditions *(increase/decrease)* passive closure time and therefore produce a *(loud/soft)* S₁.

PR
Bradycardia
increase
soft

111 In CHF there is incomplete emptying of the ventricles during systole. As a result, during diastole there is an increase in ventricular contents. This increase in contents creates an *(increased/decreased)* pressure against the AV rales, *enhancing* passive closure. Thus in the setting of CHF a *(loud/soft)* S₁ is heard.

increased

soft

112 NOTE:*Varying intensity* may indicate rhythms with a varying PR rhythm. This varying intensity is a bedside clue to the diagnosis of *CHB* and other forms of AV *dissociation.* The presence or absence of varying intensity may also aid in the differential diagnosis of VT and *supraventricular tachycardia with aberrations* (see Unit 7).

113 Let us now discuss the effects of respiration on heart sounds. Inspiration creates a *negative* pressure within the chest. This negative pressure draws blood *(into/out of)* the right side of the heart. Thus there is *increased* filling in the right side of the heart with *(inspiration/expiration)*.

into

inspiration

114 As a result of this increased filling and increased right ventricular contents, right ventricular systole is longer in duration. The *(pulmonary/aortic)* component to S₂ denoting the end of right ventricular systole is therefore delayed and separated from the aortic sound. This creates a splitting of the second heart sound.

pulmonary

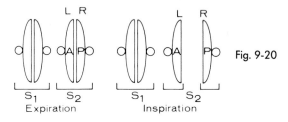

Fig. 9-20

Splitting of S₂ on inspiration, then, *(is/is not)* a normal variation of heart sounds.

is

NOTE: Splitting is loudest at the second intercostal space.

Conditions that further delay right ventricular systole may augment this normal splitting. Common conditions delaying right ventricular systole include RBBB or a left ventricular pacemaker (caused by delayed right ventricular activation).

115 Anything that delays *left ventricular* systole causes closure of the *aortic valve* to occur with delay. This delay produces a paradoxical splitting of S₂ on expiration.

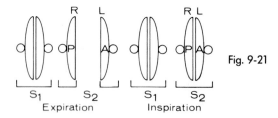

Fig. 9-21

Examples of conditions that delay left ventricular systole are:
1. Left ventricular failure
2. LBBB or a right ventricular pacemaker (caused by delayed left ventricular activation)
3. Ventricular aneurysm
4. Angina pectoris

Paradoxical splitting on expiration *(is/is not)* a normal variation of heart sounds.

is not

1. In the patient with MI, auscultate the heart with each set of vital signs and listen for:
   —Gallop sounds.
   —Murmurs, especially *(systolic/diastolic)*.   systolic
   —Changes in the intensity of S_1.
   —Paradoxical splitting of S_2 on *(inspiration/expiration)*.   expiration
2. Identify the *normal* heart sounds first!
3. When auscultating the heart, listen first *at the apex* so that the most significant changes may be heard.
4. When listening for paradoxical splitting of S_2, listen only at the second intercostal space. Do not report *normal* splitting heard on *(inspiration/expiration)*.   inspiration
5. When auscultating *gallops:*
   —Listen for both S_3 and S_4 during *(systole/diastole)*.   diastole
   —Listen for S_3 together with *(S_1/S_2)*. S_2
   —Listen for S_4 at the *end* of diastole together with *(S_1/S_2)*. S_1
   —Listen with light pressure, using the bell of the stethoscope; these are low-frequency sounds and are easily obliterated.
   —Do not expect to hear two distinct sounds; gallops often sound like mere distortions of the normal heart sound.
   —Left ventrical sounds may be augmented:
      On expiration.
      With patient in a supine position (increased venous return) on his left side (left ventricle closer to chest wall)
      With mild strain, such as coughing or squeezing the examiner's hand.

REMEMBER: The presence of an S_4 gallop without a concurrent S_3 gallop does *not* indicate CHF.

6. Report any new murmurs immediately!
   —Listen for murmurs, especially S_1 and S_2 *(systole/diastole)*, because these are the most significant in acute MI.   systole
   —If the murmur is loud and the onset is apparently sudden, watch the patient closely, checking the vital signs until the physician has checked the patient.

REMEMBER: A sudden loud murmur in the setting of acute MI may indicate _____ _____   papillary muscle rupture
_____ or _____.   VSD

Be especially concerned in the setting of *anteroseptal MI* with an old inferior MI or vice versa.
   —For complete auscultation of a murmur, note:
      Whether it is systolic or diastolic.
      If it occurs early, late, or throughout the cycle.
      Where it is heard most loudly on the chest.
      Where it radiates.

Its quality (blowing, musical).

Exactly how loud it is (usually noted on a scale of 1 to 6 with 6 being the loudest; a grade 3/6 or 4/6 murmur is a moderately loud one—a beginner should start with these).

7. When hearing *varying intensity* of S_1, look at monitor for an arrhythmia indicating a form of atrioventricular dissociation.

8. If paradoxical splitting is heard, rule out _____, _____ or _____ _____ _____, and _____ when considering it as a sign of heart failure.

aneurysm; LBBB
right ventricular pacing
angina

9. Abnormal heart sounds are frequently of very low intensity and therefore very difficult to hear. When first starting to listen, ask another nurse or physician to verify your findings. Ability to hear these changes accurately develops only with practice.

SHOCK SYNDROME

117 The shock syndrome may be defined as a state in which there is a *significant* fall in cardiac output resulting in a decreased supply of oxygenated blood to the tissues and *tissue symptoms*.

118 In the presence of heart failure resulting from acute MI, there *(is/is not)* a fall in cardiac output.

is

Therefore CHF caused by acute MI has the *potential*, if *the patient's condition* deteriorates, of leading to a *symptomatic* fall in cardiac output, or *shock*.

There are, however, other mechanisms that may lead to the shock state in the presence of acute MI. These should also be recognized and taken into consideration.

119 Shock is a clinical syndrome that occurs as a result of acute circulatory failure. The common denominator to all forms of shock is a *critical reduction* in the supply of oxygenated blood to the tissues.

REMEMBER: The demands of the tissues for oxygen are met by an adequate O_2 supply and an adequate blood supply. Tissue demands (O_2 consumption) = _____ _____ (cardiac output) × _____ _____ (O_2 content).

blood supply
O_2 supply

120 Maintenance of an adequate blood supply is dependent on the integrity of the cardiovascular system (see Fig. 9-1). The integrity of the cardiovascular system is affected by any of *four* variables:

1. Heart rate and rhythm
2. Blood _____

volume

3. Vascular resistance, or *tone*

4. Cardiac muscle _____   contractility

121 Evaluation of the *blood pressure* is a useful clinical tool for the *initial* assessment of cardiovascular function.

REMEMBER: Blood pressure = cardiac output × systemic vascular resistance.

A fall in blood pressure usually accompanies the shock state.

122 Significant alterations of any of the above four variables may cause a marked decrease in the supply of oxygenated _____ to the   blood
_____. This decrease is reflected by a significant   tissues
fall in _____ pressure, changes in cellular metabolism, and   blood
a group of characteristic symptoms. This clinical *syndrome* is known
as _____.   shock

123 A shocklike state may occur as a result of a tachyarrhythmia or a
_____ arrhythmia.   brady-

REMEMBER: Cardiac output = stroke volume × _____   heart rate
_____.

In the setting of coronary care, all possible causes of a shock state must be considered.

124 *Hypovolemic shock* may result from a severe reduction in the
_____ _____.   blood volume

Excessive diuresis and a resultant *(increased/decreased)* blood volume   decreased
may cause shock.

125 *Vasogenic shock* may result from a decrease in vascular resistance,
or _____. Drugs that produce vasodilation, such as   tone
morphine or certain sympathetic blockers, may contribute to
_____ shock (see Unit 10). The problem of sepsis   vasogenic
and endotoxic shock should also be considered when assessing *(in-*   decreased
creased/decreased) vascular tone.

126 *Cardiogenic shock* results from *severe* impairment of cardiac muscle contractility. In the setting of cardiogenic shock caused by coronary artery disease, 40% or more of the myocardium is necrotic or in-jured and as such *(does/does not)* contribute to contractility. By defini-   does not
tion, therefore, cardiogenic shock implies the presence of extensive muscle damage. The prognosis is extremely *(poor/good)*, and the mor-   poor
tality is *(high/low)*.   high

127 With early, aggressive clinical intervention, the area of myocardial infarction may be contained. Without appropriate clinical manage-ment, however, areas of *critically ischemic* tissue may subsequently become necrotic, thus extending the area of infarction. At this point, signs of heart failure may begin to evolve into *cardiogenic* _____.

shock

128 The development of shock in a cardiac patient must be assessed from all parameters: rhythm, blood _____, vascu- lar _____, and cardiac muscle _____. Ini- tial therapy should be directed toward correcting disturbances in rhythm, volume, and vascular _____. If these measures are ineffective and no *recognizable* or *treatable* cause of the shock state can be identified, the diagnosis of _____ *shock* is made.

volume

tone; contractility

tone

cardiogenic

129 Shock is a clinical syndrome that occurs as a result of acute _____ failure. The common denominator in all forms of shock is a critical reduction in the supply of _____ _____ to the tissues. This decrease results in *(adequate/inadequate)* tissue perfusion.

circulatory

oxygenated blood

inadequate

130 The clinical picture of a patient in shock is a reflection of three ma- jor occurrenes:
1. Inadequate blood supply to the body's tissues
2. Compensatory mechanisms of the body resulting in changes in the microcirculation
3. Response at the cellular level

131 When the blood supply to the tissues is inadequate, a series of compensatory mechanisms is initiated to maintain an adequate blood supply to the _____, _____, and _____. The most important compensatory mecha- nisms are:
1. *Increased/Decreased)* heart rate
   REMEMBER: One reflection of the blood supply to the tissues is the blood _____.
   BP = _____ _____ × SVR
   CO = stroke volume × _____ _____
2. Constriction of the blood vessels to the _____, ab- dominal viscera, voluntary muscles, and finally even the _____

These compensatory mechanisms occur as a result of *sympathetic* stimulation.

heart; brain

kidneys

Increased

pressure

cardiac output

heart rate

skin

kidneys

132 The symptoms of acute circulatory failure include:
1. Heart— *(increased/decreased)* heart _____
2. Skin—cool and moist (clammy)

increased; rate

3. Kidneys—urine output decreased to point of *oliguria* or *anuria*
4. Brain—lethargy, dizziness, confusion, agitation

133 The decrease supply of oxygenated blood to the tissues triggers
_____ mechanisms that cause vasoconstriction in
the _____ and _____. The skin assumes
a dusky, cool, moist appearance. The fall in cardiac output and the
vasoconstriction of the vessels to the kidneys cause *(increased/
decreased)* renal perfusion, which results in oliguria or
_____.

compensatory
kidneys; skin

decreased

anuria

134 In spite of the compensatory mechanisms, there is a(n) *(increased/de-
creased)* supply of oxygenated blood to the brain, resulting in *(in-
creased/decreased)* cerebral perfusion. Decreased perfusion to the
brain is manifested by *sensorium changes,* such as dizziness, confusion,
agitation, and lethargy. These changes may further progress to a
state of *coma.*

    The precise clinical picture of the patient in shock may vary. It is
dependent on the *cause* of the disorder and the *stage* of the shock.

decreased
decreased

135 Let us now consider the changes that occur in *microcirculation*—that
is, at the capillary level—and the response of the *cells.* In the presence of normal circulation the capillary bed is perfused. The arterial
and venous links to the capillary bed are open.

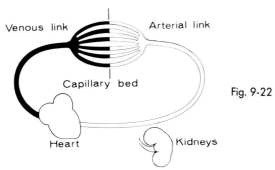

Venous link   Arterial link

Capillary bed   Fig. 9-22

Heart   Kidneys

136 With a decrease in systemic blood pressure, the compensatory
mechansims respond by releasing the sympathetic chemicals *epinephrine* and *norepinephrine.* These hormones attempt to restrict blood
flow to the tissues by *(vasoconstriction/vasodilation).* Blood is shunted
from the kidney, mesentery, and extremities to the more critical areas of the _____ and _____.

    The arterial and venous links to the capillary bed are *(constricted/
dilated).* This constriction prevents adequate circulation through the
capillary bed. This decrease in circulation implies a decrease in O$_2$
supply as well.

vasoconstriction

brain; heart
constricted

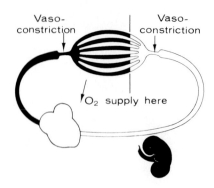

Fig. 9-23

137 The inadequate cellular perfusion causes cell *anoxia* and changes in cellular *metabolism*. During cellular anoxia, the cells are forced to metabolize glucose *(with/without)* oxygen. This abnormal metabolic process is described as *anaerobic metabolism*. As a result _____ _____ accumulates within the cell.

without
lactic acid

138 Metabolic acidosis develops, which results in a(n) *(increase/decrease)* in serum pH levels. The arterial ends of the capillary bed are not accustomed to an *(acidic/alkaline)* environment, and as a result vasodilation occurs. The venous link from the capillary bed, however, remains *(dilated/constricted)*. Therefore blood flows into the capillary bed but cannot return to the heart. Stasis and pooling of large volumes of _____ occur in the capillary bed. At this point, *cellular, tissue,* and *organ* death is imminent.

decrease

acidic

constricted

blood

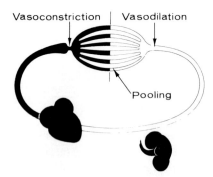

Fig. 9-24

139 Therapy for shock is based on three principles: (1) treating the underlying cause, (2) evaluating the vascular response, and (3) assisting tissue metabolism.

REMEMBER: The common denominator of all forms of shock is a critical reduction in the supply of _____ _____ to the tissues, resulting in inadequate tissue

oxygenated blood

_____. The goal of shock therapy, then, is to re- **perfusion**
store adequate tissue _____. **perfusion**

Therapy for the shock state is directed toward correcting possible causes:

1. Correcting any disturbances in _____ **rhythm**
2. Correcting disturbances in _____ **volume**
3. Increasing vascular _____ **tone**
4. Improving myocardial _____ **contractility**

140 Further management of a shock state is dependent on the stage of the shock and the ability of the blood vessels to respond. Generally shock therapy may include:

1. Administering drugs to correct disturbances in rhythm
2. Administering appropriate amounts and types of IV fluids
3. Administering drugs that increase vascular tone or promote microcirculation or both.
4. Administering drugs that improve myocardial contractility
5. Administering drugs that assist tissue metabolism
6. Monitoring various *physiological parameters:* central venous pressure, urine output, cardiac rhythm, ABG, pulmonary artery and wedge pressure, cardiac output, and SVR

Cardiogenic shock

141 LET US REVIEW: The mechanism of the shock state is determined to be cardiogenic in origin only after any problem in _____, _____, or **rhythm; volume** _____ _____ has been corrected. Ther- **vascular tone** apy for shock is based on three principles: (1) treating the _____ _____, (2) evaluating the **underlying cause** _____ response, and (3) assisting **vascular** _____ metabolism. **tissue**

142 Cardiogenic shock results from severe impairment of cardiac muscle contractility (see Frames 131 and 132). Although cardiogenic shock represents a decreased contractile state, increasing myocardial contractility is not the immediate goal of therapy.

The use of inotropic agents such as digitalis or isoproterenol (Isuprel) may be potentially hazardous because the increase in contractility is accompanied by a(n) *(increased/decreased)* O_2 consumption. **increased** The net result may be an extension of the area of infarction.

143 In cardiogenic shock caused by coronary artery disease, the impairment of contractile function results from discrepancies in myocardial O_2 supply and demand. The initial goal in the treatment of coronary cardiogenic shock is limiting or decreasing this discrepancy, thus improving myocardial oxygenation.

Therapy should be directed toward minimizing myocardial O_2 consumption demands and improving the coronary blood _____.

supply

144 *Initial* therapy is directed toward limiting the myocardial *demands*.

LET US REVIEW: The determinants of myocardial O_2 *demands* (MV O_2) are:
1. The heart's *rate*
2. The heart's *preload* or filling pressure
3. The heart's *afterload,* or the SVR
4. The myocardial *contractility*

Thus measures that limit or decrease myocardial demands include:
1. Control of heart rhythm and _____

rate

2. Limiting ventricular filling to decrease the heart's _____ (this is best accomplished while concurrently monitoring ventricular filling pressure with a Swan-Ganz catheter)

preload

3. Lowering the SVR, as with vasodilators, to decrease the heart's _____

afterload

4. Limiting or lowering *tissue* demands in an attempt to decrease demands for myocardial *contractility*

REMEMBER: *Tissue* O_2 consumption = blood supply (cardiac output) × O_2 supply.

145 Myocardial O_2 consumption *(demands)* may be lowered by the use of *vasodilator therapy*.

Coronary blood supply may be improved by:
1. Surgical revascularization
2. The use of vasoconstricting agents

All three parameters of coronary cardiogenic shock—*cardiac output,* myocardial demands, and coronary blood *supply*—may be improved by *circulatory assist* measures.

146 REMEMBER: The coronary arteries receive their blood supply during *(systole/diastole)*. Thus increasing coronary blood supply can be accomplished by *augmenting* arterial diastolic pressure.

diastole

Drugs and circulatory assist measures that increase coronary blood flow by increasing diastolic pressure are frequently referred to as modes of diastolic _____.

augmentation

147 Pharmacological *vasoconstrictors* such as norepinephrine (Levophed) increase arterial and venous SVR. Therefore they augment both anterial and venous diastolic pressure. Coronary blood flow is *(increased/decreased)*. Norepinephrine also support's the body's compensatory response by extending sites of *(vasodilation/vasoconstriction)*.

increased
vasoconstriction

424

148 Increased arterial SVR also results in an undesirable increase in the heart's *(preload/afterload)*.

afterload

The increased *venous* resistance and enhanced venous return result in an increase in the heart's filling, or *(preload/afterload)*. Thus myocardial O_2 consumption may be *(increased/decreased)*, and extension of the area of infarction may result.

preload
increased

149 Lowering of the afterload by arterial vasodilation reduces the impedence to left ventricular ejection, facilitating ventricular systole. Thus the cardiac output is *(improved/reduced)*.

improved

150 Although it does not increase the coronary blood supply, vasodilator therapy appears to have the unique advantage of improving cardiac output while at the same time *lowering* myocardial demands. However, the *ideal* mode of therapy should act to improve all *three* parameters of coronary cardiogenic shock:
1. Improve cardiac output
2. Lower myocardial demands
3. Increase coronary blood flow
Circulatory assist measures provide this beneficial threefold effect.

151 NURSING ORDERS: Shock
    1. Evaluate *underlying cause.*
      —Place patient in a flat position.
      —Treat *arrhythmias* or other abnormalities evident on ECG.
      —Check for *hypovolemia* by:
        Evaluating the patient's legs to increase venous return, then
        Checking blood pressure
        Checking CVP, pulmonary artery pressures, and wedge pressure
      —Monitor vital signs closely.
      —Remove any rotating tourniquets.
      —Have resuscitation equipment at the bedside.
      —Rule out any vasoactive mechanism such as morphine, meperidine (Demerol), nitroglycerine, or sepsis and:
        Elevate the patient's legs to increase venous return.
        Have narcotic antagonists available.
      —If possible, monitor cardiac output accurately by indicator-dilution technique; otherwise, evaluate *changes* in cardiac output by comparison of arterial and venous blood gases.
      —*If mechanism is determined to be cardiogenic and is associated with coronary artery disease*—institute measure to limit discrepancy between myocardial O_2 supply and demand.
      —Nursing action for limiting myocardial O_2 consumption:
        Rate: watch for and correct any significant arrhythmias quickly.

Preload: monitor fluid intake and output carefully; administer diuretics as ordered; check wedge pressure for effectiveness.

Afterload: correct any hypertensive state; relieve stress factors, such as pain or anxiety.

Contractility: correct any acid-base or electrolyte abnormalities quickly; limit peripheral demands by providing and investigating and/or managing any other systemic diseases such as diabetes, chronic lung disease, sepsis; if inotropic agents are ordered, monitor vital signs and other hemodynamic parameters carefully for patient deterioration.

— Nursing action for increasing O_2 supply:

Administer supplementary oxygen; be sure to document effectiveness on ABG samples.

2. Evaluate *vascular response:*

— Monitor vasoactive drugs carefully (norepinephrine [Levophed], metaraminol [Aramine], dopamine) (see Unit 10).

— Determine end point of therapy with physician.

3. Evaluate and assist *tissue metabolism.*

— Monitor blood gases for metabolic acidosis.

— Watch for Kussmaul-type respirations as sign of respiratory compensatory efforts.

— Evaluate patient symptoms of tissue perfusion; watch for deterioration, such as deepening of sensorium changes.

— Administer and monitor effects of drugs that may aid in stabilizing tissue metabolism, such as steroids or osmotic diuretics.

Circulatory assist: intraaortic balloon pumping

152 Circulatory assist devices are used to assist the coronary circulation. They are indicated in those clinical situations when there is a critical imbalance between myocardial oxygen supply and demand and usual pharmacologic means of restoring this balance are ineffective.

153 The *intra-aortic balloon pump* (IABP) is the most common mode of circulatory assist being used in the coronary care unit because of ease of insertion in acute situations and ease of operation.

The *intra-aortic balloon catheter* is usually inserted percutaneously under fluroscopy through the femoral artery and positioned in the descending aorta just below the origin of the left subclavian artery. The balloon is connected to a *console* that controlls the balloon infation and deflation, or pump action (see Fig 9-25, A and B).

154 *Inflation* of the balloon at the beginning of diastole displaces the blood proximally into the coronary and cerebral arteries and distally

into the renal arteries and other peripheral vessels and *(raises/lowers)*   raises
the aortic diastolic pressure. Coronary blood flow and myocardial O_2
(supply/demands) are subsequently increased.   supply

INTRAAORTIC BALLOON PUMP

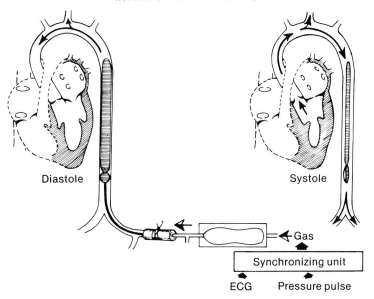

A

Diastole   Systole

Fig. 9-25

← Gas

Synchronizing unit

ECG   Pressure pulse

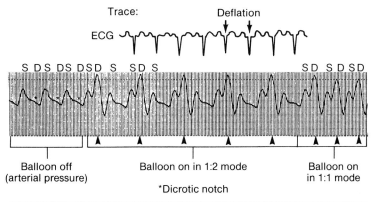

Trace:

Deflation

ECG

S D S DS DSD S   SD S   S D S D SD

Balloon off   Balloon on in 1:2 mode   Balloon on
(arterial pressure)   in 1:1 mode
              *Dicrotic notch

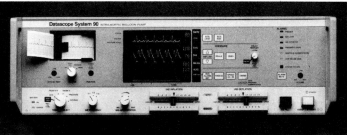

B

The usual volume of gas required to inflate the balloon is *40 ml.* The balloon console is checked prior to insertion of the catheter by nursing or technical personnel. CO_2 was formerly used but presented problems when the balloon was used during tachycardias because of slow balloon filling times. Helium is the gas currently used most often.

155 *Deflation* of the balloon just prior to systole decreases the aortic root pressure, thus facilitating systolic emptying and decreasing the *(preload/afterload)* of the left ventricle. The cardiac output is *(increased/decreased)*.

afterload

increased

NOTE: The deflation action of the balloon exerts almost a "sucking" effect when the left ventricle effects its contents.

Use of the intraaortic balloon may reverse the shock state or serve to stabilize or "buy time" for the critical patient in preparation for cardiac catherization, cardiac surgery, or cardiac transplantation. It is contraindicated in patients with aortic insufficiency, aortic aneurysm, or aortic wall abnormalities. It should be used with caution in patients with known peripheral vascular disease because of potential compromise of left blood flow with catheter placement.

156 Either the ECG or the arterial wave form may be used as the initial signal or "trigger" for balloon inflation and deflation. Although the ECG is the automatic initial signal or _____, optimal timing is subsequently adjusted manually using the arterial line trace. Thus *both* a clear ECG and arterial line trace should be obtained prior to beginning counterpulsation. Ideally, the ECG and arterial line trace should be simultaneously displayed on both the bedside monitor and IABP console.

trigger

When the arterial line trace is dampened, the ECG becomes the sole trigger and the timing *(may/may not)* be manually adjusted.

may not

157 More specifically, the dominant QRS deflection of the ECG (loosely referred to as the "R wave") triggers balloon *deflation*. To determine balloon *inflation* time, the IABP console senses the average R-R cycle length to determine the exact onset of diastole. The onset of diastole usually corresponds approximately with the end of the T wave on the ECG complex.

When the patient requires single chamber pacing, the pacing spike will usually act as an effective ECG trigger. However, if the patient requires single chamber atrial or dual chamber pacing, the initial atrial spike may trigger premature deflation and distort inflation timing.

REMEMBER: The balloon should deflate during _____ diastole. Delation of the balloon is triggered by the major *(ECG/pulse wave)* deflection.

end

ECG

Manual adjustment of timing

158 Although the automatic trigger for inflation and deflation of the balloon is the ECG, fine tuning of the timing is controlled manually by the pump operator using the patient's _____ wave form.   *pressure*

Timing is adjusted using slide controls located on the front of the balloon console. Accurate timing of inflation and deflation is critical for optimal augmentation (Fig. 9-25). Manual timing may be difficult or impossible in the settings of rapid or grossly irregular rhythms. Automatic timing, although not necessarily more effective, is the only alternative in these settings.

159 Balloon pump manufacturers provide options for balloon assist that range from augmentation of every beat to augmentation of every eighth beat (i.e., 1:1 to 1:8). This allows the nurse to make adjustments in the assist rate for different clinical conditions and allows for a gradual decrease in augmentation as the patient is weaned from the balloon pump. There are some patients who may benefit more from a 1:2 or 1:3 assist mode than from the 1:1 mode. This judgement is based on clinical parameters, such as the patient's B.P., heart rate and rhythm, and requirements for pharmacologic support.

160 Adjustment of balloon inflation and deflation timing should always be done when the balloon pump is in the 1:2 assist mode or less to allow for comparison between the patient's *normal* arterial pressure tracing and the *assisted* arterial pressure tracing.

Optimal timing of balloon inflation and deflation is adjusted using the _____ _____ _____.   *arterial wave form*
The goal of timing is to augment _____ blood flow   *coronary*
and maximize _____ reduction for the left ventricle.   *afterload*

Augmentation of coronary blood flow is a function of balloon *inflation*. Afterload reduction is a function of balloon *deflation*.

161 Inflation is typically adjusted first. *Inflation* of the balloon should start at the onset of diastole or the *dicrotic notch* on the arterial waveform (see Fig. 9-25A).

The inflation upstroke should form a "v" when allligned with the arterial wave form. Balloon inflation pressure, known as *augmentation pressure* or *peak diastolic augmented pressure* is usually higher than *peak systolic pressure* (PSP). The PSP is the pressure reached at the height of _____.   *systole*

162 *Late inflation* occurs when the dicrotic notch is visible before inflation begins. There is no danger to the patient with late inflation, but optimal augmentation is not achieved since some of the aortic volume has already been dispersed before inflation begins. Late inflation can be corrected by moving the inflation slide control to the left.

With *early inflation* the balloon waveform is superimposed on the patient's arterial waveform. Early inflation is detrimental to the patient because it increases the afterload of the LV and actually increases resistance to left ventricular emptying. Early inflation can be corrected by moving the inflation slide to the right.

163 LET US REVIEW: Augmentation of coronary blood flow is a function of balloon *(inflation/deflation)*. Inflation should be timed to begin with the _____ notch on the arterial waveform, which marks the beginning of *(systole/diastole)*.

Late inflation *(is/is not)* dangerous to the patient and is recognized by visualizing the dicrotic notch before inflation. Early inflation *(is/is not)* dangerous to the patient because it increases the _____ of the left ventricle.

inflation
dicrotic
diastole

is not

is
afterload

164 *Deflation* of the balloon is adjusted to occur exactly at the end of diastole or just prior to systole to maximize the assist to the left ventricle.

REMEMBER: As the balloon deflates, aortic root pressure is decreased thereby reducing systemic vascular resistance or the _____ of the left ventricle.

With proper deflation, the balloon aortic (Ao) end-diastolic pressure (BAoEDP) should be lower than the patient's end-diastolic pres-

afterload

1. Patient aortic end diastolic pressure (PA$_o$EDP)
2. Peak systolic pressure (PSP)
3. Augmentation pressure (balloon inflation)
4. Balloon aortic end diastolic pressure (BA$_o$EDP)
5. Balloon assisted peak systolic pressure (BAPSP)

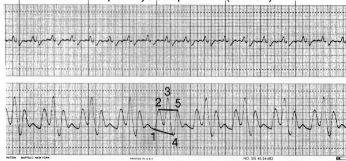

NOTE: The assisted systole is the one after balloon deflation (5). The unassisted systole is the one before balloon inflation (2).

Fig. 9-26

sure (PAoEDP) (see Fig. 9-26). Both the *patient aortic* (Ao) *end* diastolic pressure and the BAoEDP are the lowest pressures before the upstroke of systole. The PAoEDP is determined from the non-assisted pulses while the BAoEDP is determined from the _____ pulses.

assisted

REMEMBER: Adjustment of balloon inflation and deflation timing should always be done when the balloon pump is in the _____ assist mode (see Fig. 9-26).

1:2

165 This reduction in left ventricular afterload assists the ejection of blood with the systole, which follows balloon deflation. The arterial waveform following balloon deflation is thus known as the *assisted systole* or *balloon assisted peak systolic pressure*. This pressure should be equal to or lower than the unassisted systole, reflecting the afterload reduction (see Fig. 9-26).

Late deflation of the balloon results in an increased afterload for the left ventricles as it is trying to eject its contents against a *higher than normal* diastolic pressure. This is evident on the balloon tracing by the absence of a drop or an actual rise in the BAoEDP. Late deflation can be corrected by moving the deflation slide control *to the left* until a proper waveform is achieved.

166 *Early deflation* is recognized by a "u" shaped or plateau effect in the deflation curve rather than the normal sharp "v shape." Early deflation minimizes the assist to the left ventricle and may allow for retrograde flow from the coronary arteries into the aortic root, thereby jeopardizing coronary flow. With early deflation the balloon assisted peak systolic pressure is not lowered. Correction of this problem can be accomplished by moving deflation slide control *to the right* and observing the waveform.

167 LET US REVIEW: Reduction of afterload by the intra-aortic balloon is a function of *(inflation/deflation)*. Deflation of the balloon should occur at the end of _____ or just prior to _____. With proper timing of deflation, balloon assisted aortic end diastolic pressure (BAoEDP) should be *(greater than/ less than)* patient aortic end diastolic pressure (PAoEDP).

deflation
diastole
systole
less than

Patient assessment/problem solving

168 The three major complications associated with the use of the IABP are: 1) impaired peripheral circulation, 2) infection, and 3) bleeding.

Close monitoring of sensation, temperature, and pulses in the affected limb is the high priority with nursing assessment. It is not unusual to have some decrease in pulse amplitude in the affected limb and perhaps some slight difference in temperature, but any perceived significant loss, such as total loss of pulses or acute pain or other sensory abnormalities, should be reported immediately.

169 Scrupulous use of sterile technique when dressing the insertion site and care to prevent cross contamination with other patients in the CCU is imperative. This is especially important when managing patients awaiting cardiac transplant who may already be in a seriously debilitated state, and infection will mean they are no longer a candidate for transplant. Special instructions and precautions to visitors are also indicated.

Anticoagulant therapy is required during intra-aortic balloon therapy to prevent clot formation on the balloon catheter. Both heparin and low molecular weight dextran have been used. For this reason as well as a high occurrence of stress ulcers, close monitoring of coagulation studies, testing N/G and stool for occult blood, and instituting measures to reduce physiologic and psychologic stress are also very important in this group of patients. Histamine 2 antagonists, antacids, or similar preparations should probably be given to all patients who require IABP support to prevent stress bleeds.

170 Other problems that may occur with patients requiring IABP support are (1) compromise of renal, cerebral, and left arm circulation due to malposition of the balloon catheter, (2) alteration in sleep patterns due to the critically ill state and sounds of the balloon pump, and (3) alteration in nutritional status.

The patient requiring the IABP is usually critically ill and requires intensive monitoring by both nursing and medical personnel. Titration of pharmacological support is correlated with hemodynamic profiles and the balloon timing.

Problems related to the balloon catheter or the balloon console include kinking of the balloon catheter, slow gas leaks, improper timing, balloon rupture, and console failure. Newer balloon pumps have sophisticated alarm systems that alert the operator to all of these problems except improper timing. Most manufactuerers provide troubleshooting guidelines for dealing with these common problems. Only nurses trained in the operation of the balloon pump should assume responsibility for this device. A backup plan in the event of console failure should always be delineated.

171 LET US REVIEW: The major complications associated with the use of the IABP are compromise or _____ of leg circulation, infection, and _____. Checks of the _____, _____, and _____ in the affected leg are a critical part of the nursing assessment.

Malposition of the balloon catheter could potentially result in compromise of circulation to the _____ arm, the _____, and the _____.

disruption
bleeding
pulses; temperature
sensation

left
brain; kidney

432

Patient temperature should be monitored closely when the patient requires the IABP support to detect the earliest signs of

_____.   infection

Stress bleeds can be prevented by close monitoring of
_____ studies and administering   coagulation
_____ and/or H$_2$ antagonists as prescribed.   antacids

172 NURSING ORDERS: Circulatory assist with the intraaortic balloon
  1. Explain to the patient and family the purpose for balloon insertion and what to expect with balloon insertion and operation; obtain signed consent.
    — Equipment (console, balloon catheter, A-line)
    — Discomfort, premedication, anesthesia
    — Sensations associated with balloon function
    — Activity limitations
  2. Record baseline signs and clinical observations regarding pulses, temperature, and skin color of legs before balloon insertion; intraaortic balloon should be inserted only in a patient with a patent artery and good collateral flow.
  3. Guard against sepsis; following insertion, apply sealed sterile dressing to insertion site and inspect frequently for bleeding; change dressing every 24 hours or as ordered.
    — Maintain nutritional support.
    — Use scrupulous aseptic technique with invasive lines.
    — Request blood cultures for patients with a temperature greater than 38° C (101° F).
    — Monitor WBC and differential blood count.
  4. Evaluate timing and effectiveness of counterpulsation.
    — Compare pressure waveform with ECG to determine if augmentation is timed appropriately. Does inflation begin at the dicrotic notch? Is BAoEDP less than PAoEDP? Is presystolic dip present?
    — Correlate wedge pressure, cardiac output, arterial pressure, and SVR with clinical parameters such as neurological status, respiratory status, and renal function.
    Are these parameters improving with augmentation? If so, can augmentation be decreased to every second or third beat (2 to 1 or 3 to 1 as opposed to 1 to 1)?
    — Titrate vasoactive drugs as indicated.
  5. Check blood flow to areas potentially involved with balloon insertion.
    — Verify balloon position by *x-ray* examination.
    — Check pulses, temperature, and color of leg and foot distal to insertion; compare with noninvolved leg.
    Report any pain, numbness, temperature or color change; loss of motor function in the involved leg is a medical

emergency requiring immediate removal of the balloon.

—Check pulses, temperature, and color of arms, especially *left* arm, to rule out balloon occlusion of *left* subclavian artery, particularly if there is a loss of radial artery tracing.

—Monitor neurological status to rule out embolic phenomena or occlusion of left carotid artery by the balloon.

—Monitor renal status; if urine output diminishes rather than improves with balloon function, check for possible occlusion of renal artery by balloon.

—Avoid raising head of bed greater than 45 degrees to prevent displacement of balloon.

6. Administer anticoagulants as ordered to prevent platelet aggregates and/or fibrin deposition on the balloon. Monitor coagulation studies.

7. Avoid unnecessarily flexing the patient's leg at the groin to prevent kinking of balloon catheter; the patient may be up in a chair but should have his or her leg elevated to avoid sustained flexion of the leg. Periodically inspect balloon catheter for kinking, cracking, disconnections, or leaks.

8. Assess laboratory values relating to balloon function.

—RBC count; anemia may result from hemolysis (rare).

—Platelet count; thrombocytopenia may result from mechanical destruction (rare).

9. In the patient with an intraaortic balloon anticipate high stress levels caused by critical physiological state, sensory overload, activity restriction, and discomfort.

—Provide consistent personnel and optimum emotional support.

—Maintain family contact as much as possible.

—Administer antacids or agents that decrease acid levels rising in response to stress.

10. If balloon shut-off is required, notify patient to allay anxiety; if balloon console breaks and back-up unit is not available, patient support is imperative. Psychological dependence on the balloon may predispose the patient to physiological crisis if abruptly withdrawn.

    NOTE: The balloon should be manually inflated every ten minutes to prevent clot formation on the balloon.

11. Wean the patient from balloon according to planned protocol, with frequent observation of cardiac hemodynamic profile.

In summary:

Table 12. Intervention in hemodynamic imbalance of patients with congestive heart failure or shock

Management goal	Intervention
1. Preload	
To decrease preload (with pulmonary or systemic congestion)	*Decrease venous return*
	High Fowler's postition with legs dangling
	Rotating tourniquets
	Morphine sulfate
	Furosemide (Lasix)
	Nitroglycerin/isosorbide (Isordil) (decreased afterload also)
	PEEP
	Decrease circulating blood volume
	Phlebotomy *plasmaphoresis)
	Furosemide (Lasix) and other diuretics
	Decrease of IV fluids
To increase preload (with decreased cardiac output and wedge pressure)	*Increase volume*
	Crystalloids
	Dextran
2. To decrease afterload	Nitroprusside (Nipride)
	Hydralazine (Apresoline)
	Captopril (Capoten)
	IABP
3. To increase contractility	Dopamine
	Dobutamine
	Amrinone
	Digitalis
	Repair of mechanical defects
4. To increase O$_2$ supply and decrease O$_2$ demands	Oxygen
	Psychological support
	Rest
	Morphine sulfate
	Defoaming agents
	IABP
	Coronary bypass
	Decrease of preload/afterload
5. To support tissue metabolism	Hyperalimentation
	Steroids
	Mannitol

SUGGESTED READINGS
Congestive heart failure and shock

Ayres SM: The prevention and treatment of shock in acute myocardial infarction, Chest (Suppl) 94(1):17S, 1988.

Billhardt RA and others: Cardiogentic and hypovolemic shock, Med Clin North Am 70(4):853, 1986.

Bobb J: What happens when your patient goes into shock, RN pp. 26-29, March, 1984.

Borden R and others: Right ventricular infarction, Cardiovasc Nurs 19:7, 1983.

Braunwald E, editor: Heart disease: a textbook of cardiovascular medicine, ed. 3, Philadelphia, 1988, WB Saunders Co.

Chatterjee K: Myocardial infarction shock, Crit Care Clin 1:563, 1985.

Chernow B and others: Pharmacologic manipulation of the peripheral vasculature in shock: clinical and experimental approaches, Circ Shock 18(2):141, 1986.

Doenges ME and others: Nursing care plans: nursing diagnoses in planning patient care, Philadelphia, 1984, FA Davis Co.

Francis GS: Neurohumoral mechanisms involved in congestive heart failure, Am J Card 55:15A, 1985.

Francis GS: Development of arrhythmias in the patient with congestive heart failure: pathophysiology, prevalence, and prognosis, Am J Cardiol 57(3):3B, 1986.

Franciosa JA: Epidemiologic patterns, clinical evaluation, and long-term prognosis in chronic congestive heart failure, Am J Med 80(2B):14, 1986.

Genton R and Jaffe AS: Management of congestive heart failure in patients with acute myocardial infarction, JAMA 256:2556, 1986.

Goldberger JJ and others: Prognostic factors in acute pulmonary edema, Arch Intern Med 146(3):489, 1986.

Groer ME and Sheckleton ME: Basic pathophysiology: a conceptual approach, St. Louis, 1983, The CV Mosby Co.

Groeger JS: Opiod antagonists in circulatory shock, Crit Care Med 14(2):170, 1986.

Guyton AC: Textbook of Medical Physiology, Philadelphia, 1986, WB Saunders Co.

Hoagland P: Right ventricular infarction, CCQ 7(4):19, 1985.

Hurst WJ and Logue RB, editors: The heart, arteries, and veins, ed. 6, New York, 1986, McGraw-Hill Inc.

Jafri SM: Prevalence of congestion in chronic heart failure, Chest 90(3):311, 1986.

Killip T: Epidemiology of congestive heart failure, Am J Cardiol 56:2A, 1985.

Klein DM: Shock: physiology, signs, and symptoms, Nursing 14(9):44, 1984.

Lewis BS and others: The hyperacute phase of right ventricular infarction, Heart Lung 13(6):682, 1984.

Mac Intyre E and others: Fluid replacement in hypovolemia, Intensive Care Med 11(5):235, 1985.

Massie B: Updated diagnosis and management of congestive heart failure, Geriatrics 73(2):257, 1986.

MC Cauley K: Probing the ins and outs of congestive heart failure, Nursing 12(11):60, 1982.

Parmley WW: Congestive heart failure and arrhythmias: an overview, Am J Cardiol 57(3):34B, 1986.

Parmley WW: Pathophysiology of congestive heart failure, Am J Cardiol 56:7A, 1985.

Parmley WW: Pathophysiology of congestive heart failure, Am J Cardiol 55:9A, 1985.

Porth C: Pathophysiology, concepts of altered health, ed. 2, Philadelphia, 1986, JB Lippincott Co.

Remme WJ: Congestive heart failure—pathophysiology and medical treatment, J Cardiovasc Pharmacol Suppl 8(1):S36, 1986.

Roberts N and others: Right ventricular infarction with shock but without significant left ventricular infarction: a new clinical syndrome, Am Heart J 110(5):1047, 1985.

Ruggie N: Congestive heart failure, Med Clin North Am 70(4):829, 1986.

Ryan AM: Stopping CHF while there's still time, RN 49(8):28-36, 1986.

Sanders J and others: A comparison of plasma renin activity levels in patients with and without congestive heart failure after myocardial infarction, Heart Lung 14(1):1, 1985.

Smith WM: Epidemiology of congestive heart failure, Am J Cardiol 55:3A, 1985.

Srebro J and others: Congestive heart failure, Curr Probl Cardiol 11(6):30, 1986.

Stanley M: Helping an elderly patient live with CHF, RN 49(9): 35-7, 1986.

Sturm JA and others: Fluid resuscitation of hypovolemia, Intensive Care Med 11(5):231, 1985.

Textbook of Advanced Cardiac Life Support, 1987, American Heart Association.

Van Paris E: Assessing the failing state of the heart, Nursing 17(2):42, 1987.

Weber KT and others: Pathophysiology of cardiac failure, Am J Cardiol 56:3B, 1985.

Auscultation

Bates B: A guide to physical examination, ed. 4, Philadelphia, 1987, JB Lippincott Co.

Braunwald E, editor: Heart disease: a textbook of cardiovascular medicine, ed. 3, Philadelphia, 1988, WB Saunders Co.

Dennison R: Cardiopulmonary assessment: how to do it better in 15 easy steps, Nursing 16:4, 1986.

Erickson BA: Detecting abnormal heart sounds, Nursing 16(1):58, 1986.

Erickson B: Heart sound and murmurs—A practical guide, St. Louis, 1987, The CV Mosby Co.

Malasanos L and others: Health assessment, ed. 3, St. Louis, 1986, The CV Mosby Co.

Miracle VA: Anatomy of a murmur, Nursing 16(7):26, 1986.

Saul L: Heart sounds and common murmurs, AJN 83(12):1680, 1983.

Taylor DL: Assessing heart sounds, Nursing, 15(1):51, 1985.

Tilkian AG and Conover MB: Understanding heart sounds and murmurs, ed. 2, Philadelphia, 1984, WB Saunders Co.

Yacone LA: Cardiac assessment: what to do, how to do it, RN 50(5):42, 1987.

Hemodynamics

Ahnve S and others: Limitations and advantages of the ejection fraction for defining high risk after acute myocardial infarction, Am J Cardiol 58:872, 1986.

Bodai BI and Halcroft J: Use of the pulmonary arterial catheter in the critically ill patient, Heart Lung 11:406, 1982.

Brantigan C: Hemodynamic monitoring: interpreting values, AJN pp. 86-89, Jan, 1982.

Bullas J and others: Hemodynamic assessment, Crit Care Nurse 5(4):73, 1985.

Campbell M and Greenberg CA: Reading pulmonary artery wedge pressure at end-expiration, Focus Crit Care 15(2):60, 1988.

Daily EK and Schroeder : Techniques in bedside hemodynamic monitoring, ed. 3, St. Louis, 1984, The CV Mosby Co.

Daily EK and Schroeder : Hemodynamic wave forms: exercises in identification & management, St. Louis, 1983, The CV Mosby Co.

Darovic GO: Hemodynamic Monitoring: invasive and noninvasive clinical applications, Philadelphia, 1987, WB Saunders Co.

Eisenberg P and others: Clinical evaluation compared to pulmonary artery catheterization in the hemodynamic assessment of critically ill patients, Crit Care Med 12(7):549, 1984.

Epstein SE and others: Hemodynamic principles in the control of coronary blood flow, Am J Cardiol 56(9):4E-10E, 1985.

Fraulin KE and others: Action stat: dislodged PA catheter, Nursing 15(10):33, 1985.

Jastremski M and Levy H: Hemodynamic monitoring, Fam Prac Recertification 6(1):89, 1984.

Kleinhenz TJ: The inside story on preload and afterload, Nursing 15(5):50, 1985.

Lough ME: Introduction to hemodynamic monitoring, Nurs Clin North Am 22(1):89, 1987.

Morra L: Troubleshooting pulmonary artery catheters, RN 50(2):46, 1987.

McGrath RB: Invasive bedside hemodynamic monitoring, Prog Cardiovasc Dis 29(2):129, 1986.

Marino P and Krasner J: An interpretive computer program for analyzing hemodynamic problems in the ICU, Crit Care Med 12(7):601, 1984.

Muncas EJ and Woods SL: Normal fluctuations in pulmonary artery and pulmonary capillary wedge pressure in acutely ill patients, Heart Lung 11:393, 1982.

Price D: Hemodynamic monitoring for critical care, Norwalk, 1986, Appleton-Century-Crofts.

Scordo K: Hemodynamic monitoring: learning to read the waves, Nursing 15(7):40, 1985.

Shoemaker W and others: The society of critical care medicine textbook of critical care Philadelphia, 1984, WB Saunders.

Spangler R: Hemodynamic monitoring: using the pulmonary artery catheter, Cardiothoracic Nurse 5(3):3, 1987.

(See also Unit 3: Oxygenation)

Intraaortic balloon (circulatory assist)

Birkholz G: IABP: legal and ethical issues, DCCN 4:285, 1985.

Bolooki H: Clinical application of intra-aortic balloon pump, Mount Kisco, New York, 1984, Futura Publishing Co Inc.

Bolooki H: Current status of circulatory support with an inta-aortic balloon pumping, Cardiol Clin 3(1):123, 1985.

Bullas JD: Care of the patient on the percutaneous intra-aortic counterpulsation balloon, Crit Care Nurse 2(4):40, 1982.

Chenevey B and Sexton-Stone K: Lower limb ischemia: an iatrogenic complication of IABP, DCCN 4:264, 1985.

Goldberger M and others: Clinical experience with intra-aortic balloon counterpulsation with 112 consecutive patients. Am Heart J 111(3):497, 1986.

Haak SW: Intra-aortic balloon pump techniques, DCCN 2:196, 1983.

Kratz JM: IABP timing using temporary myocardial pacing wires, Ann Thorac Surg 42(1):120, 1986.

Moulopoulos S and others: Intraaortic balloon assistance in intractable cardiogenic shock, Eur Heart J 7(5):396, 1986.

Nursing care of patients in shock: fluids, oxygen, and the intra-aortic balloon pump (programmed instruction), AJN 82(9):1401, .

Purcell JA and others: Intra-aortic balloon pump therapy, AJN 83:775, 1983.

Sanfelippo PM and others: Experience with intraaortic balloon counterpulsation, Ann Thorac Surg 41(1):36, 1986.

Scheidt S and others: Mechanical circulatory assistance with the intraaortic ballon pump and other counterpulsation devices, Prog Cardiovasc Dis 25(1):55, 1982.

Quaal SJ: Comprehensive intra-aortic balloon pumping. St. Louis, 1984, The CV Mosby Co.

Pharmacological Intervention in Coronary Artery Disease

---

1 Problems related to both *structural* and *functional* cardiovascular disorders complicate coronary artery disease (angina or MI).

The three major life-threatening problems complicating coronary artery disease are *general functional disorders,* which may also occur in other forms of heart disease (see Fig. 10-1). They include the following:

1. *Arrhythmias* caused by alterations in _____ activity

2. *Heart failure* caused by alterations in _____ activity

3. *Shock* caused by alterations in either _____ or _____ activity

electrical

mechanical

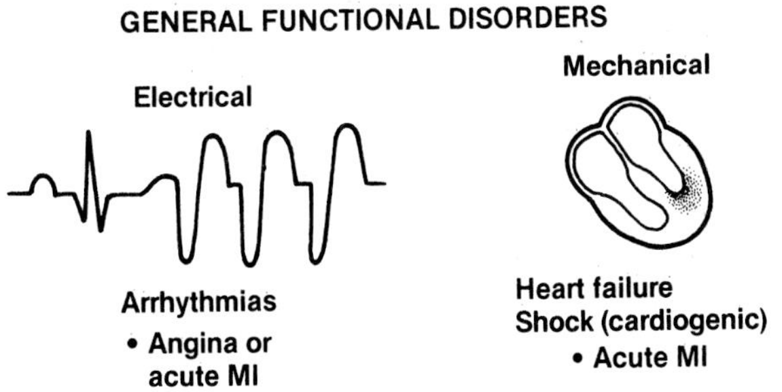

electrical
mechanical

GENERAL FUNCTIONAL DISORDERS

Electrical

Mechanical

Fig. 10-1

Arrhythmias
• Angina or acute MI

**Heart failure
Shock (cardiogenic)**
• Acute MI

Arrhythmias may occur during *either* angina or acute MI. However, the disorders of mechanical activity are more typically related to the permanent structural changes in the muscle wall associated with acute MI. When these disorders (electrical or mechanical) occur in other forms of heart disease, they are often also treated in a coronary care unit with the same pharmacological agents. Because of their significance and scope, the use of pharmacological agents in the management of these general functional problems is discussed in the early part of this unit.

Another general functional disorder that may also occur in patients with coronary artery disease is hypertension. Hypertension usually represents altered mechanical activity in both the heart and the vascular bed. Although it may not be directly life threatening, it can aggravate heart failure and/or precipitate the fourth major problem occurring in these patients—coronary chest pain. Although the pharmacological therapy of hypertension is not separately dealt with, most of the agents currently used are included within the discussions relating to the management of either heart failure or chest pain.

2 A fourth major problem occurring in the patient with coronary artery disease is *chest pain*. Chest pain is usually the initial presenting problem in both angina and acute MI. It contributes significantly to both patient discomfort and a stress response, further aggravating the problem. However, it is not directly life threatening. Chest pain is most significant in the context of structural coronary artery disease because of the potential for a life-threatening functional disorder (see Frame 1). It is treated differently in this context than when associated with other forms of heart or lung disease.

Chest pain, when in the context of *structural* coronary artery changes, usually represents acute, often temporary, *coronary system failure*. This suggests a more specific functional disorder closely linked to structural changes in the vessels and/or muscle wall (Fig. 10-2).

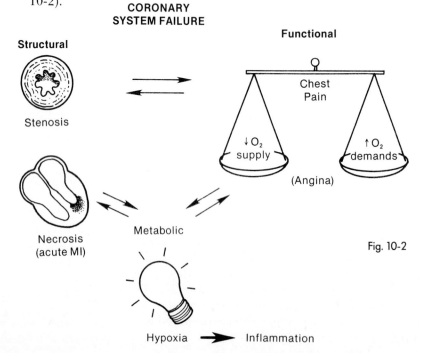

CORONARY SYSTEM FAILURE

Structural

Functional

Stenosis

Chest Pain

$\downarrow O_2$ supply

$\uparrow O_2$ demands

(Angina)

Necrosis (acute MI)

Metabolic

Fig. 10-2

Hypoxia ➔ Inflammation

3 Coronary chest pain is thus related to specific, closely linked _____ and _____ changes. This chest pain may be relieved by direct suppression of the pain by the reversal of the related structural, functional, and/or metabolic changes.

structural; functional

REMEMBER: Chest pain occurs because of metabolic toxins released in the presence of coronary _____ (*structural* change), ischemia, and myocardial _____ (*functional* changes). These changes may result in permanent *structural* damage to the muscle wall. The use of pharmacological agents in the management of chest pain is discussed in the latter part of this unit.

stenosis

hypoxia

Drugs reversing the structural, functional, and/or metabolic changes associated with coronary artery disease may prevent or minimize the structural damage to the muscle wall associated with *(angina/acute MI)*. They may also be used to prevent death following acute myocardial infarction. This application of these agents is discussed in the section about preserving ischemic myocardium (Frames 217 to 219).

acute MI

Following this section, the current role of drugs altering the clotting process is discussed in relation to the arterial structural changes and venous complications of coronary artery disease.

4 Cardiac arrest is usually a manifestation of an extreme functional disorder associated with hypoxic metabolic complications. Therefore the drugs used in the setting of cardiac arrest include agents to manage arrhythmias, chest pain, heart failure, and shock, as well as additional agents used to manage related metabolic complications. These drugs are summarized at the end of the chapter and are correlated to previous discussions (see Table 16).

DRUG THERAPY IN THE MANAGEMENT OF ARRHYTHMIAS

5 Generally arrhythmias may be considered as resulting from disturbances in _____ and _____, which contribute to electrical instability. The three major types of arrhythmias we consider are:

automaticity; conduction

    1. ventricular tachyarrhythmias
    2. Supraventricular tachyarrhythmias
    3. Bradyarrhythmias

Drugs for ventricular tachyarrhythmias

6 Ventricular arrhythmias are a manifestation of electrical instability in the _____.

ventricles

Electrical instability in the ventricles may result in PVCs, VT, or _____.

VF

REMEMBER: Initial therapy in the management of ventricular arrhythmias is directed toward depressing ectopic impulse formation in the _____.

The drugs used to manage arrhythmias caused by electrical instability are known as the antiarrhythmic drugs. These drugs depress ectopic impulse formation in the ventricles. Some also depress ectopic impulse formation in the atria and/or AV node (junction). The focus of this discussion is the use of antiarrhythmic drugs in the management of ventricular arrhythmias.

7 Antiarrhythmic drugs depress ventricular ectopic impulse formation (electrical instability) by (1) directly depressing automaticity, (2) altering conduction and repolarization so that reentry circuits are broken, or (3) both of these (see Unit 7, Frames 21 to 51).

REMEMBER: Automaticity is the ability to _____ impulses spontaneously; it is a property of electrical *(stable/unstable)* cells. Antiarrhythmic drugs depress automaticity by altering the permeability of the cell membrane to those ions moving *into the cells* during _____ depolarization. They may also act on autonomic receptors and/or chemicals that facilitate this ion movement (see Frames 10 to 12 and Fig. 10-3).

8 Disturbances in conduction produce ectopic impulses and generate tachyarrhythmias by the process known as _____ (see Unit 7, Frames 27 to 39). Antiarrhythmic drugs prevent or break reentry circuits by either altering the movement of ions *into the cell* during depolarization (conduction) or *out of the cell* during _____. They thus promote *uniform* and *synchronous* _____ _____ and stabilize the rhythm.

REMEMBER: Depolarization (spontaneous or activated) is controlled by the movement of Na^+ ions via fast channels and/or Ca^{++} ions via _____ channels. These ion movements *(into/out of)* the cell may contribute to either automaticity or reentry.

Both ventricular Purkinje and myocardial depolarization *primarily* depend on *(Na^+/Ca^{++})* movements via *(slow/fast)* channels. Ventricular ectopic activity is therefore most effectively suppressed by altering the movement of *(Na^+/Ca^{++}) into the cell.*

9 The antiarrhythmic drugs are most commonly grouped into four classes according to the system proposed by Singh and Vaughn-Williams. These classes and the currently available agents are as follows:

Class I agents: Suppress Na^+ channels
- Quinidine sulfate (Quinidine)
- Procainamide HCl (Pronestyl)

ventricles	
initiate	
unstable	
spontaneous	
reentry	
repolarization	
conduction (depolarization)	
slow; into	
Na^+; fast	
Na^+	

- Disopyramide phosphate (Norpace)
- Lidocaine HCl (Xylocaine)
- Phenytoin sodium (Dilantin)
- Tocainide HCl (Tonocard)
- Mexiletine HCl (Mexitil)
- Flecainide acetate (Tambocor)
- Encainide (Enkaid)

Class II agents: Block sympathetic receptors and/or chemicals (beta blockers)
- Propranolol HCl (Inderal)
- Others (see Frames 191-203)

Class III agents: Act selectively on repolarization and reentry circuits and are most effective in abolishing ventricular fibrillation
- Bretylium tosylate (Bretylol)
- Amiodarone HCl (Cordarone)

Class IV agents: Suppress Ca^{++} channels
- Verapamil (Isoptin, Calan)
- Diltiazem (Cardizem)

NOTE: All antiarrhythmic drugs are depressants and should be administered with caution when signs of either electrical or mechanical depression are evident.

Although the exact mechanism of each drug's action may differ, as a group these drugs act to suppress ectopic impulse formation in the _____. Some also suppress ectopic formation in the _____ and/or the _____ _____ (junction).

ventricles

atria; AV node

Verapamil is included in this classification because of its ability to suppress, potentially, selected forms of ventricular arrhythmias. However, unlike the other agents listed, it is used *primarily* in therapy of supraventricular tachyarrhythmias because of its more significant effect on the AV node (see Frames 69 to 81).

THE ANTIARRHYTHMICS

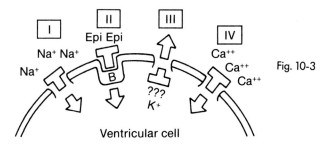

Fig. 10-3

443

10 Ventricular arrhythmias are usually most effectively managed by agents that suppress *(Na⁺/Ca⁺⁺* channels or Class _____ agents. The most common, traditionally used antiarrhythmic agents belong to this category.

Na⁺; I

The specific effects of Class I agents differ with regard to depolarization and repolarization. Class I agents may be further divided into Class IA, IB, and IC according to these differences.

Class IA antiarrhythmic drugs

11 Class IA agents prolong both depolarization and _____. Prolongation of depolarization results in widening of the _____ complex at toxic levels. Prolongation of repolarization results in prolongation of the _____ interval with an accompanying risk of producing _____ (see Unit 12, Frames 13-23). These agents are effective in both ventricular and atrial arrhythmias, and include quinidine, procainamide, and disopyramide.

repolarization

QRS

Q-T(U)

torsades; de pointes

Class IB agents have _____ effects on depolarization and _____ repolarization. These agents, as a group, are primarily effective in _____ arrhythmias, and include lidocaine, phenytoin, tocainide, and mexiletene.

minimal

shorten

ventricular

Class IC agents prolong _____, which may result in widening of the _____ complex, but have no effect on _____. They, therefore,*(are/are not)* associated with torsades de pointes.

depolarization

QRS

repolarization; are not

12 The antiarrhythmic drug used most commonly in the management of acute ventricular arrhythmias is the Class IB agent lidocaine. Lidocaine is ideal for use in the setting of acute MI because of two characteristics: its rapid onset of action and its relative lack of toxic effects on the heart.

All antiarrhythmic agents (Classes I-IV) may potentiate or generate the very ventricular arrhythmias they are designed to suppress or abolish. This effect is referred to as their *proarrhythmic* actions (see Unit 12, frame 10). The incidence, specific characteristics of the arrhythmias produced, and the corresponding dose range, however, vary with the specific agents (see Frames 13-52).

13 The class IA antiarrhythmic agents include quinidine sulfate (_____), procainamide HCl (_____), and disopyramide phosphate (_____). These agents, although pharmacologically different, have certain common actions—especially in _____ and _____. Quinidine, procainamide, and disopyramide depress ectopic impulse forma-

quinidine

Pronestyl

Norpace

repolarization; conduction

Table 12 Class I antiarrhythmics: Major differences

	Class IA	Class IB	Class IC
Depolarization (QRS)	prolonged	minmial effect	prolonged
Repolarization (Q-T/U)*	prolonged	shortened	no effect
Spectrum of activity	A/V	V	A/V/AV re-entry

*torsades de pointes is most typically produced by agents which prolong the QT(U) interval

tion in both the atria and ventricles. Therefore these drugs may be used in the management of both acute and chronic atrial and _____ arrhythmias. These are also effective in the atrial fibrillation of WPW (see Unit 12, Frame 45). In addition to *(enhancing/suppressing)* automaticity, the Class IA drugs have specific effects on repolarization and _____ that may affect _____ circuits. These effects include (1) prolongation of the refractory period, thus *(shortening/prolonging)* repolarization, and (2) dose-related showing of AV junctional as well as intraventricular conduction.

ventricular

suppressing
conduction
reentry
prolonging

14 Class IA drugs at therapeutic blood levels show AV conduction. However, with initial administration they may accelerate AV conduction. This transient vagolytic effect of Class IA agents necessitates the administration of digitalis before using these agents in the initial therapy of supraventricular arrhythmias, such as atrial fibrillation.

15 Class IA agents affect intraventricular conduction both therapeutically and toxically. The toxic effect of Class IA drugs on intraventricular conduction is seen by analyzing the *(P waves/QRS complexes)* of the normal beats.

QRS complexes

Widening of the normal QRS complexes is a toxic manifestation of these drugs and *(is/is not)* an indication for discontinuing therapy. Class IA drugs should be administered with caution to patients who have normally wide QRS complexes, indicating preexisting intraventricular conduction abnormalities. Examples include patients with complete bundle branch blocks and periinfarction blocks. Class IA agents are also contraindicated in the presence of hyperkalemia.

is

REMEMBER: Potassium is a cardiac *(depressant/stimulant)*.

depressant

16 Class IA drugs abolish intraventricular reentry circuits (therapeutic effect) by (1) slowing conduction in ischemic tissue so that the impulse is extinguished, or (2) prolonging the refractory period of the ischemic cells within the circuit so that the impulse is blocked from reentering the ischemic area (see Fig. 10-4).

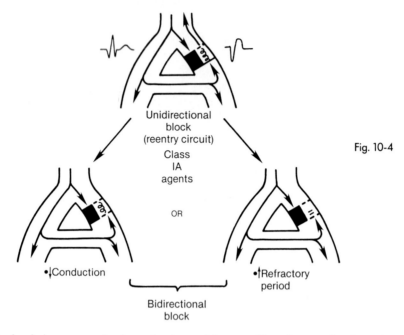

Fig. 10-4

17 In both instances the impulse is unable to utilize the conduction circuit to reenter the heart in the opposite direction, producing bidirectional block. Impulse conduction therefore again becomes uniform.

REMEMBER: Reentry occurs when an impulse is blocked in one direction within a circular conduction pathway. This phenomenon is referred to as _____ _____.   unidirectional block
The antiarrhythmic drugs convert. unidirectional block to _____ block,thus preventing reentry from occurring.   bidirectional

18 Quinidine, procainamide, and disopyramide *(shorten/prolong)* the refractory period of cardiac cells, thus *(shortening/prolonging)* repolarization. Prolonged or delayed repolarization may be manifested on the EG by the appearance of a U wave, TU fusion, and "pseudo" QT prolongation. This ECG manifestation of the group IA antiarrhythymic drugs mimics the ECG pattern of *(hypokalemia/hyperkalemia)*. It is often referred to as the "quinidine effect" and does not usually represent a toxic effect of these drugs. However, toxic levels of group I agents may result in severe prolongation of the refractory period, with extreme distortion of the QT interval and enhancement—rather than suppression—of ectopic activity. Repolarization is so prolonged that recovery in adjacent cells becomes *(more/less)* uniform. VT or VF can occur, producing what has   prolong
prolonging

hypokalemia

less

been referred to as quinidine syncope. This ventricular arrhythmia has also been reported as a toxic effect of disopyramide therapy. It is also known as *torsades de pointes*, since it gives the appearance of twisting around a central point (baseline). The ECG pattern can mimic both VT and VF (see Unit 12, Frames 13). This is the most typical proarrhythmic effect of this class and can occur with initial doses.

19 LET US REVIEW: Class IA drugs depress ectopic activity in both the _____ and _____. Electrophysiological effects include showing of _____ _____ and _____ conduction and *(prolongation/shortening)* of the refractory period, in addition to *(increased/decreased)* automaticity.

atria; ventricles
AV junctional
intraventricular; prolongation
decreased

With initial administration Class IA drugs may accelerate _____ conduction. Widening of the QRS complex is a *(therapeutic/toxic)* effect of group I drugs and *(is/is not)* an indication for discontinuing the drug.

AV
toxic; is

Another toxic manifestation of therapy with Class IA drugs is VT and VF associated with severe distortion of the _____ interval. TU fusion *(does/does not)* usually represent toxic levels of these agents.

QT
does not

20 Class IA drugs also have hemodynamic side effects. Quinidine, procainamide, and disopyramide depress myocardial mechanical function. They may cause a rise in LVEDP (filling pressure) and a fall in cardiac output and must therefore be administered cautiously to the patient with heart failure.

The effects of disopyramide are the most pronounced. Caution should be used when this agent is administered in conjunction with other myocardial depressants, particularly beta blockers and calcium blockers.

Procainamide is a peripheral vasodilator and therefore may cause *(hypotension/hypertension)*. This drug is the only group IA agent commonly administered by the IV route. It is therefore used more often in the *(acute/chronic)* management of ventricular arrhythmias than are disopyramide or quinidine. Toxic side effects are potentially more pronounced when the IV route of administration is used. Intravenous procainamide should be administered slowly (no more than 20 mg/minute) to allow for close ECG monitoring for QRS widening and prevent marked vascular effects (that is, hypotension).

hypotension

acute

21 Other side effects have also been reported following the administration of group I agents. Class IA drugs may cause GI disturbances, such as nausea and vomiting. This can be minimized by concurrent administration with milk or meals. Quinidine frequently causes diarrhea. A side effect specifically associated with disopyramide therapy is urinary retention. Dryness of the mouth has also been reported. Other side effects associated with specific Class IA drugs include thrombocytopenia and hemolytic anemia (associated with quinidine therapy) and the reversible lupuslike syndrome (commonly seen with chronic procainamide therapy). Quinidine administration has also been linked with the occurrence of a cinchonism—a syndrome associated with the administration of cinchoma bark derivatives such as quinine and quinidine. The syndrome is associated with the following symptoms: tinnitus, blurring of vision or diplopia, loss of hearing, headache, and confusion.

Concurrent administration of quinidine and digitalis has been known to raise serum digitalis levels, most likely by displacing digitalis bound to serum proteins. The potential for digitalis toxicity is thus enhanced in this setting.

22 The antidote for the QRS widening associated with toxicity from Class IA drugs is sodium bicarbonate or sodium lactate. The sodium ion acts as a stimulus to the heat. Alkalinization promotes binding of the drug to serum proteins, thus lowering toxic levels.

REMEMBER: Sodium plays a major role in depolarization.

LET US REVIEW: Class I drugs may cause a rise in _____ LVEDP
and a fall in _____ output. When administering cardiac
procainamide intravenously one should watch specifically for widening of the _____ _____ and *(hypotension/* QRS complex; hypotension
hypertension). A side effect commonly associated with disopyramide
therapy is _____ _____. The an- urinary retention
tidote for toxicity of group IA drugs is _____ sodium bicarbonate
_____ or _____ sodium lactate
_____.

23 NURSING ORDERS: Patients receiving Class IA drugs for management of ventricular arrhythmias

1. Quinidine, procainamide, and disopyramide are cardiac *(stim-* depressants
ulants/depressants). In toxic dosages they may produce widening QRS complex
of the _____ _____. The antidote sodium bicarbonate
for toxicity of Class IA drugs is _____
_____.

2. When administering provainamide intravenously, watch for
the development of _____ and widening of hypotension
the _____ complex. QRS
—Administer slowly (no more than _____). 20 mg/minute
—Procainamide "boluses" may be followed by continuous IV
infusion in dosages similar to those for lidocaine.

3. GI disturbances, such as _____ and nausea
_____, may occur with the administration of vomiting
Class IA drugs. Administration with _____ or milk

_____ can minimize these effects. Watch for
the development of _____ with quinidine
therapy.

food
diarrhea

4. Watch for the development of urinary
_____ with _____ therapy.

retention; disopyramide

5. REMEMBER: Class IA agents *(would/would not)* be the initial drugs
used to treat a supraventricular tachyarrhythmia. Class IA
drugs may *(accelerate/slow)* AV conduction with initial
administration.

would not

accelerate

Class IB antiarrhythmic drugs

24 The current Class IB agents include lidocaine HCl
(_____), phenytoin sodium (_____),
tocainide HCl (_____), and mexiletine
(_____). Another Class IB agent still under
investigation is Ethmozine (Moricizine). These agents share certain
common mechanisms of action that allow them to be grouped
together. However, the clinical effectiveness differs significantly. For this reason, we will discuss phenytoin separately from the
others.

Xylocaine; Dilantin
Tonocard

Mexitil

Lidocaine, Tocainide, Mexiletine

25 The antiarrhythmic drug most commonly used in the management of acute ventricular arrhythmias is the Class IB agent,
_____.

lidocaine

Lidocaine is ideal for use in the setting of acute MI because of
two characteristics: its rapid onset of action and its relative lack of
toxic effects on the heart.

The route of lidocaine administration in the acute setting is intravenous. It may be given in a single bolus of 1mg/kg (usually 50-100
mg) or by a continuous infusion drip 2-4 mg/min. When an infusion
drip is started, a bolus should be given simultaneously to ensure that
adequate blood levels are achieved rapidly.

NOTE: The use of prophylactic lidocaine in the first 24 to 48 hours
of acute MI has been advocated by many practitioners.

26 The more recently approved agents mexiletine and tocainamide are
administered by the oral route, and, therefore, *(do/do not)* have the
same rapid onset of action. Their mechanisms of action and spectrum of activity is very similar to lidocaine. Unlike lidocaine, however, they may be used in the management of both acute and
_____ arrhythmias.

do not

chronic

REMEMBER: Class IB agents as a group are primarily effective in
the management of _____ arrhythmias. Supraven-
tricular arrhythmias may in fact be aggravated at times by the use of
lidocaine (see Frame 31).

ventricular

27 Class IB agents suppress arrhythmias resulting from either enhanced automaticity or reentry mechanisms.

Class IB agents depress ventricular automaticity by decreasing (Na^+/Ca^{++}) influx during phase _____ of unstable cells.

REMEMBER: Both stable and unstable ventricular cells depend on Na^+ influx for depolarization.

Na^+; 4

28 Class IB agents break reentrant circuits by producing a bidirectional block. Lidocaine has been said to act preferentially on ischemic myocardium. Mexiletine and tocainide are believed to act similarly. A bidirectional block is produced when lidocaine selectively prolongs the refractory period in ischemic cells. These effects are similar to the effects of the Class IA agents, but are more selective on _____ myocardium. Depressed conduction within the circuit may also extinguish the impulse.

ischemic

REMEMBER: The effects of Class IB agents on normal cardiac cells is to only _____ prolong _____ (i.e., depress conduction) and shorten _____. Therefore, these agents (do/do not) widen the QRS complex or prolong the QT(U) interval.

minimally; depolarization
repolarization
do not

These agents may actually shorten the QT interval slightly and have been, therefore, suggested as therapy for torsades de pointes or as alternate antiarrhythmics in patients with pre-existing borderline or prolonged _____ intervals.

Q-T(U)

29 The Class IB agents rarely cause adverse cardiac effects. They have the least negative inotropic effects of all the antiarrhythmic agents and minimal proarrhythmic effects. The most common cardiovascular side effect is hypotension, but this is uncommon except with IV Lidocaine. Lidocaine also has potential deleterious effects in aberrant conduction and ventricular escape rhythms (see frames 31, 32).

Mexiletine and tocainide can be less effective than lidocaine or other antiarrhythmics especially in VT or VF unless combined with a Class IA agent. Class IB agents are ideal for combination therapy because of their (minimal/extensive) cardiotoxicity. Lower doses of both the Class IB and Class _____ agent may be used.

minimal
IA

30 Lidocaine, mexiletine, and tocainide share similar neurologic side effects. These include tremors, hot and cold flashes, dysarthria, diplopia/blurred vision, confusion, atazia, dizziness, paresthesias, and numbness. Seizures have been reported with both mexiletine and lidocaine. Nausea and vomiting can also occur, but may be minimized by taking the drug with food. Cases of agranulocytosis, severe neutropenia, and pulmonary fibrosis have been reported with tocainide. These agents are predominantly metabolized in the liver with some renal excretion with tocainide. Drug dosages should be lowered in patients with renal or _____ failure or hepatic congestion secondary to CHF.

hepatic

31 Let us now consider the effects of lidocaine on other cardiac tissue.

Lidocaine does not appear to have a significant direct effect on either AV node refractoriness or conduction. However, lidocaine may decrease the ectopic rates of atrial flutter and atrial fibrillation, thus indirectly facilitating AV conduction and aberrant conduction. This effect should be considered when administering a therapeutic trial of lidocaine in the presence of suspected aberrant conduction; however, this potential effect does not minimize the value of a lidocaine trial in differentiating ventricular ectopy from aberrant conduction.

If bursts of ectopic beats decrease in frequency or are abolished following the administration of lidocaine, the beats are very *(likely/unlikely)* to be ventricular.

likely

If the ectopic beats seem to increase after the administration of lidocaine, they are *(more/less)* likely to be ventricular in origin, and the possibility of aberrant conduction should be considered.

less

32 Lidocaine also does not significantly affect automaticity and conduction in the SA node. Therefore lidocaine is relatively safe to use in the setting of sinus bradycardia. However, it is recommended that atropine be readily available as a precaution.

Lidocaine should *never* be administered in the presence of a sustained idioventricular rhythm. Asystole may occur, caused by elimination of this compensatory ventricular ectopic rhythm.

LET US REVIEW: Lidocaine *(is/is not)* indicated in the therapy of supraventricular rhythms with aberration. It *(may/may not)* be used to prevent the recurrence of VF. Toxic effects of lidocaine include *(hypotension/hypertension)*, sensorium _____, and _____ or _____. Lidocaine should never be given in the presence of sustained _____ _____.

is not
may

hypotension; changes
paresthesias; tremors

intraventricular rhythm

33 NURSING ORDERS: Patients receiving Class IB drugs (lidocaine, mexiletine, tocainide) for ventricular arrhythmia
1. Analyze the need for the drug within the clinical context of the arrhythmia, especially prior to administering IV Lidocaine.
    —Is the underlying rhythm fast or slow?
    —Is the arrhythmia acutely life threatening?
    —Is the arrhythmia a precursor to ventricular fibrillation?
    REMEMBER: Lidocaine may also be used to prevent the recurrence of _____.

VF

2. Evaluate the possible causes of ventricular arrhythmia.

3. Monitor cardiac status, BP, respiratory status, and sensorium during IV infusion of lidocaine.
   —Evaluate the response of the rhythm to the drug; has the lidocaine therapy suppressed the arrhythmia?
   —Observe the patient for these signs of lidocaine toxicity: *(hypotension/hypertension)* and changes in _____. If these occur, stop the infusion, have the patient lie flat and raise the patient's legs.

   hypotension

   sensorium

4. Monitor for neurologic and GI side effects with tocainide and mexiletine. Administer with food.
5. If the patient has liver failure or congestion secondary to CHF, consider small amounts of the drug for initial administration.

Phenytoin sodium

34 Unlike the other Class IB agents, phenytoin sodium depresses ectopic impulse formation in both the _____ and _____. It also depresses ectopic impulse formation in the AV junctional tissue. It *(accelerates/slows)* AV conduction and *(prolongs/shortens)* the refractory period.

atria

ventricles

accelerates

shortens

Phenytoin sodium may be used in the management of acute and chronic ventricular _____. It is effective primarily in the management of digitalis-induced arrhythmias, both ventricular and supraventricular. It is especially effective in the presence of junctional tachycardia caused by digitalis toxicity.

arrhythmias

NOTE: The arrhythmias of digitalis toxicity represent increased automaticity in the presence of decreased conduction. Phenytoin sodium *(increases/decreases)* automaticity and *(increases/decreases)* conduction, thus reversing the toxic effects of digitalis.

decreases; increases

Phenytoin sodium does not produce significant hemodynamic alterations. In toxic dosages it can produce bradyarrhythmias and cardiac standstill. Respiratory depression can also be a toxic manifestation of phenytoin sodium therapy. The degree of cardiac and respiratory depression produced appears to be related to the dose and speed of administration. Other side effects that may be associated with phenytoin sodium therapy are visual disturbances, gingivitis, and an autoimmune blood dyscrasia known as Stevens-Johnson syndrome, manifested dermatologically be the sloughing of tissues.

35 LET US REVIEW: Phenytoin sodium acts by depressing ectopic impulse formation and accelerating _____ conduction. It *(may/may not)* be used in the treatment of VT. It *(may/may not)* be used in the treatment of arrhythmias associated with digitalis toxicity, especially _____ tachycardia. When administering it, the nurse should observe for both respiratory and cardiac electrical _____. Other side effects as-

AV

may; may

junctional

depression

sociated with phenytoin sodium are _____ disturbances and _____.

visual
gingivitis

1. Incompatibilities with D_5W and/or saline are prevented by IV push administration at a rate not to exceed 50 mg/minute. Flush the glucose solution with a saline bolus before and after administration.

2. With IV administration, watch for the development of brady-arrhythmias, which may progress to _____ _____; also observe for the development of respiratory _____.

cardiac standstill

deprerssion

3. Observe for disturbances in _____, _____, and Stevens-Johnson syndrome.

vision
gingivitis

Class IC antiarrhythmic drugs:

36 The two currently available Class IC agents are flecainide acetate (_____) and encainide (_____). By the time this edition is published, a third Class IC agent propafenone (Rhytmonorm) will probably have been released. This agent has beta blocking and calcium blocking effects also, actually combining three classes in one drug. Other Class IC agents still under investigation include lorcainide and indecainide.

Tambocor; Enkaid

These agents have a *(narrow/broad)* spectrum of activity affecting most areas of the heart. Therefore, these drugs are effective in the control of both atrial and _____ arrhythmias. They are also the only Class I agents effective in both the PAT and atrial fibrillation of WPW due to effects on both the AV node and accessory pathway (see Unit 12, Frame 42).

broad

ventricular

These agents are highly effective in the control of ventricular arrhythmias since they are the most potent Class I agents. They are usually indicated when Class IA and/or Class IB agents have been ineffective or toxic effects have limited their use. However, they possess significant proarrhythmic effects, ironically more when used with malignant, complex ventricular arrhythmias, such as VT or VF, where they are also most effective. Flecainide also produces significant negative inotropic effects.

37 In addition to *(enhancing/suppressing)* automaticity, Class IC agents abolish intraventricular reentry circuits by _____ conduction so that the impulse is extinguished. This action is due to prolongation of *(depolarization/repolarization)* similar to *(Class IA/Class IB)* agents. However, unlike Class IA agents, Class IC agents have no effect on _____ and the refractory periods of reentry circuits. Since these agents *(do/do not)* prolong the Q-T(U) interval (beyond the QRS complex), they may be used in patients at risk for torsades de pointes. These agents *(do/do not)* have selective effects on ischemic tissues like the Class IB agents.

suppressing
depressing

depolarization; Class IA

repolarization
do not

do not

38 Because of their profound effect on conduction, widening of the QRS complex may occur therapeutically with these drugs and *(is/is not)* necessarily an indication for discontinuing therapy. Other cardiac side effects include *(positive/negative)* inotropic effects most pronounced with *(encainide/flecainide)*. Patients should be monitored for signs of congestive _____ _____. The newest agent propafenone possesses slight negative inotropic effects. Patients with significant preexisting heart failure should not receive flecainide. Additive effects can occur when these agents are combined with beta blockers, calcium channel blockers, or disopyramide. Class IC agents may also significantly suppress SA and AV node function when combined with agents, such as digitalis, the calcium channel blockers, or beta blockers.

is not

negative
flecainide

heart failure

39 NURSING ORDERS: The patient receiving a Class IC agent for arrhythmias

1. Flecainide and encainide are cardiac *(stimulants/depressants)*. They may produce widening of the _____, which may not necessarily indicate toxicity.

depressants
QRS

2. Monitor for increasing signs of CHF with flecainide—i.e., increase in rales, new S_3 gallop.
3. Monitor for any increase rather than decrease in ventricular arrhythmias.
4. Monitor for CNS and visual side effects with both agents and metallic taste with _____.

encainide

Class II antiarrhythmic drugs

40 Sympathetic (beta-) blocking drugs, such as propranolol (Inderal), can also act as antiarrhythmic agents by depressing ectopic formation in the ventricles. They are currently used in the *chronic* management of ventricular arrhythmias as a backup or alternative to Class I agents with the exception of the recently released beta blocker esmolol (Brevibloc), which is used exclusively in the management of acute supraventricular arrhythmias.

Beta blockers are most effective in suppressing automaticity (whether mediated by Na^+ or Ca^{++}) and reentry circuits that are catecholamine induced (see Frames 7 and 8). These include arrhythmias that are either stress-related or triggered-sustained by _____ nervous system activity stimulation.

sympathetic

Beta blockers such as propranolol also significantly depress impulse formation in the SA node, slow AV conduction and depress myocardial contractility. Because of their effect on AV junctional node automaticity and conduction, beta blockers are also useful in the management of supraventricular arrhythmias. A thorough discussion of the beta blockers is presented in Frames 61, 94 to 100, and 191 to 203.

Class III antiarrhythmic drugs

41 The two currently available Class III antiarrhythmic agents are bretylium tosylate (_____) and amiodarone (_____). Agents within this category that are still under investigation include bethanidine, clofilium, and sotalol (Sotacor).

    REMEMBER: Class III agents act on (*depolarization/repolarizaton*) and _____ circuits and are most effective as a group in abolishing _____ _____.

    Prolongation of repolarization and refractory periods prevents or interrupts re-entry circuits by producing _____ block (see Class IA agents, Frames 16 to 19, Fig. 10-4). Bretylium also promotes homogeneity between normal and ischemic cells due to a differential effect on ischemic tissues simlar to Xylocaine and the other Class IB agents. Class III agents also raise the VF threshold.

Bretylol

Cordarone

repolarization

reentry

ventricular fibrillation

bidirectional

42 The indications for, spectrum of activity, and side effects of these two agents vary significantly. Amiodarone has a diffuse effect on the heart affecting all conduction structures and is associated with many significant cardiac and extracardiac side effects. In contrast, bretylium acts selectively on ventricular fibers and is associated with fewer side effects.

    Bretylium is used primarily in the management of recurrent VF, when defibrillation or Xylocaine are ineffective. It may also be used to manage ventricular arrhythmias—principally VT and VF—that are unresponsive to other antiarrhythmic drugs. Bretylium generally antagonizes the effects of quinidine and has been used to treat ventricular arrhythmias secondary to quinidine toxicity.

43 Bretylium is a sympathetic blocking drug that causes an initial displacement of norepinephrine from nerve terminals with subsequent depletion of this chemical mediator.

Since bretylium initially displaces _____ (a sympathetic chemical transmitter) from nerve terminals, it may cause a transient increase in automaticity with tachycardia, hypertension, increased ventricular ectopic activity, or all of these. For this reason it is not indicated in the initial therapy for single, malignant PVCs. Thus bretylium (*is/is not*) a first-line agent in the management of all malignant ventricular arrhythmias. Because of this transient increase in norepinephrine release, bretylium may also potentiate the effects of digitalis toxicity. Thus it should be administered to a patient receiving digitalis only when the ventricular arrhythmias do not appear to be related to digitalis toxicity.

norepinephrine

is not

44 When used in therapy for VF, bretylium is given as an undiluted rapid bolus of 5-10 mg/kg (usually 250-700 mg). (Hypotension, nausea, and vomiting may occur with rapid IV administration when given in a setting other than VF.) The effect of bretylium in *(raising/ lowering)* the VF threshold is usually seen rapidly.

    raising

    Unlike lidocaine and procainamide, bretylium has a long half-life (6 to 8 hours). Therefore initiation of continuous IV infusion therapy can often be postponed for several hours without a significant drop in blood levels. When used to manage VT or other ventricular arrhythmias, bretylium is given diluted by IV Soluset or intramuscularly. In this setting the effect is seen less rapidly, usually within 20 minutes to 2 hours after administration. Although it may produce *(hypotension/hypertension)* bretylium does not appear to affect LVEDP or cardiac output adversely. In fact, it is thought to stimulate cardiac contractility (positive inotropic effect). Other side effects reported with the use of bretylium include vertigo, light-headedness, and dizziness.

    hypotension

45 LET US REVIEW: Bretylium rapidly raises the _____ threshold. When used in therapy for recurrent VF, it is given as an undiluted _____. Bretylium is a peripheral *(vasodilator/vasoconstrictor)* and thus may cause _____. It *(is/is not)* indicated in the initial therapy for single, malignant ventricular arrhythmias.

    VF

    bolus; vasodilator

    hypotension; is not

46 Amiodarone has a *(localized, diffuse)* effect on the cardiac conduction structures; it is not limited to the ventricular myocardium. It prolongs the refractory period of the SA node, AV node, atria, and accessory bypass tract tissues, as well as the ventricular Purkinje fibers and myocardium. It is most useful in the WPW syndrome, recurring VT and VF, and where a variety of arrhythmias, unresponsive to standard antiarrhythmic therapy are present. Amiodarone has a slow onset of action (averaging 4 to 10 days) and is therefore *not* indicated in the acute management of ventricular arrhythmias.

    diffuse

    Significant therapeutic effects may be delayed for weeks. The use of loading doses can provide antiarrhythmic effects within a few days. Because of this delayed onset of action and *(signifcant/minimal)* side effects, 2-3 weeks of in-hospital monitoring may be initially required. Although amiodarone may be administered intravenously. It is currently approved only in oral form.

    significant

47 Amiodarone produces significant cardiotoxicity. Its significant negative inotropic effects have been associated with aggravation of congestive _____ _____. Its proarrhythmic effects are related to significant prolongation of the refractory periods and _____ interval. This toxic effect may be minimized by maintaining normal serum K^+ levels.

    heart failure

    Q-T(U)

REMEMBER: Significant prolongation of the Q-T(U) interval is associated with _____ _____ torsades de pointes
_____, which mimics VT and VF and is unresponsive to conventional modes of therapy for these (see Unit 12, Frame 13).

Ironically, bretylium does not share this toxic effect and may actually be beneficial in the therapy of torsades. This may be explained by its differential, more selective effect on *(normal/abnormal)* conduction tissue. abnormal

AV block and bradycardia have also been reported as complications of amiodarone therapy due to its effects on the _____ and _____ nodes. SA; AV

48 Extracardiac side effects include corneal microdeposits, neurologic toxicity, GI symptoms, skin photosensitivity and gray or blue discoloration (pseudocyanosis). The corneal deposits may cause blurring of vision or orange and yellow halos at night or in dim light. Administration of artificial tears can help decrease these. Neurologic toxic effects include tremors, insomnia, ataxia, peripheral polyneuropathy, and thigh muscle weakness. GI symptoms include nausea, vomiting, and constipation.

Both hypo and hyperthyroidism can occur due to a release of high levels of iodine from amiodarone metabolism. Pulmonary toxicity, including pulmonary fibrosis, is the most common serious toxic effect. Hepatic and renal toxicity have also been reported. Asymptomatic abnormalities in liver function tests occur more commonly.

49 Most of the extracardiac side effects of amiodarone are reversible, but due to the *(short/long)* duration of action, these, as well as the long electrophysiologic effects, may continue for 3 months up to 1 year after cessation of therapy. The pulmonary fibrotic changes are the least likely to revert.

Interactions with Coumadin, digitalis, quinidine, and Pronestyl have been reported.

50 NURSING ORDERS: The patient receiving a Class III agent for arrhythmias
1. Assess for neurologic side effects including both motor and sensory deficits.
2. Administer artificial tear solution to minimize corneal microdeposits.
3. Instruct the patient to avoid sun exposure—cover exposed areas with clothing; use sunscreen.
4. Instruct the patient to report new onset of cough, fever, or shortness of breath immediately.

5. Assess for and report any signs of possible hyper or hypothyroidism including tremors, weight loss or gain, lethargy, palpitations.

6. Monitor for increased sensitivity to digitalis, calcium blockers, beta blockers, Class IA agents, and warfarin.

7. Assess the Q-T(U) interval for risk of torsades de pointes.

8. Ausculate the heart and lungs for signs of increased CHF—i.e., rales, new S_3 gallop.

9. Obtain baseline liver and pulmonary function tests and thyroid profile prior to initiating therapy and monitor regularly thereafter.

Class IV antiarrhythmic drugs:

51 Class IV agents act by suppressing (Na^+/Ca^{++}) channels. They are therefore referred to as calcium-channel blockers or calcium antagonists. The two currently available Ca^{++} antagonist with significant electrophysiological effects in verapamil (Isoptin or Calan) and diltiazem (Cardizem). However, the effects of verapamil are more pronounced.

Ca^{++}

REMEMBER: Although ventricular ectopic beats are typically caused by Na^+-dependent (fast) cells, fast cells may be converterd to _____ cells in the presence of selected _____. These slow cells may contribute to either enhanced automaticity or conduction blocks, resulting in reentry (see Unit 7, Frames 21 to 51).

slow
pathologies

52 Arrhythmias that are unresponsive to usual antiarrhythmic therapy (Class I and/or II agents) may be produced by Ca^{++}-dependent (slow) cells rather than Na^+-dependent (fast) cfells. Ca^{++} channel antagonists such as verapamil may be more effective. Verapamil has also proved effective in the control of ventricular arrhythmias related to coronary spasm (see Frames 200 to 216).

However, the significant depressant effect of verapamil on the AV node limits its application in ventricular arrhythmia unless a temporary or permanent pacemaker is inserted.

Verapamil is used primarily in the management of _____ tachyarrhythmias. A thorough discussion of the use of verapamil in arrhythmias is presented in Frames 66 to 78.

supraventricular

Drugs for supraventricular tachyarrhythmias and bradyarrhythmias
Role of sympathetic/parasympathetic nervous systems

53 Before continuing our discussion of the pharmacological management of problems associated with acute coronary artery disease, it is necessary to discuss a classification of drugs that is based on the effects of the parasympathetic and sympathetic (autonomic) nervous systems. Drugs that mimic, support, or block the effects of the sympathetic and parasympathetic nervous systems on the heart and blood vessels are commonly used in the pharmacological management of:

1. Supraventricular tachyarrhythmias
2. Bradyarrhythmias
3. Heart failure
4. Shock
5. Chest pain
6. Hypertension
7. Cardiomyopathy
8. Mitral prolapse

For the use of these agents in cardiomyopathy and mitral prolapse, see Unit 12.

54 The cardiovascular system is richly innervated by the autonomic nervous system, which includes both the _____ and _____ nervous systems. Sympathetic and parasympathetic receiving, or receptor, sites line the surface of cardiac electrical and muscle cells. Certain chemicals in the body act as mediators, or "messengers," carrying sympathetic and parasympathetic information from the nerves and CNS to the receptor sites. Chemical mediators of the sympathetic nervous system are norepinephrine (noradrenalin) and epinephrine (adrenalin). The chemical mediator of the parasympathetic nervous system is acetylcholine. The receptors act as doors, allowing the chemical mediators, or messengers, to enter the cell.

sympathetic
parasympathetic

AUTONOMIC NERVOUS SYSTEM

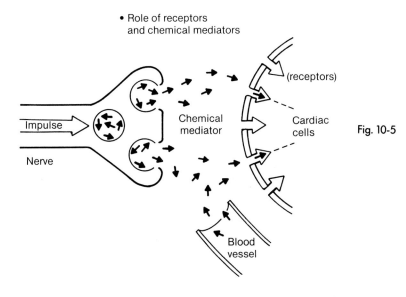

• Role of receptors
  and chemical mediators

Fig. 10-5

55 Let us first consider the effects of the sympathetic chemicals in more detail. The sympathetic nervous system exerts its major influence on the blood vessels, heart, and lungs. The chemical mediators of the sympathetic nervous system are _____ and _____. They are both produced within the adrenal medulla and are released into the bloodstream following sympathetic stimulation. Norepinephrine is also produced and stored in granules at sympathetic nerve endings and within the CNS. Because of their common production site within the _____ medulla, these sympathetic chemicals—and other synthetic sympathetic drug agents that mimic their action—are commonly referred to as "adrenergic." Still another term used when referring to norepinephrine and epinephrine is "catecholamines" (named after their similar chemical core—a cathechol ring). The receptors act as _____, allowing these chemical messengers to enter the cells.

epinephrine
norepinephrine

adrenal

doors

56 The sympathetic nervous system has two types of receptors: alpha (α) and beta (β). Alpha receptors are primarily located in the peripheral and coronary blood vessels. Beta receptors are primarily located in the heart and lungs but are also located in the blood vessels. Norepinephrine (more commonly known by its trade name, Levophed) is primarily attracted to alpha-receptor sites, but can also stimulate beta receptors to some extent. It is therefore referred to as an alpha-adrenergic agent. The effect of norepinephrine is primarily on the _____ _____. Epinephrine is primarily attracted to beta sites but can also stimulate the alpha receptors to some extent; it is therefore referred to as a _____ agent. The effect of epinephrine is primarily on the _____ and _____.

blood vessels

beta-adrenergic
heart
lungs

57 Stimulation of the alpha receptors results in vasoconstriction. Beta receptor sites can be further differentiated into B_1 sites on cardiac muscle and conduction structures and B_2 sites on bronchial smooth muscle. Stimulation of the B_2 receptors results in bronchodilation; stimulation of B_1 receptors affects the _____.

heart

The effects of autonomic stimulation on the heart may be classified as (1) chronotropic—affeting heart rate, (2) dromotropic—affecting conduction through the AV junctional tissue, or (3) inotropic—affecting contractility. To describe these responses of the heart to a drug, the terms *positive* and *negative* may be used. A drug that increases contractility has a *(positive/negative)* inotropic effect.

positive

NOTE: The peripheral and coronary vascular smooth muscles also contain B_2-receptor sites. Stimulation of these receptor sites results in relaxation, offsetting the effects of alpha-receptor stimulation.

These effects are mediated by the opening and/or closing of the vascular calcium channels (see Unit 4, Frame 99).

58 Responses to B_1 receptor stimulation include:
1. Increase in heart rate (positive _____ effect)   chronotropic
2. Increase in AV conduction (positive _____ effect)   dromotropic
3. Increase in contractility (positive _____ effect)   inotropic
4. Increase in automaticity
REMEMBER: Sympathetic fibers supply the _____ node, the   SA
_____, the _____ _____ tissue,   atria; AV junctional
and the _____ system (see Fig. 10-6).   His-Purkinje

59 Drugs affecting the sympathetic nervous system are classified into (1) alpha-adrenergic stimulators or alpha-adrenergic blockers and (2) beta-adrenergic stimulators or beta-adrenergic blockers. Let us first consider the drugs that stimulate the beta receptors. These drugs are also referred to as beta- _____ agents.   adrenergic
REMEMBER: Beta receptors are primarily located in the _____ and _____. Drugs that   heart; lungs
stimulate beta receptors therefore act on the _____   heart
and _____.   lungs

Selective B_2 (lung) agents are commonly available for use in patients with pulmonary disorders. These agents have only weak B_1 (heart) effects. However, many sympathetic drugs that significantly affect the heart have significant lung effects as well. Thus these drugs usually have both B_1 and _____ effects. B_2

60 LET US REVIEW: In the heart, beta stimulation produces:
1. A (positive/negative) chronotropic effect.   positive
2. A (positive/negative) dromotropic effect   positive
3. A (positive/negative) inotropic effect   positive
4. (Increased/Decreased) ventricular automaticity   Increased

Therefore it can be expected that beta stimulation will produce a(n) (increased/decreased) heart rate, (accelerated/depressed) AV conduciton,   increased; accelerated
(increased/decreased) contractility, and increased   increased
_____ ectopic beats. Because of its effect on heart   ventricular
rate and contractility, beta stimulation (increases/decreases) myocardial   increases
O_2 consumption. In the lungs beta stimulation causes
_____.   bronchodilation

61 Just as the beta receptors may be stimulated, they may also be blocked. Drugs that block the beta receptors produce effects opposite from those of beta stimulators. In the heart, beta blockers produce:

SITES OF ACTION/EFFECTS

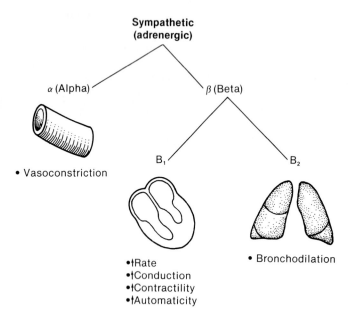

**Sympathetic
(adrenergic)**

α (Alpha) β (Beta)

• Vasoconstriction

B₁   B₂

•↑Rate   • Bronchodilation
•↑Conduction
•↑Contractility
•↑Automaticity

Fig. 10-6

• • • • • • • • • •

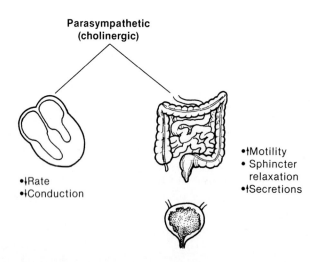

**Parasympathetic
(cholinergic)**

•↓Rate   •↑Motility
•↓Conduction   • Sphincter
                  relaxation
                •↑Secretions

NOTE: Illustrated here are major effects of sympathetic
and parasympathetic *stimulation*. Sympathetic and/or
parasympathetic blockade can be expected to produce
the exact opposite effects.

1. A *(positive/negative)* chronotropic effect   negative
2. A *(positive/negative)* dromotropic effect   negative
3. A *(positive/negative)* inotropic effect   negative
4. *(Increased/Decreased)* ventricular automaticity   Decreased

    Therefore it can be expected that beta blockers will cause a(n) *(increased/decreased)* heart rate, *(accelerated/depressed)* AV conduction, *(increased/decreased)* myocardial contractility, and decreased ventricular _____ beats. Because of their effects on heart rate and contractility, beta blockers *(increase/decrease)* myocardial O_2 consumption. In the lungs beta blockers cause bronchial *(dilation/constriction)*.

> decreased; depressed
> decreased
> ectopic
> decrease
> constriction

62 Alpha receptors may also be both stimulated and blocked.

    REMEMBER: Alpha receptors are primarily located in the peripheral _____ _____ but are also located in coronary vessels. Drugs that stimulate the alpha receptors therefore act on peripheral and coronary _____ _____.

> blood vessels
>
> blood vessels

    Alpha stimulation produces vasoconstriction and coronary spasm. Drugs that block the alpha receptors produce an effect opposite from that of the alpha stimulators. Therefore alpha blockers produce *(dilation/constriction)* of the peripheral blood vessels and relax or reverse coronary spasm.

> dilation

63 Let us now consider the effects of parasympathetic chemicals in more detail. The parasympathetic nervous system exerts a major influence on the heart, smooth muscles of the GI and genitourinary (GU) tracts, and respiratory system, as well as on GI secretions. The chemical mediator of the parasympathetic nervous system is _____. For this reason, this parasympathetic chemical and other synthetic parasympathetic drug agents that mimic or enhance its action are commonly referred to as "cholinergic." The major nerve of the parasympathetic nervous system is the vagus nerve (cranial nerve X). Therefore parasympathetic agents are also often referred to as "vagomimetic."

> acetylcholine

64 In the heart, parasympathetic stimulation produces:
1. A negative chronotropic effect
2. A negative dromotropic effect
3. No effects on inotropy or ventricular automaticity

    Therefore it can be expected that parasympathetic stimulation will cause a(n) *(increased/decreased)* heart rate and *(accelerated/depressed)* AV conduction.

> decreased; depressed

    REMEMBER: Parasympathetic fibers supply the _____ node, the _____, and AV _____ tissue. Parasympathetic stimulation produces essentially no effects on inot-

> SA
> atria; junctional

ropy or ventricular automaticity because there are few parasympathetic fibers in the ventricles.

In the GI and GU tracts, parasympathetic stimulation increases the motility and relaxes the sphincter muscle, thus *(facilitating/inhibiting)* emptying. In the GI and respiratory tracts, parasympathetic stimulation *(increases/decreases)* the secretions.

facilitating

increases

65 Just as parasympathetic fibers may be stimulated, they may also be blocked. Drugs that block or inhibit the effects of the parasympathetic nervous system may be referred to as anticholinergic, or vagolytic. In the heart, parasympathetic blockers produce:
1. A *(positive/negative)* chronotropic effect
2. A *(positive/negative)* dromotropic effect

Therefore parasympathetic blockers will cause a(n) *(increased/decreased* heart rate and *(accelerated/depressed)* AV conduction. In the GI and GU tracts, parasympathetic blockade _____ motility and _____ the sphincter muscle, thus *(facilitating/inhibiting)* emptying. In the GI and respiratory tracts, parasympathetic blockade *(increases/decreases)* secretions. (See Fig. 10-6.)

positive
positive
increased
accelerated
decreases
contracts; inhibiting

decreases

Drugs for supraventricular tachyarrhythmias

66 With this background, let us consider the problem of supraventricular tachyarrhythmias.

REMEMBER: Initial therapy in the management of fast supraventricular arrhythmias is directed toward *(increasing/decreasing)* the ventricular rate. The drugs that are capable of decreasing the ventricular rate include (1)calcium antagonists, (2) beta blockers, (3) parasympathetic stimulators, and (4) alpha stimulators.

decreasing

67 The drugs *most commonly* used in the current management of acute supraventricular arrhythmias are digitalis (a parasympathetic stimulator) and verapamil (a calcium antagonist). A third agent more recently introduced is esmolol (a beta-adrenergic blocker). The drug indicated by the American Heart Association (1987) for the *emergency* treatment of supraventricular tachyarrhythmias is the calcium antagonist, verapamil (Isoptin or Calan).

68 Verapamil is ideal for the critically ill patient because of two characteristics: its rapid onset of action, and its relative lack of toxic effects on the heart and lungs. Its use in supraventricular arrhythmias parallels the use of _____ in ventricular arrhythmias. Digitalis is currently more commonly used in the *chronic* management of supraventricular arrhythmias. The antiarrhythmic agents quinidine and procainamide are also commonly used in the chronic management of supraventricular arrhythmias in combination with a rate suppressant; they act to prevent or abolish the arrhythmias.

lidocaine

Verapamil (calcium antagonist)

69 Calcium antagonists act by blocking the entry of extracellular calcium into cardiovascular cells. They are therefore also referred to as Ca^{++}_____ blockers and *(do/do not)* alter total serum calcium.

REMEMBER: Cardiovascular cells depend on *(intracellular/extracellular)* Ca^{++} sources caused by poor intracellular stores (see Unit 4).

channel; do not

extracellular

70 Calcium has significant, distinct electrical roles in the heart. Depolarization can be either sodium (Na^+) dependent or _____ dependent. However, depolarization of the _____ and _____ nodes is calcium dependent.

Ca^{++}
SA
AV

Two currently available Ca^{++} antagonists have potentially significant electrophysiological effects. These two agents are verapamil (Isoptin or Calan) and diltiazem (Cardizem). However, the only Ca^{++} antagonist currently approved for use in supraventricular arrhythmias is _____.

verapamil

71 Verapamil acts by suppressing *(fast/slow)* channel activity.

slow

REMEMBER: Depolarization via Ca^{++} channels occurs more slowly than Na^+-dependent depolarizaton. Therefore this type of electrical activity is referred to as _____. The SA node and AV nodes, which normally utilize this type of electrical activity, are referred to as _____ cells.

slow

slow

72 The potential actions of a calcium antagonist such as verapamil on the electrical structures of the heart include (1) SA block, (2) AV block, and (3) suppression of slow cell ectopy (supraventricular or ventricular).

These actions are related to depressed automaticity within the SA and AV node and prolongation of SA and AV node refractory periods and conduction time. The calcium antagonists may also influence the abnormally slow conduction within the ischemic zone of selected reentry circuits.

73 The clinical effects of verapamil in supraventricular tachyarrhythmias are (1) decreased ventricular rate and/or (2) conversion or prevention of supraventricular arrhythmias with an AV node reentry circuit.

Supraventricular arrhythmias such as PAT typically use an AV node reentry circuit. Therefore the effects of verapamil in PAT are _____ and _____. Supraventricular arrhythmias such as atrial flutter or fibrillation *(do/do not)* use AV node reentry circuits. However, AV node refractory periods and conduction time determines the ventricular rate of these arrhyth-

conversion; prevention
do not

mias. Therefore the effect of verapamil in atrial flutter and/or fibrillation is primarily to decrease the _____   ventricular rate
_____.

SUPRAVENTRICULAR TACHYARRHYTHMIAS
(action of verapamil)

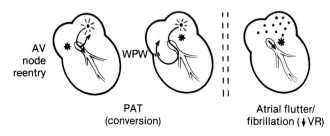

Fig. 10-7

The supraventricular arrhythmias occurring in the WPW syndrome constitute a special category in which extra precautions must be taken before verapamil can be safely administered.

74 Toxic effects of verapamil occur infrequently. They include hypotension caused by peripheral vasodilation, bradycardia, and constipation. Bradycardia occurs primarily in the presence of preexisting SA or AV node disease. Therefore verapamil is contraindicated   sinus
in sick _____ syndrome, second-degree or third-degree   hypotension
AV block, and severe *(hypertension/hypotension)*.

75 Atropine or dopamine may be used as indicated to manage these adverse reactions. The use of calcium should be avoided, since it may unnecessarily increase the total serum calcium.
   REMEMBER: The calcium antagonists are actually calcium
_____ blockers and *(do/do not)* act by altering total   channel; do not
serum calcium.

76 Intravenous verapamil should be administered slowly to minimize these side effects. Boluses of 5 to 10 mg are administered over a 2-minute period. A 3-minute period is recommended for patients over 55 years of age. Maximal-dose boluses should be separated by 30 minutes. Continuous IV drip is not required and may be difficult to monitor.
   Sustained control of the ventricular rate may be accomplished by the concurrent administration of intravenous or oral digitalis. Oral verapamil may later be added if digitalis is not effective. However, the digitalis dosage should then be reduced, since chronic verapamil therapy increases serum digoxin levels from 50% to 70% and may

466

increase the risk of digitalis toxicity. Subsequent serum digitalis levels should be monitored carefully.

77 LET US REVIEW: Continuous IV drip verapamil usually *(is/is not)* required. Maximal dose boluses should be separated by _____ minutes and should be given *(rapidly/slowly)*.

is not

30; slowly

When oral verapamil and digitalis are administered together, the digitalis dosage should be *(increased/decreased)*.

decreased

78 In doses used for arrhythmia control, verapamil produces only minimal effects on myocardial calcium transport. These effects are usually offset by the vasodilating actions and decreased heart rate, and should not aggravate CHF. However, according to its manufacturer, verapamil is contraindicated in *severe* CHF unless it is secondary to a supraventricular tachyarrhythmia. Myocardial depression may also be magnified when this agent is used in combination with either disopyramide or *intravenous* propranolol. Disopyramide should not be administered within 48 hours before or 24 hours after verapamil. Concurrent administration of intravenous verapamil and intravenous propranolol produces significant electrical and mechanical depression and is contraindicated. Combined oral use of these agents does not usually produce these effects but probably should be avoided in situations in which electrical and/or mechanical function is already significantly depressed.

79 LET US REVIEW: Verapamil is a *(sodium/calcium)* antagonist that acts primarily on *(fast/slow)* cells. It is most effective against *(ventricular/supraventricular)* arrhythmias.

calcium
slow; supraventricular

Toxic effects include *(bradycardia/tachycardia)*, and *(hypotension/hypertension)*. These adverse reactions may be treated with _____ or _____. Oral verapamil therapy is also associated with *(constipation/diarrhea)* and may be treated with laxatives. Verapamil is contraindicated in severe _____ sick _____ syndrome, and second-degree or third-degree _____ block. Myocardial depression may be magnified when this agent is used in combination with either _____ or intravenous _____.

bradycardia; hypotension

atropine; dopamine
constipation

CHF; sinus
AV

disopyramide; propranolol

80 Ca^{++} antagonists are also used in the treatment of angina and hypertension (see Frames 200 to 216). These agents may also be used after aneurysmectomy and in other cardiovascular disorders, such as migraine headaches, cerebrovascular spasm, peripheral vascular spasm (Raynaud's disease), pulmonary hypertension, hypertrophic cardiomyopathy, or coronary spasm associated with angioplasty. They may also be effective in disorders of the GU or GI smooth muscle and bronchial smooth muscle (i.e., asthma).

81 NURSING ORDERS: Patient receiving verapamil for a supraventricular tachyarrhythmia:

1. Do not administer in patients with severe hypotension, CHF, sick sinus syndrome, or severe AV block. (Check pulse before administering.)
2. Administer slowly when given intravenously (that is, 5 mg over _____ minutes). If more than 15 mg are required, wait 30 minutes between doses. An IV infusion is not typically used. Request follow up orders for digitalis, oral verapamil, or beta blockers.

   2 to 3
3. Watch for bradycardia, hypotension, or constipation. Have atropine and dopamine available.
4. Never administer IV verapamil and IV propranolol together.

Digitalis (parasympathetic stimulator/Na⁺-K⁺ pump inhibitor)

82 Digitalis is commonly used in the management of supraventricular tachyarrhythmias.

REMEMBER: The drugs most commonly used in the current management of acute supraventricular arrhythmias are verapamil and

_____.

digitalis

Digoxin (Lanoxin) is, by far, the most commonly prescribed digitalis glycoside due to its onset and duration of action, stability, and ease of administration.

83 The mechanism of action of digitalis on cardiovascular cells is probably dual; it includes (1) parasympathetic stimulation and (2) local cellular metabolic action.

REMEMBER: Drugs that stimulate the parasympathetic nervous system produce these effects on the heart: *(increased/decreased)* heart rate and *(accelerated/depressed)* AV conduction.

decreased
depressed

The primary clinical effect of digitalis in supraventricular tachyarrhythmia is to *(increase/decrease)* the ventricular rate.

decrease

84 Another therapeutic effect of digitalis is its positive inotropic effect, or its ability to increase myocardial _____. This action of digitalis is caused by a direct effect on the myocardial cells and is independent of its parasympathetic action. Digitalis enhances contractility by partial inhibition of the Na⁺-K⁺ pump. The accumulation of intracellular Na⁺ triggers the uptake of Ca⁺⁺, which activates the contractile proteins.

contractility

Improved contractility may result in further reductions in rate or prevent atrial arrhythmias caused by CHF.

85 Inhibition of the Na⁺-K⁺ pump also results in a deficit of intracellular K⁺.

The deficit in intracellular K^+ produces electrical instability by enhancing automaticity. This effect is magnified in the presence of hypokalemia. Thus the arrhythmias of digitalis toxicity are magnified in the presence of _____. The arrhythmias of digitalis toxicity are also enhanced in the presence of a low serum Mg^{++} level.

 REMEMBER: Mg^{++} is necessary to activate the _____ _____.

                      hypokalemia

                      Na^+-K^+ pump

86 In therapeutic dosages digitalis has these effects on the heart:
1. *(Increased/Decreased)* heart rate   Decreased
2. *(Accelerated/Depressed)* AV conduction   Depressed
3. *(Increased/Decreased)* myocardial contractility   Increased
 Therefore digitalis can be said to produce:
1. A *(positive/negative)* chronotropic effect   negative
2. A *(positive/negative)* dromotropic effect   negative
3. A *(positive/negative)* inotropic effect   positive

87 Toxic effects of digitalis therapy include anorexia, nausea, vomiting, fatigue, yellow-green halos around visual images, disturbances in red-green color perception, and the digitalis-toxicity arrhythmias. Hyperkalemia has also been reported with severe digitalis toxicity.

 REMEMBER: Digitalis enhances contractility by partially inhibiting the _____ pump. The Na^+-K^+ pump actively pumps Na^+ out of the cell and K^+ _____ the cells, maintaining the concentration _____ for each ion (see Unit 4, Frames 71 to 75). Thus suppression of this pump leaves more K^+ _____ of the cell, *(raising/lowering)* the serum K^+.

                      Na^+-K^+

                      into

                      gradient

                      out; raising

88 The arrhythmias of digitalis toxicity are a manifestation of either enhanced _____, or depressed _____, or both. Digitalis has the ability to increase automaticity in the atria, AV junctional tissue, and ventricles. In the presence of digitalis toxicity, this property may lead to the development of the following arrhythmias (Fig. 10-8):
1. PAT with block
2. Nodal or junctional tachycardia
3. Ventricular arrhythmias, especially ventricular bigeminy
 NOTE: A fourth arrhythmia, which occurs much less commonly but is also characteristic of digitalis toxicity arrhythmias, is birectional ventricular tachycardia, which gives the initial ECG appearance of a bigeminal rhythm (see Fig. 10-8, B).

                      automaticity

                      conduction

89 The ventricular arrhythmias of digitalis toxicity may be treated with lidocaine but may also respond to diphenylhydantoin. Symptomatic junctional tachycardia may be treated with either diphenylhydantoin or propranolol. The ventricular rates of PAT with block are usually not rapid, and therefore aggressive therapy is rarely indicated. Cessation of the digitalis and/or electrolyte replacement as needed may suffice.

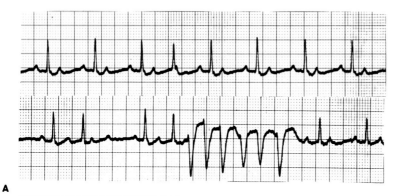

A

Fig. 10-8

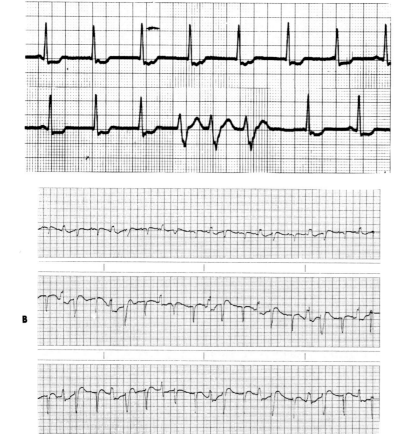

B

NOTE: Leads I, II, and III taken simultaneously.

90 Severe, potentially life-threatening digitalis toxicity may also be treated with the recently approved Digoxin Immune Fab (Digibind), which has been under investigation since the 1970s.

Digibind consists of fragments of digoxin-specific antibodies obtained from sheep serum. The key antigen binding fragments, referred to as "Fab", bind to the digoxin, inactivating it and facilitating its excretion through the kidney. Antibody fragments are less antigenic and allow for an earlier onset of action than a complete antibody. Allergic reactions have not been reported. The dose is determined from the serum level or the amount of tablets ingested (with overdose).

A therapeutic effect of arrhythmia control may be seen within minutes of administration. Resolution of all toxic effects is usually seen within 2-3 hours. Serum digitalis levels typically rise following the administration of Digibind and remain distorted for up to one week. This increase in digitalis concentration includes the bound fragments which have been inactivated and *(should/should not)* be of concern.

should not

When reversal of toxicity occurs too rapidly, *(hyperkalemia/ hypokalemia)* may occur. For this reason, serum and ECG effects should be monitored during the administration of Digibind.

hypokalemia

Other arrhythmias associated with digitalis toxicity are related to depressed automaticity in the SA node and depressed conduction (for example, sinus bradycardia and AV block).

91 The AV blocks most typically asiocated with digitalis toxicity include first-degree, second-degree (Wenkebach or Mobitz I), and third-degree AV block with an *(idiojunctional/idioventricular)* response.

idiojunctional
AV node

REMEMBER: These forms of AV block are associated with *(AV node/ bundle branch)* block (see Unit 7, Frames 153 to 162 and 171 to 176). Symptomatic AV block caused by digitalis is usually responsive to atropine therapy. However, isoproterenol and/or temporary pacing may also be used if necessary. For severe AV block unresponsive to these measures, Digibind may be used.

92 Digitalis also has an effect on the ECG that is not necessarily associated with toxicity, and may appear only during exercise, making it difficult at times to distinguish from ischemic changes.

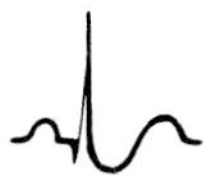

DIGITALIS EFFECT

Fig. 10-9

REMEMBER: The electrolyte that affects contractility is
_____. Ca^{++} affects the _____ segment on the   calcium; ST
ECG. The effect of digitalis on the ECG is to shorten the
_____ segment. Digitalis also causes sagging of the ST seg-   ST
ment. Ischemic changes do not typically shorten the ST segment.

NOTE: Another parasympathetic stimulator that may be used in
some settings to manage rapid supraventricular arrhythmias is edro-
phonium chloride (Tensilon).

93 NURSING ORDERS: Patients receiving digitalis for fast supraventricular
arrhythmia

1. Observe for the therapeutic effects of digitalis.
   NOTE: Digitalis may slow the heart rate simply by improving
   myocardial function.
   —Is heart failure improving?
   —Is heart rate slowing?
2. Observe for the development of anorexia.
   NOTE: This development is often the first sign of digitalis intol-
   erance.
3. Watch for the development of nausea and vomiting.
4. Monitor the patient carefully for development of arrhythmias:
   —PAT with block
   —Junctional _____   tachycardia
   —Ventricular   arrhythmias,   especially   ventricular
   _____, and bidirectional VT   bigeminy
   —Sinus bradycardia
   —AV block
5. Check serum potassium levels.
6. Elevate renal function.
   For further information on digitalis see Frame 140.
7. When administering Digibind for severe digitalis toxicity,
   monitor for high temperature or low BP due to allergic reactions, and ECG for K$^+$ effects.

Esmolol (beta blocker)

94 The sympathetic beta-blocking drug esmolol (Brevibloc) was recently introduced for the acute management of supraventricular tachyarrhythmias. It is shorter acting than the prototype beta-blocking
agent propanolol (Inderal) and is more selective in its action.

Prior to the availability of the Ca^{++} channel blocker verapamil,
propranolol was commonly used in the management of acute supraventricular tachyarrhythmias. Propranolol and the other beta-
blocking agents are currently used primarily in the chronic management of both supraventricular and ventricular arrhythmias. Beta
blockers, such as esmolol and propranolol, are particularly effective
in controlling arrhythmias, which are stress-related.

REMEMBER: Drugs that block the beta receptors of the sympathetic nervous system produce these effects on the heart and lungs:
1. Decreased heart rate (negative _____ effect)   chronotropic
2. Depressed AV conduction (negative _____ ef-   dromotropic
   fect)
3. Decreased myocardial contractility (negative
   _____ effect)   inotropic
4. Depressed automaticity (ventricular, atrial, junctional)
5. Bronchoconstriction

95 The actions of beta blockers in supraventricular arrhythmias are the following:
    1. To slow _____ conduction   AV
    2. To depress ectopic formation in the _____ or AV   atria
       _____. Therefore it will slow the ventricular   junction
       _____ of these arrhythmias and convert or prevent   rate
       them from occurring. Propranolol may also be used in the man-
       agement of _____ arrhythmias.   ventricular

96 Major toxic effects of beta-blocker therapy include bronchospasm
    and heart failure as well as (hypertension/hypotension) and (bradycardia/ hypotension; bradycardia
    tachycardia)
        Esmolol is cardioselective, producing less toxic effects on the
    lungs and vascular bed, and mimicking most closely the action of the
    beta blocking agent metoprolol (Lopressor).
        Unlike metaprolol, however, esmolol is available for IV use only.
    Its onset and duration of action is also shorter than metoprolol.

97 Esmolol is administered as an IV drip only. Titration is complex, be-
    ginning at an initial loading dose of 500 mcg/kg/min. for 1 minute
    followed by an infusion of 50 mcg/kg/min. for 4 minutes. This se-
    quence is repeated q5min, increasing the second dose by 50 mcg/kg/
    min until a response is seen or a dose of 200 mcg/kg/min. is reached.
    A maintenance infusion may be continued at the second dose range
    minus 25 mcg/kg/min. The drug is more effective in patients receiv-
    ing concurrent digitalis therapy. The drip is discontinued over 1 ½
    hrs as new oral agents are introduced or the doses of these are in-
    creased.
        Esmolol has been shown to be equally effective as IV propanolol
    in controlling supraventricular tachyarrhythmias. The major adverse
    reaction reported is hypotension—usually asymptomatic and resolv-
    ing within 30 minutes of discontinuing the drug. This side effect oc-
    curs more often than with IV propanolol. Merely lowering the dose
    range may also be effective. Bradycardia, dose-related bronchos-
    pasm and CHF, and nausea have also been reported in other stud-
    ies. If these occur, rapid recovery is possible.

98 LET US REVIEW: Esmolol is an IV *(sympathetic/parasympathetic)* blocking agent, which may be used in the initial management of *(ventricular/ supraventricular)* arrhythmias. Esmolol is *(short/long)* acting, and produces blockade of the *(alpha/beta)* receptors with _____ selectivity. The major reported side effect is _____.

sympathetic
supraventricular
short
beta; cardio
hypotension

99 Only one study is currently available comparing the efficacy of esmolol to verapamil. This study reported a greater effectiveness with esmolol. Esmolol also has a shorter duration of action and may be less potent a suppressant on the AV node than verapamil. For these reasons, some physicians choose this agent in lieu of verapamil for the initial therapy of *(ventricular/supraventricular)* tachyarrhythmias, using verapamil only in patients unresponsive to esmolol.

supraventricular

However, to date, esmolol remains less popular than verapamil. It is the authors' opinion that this is due to the greater complexity in preparing and administering this agent, in spite of shortcuts provided by the manufacturer.

Although the administration of verapamil may follow esmolol, the converse is not true due to the longer half-life of verapamil.

100 NURSING ORDERS: Patients receiving esmolol for a fast supraventricular arrhythmia
1. Thirty minutes following the administration of an oral agent, reduce the Brevibloc infusion rate by one-half. Discontinue the infusion one hour after the second dose.
2. If hypotension occurs, decrease or stop the infusion.
3. Monitor breath sounds (wheezes/rales) and heart rate, especially at higher dose ranges.
4. Avoid in patients with renal failure.
5. Do not administer IV verapamil following Brevibloc.

Vasopressor agents

101 Another group of drugs that may be used in the management of rapid supraventricular arrhythmias is the vasopressor drugs. Drugs such as norepinephrine (Levophed), metaraminol bitartrate (Aramine), and phenylephrine hydrochloride (Neo-Synephrine) have both alpha and beta properties. They act as alpha stimulators on the blood vessels and cause *(vasoconstriction/vasodilation)*. These drugs have some beta-stimulating properties on the heart and cause a slight positive intropic effect and a(n) *(increase/decrease)* in heart rate. Norepinephrine, metaraminol, and phenylephrine exhibit predominantly _____ adrenergic effects. These drugs can temporarily elevate the blood pressure above normal limits by constricting the _____ _____ and increasing the peripheral _____ resistance.

vasoconstriciton

increase

alpha-

blood vessels
vascular

REMEMBER: In the presence of a high blood pressure, the

_____ receptors are activated, causing a _____, or _____, response. Subsequent _____ of the heart rate occurs. Carotid sinus pressure may also be more effective in the presence of this pressoreceptor response.

presso-; vagal
parasympathetic
slowing

102 NURSING ORDERS: Patients receiving norepinephrine, metaraminol, or phenylephrine, for rapid supraventricular arrhythmia
1. Monitor BP and cardiac status closely.
—Avoid severe increase in BP.
—Watch for development of PVCs.
2. Avoid infiltration into subcutaneous tissue; norepinephrine may cause severe tissue sloughing.
NOTE: The antidote used to counteract the effects of norepinephrine on the subcutaneous tissue is phentolamine (Regitine).
3. Patients receiving these drugs will probably have cold, clammy skin.

Drugs for bradyarrhythmias

103 Let us now consider the problem of bradyarrhythmias.
REMEMBER: The initial therapy in the management of bradyarrhythmias is directed toward increasing the _____ _____. The mechanisms by which the ventricular rate may be accelerated are the following:
1. Increasing the sinus rate
2. Accelerating AV conduction
3. Stimulating AV junctional automaticity
4. Stimulating ventricular automaticity
The drugs that are capable of increasing the ventricular rate are (1) the parasympathetic blockers and (2) the beta stimulators.

ventricular rate

Atropine (parasympathetic blocker)

104 An example of a drug that blocks the parasympathetic nervous system is atrophic. The parasympathetic nerve that innervates the heart is the vagus nerve; therefore, atropine is also known as a vagolytic drug.
REMEMBER: Drugs that block the parasympathetic nervous system have these effects of the heart: *(increased/decreased)* heart rate and *(accelerated/depressed)* AV conduction. Atropine has the ability to stimulate the sinus rate and accelerate AV conduction and thus to increase the ventricular rate.
REMEMBER: Bradyarrhythmias may result in a symptomatic fall in cardiac output. In this setting acceleration of the ventricular rate *(is/ is not)* indicated. Selected studies indicate that caution must be used when one accelerates the heart rate in a recently injured ischemic

increased; accelerated

is

myocardium. One should accelerate the ventricular rate gradually, using small increments of atropine until the patient's symptoms disappear. Acceleration, even moderate acceleration, has been shown to increase myocardial O_2 consumption in the ischemic areas, causing an unfavorable, relation between myocardial O_2 supply and demand. A manifestation of this increase in O_2 consumption may be ventricular arrhythmias associated with ischemia.

105 Another undesirable effect of atropine is its ability to produce urinary retention. The bladder is innervated by parasympathetic fibers; thus blockage of these nerves may lead to difficulty in voiding for some patients. Prolonged atropine therapy may cause mental confusion, which has been labeled "atropine madness" or "atropine psychosis." Additional side effects associated with atropine therapy include dryness of the mouth, flushing of the face, and dilation of the pupils.

NOTE: Atropine is generally contraindicated in patients with glaucoma; however, in emergency settings it may be used if mitotic eye drops are concurrently administered.

106 LET US REVIEW: Atropine is classified as a *(parasympathetic/sympathetic)* _____. Therapeutic effects of atropine include (1) an *(increased/decreased)* sinus rate and (2) *(accelerated/depressed)* AV conduction. Undesirable side effects of atropine include (1) urinary _____ and (2) mental _____. Other side effects associated with atropine include (1) _____ of the mouth, (2) _____ of the face, and (3) _____ of the pupils.

parasympathetic
blocker
increased; accelerated

retention; confusion

dryness; flushing
dilation

107 NURSING ORDERS: Patient receiving atropine for bradyarrhythmia
1. Monitor the heart rate for the therapeutic response when administering atropine.
2. Watch for the development of urinary retention.
3. With prolonged atropine therapy, watch for changes in sensorium.
4. Atropine is generally contraindicated in patients with _____.

glaucoma

Isoproterenol (sympathetic stimulator)

108 An example of a pure beta stimulator is isoproterenol hydrochloride (Isuprel).

REMEMBER: Drugs that stimulate the beta receptors of the sympathetic nervous system produce these effects on the heart, lungs, and blood vessels.
1. Increased heart rate (positive _____ effect)

chronotropic

2. Accelerated _____ conduction (positive _____ effect)

    AV
    dromotropic

3. Increased myocardial _____ (_____ effect)

    contractility
    inotropic

4. Increased AV junctional automaticity

5. Increased ventricular _____

    automaticity

6. *(Bronchoconstriction/Bronchodilation)*

    Bronchodilation

7. Peripheral vasodilation

Isoproterenol has the ability to *(increase/decrease)* the sinus rate, *(accelerate/depress)* AV conduction, *(increase/decrease)* AV junctional automaticity, and *(increase/decrease)* ventricular automaticity. Therefore it may be used in the management of bradyarrhythmias.

    increase; accelerate
    increase
    increase

Isoproterenol is currently considered a second-line agent in this setting, its use being limited to those bradyarrhythmias refractory to atropine only when an external (transthoracic) pacemaker is not available (see Unit 11, Frames 65 to 66).

109 Isoproterenol is given as a continuous intravenous infusion and must be titrated carefully to prevent tachyarrhythmias and ventricular arrhythmias.

NOTE: These side effects may also be noted when isoproterenol is used in respiratory therapy as a bronchial _____.

    dilator

The peripheral vasodilating actions of isoproterenol may potentiate bleeding. Epinephrine may be used as an alternate drug in these settings because of its additional alpha-stimulating effects.

110 LET US REVIEW: Isoproterenol is classified as a pure *(alpha/beta)* _____.

    beta stimulator

Therapeutic effects of isoproterenol include the following:

1. *(Increased/Decreased)* heart rate

    Increased

2. *(Accelerated/Depressed)* AV conduction

    Accelerated

3. *(Increased/Decreased)* myocardial contractility

    Increased

4. *(Increased/Decreased)* AV junctional automaticity

    Increased

5. *(Increased/Decreased)* ventricular automaticity

    Increased

6. Bronchial *(constriction/dilation)*

    dilation

On the peripheral blood vessels, isoproterenol acts as a *(vasodilator/vasoconstrictor)*.

    vasodilator

NOTE: Isoproterenol, like other inotropic agents, also causes increased O_2 consumption by the heart. For this reason and its effect on electrical instability, isoproterenol is not indicated in the management of shock.

NURSING ORDERS: Patient receiving isoproterenol for bradyarrhythmia

    1. Monitor BP and cardiac status closely.

    2. Watch for the development of tachyarrhythmias and ventricular arrhythmias with isoproterenol.

DRUG THERAPY IN THE MANAGEMENT OF HEART FAILURE

111 Heart failure has been defined as inadequate cardiac output to meet the _____ of the tissues, with the _____ being the direct cause of the imbalance. Heart failure is distinguished from cardiogenic shock by the absence of direct _____ _____ of hypoxia (see Unit 9). The major goals in the pharmacological management of heart failure are (1) to decrease pulmonary and systemic congestion and/or (2) to improve cardiac output. Pulmonary congestions is decreased by decreasing _____ return. Cardiac output may be improved by either directly stimulating the myocardium or reducing the cardiac _____ _____.

demands; pump

tissue symptoms

venous

work load

112 Initial therapy in the management of heart failure in acute MI was formerly directly toward stimulating myocardial contractility with digitalis. The current emphasis on preservation of ischemic myocardium has discredited the routine use of inotropic agents, such as digitalis, that also increase myocardial O_2 consumption, or MVO_2. Drugs that reduce cardiac work load (unload the heart), such as diuretics and vasodilators, are currently emphasized in the initial management of heart failure in acute MI.

Intravenous inotropic agents such as dopamine hydrochloride (Intropin) or dobutamine hydrochloride (Dobutrex) are used in the management of severe CHF. These agents are now commonly used in combination with vasodilators and diuretic therapy. Digitalis must be used with caution in the setting of acute MI and is not the preferred agent in this setting. The arrhythmogenic activity of digitalis may further complicate the situation.

113 LET US REVIEW: In the presence of left ventricular failure events occur that lead to the accumulation of fluid in the _____ and an increased cardiac work load (Fig. 10-3). See also Unit 3, frames 36 and 37, Fig. 4-9. These events include an *(increase/decrease)* in renal perfusion, which is caused by the _____ receptors ultimately resulting in the release of renin, angiotensin and _____.

This vicious cycle may be broken by unloading the heart (lungs) with the use of agents such as _____ and _____ and by supporting the contractile state with _____ agents. Pharmacological intervention for CHF caused by acute MI includes the use of the following agents, listed in the order of priority:
1. Diuretic agents
2. Vasodilators
3. Inotropic agents

lungs

decrease

presso

aldosterone

diuretics

vasodilators

inotropic

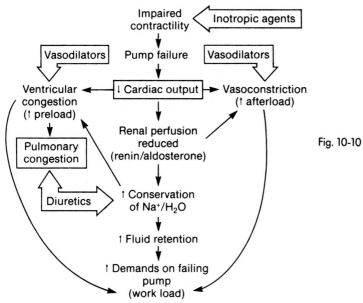

Fig. 10-10

Diuretic agents

114 Let us now discuss the role of diuretic agents in the pharmacological management of heart failure in acute MI. The primary goals in the management of heart failure are to decrease _____ _____ and to improve cardiac _____. Diuretic agents act principally to decrease pulmonary congestion. They also improve cardiac output by decreasing cardiac work load.

    REMEMBER: Cardiac work load, or mycoardial O_2 consumption, is a function of (1) heart rate, (2) preload (radius) or _____ return, (3) afterload, and (4) contractility. Diuretics decrease pulmonary congestion and cardiac work load by decreasing volume and venous return. Diuretics thus decrease the radius of the heart during diastole and lower the _____.

pulmonary congestion

output

venous

preload

115 Diuretics are classified according to their mechanism of action and site of action in the nephron of the kidney. The action common to most diuretic agents is to inhibit tubular reabsorption of Na^+. Diuretics may also act by increasing renal blood flow or altering hormonal effects on the kidney tubules.

    REMEMBER: Water usually moves with Na^+. Thus, as Na^+ is excreted, so is _____. Excretion of water acts to decrease circulating _____ and thus decrease _____ return, *(preload/afterload),* and _____ congestion.

water

volume

venous; preload

pulmonary

The focus of this discussion is on those diuretic agents commonly used in acute coronary settings. These include the loop diuretics, osmotic agents, and the selective renovascular dilator dopamine. Other commonly used diuretic agents are referred to in Table 12 and include the thiazides, potassium-sparing agents, and carbonic anhydrase inhibitors.

Loop diuretics

116 Furosemide (Lasix), bumetanide (Bumex), and ethacrynic acid (Edecrin), are classified as loop diuretics because they act primarily by inhibiting sodium reabsorption in the ascending loop of Henle. Furosemide has other characteristics that add to its usefulness in acute settings. It decreases _____ congestion and reduces cardiac work load by at least two mechanisms.

pulmonary

IV furosemide is usually the diuretic of choice for severe congestive heart failure due to its immediate venodilating effect and effectiveness even in the presence of a low renal blood flow. The venodilating effect decreases the venous return to the heart and lungs and reduces the *(preload/afterload).*

preload

The left ventricular filling (wedge) pressure *(rises/falls).* Furosemide also reduces circulating blood volume by its diuretic effect. The immediate fall in LVEDP with IV furosemide may precede the diuretic effect and provide immediate symptomatic relief.

falls

117 Bumetanide differs from furosemide primarily in its potency allowing for small doses to be effective, even in patients not responsive to furosemide. Ototoxicity is less but renal toxicity is greater (see frame 118).

Therapy with potent diuretics, such as furosemide or ethacrynic acid, may result in hypovolemia and electrolyte depletion. Hypovolemia may result in hypotension from the reduction of circulating _____ _____. The most common electrolyte disturbance associated with the use of furosemide is *(hypokalemia/hyperkalemia).* Chloride (Cl^-), an anion, is frequently lost with the K^+. When an anion, in this case Cl^-, is lost, the body attempts to compensate by retaining another anion, _____. This may eventually cause a metabolic *(acidosis/alkalosis).* Loss of H^+ may also contribute to the alkalosis. Potassium replacement solutions must also contain chloride if metabolic *(acidosis/alkalosis)* is to be prevented.

blood volume
hypokalemia

HCO_3
alkalosis

alkalosis

118 Reports of deafness (ototoxicity) and abnormal liver function tests after large doses of ethacrynic acid have discouraged routine use of this diuretic. An additional limitation is the preparation time. However, in an occasional patient refractory to furosemide therapy, it may produce significant diuresis and thus be clinically useful. Ototoxicity has also been reported with the use of furosemide but is more transient than that caused by ethacrynic acid therapy.

119 LET US REVIEW: Diuretics that initiate Na^+ reabsorption in the ascending loop of Henle are known as _____ diuretics.

loop

The most commonly used loop diuretic in the CCU is _____. IV furosemide decreases pulmonary congestion by producing _____ dilation and decreasing _____ volume. Furosemide decreases the cardiac work load by decreasing the _____.

furosemide
venous
circulating
preload

As a result of the effects on venous return and preload, furosemide also *(increases/decreases)* LVEDP. The immediate decrease in LVEDP and symptomatic relief following an IV bolus of furosemide may precede the _____ effect. The most common electrolyte disturbance associated with the use of furosemide is _____. Ototoxicity has been reported with the use of _____ and _____ _____.

decreases

diuretic

hypokalemia
furosemide; ethacrynic acid

Osmotic diuretics: mannitol

120 The osmotic diuretic most commonly used in patients with coronary artery disease is mannitol. Albumin (25%), although not specifically classified as a diuretic, has osmotic diuretic effects similar to those of mannitol.

NOTE: The increased concentration of glucose in GIK solutions may also exert an osmotic diuretic effect. Osmotic diuretics increase urine flow by (1) increasing plasma tonicity (osmolality) and thus mobilizing excess fluid from the cells and interstitial spaces and (2) increasing the osmolality of the glomerular filtrate.

121 Mannitol is a hypertonic solution, compared with the body fluids.

REMEMBER: A hypertonic solution has a *(greater/lesser)* concentration of dissolved particles than another solution, for example, the interstitial or intracellular fluid. Mannitol is given only by the IV route. Administration of a hypertonic agent into the plasma causes fluid to move from the _____ and _____ spaces into the vascular space. Hypertonic agents produce an immediate *(increase/decrease)* in circulating blood volume.

greater

intracellular
interstitial
increase

122 Subsequent increased fluid flow to the kidneys promotes diuresis.

REMEMBER: The ability of hypertonic solutions to expand circulating blood volume rapidly requires that one exercise caution when using them in the presence of fluid overload. If diuresis does not occur, the nurse should rapidly assess the patient for an increase in heart failure caused by fluid overload. Administration of mannitol is less hazardous in the treatment of local fluid accumulation, such as cerebral or myocardial edema caused by hypoxic injury.

123 After IV administration mannitol is freely filtered by the kidneys but cannot be reabsorbed. It thereby increases the osmolality (tonicity) of the glomerular filtrate and promotes Na^+ and water loss, primarily through the proximal tubules of the nephrons. The major diuretic effect of mannitol is probably by means of this mechanism.

Mannitol is most commonly used in coronary care to establish urine flow in oliguria with suspected impending acute tubular necrosis or in refractory pulmonary edema. Mannitol may also be used to confirm the presence of prerenal, as opposed to intrarenal, mechanisms in states of low urine output. Mannitol is generally not used in the acute management of heart failure because of its initial effect of increasing _____ volume. Potential complications of therapy with mannitol include cellular dehydration and worsening of heart failure.

circulating

124 LET US REVIEW: Administration of an osmotic diuretic such as mannitol causes fluid to move from the _____ and _____ fluid into the _____ space. Subsequent increased fluid flow to the kidneys promotes _____. Mannitol is freely filtered in the nephrons of the _____ but cannot be _____. The osmolality of the _____ _____ is thus (increased/decreased), and Na^+ and _____ are lost, resulting in diuresis. Potential complications of mannitol therapy include _____ dehydration and the worsening of _____ _____.

cells
interstitial; vascular

diuresis
kidneys
reabsorbed
glomerular
 filtrate; increased
water
cellular
heart failure

Albumin (25%)

125 Albumin, a plasma protein, is not classified as a diuretic. However, it may be used to mobilize edema fluid because of its influence on oncotic as well as osmotic pressure (see Unit 4).

REMEMBER: One major force is responsible for holding fluid within the vascular compartment—serum _____ osmotic pressure (oncotic pressure). This force is exerted by the largely nondiffusible plasma _____, the primary one being _____.

colloid

proteins
albumin

126 When hypoalbuminemia is present because of such things as stress, liver disease, or malnutrition, oncotic pressure (increases/decreases). As a result, fluid moves more easily from the vascular compartment into the _____ spaces. Albumin increases plasma on-

decreases

interstitial

cotic pressure and promotes fluid movement back from the interstitial spaces to the _____.

plasma

127 Because of its ability to increase circulating blood volume, albumin (25%) should be administered very slowly in patients with heart failure. Close monitoring of hemodynamic parameters—such as pulmonary artery pressures, PCWP, arterial pressure, and cardiac output profiles—is desirable to prevent worsening of heart failure.

Albumin may be used for purposes similar to those of mannitol in the patient with coronary artery disease.

Selective renovascular dilator: dopamine

128 Dopamine (Intropin) is a sympathomimetic drug that has both alpha-stimulating and beta-stimulating properties and selective renal actions in specific dose ranges. It is used primarily for its B_1-stimulating effects or its action on the *(heart/kidney)* and is most commonly known as a positive inotropic agent (see Frames 147 to 153).

heart

REMEMBER: A drug that has a positive inotropic effect increases _____. The ability of dopamine to induce diuresis is related to both its cardiac action and its ability to dilate the _____ arteries selectively at low dosages, thus *(increasing/decreasing)* renal blood flow.

contractility

renal; increasing

129 When administered at low dosages, dopamine selectively dilates the renal arteries, thereby promoting renal blood flow and inducing _____. When administered in moderate to high dosages, the cardiotonic effects predominate. Improvement in cardiac output by these effects also enhances renal blood flow and thus induces _____. A more thorough discussion of dopamine and nursing orders relating to its administration are presented in the section on inotropic agents (see Frames 143 to 149).

diuresis

diuresis

LET US REVIEW: Cardiotonic agents such as dopamine may induce diuresis by improving _____ _____ or by direct effects on the _____. Dopamine selectively dilates the _____ arteries at *(low/high)* dosages and thereby promotes _____.

cardiac output

kidneys
renal; low
diuresis

130 NURSING ORDERS: Patient receiving diuretic agents for management of heart failure.
  1. Observe for therapeutic effects following administration.
     —Is there an increase in urine output?
     —Is heart failure improving?
     —Is symptomatology diminishing?

—Is wedge pressure decreasing?
—Are rales diminishing:
2. Accurately record intake and output.
3. Watch for the development of complications.
—Hypovolemia and hypotension: assess hydration status.
—Hypokalemia: check serum K^+ levels; note whether patient is receiving potassium chloride supplements.
—Metabolic alkalosis: check arterial pH and HCO_3^- levels on ABG samples, check total carbon dioxide on serum electrolytes.
—Hypomagnesemia: check serum Mg^{++} levels.
4. Monitor daily serum electrolytes, BUN, and creatinine.
5. With administration of furosemide and ethacrynic acid, watch for symptoms of ototoxicity (tinnitus, deafness).
6. With albumin (25%) and mannitol administration, watch for worsening of heart failure caused by initial increase in circulating blood volume.

Table 13. Summary chart: diuretics

Classifications	Common agents	Chief site of action*	Primary complications
Loop diuretics	Furosemide (Lasix) Bumetanide Ethacrynic (Edecrin) (Bumex)	Ascending limp; loop of Henle	Hypokalemia; hypovolemia; metabolic alkalosis ototoxicity
Thiazides and related agents	Chlorothiazide (Diuril); hydrochlorothiazide (HydroDiuril, Esidrix, Oretic); Chlorthalidone (Hygroton)	Distal tubule	Hypokalemia; metabolic alkalosis, hyperglycemia uric acid cholesterol
Renovascular dilator	Dopamine (Intropin) (in low dosage)	Increased cardiac output Selectively dilates renal arteries in low doses	Tachyarrhythmias
Osmotic agents	Mannitol; albumin (25%); glucose	Proximal tubule	Cellular dehydration; worsening of heart failure
Potassium-sparing agents	Spironolactone (Aldactone); triamterene (Dyrenium)	Distal tubule; collecting duct	Hyperkalemia
Carbonic anhydrase inhibitors	Acetazolamide (Diamox)	Proximal tubule	Hyperchloremia; metabolic acidosis

*The site of actions of most diuretic agents is multiple. The chief site listed is a general consensus derived from several texts.

Vasodilators

131 Another group of drugs currently being used in the management of heart failure is the *vasodilators*. They are most typically indicated in severe CHF when either diuretic or digitalis or both have been

ineffective. These agents are also being used in acute settings to treat angina and hypertension and to preserve ischemic myocardium. The general effect of the vasodilators is to *decrease the cardiac work load* or unload the heart by acting on either preload, afterload, or both. *Pulmonary congestion* and *cardiac output* may also improve. Certain vasodilators produce a greater improvement in cardiac output, whereas others primarily decrease _____   pulmonary congestion
_____. These selective actions are related to the dilating effects of the agents on either the *arterial* or *venous* systems or on both.

132 The major categories of vasodilators currently used in the management of CHF include: 1) the direct vasodilators, such as nitroprusside, the nitrates, and hydralazine; 2) the alpha-adrenergic blocking agents, such as prazosin; and 3) angiotensin-converting enzyme (ACE) inhibitors, such as captropril and enalapril.

NOTE: Calcium channel blockers (a subcategory of direct vasodilators) may also be effective, but need to be used with caution due to a potentially significant negative inotropic effect. Nifedipine is preferred.

133 Dilation of the venous bed increases venous capacity and decreases venous return, thus reducing ventricular *(preload/afterload)*. Reduction of preload reduces LVEDP and will *(increase/decrease)* pulmonary congestion. Cardiac output may also improve, since the heart is able to function more efficiently at optimal filling pressures. Dilation of the arterial bed decreases arteriolar resistance and thus primarily reduces *(preload/afterload)*. Reduction of afterload decreases resistance to left ventricular emptying, thus facilitating left ventricular ejection. As a result the cardiac output *(increases/decreases)*.

    preload
    decrease

    afterload

    increases

134 In the normotensive patient with heart failure the SVR is typically *(high/low)*. In this setting the cautious use of vasodilators affecting the arterial bed facilitates left ventricular ejection and improves the cardiac output.

    high

REMEMBER: In patients with acute MI and left ventricular failure an initial *(symptomatic/asymptomatic)* fall in cardiac output is associated with a reflexive rise in SVR, which may further impede and actually lower the cardiac output. However, the blood pressure may remain normal because blood pressure is a product of both _____ _____ and _____.

    asymptomatic

    cardiac output
    SVR

In this setting reduction of SVR with vasodilators may produce little or no change in the arterial pressure while improving the cardiac output. That is because the improvement in cardiac output usually offsets the reduction in SVR. However, as a precaution in this setting, these drugs are initially administered slowly and in small doses. Their effects on hemodynamic parameters are also carefully monitored.

135 Larger doses are usually required in the hypertensive patient with heart failure caused by severe, chronically sustained elevation in _____. This increase in SVR also compromises the _____ _____. However, administration of vasodilators in this setting is less hazardous and may not rerquire such aggressive hemodynamic monitoring. The arterial blood pressure must still be frequently checked, and invasive hemodynamic monitoring is preferred.

 Because of their effect on the preload, or the *(venous/arterial)* bed, the use of venous vasodilators in patients with normal or low filling pressurers may result in hypotensive episodes and reflexive tachyarrhythmias. The systemic pressoreceptors are activated, resulting in a compensatory tachycardia.

SVR
cardiac output

venous

136 The vasodilators most commonly being used in the management of acute MI complicated by CHF are the nitrates and nitroprusside since they may both be administered intravenously. The general effect of these agents is to _____ the heart by reducing _____ or _____ or both. Cardiac output and tissue perfusion may also improve.

unload
preload; afterload

Nitroprusside

137 Sodium nitroprusside (Nipride) acts directly on the smooth muscle blood vessels, dilating both the venous and arterial beds. It reduces preload by producing *(arterial/venous)* dilation and afterload by producing _____ dilation. Nitroprusside may help preserve ischemic myocardium by reduction of both _____ and _____. Its effects on preload and afterload reduction are balanced, so that neither effect predominates. Thus the hemodynamic improvements seen with nitroprusside therapy are related to both preload and _____ reduction. Reduction in preload reduces LVEDP and thereby decreases _____ congestion. Reduction in arterial resistance, or _____, reduces impedance to left ventricular emptying and thus *(increases/decreases)* cardiac output. Improvement in cardiac output is usually the major goal in nitroprusside therapy.

venous
arterial

afterload; preload

afterload
pulmonary
afterload
increases

138 Nitroprusside is administered only by the IV route and thus is used only in an acute setting. When used in *normotensive* patients, it should be administered only in intensive cardiac care units capable of hemodynamic monitoring. Factors such as pulmonary artery pressures, wedge pressure, arterial pressure, and cardiac output profiles should be monitored.

In the normotensive patient with heart failure, excessive reduction of afterload (mean arterial pressure) may significantly compromise coronary filling and jeopardize ischemic myocardium.

LET US REVIEW: The major goal of nitroprusside therapy is usually _____ in _____ _____. This effect is currently best evaluated by *(invasive/noninvasive)* monitoring of cardiac output. The major complications of nitroprusside administration are:

improvement; cardiac output

invasive

1. Excessive reduction in preload
2. Excessive reduction in afterload
3. A fall in cardiac output

139 Excessive preload reduction can be detected by monitoring _____ pressures; excessive afterload reduction can be detected by monitoring _____ pressures. Thus before and immediately after initiating nitroprusside therapy—especially in the normotensive individual—measurements of at least _____ pressure and _____ pressure should be obtained. Measurement of cardiac output, SVR, and PVR is also preferred. These parameters should be measured at regular intervals throughout the course of the therapy.

wedge

arterial

arterial; wedge

140 Nitroprusside contains cyanide as a part of its molecular structure. Metabolism of nitroprusside by the liver results in the release of cyanide, which is subsequently converted to thiocyanate. Long-term therapy with nitroprusside may result in cyanide or thiocyanate toxicity, which impairs tissue O_2 utilization. Renal dysfunction increases the risk of toxicity because these metabolic end products are excreted by the kidneys. If patients require therapy with nitroprusside for longer than 3 days, it is recommended that blood levels of cyanide and thiocyanate be evaluated.

Nitroprusside has also been shown to interfere with platelet function. This may contraindicate its use in certain patients.

NOTE: Signs of thiocyanate toxicity include tinnitus, blurred vision, and delirium. Signs of cyanide poisoning include coma, imperceptible pulse, absent reflexes, dilated pupils, pink color, hypotension, and shallow breathing. When signs of cyanide toxicity are present, amyl nitrite inhalations should be administered for 15 to 30 seconds each minute until 3% sodium nitrate solution can be prepared for IV administration.

141 LET US REVIEW: Nitroprusside produces a balanced reduction in _____ and _____.

preload; afterload

Reduction of preload reduces left ventricular _____ and thereby reduces _____ _____.

Reduction of afterload reduces _____ to left ventricular ejection, thereby increasing _____ _____. Reduction of both preload and afterload *(increases/decreases)* the cardiac work load and can also serve to preserve _____ _____.

Patients requiring therapy with nitroprusside for longer than 3 days should have _____ and _____ levels evaluated.

Cyanide poisoning interferes with _____ oxygenation. Nursing orders for the administration of nitroprusside are presented in Frame 142.

Nitroglycerin

142 Nitroglycerin, a nitrate, is commonly used in the acute and chronic management of heart failure. It is also used in the management of chest pain (see Frames 181 to 187). Nitroglycerin acts directly on the smooth muscle of the vascular bed. It reduces preload by producing *(venous/arterial)* dilation and reduces afterload by producing arterial _____. The predominant effect of nitroglycerin is on the venous bed. Therefore the beneficial hemodynamic effects seen with nitroglycerin therapy are primarily a result of reduction in *(preload/afterload)*.

SMALL-CAPS REMEMBER: Reduction of preload reduces LVEDP and thereby decreases _____ _____. There may also be an improvement in cardiac output, since the heart is able to function more efficiently at optimal filling pressure.

Reduction in diastolic filling pressure also decreases impedance to coronary filling and thus may improve coronary flow.

143 Nitroglycerin may also improve perfusion of ischemic areas by increasing blood flow in collateral vessels and/or relaxing spasm. Because of these effects on coronary blood flow, in the setting of acute MI or unstable angina nitroglycerin may be more ideally used than nitroprusside. Nitroglycerin may be administered sublingually, intravenously, orally, or topically. In the therapy of heart failure in an acute setting, it is usually administered by the IV, topical, or sublingual route.

144 As with other vasodilators, nitroglycerin administration may result in hypotension and reflexive tachyarrhythmias in patients with normal or low filling pressures. These effects are uncommon when nitroglycerin is used in the management of heart failure. The

end-diastolic pressure

pulmonary congestion
resistance
cardiac output
decreases

ischemic myocardium

cyanide
thiocyanate
tissue

venous
dilation

preload

pulmonary congestion

488

use of a Swan Ganz catheter has not proven to be critical even during continuous intravenous therapy. Frequent checking of arterial BP via cuff or arterial line is usually adequate (see Frame 185).

LET US REVIEW: The predominant effect of nitroglycerin is to dilate the *(veins/arteries)* and thereby reduce _____. Subsequent reduction of LVEDP (wedge pressure) decreases _____ _____. Nitroglycerin may also increase perfusion of critically ischemic areas by improving blood flow through _____ _____. The nursing orders for the patient receiving intravenous nitroglycerin for the management of heart failure are presented in combination with the orders for nitroprusside in Frame 142. Nursing orders for sublingual or topical nitroglycerin use are included in the management of chest pain (see Frame 187).

veins; preload

pulmonary congestion

collateral vessels

145 NURSING ORDERS: Patients receiving IV vasodilators in the management of heart failure

1. Monitor hemodynamic parameters, such as pulmonary artery pressures, wedge pressures, arterial pressure, cardiac output, SVR, and PVR, during infusion of IV vasodilators in the normotensive individual.
2. Determine with the physician the critical LVEDP (wedge pressure) and arterial pressure to be achieved.
3. Prepare prescribed dose of medication.
   —Preparation of nitroprusside:
   Protect from deterioration by light by wrapping the bottle in foil or other opaque material.
   Infuse only with microdrip or infusion pump.
   Change the solutions q 4 hours.
   Do not add other medications to IV solutions containing Nipride.
   —Preparation of nitroglycerin: nitroglycerin infusions should be mixed in glass containers to avoid adherence to plastic containers.
4. Monitor wedge pressure or PAEDP and arterial pressure frequently during the infusion.
   REMEMBER: Nitroprusside produces a balanced reduction in preload and afterload. Nitroglycerin, however, predominantly affects _____.

   preload

5. With nitroprusside therapy, determine the thiocyanate and cyanide levels after _____ hours. Nitroprusside may also inhibit _____ function. Thus one should monitor patients with bleeding tendencies carefully if they are receiving nitroprusside.

   72
   platelet

Isosorbide dinitrate

146 Isosorbide dinitrate (Isordil), a nitrate, acts directly on the smooth muscle of the vascular bed. It reduces preload by producing *(venous/arterial)* dilation and reduces afterload by producing *(venous/arterial)* dilation. As with nitroglycerin, the predominant effect of isosorbide is on the venous rather than on the arterial bed. Therefore the hemodynamic benefits seen with isosorbide therapy are primarily related to a reduciton in left ventricular filling pressure or *(preload/afterload)*. By reducing LVEDP or left ventricular filling pressure, one reduces pulmonary congestion, and accompanying symptoms are relieved. Isosorbide may be given sublingually or orally; a sustained effect may be achieved by either route. Nursing orders for the patient receiving isosorbide are presented in the section on chest pain (see Frame 187).

venous
arterial

preload

Captopril/Enalapril

147 Captopril (Capoten) and enalapril (Vasotec) are both classified as angiotensin converting enzyme (ACE) inhibitors. The ACE inhibitors dilate both the arterial and venous beds resulting in a reduction in both preload and _____. These agents *inhibit* the renin-angiotensin system.

REMEMBER: Renin is secreted in CHF in response to a _____ in cardiac output and ultimately results in an increased secretion of _____ and intense *(vasodilation/vasoconstriction)*. Inhibition of this response results in excretion of sodium and _____, retention of _____, and _____.

afterload

fall
aldosterone; vasoconstriction

water; K^+
vasodilation

148 These agents are often the vasodilators of choice in CHF since they effect both the hormonal and vascular responses in CHF. Unlike prazosin, tolerance does not develop—making these agents ideal for both acute and long-term therapy. These agents are also effective in the management of hypertension, particularly when associated with high renin levels.

They are ideally combined with non-K^+ sparing diuretics, such as the loop and thiazide diuretics, because of their K^+ retaining effects.

149 Two major groups of side effects that occur with ACE inhibitors are renal and immune effects. Drug-induced hyper _____ may further compromise patients with borderline renal function. Immune effects include loss of taste, rash, and neutropenia.

Contraindications for use include renal failure or severe renal disease and concomitant use with other agents that can potentially alter immune function, such as procainamide, hydralazine, tocainide, and probenecid.

kalemia

Hydralazine

150 Hydralazine hydrochloride (Apresoline) is another peripheral dilator being used in the management of both acute and chronic heart failure. The predominant effect of hydralazine is to dilate the arteral bed and thus reduce *(preload/afterload)*. As a result SVR *(increases/decreases),* and cardiac output *(increases/decreases).* Hydralazine may be used in combination with a nitrate to achieve a more balanced effect on preload and afterload reduction, particularly in patients with signs of congestion. A major disadvantage is the development of tolerance through long-term therapy.

afterload; decreases
increases

151 Side effects associated with the use of hydralazine include intractable headache, nausea, abdominal pain, and potentiation of ischemic events. Potentiation of ischemia without CHF may be caused by a reflexive tachycardia. However, in the management of CHF, dilators usually *(do/do not)* induce a reflexive tachycardia. Potention of ischemic events in this setting has been shown to be caused by a decrease in coronary perfusion gradient induced by the marked afterload reduction. Autoimmune symptoms, such as lupus, have been reported. An increase in renin may occur secondary to vasodilation resulting in Na^+ and fluid retention.

do not

Prazosin

152 Prazosin hydrochloride (Minipress) exerts a vasodilator action either by blocking the alpha receptors of the sympathetic nervous system.
REMEMBER: The alpha-adrenergic receptors are found primarily in the *(lungs/blood vessels).* Prazosin dilates both the venous and arterial beds and produces a balanced reduction in preload and afterload, as IV nitroprusside does.

blood vessels

Prazosin is currently in use as an oral antihypertensive agent and is being clinically investigated in the management of heart failure as-

Table 14. Summary of the vasodilators used in CHF

| Vasodilator drug | Predominant effect | | Effect on cardiac output |
	Afterload reduction (arterial bed)	Preload reduction (venous bed)	
Nitroprusside (Nipride)	X	X	Increase
Nitroglycerin		X	Slight increase or no change
Isosorbide (Isordil)		X	Slight increase or no change
Hydralazine (Apresoline)	X		Increase
Prazosin (Minipress)	X	X	Initial increase
Captopril (Capoten)	X	X	Increase
Enalapril (Vasotec)	X	X	Increase

sociated with acute MI, especially as a potential alternative to IV nitroprusside. Hemodynamic responses to initial doses of prazosin used in the management of heart failure hae been shown to be favorable. However, rapid development of drug tolerance and complete loss of favorable effects may occur with longer therapy. Further clinical studies will determine if prazosin has a role as a vasodilator in the management of heart failure. Reported side effects include dizziness, headache, nausea, and palpitations.

Inotropic agents

153 Inotropic agents may be administered to patients with CHF to stimulate myocardial _____ and thus to improve cardiac output. However, positive inotropic agents also *(increase/decrease)* myocardial O_2 consumption and may prove harmful to ischemic myocardium, resulting in further myocardial necrosis. Thus these agents must be used with caution in the setting of acute MI and are usually used in conjunction with unloading agents. Their use is limited to cases of severe left ventricular failure. The most common inotropic agents currently used in the management of CHF include digitalis, dopamine, dobutamine, and amrinone. The milder inotropic agents, dopamine, dobutamine, and amrinone are associated with fewer deleterious effects on ischemic myocardium as well as fewer arrhythmogenic effects. Thus these agents are currently preferred over digitalis in the acute, short-term management of *(mild/ severe)* CHF caused by MI.

contractility
increase

severe

Digitalis

154 REMEMBER: The major goals in the management of heart failure are to decrease _____ _____ and improve _____ _____. This may be accomplished by directly stimulating the _____ or reducing cardiac _____ _____.

pulmonary congestion
cardiac output
myocardium
work load

Digitalis may be indicated in the management of heart failure because it has a *(positive/negative)* inotropic effect and thus *(stimulates/depresses)* myocardial _____. However, inotropic agents also *(increase/decrease)* myocardial O_2 consumption. Therefore, when there is already a critical reduction in O_2 supply to the heart, digitalis must be used with _____. In the setting of acute MI, digitalis may cause extension of the infarcted area. The ischemic myocardium is also more sensitive to the effects of digitalis toxicity. Thus digitalis is not the drug of choice in the initial management of heart failure caused by MI. However, it may be indicated in the management of CHF that persists or is caused by other mechanisms.

positive; stimulates
contractility
increase

caution

155 REMEMBER: The undesirable side effects associated with digitalis therapy are (1) anorexia, (2) nausea and vomiting, (3) arrhythmias such as _____ with block, AV _____ tachycardias, ventricular arrhythmias, AV blocks, and sinus bradycardia. These effects are aggravated in the presence of hypoxia, hypokalemia, and hypomagnesemia and if severe may be reversed with Digibind (see Frame 90).

PAT; junctional

Dopamine and dobutamine

156 Dopamine hydrochloride (Intropin) may be indicated in some forms of severe CHF in preference to digitalis. Dopamine, within carefully controlled dose ranges, has the unique ability to produce an increase in myocardial contractility selectively, without significant increases in rate or arrhythmia formation.

REMEMBER: Dopamine is a *(sympathetic/parasympathetic)* chemical mediator with both _____ and _____ stimulating properties within specific dose ranges. It is a naturally existing _____ that acts as a precursor to _____ and is used by the body predominantly for its _____ effects (see Frame 111). In a moderate dose range (2 to 10 g/kg/minute) selective B_1 stimulation occurs. B_1 receptors line the *(cardiac/pulmonary)* musculature. Stimulation of B_1 receptors routinely produces an increase in heart _____ (chronotropic effect), an increase in _____ (dromotroptic effect), an increase in _____ (inotropic effect), and enhanced _____. However, the beta effects on dopamine are initially _____. Thus in this dose range only the inotropic effects are seen.

sympathetic
alpha-; beta-

catecholamine
norepinephrine
alpha

cardiac
rate
conduction
contractility
automaticity
selective

In dosages exceeding 10 μg/kg/minute, other B_1 properties begin to appear. These affects are seen in the form of tachycardia or ventricular arrhythmias or both.

REMEMBER: Tachycardias *(increase/decrease)* myocardial O_2 consumption and may further compromise an ischemic myocardium.

increase

In dosages exceeding 10 to 20 μg/kg/minute, alpha-adrenergic properties appear.

REMEMBER: Dopamine is a precursor to the alpha-adrenergic chemical _____ (Levophed). Alpha-adrenergic receptors line the _____ _____. Stimulation of these receptors produces _____ and increases the _____ _____ and *(preload/afterload)* on the heart. This effect further increases myocardial O_2 consumption and may counterbalance any benefits obtained by dopamine administration. Necrosis and sloughing off of tissues may also occur in the presence of IV infiltration, particularly in these dose ranges. Phentolamine (Regitine)—an alpha blocker—may be administered subcutaneously to treat the infiltration.

norepinephrine
blood vessels
vasoconstriction
blood pressure; afterload

157 Careful calculation of the dose range is critical in determining the beneficial effects and preventing the potential toxic effects of dopamine administration. Concurrent monitoring of both cardiac output and wedge pressure can provide documentation of either improvement or deterioration in left ventricular function. The wedge pressure typically rermains unchanged or decreases slightly as the cardiac output increases and left ventricular emptying improves. Thus an increase in wedge pressure indicates a *(normal/toxic)* response, possibly related to increased MV_{O_2}. Dopamine is commonly used in conjunction with the afterload-reducing agent nitroprusside to facilitate any improvement in cardiac output and to minimize any increase in O_2 consumption. Dopamine may also be used in conjunction with intropic agents having arterial vasodilating effects, such as dobutamine (Dobutrex) on amrinone (Inocor) for similar reasons.

    toxic

158 In low dosage ranges (less than 2.5-3 μg/kg/min.) dopamine has the unique ability to produce vasodilation selectively in certain vascular beds, such as the renal, superior mesenteric, celiac, and intracerebral arteries. Dopamine enters the renal vessels via special _____ receptors and may be indicated to improve renal blood flow, prevent renal failure, and increase urine output in low-output states, such as CHF.

    dopamine

    REMEMBER: In the presence of CHF the fall in cardiac output produces a(n) *(increase/decrease)* in real perfusion, with a corresponding fall in _____ output. In high dosage ranges, renal blood flow and urine output may actually decrease as the _____ adrenergic effects on the renal vessels dominate.

    decrease
    urine
    alpha-

159 Dobutamine hydrochloride (Dobutrex) is a synthetic catecholamine with inotropic properties similar to those of dopamine, also mediated by B_1 receptors. Its inotropic action begins at the same dosage of dopamine (2.5-20 μg/kg/min.) but continues up to higher ranges. However, dobutamine appears to be slightly less chronotropic and has a more significant effect in lowering wedge pressures. Thus pulmonary congestion may decrease as the cardiac output increases.

    In contrast to dopamine, dobutamine does not have a direct renal vasodilating effect and has mild vasodilating effects resulting in a reduction of both preload and afterload although the exact mechanism is unclear. Therefore, dobutamine appears to possess the unique ability to combine the benefits of both inotropic and vasodilator therapy.

    Unlike dopamine, dobutamine may also be administered by intermittent infusion for the management of chronic congestie heart failure and is associated with an unexplained prolonged duration of action.

Amrinone

160 Amrinone lactate (Inocor) is an intravenous inotropic agent with effects similar to dobutamine but with a totally different mechanism of action. It is commonly referred to as a non-glycoside, non-catecholamine inotropic agent. The usual therapeutic range is 5-10 mcg/kg/min.

Amrinone acts as a phosphodiesterase inhibitor (similar to the bronchodilator aminophylline) resulting in an increased level of cAMP, an intracellular sympathetic messenger. However, it's action is more selective than aminophylline, acting primarily in cardiovascular tissues to produce an *(increase/decrease)* in contractility and *(vasodilation/vasoconstriction)*.

increase

vasodilation

161 Tachyarrhythmias are uncommon, but can occur at higher dose ranges. Thrombocytopenia has also been reported. The incidence of nausea and vomiting associated with oral administration has limited its long-term use.

Experimental agents within this classification system include milrinone, fenoximone, and sulmazol.

162 NURSING ORDERS: Patients receiving intravenous inotropic agents for heart failure
   1. Monitor the wedge pressure and cardiac output before and immediately after onset of therapy; continue to evaluate them at regular intervals thereafter.
   2. Determine the patient's weight and calculate the dosage accordingly.
   3. Look for toxic effects, depending on dosage:
      —Tachycardias/ventricular arrhythmias
      —Increased blood pressure
      —Decreased urine output
      —Increased wedge pressure
      —Sloughing of tissues (antidote is phentolamine)
   4. Document the improvement in urine output with a low dosage range (dopamine only).
   5. Administer with an infusion pump.
   6. Avoid the peripheral line; watch for necrotic areas.
   7. Do not administer with sodium bicarbonate or other alkaline solutions. Mix amrinone only with saline solutions.
   8. Monitor for thrombocytopenia when administering amrinone.

DRUG THERAPY IN THE MANAGEMENT OF SHOCK

163 Shock is a syndrome reflecting tissue hypoxia caused by a critical fall in
_____ _____ (see Units 3 and 9).

cardiac output

Therapy is directed toward the following:
1. Treatment of the underlying cause
2. Evaluation of the _____ response   vascular
3. Support of the hypoxic tissues

LET US REVIEW: The shock state may be produced by primary disturbances in _____, _____,   rhythm; volume
_____ tone, or myocardial   vascular
_____. Significant disturbances in rhythm—   contractility
whether slow, fast, ventricular—may be corrected with the use of antiarrhythmic, adrenergic, or cholinergic agents previously mentioned. Hypovolemic shock can be corrected by rapid volume replacement with crystalloids.

164 Vasopressors may be used in the management of shock in acute MI because they may increase coronary perfusion by raising diastolic pressure. However, if the mean arterial pressure remains above 80 mm Hg, asodilators may also be used to lower the compensatory increase in ventricular resistance accompanying cardiogenic shock.

REMEMBER: The compensatory increase in vascular resistance occurring in response to a fall in cardiac output produces an increased *(afterload/preload)*, which further impedes cardiac output.   afterload

165 The inotropic agents discussed in the management of CHF may also be used in the therapy of cardiogenic shock. Thus the major drugs currently used in the management of cardiogenic shock are (1) the vasodilators and (2) the inotropic agents. These drugs are also used in therapy for severe _____ and have already been thoroughly discussed.   CHF

166 A few drugs are currently restricted to use in the management of the shock state. These agents primarily support the hypoxic tissues. Their effectiveness in cardiogenic shock is still under investigation. They include mannitol, steroids such as hydrocortisone (Solu-Cortef), methylprednisolone (Solu-Medrol), and various metabolites. The administration of GIK solution may also be beneficial to hypoxic tissues—especially the hypoxic myocardium (see Unit 6 and Frames 223 and 224). However, its use is not primarily in the management of the shock state.

DRUG THERAPY IN THE MANAGEMENT OF CHEST PAIN

167 Chest pain is most significant when it is closely related to specific changes in coronary artery _____ and   structure
_____.   function

LET US REVIEW: The specific function of the coronary arteries is to provide an adequate blood and _____ supply to meet the O_2

cellular energy or _____ demands of the cardiac structures (see Frames 2 and 3 and Units 1 and 6).   metabolic

168 When the coronary blood supply is inadequate in meeting myocardial O_2 demand, a critical O_2 imbalance occurs, resulting in hypoxia. Hypoxia produces cellular metabolic changes that irritate pain reeptors and alter cellular function and can cause death of cells. This process suggests specific _____   coronary system
_____ failure (see Frame 2). Coronary blood supply is diminished and/or interrupted in the patient with acute MI or angina due to a process of coronary narrowing, or _____. This structural decrease in blood and O_2 stenosis
supply may be further aggravated by increases in myocardial O_2
_____, producing a critical functional   demand
_____. Temporary or sustained period of hypoxia   imbalance
result, compromising metabolism.

169 The structural coronary changes occurring in acute MI and angina are the *(same/different)*. Therefore the initial clinical presentaton of   same
both may be similar.
   REMEMBER: The characteristic presentng symptom of both angina and acute MI is _____ _____ (see Unit 6, Frame   chest pain
7). This chest pain occurs caused by metabolic toxins released in the presence of coronary _____ (narrowing), ischemia   stenosis
(decreased blood supply), and _____.   hypoxia

170 Angina and acute MI differ in their functional impact.
   Angina represents a transient O_2 imbalance that can occur either at rest or during exertion.
   Acute MI is associated with a more severe, extended O_2 deficit—eventually resulting in the death of tissue (necrosis or _____).   infarction
   The chest pain of both angina and evolving MI represents an "energy crisis" secondary to coronary artery changes. The pain is similar in quality and location, but it differs in duration, precipitating or triggering factors, and specific modes of relief.
   Coronary chest pain may be relieved by direct suppression of the pain or by reversal of the related structural or _____ changes (see Fig. 10-2 and Frames 1 and 2).   functional

171 The three most common mechanisms of large-vessel coronary stenosis or occlusion are the following:
1. Lipid infiltration (atherosclerosis)
2. Platelet aggregation
3. Coronary spasm
   Large-vessel coronary stenosis may result in either acute MI

or _____. Occlusion is more typically associated with acute transmural MI. Angina represents a _____ myocardial O_2 imbalance that may occur either at rest or during _____. It is typically triggered by an increased O_2 demand, coronary spasm, or a combination of the two.

angina

transient

exertion

172 Angina triggered by exertion or temporary increases in myocardial O_2 demands is thought to be caused by atherosclerotic vessel narrowing (fixed disease) with secondary platelet aggregation. This syndrome is also referred to as classic exertional or effort angina or chronic stable angina. It is often associated with transient ST depression (see Unit 6).

The chest pain of effort angina is usually effectively treated by rest or drugs that *(raise/lower)* O_2 demands, such as the nitrates or beta blockers. Calcium antagonists may also act to lower O_2 demands, but this effect varies according to the specific agent. They may be added to the therapeutic regimen in patients unresponsive to both nitrates and beta blocker therapy.

lower

173 Angina not triggered by exertion—occurring at _____—has been recognized for many years but has received renewed attention in recent years. The syndrome of rest angina associated with transient ST elevation is also referred to as Prinzmetal, or variant, angina and is thought to be caused by coronary spasm without significant atherosclerosis.

The chest pain of angina at rest or angina caused by _____ _____ is effectively treated by vasodilators, such as the calcium antagonists or nitrates. These drugs increase coronary blood supply by relieving spasm, thus restoring O_2 _____. The calcium antagonists are currently considered first-lijne agents in the management of this syndrome. Beta blockers can aggravate spasm and are therefore best avoided in the therapy of rest angina.

rest

coronary spasm

balance

174 Coronary spasm has also been documented in exertional angina associated with transient ST depression. In this setting the coronary spasm is probably superimposed on the fixed atherosclerotic lesion, further occluding the lumen. These patients may have a history of both effort and rest angina or unstable angina (see Frame 171).

Angina caused by a mixture of both fixed disease and spasm is most effectively treated *first* with drugs that lower demands without aggravating spasm such as the _____ or _____ _____. The nitrates are currently considered first-line agents in the management of mixed angina syndromes.

nitrates

calcium antagonists

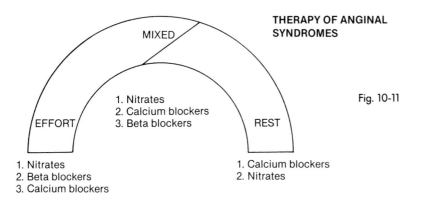

MIXED

THERAPY OF ANGINAL SYNDROMES

1. Nitrates
2. Calcium blockers
3. Beta blockers

Fig. 10-11

EFFORT

REST

1. Nitrates
2. Beta blockers
3. Calcium blockers

1. Calcium blockers
2. Nitrates

Beta blockers or calcium antagonists may be added or substituted as needed. These agents may provide added benefits _____ _____.

lowering demands

175 LET US REVIEW: Angina represents a temporary _____ between O_2 supply and demand or _____ _____ failure. The chest pain of angina can be treated with drugs that either increase coronary blood flow and O_2 _____ or lower _____.

imbalance
coronary system

supply
demands

The major drugs currently used in the therapy of angina are the _____, _____ _____, and _____ _____. Rest angina is most effectively relieved by drugs that relieve _____ _____, thus increasing the coronary blood flow and O_2 _____. Therefore the chest pain of angina at rest is best treated by either _____ or _____ _____ and may be aggravated by _____ _____.

nitrates; beta blockers
calcium antagonists
coronary spasm

supply
nitrates; calcium
 antagonists
beta blockers

176 The chest pain of effort and/or mixed angina syndromes is best treated by agents that *(increase supply/lower demands)*. The agents most effective in lowering demands are the _____ and _____ _____. However, the _____ are best used initially in the management of _____ angina syndromes, since they also relieve _____. The action of the nitrates and beta blockers in effort or mixed angina may be complemented by the addition of the _____ _____ (see Fig. 10-13).

lower demands
nitrates
beta blockers
nitrates
mixed
spasm

calcium antagonists

The chest pain associated with evolving MI is usually *not* effectively suppressed by drugs that either reduce demands or reverse coronary changes, unless these drugs are injected directly into the coronary arteries (see Frame 221).

REMEMBER: Acute MI is associated with a more _____, _____ O_2 deficit, eventually resulting in _____ of tissue. Relief of chest pain in this setting usually requires direct suppression of CNS pain receptors with narcotic analgesics.

severe

extended

death

177 Impending myocardial infarction is suspected in patients with an accelerated change in pattern of effort angina or new onset of rest angina. This syndrome is also referred to as _____, or _____, angina. These patients are most likely to have a mixture of severe, fixed disease and spasm.

unstable

crescendo

The contribution of spasm to coronary obstruction is thought to be significant in this stage, regardless of its previous role.

The chest pain of unstable angina is best treated with IV nitrates.

REMEMBER: Nitrates act to *both* decrease O_2 demand and increase _____ _____ by relieving _____. The addition of calcium antagonists may complement this action. The use of oral beta blockers in unstable angina is also well established. Control of chest pain in this setting may ultimately require suppression by narcotic analgesics.

O_2 supply; spasm

Narcotic analgesics

178 The drugs most commonly used in the management of the chest pain of acute MI are the narcotic analgesics. Therapy is directed toward relieving the discomfort rapidly and effectively, with as few side effects as possible. The two narcotics probably used most commonly in the setting of coronary care are morphine sulfate and meperidine hydrochloride (Demerol). Narcotic analgesics act by blocking CNS pain perception. The concurrent use of beta blockers may decrease the need for narcotics.

Morphine

179 Morphine sulfate is a CNS depressant that exerts a narcotic effect. A drug that exerts a narcotic effect may produce sleep as well as analgesia. Another manifestation of the narcotic effect may be changes in sensorium. Because of its ability to relieve pain rapidly and effectively when administered intravenously, morphine is commonly used in the management of chest pain associated with acute MI.

180 Another manifestation of the effect of morphine on the CNS may be vasodilation caused by depression of sympathetic pathways. Thus morphine administration may result in *(hypotension/hypertension)*.

hypotension

Morphine has been shown not only to decrease arteriolar constriciton but also to produce venodilation. Venodilation results in peripheral pooling and thus reduces *(preload/afterload)*. This effect on preload is desirable in the relief of pulmonary edema.

preload

Another effect of morphine that is beneficial in the management of pulmonary edema is its ability to decrease the respiratory rate and anxiety.

181 Morphine has also been shown to slow the heart rate in some settings by creating autonomic imbalance. Therefore morphine should be administered with caution in patients with bradycardias or enhanced vagal tone, such as occurs in *(AWMI/IWMI)*.

IWMI

Morphine decreases the sensitivity of the respiratory center to arterial CO_2 levels, thereby *(depressing/stimulating)* respirations. The administration of morphine to patients known to have limited respiratory reserves must therefore be approached with caution. Respiratory depression may be reserved by a narcotic antagonist such as naloxone hydrochloride (Narcan).

depressing

Meperidine

182 Meperidine hydrochloride (Demerol), another narcotic analgesic, is structurally different from morphine but has a similar mechanism of action. Because of its ability to relieve pain rapidly and effectively when administered intravenously, it is also commonly used in the management of chest pain associated with acute MI.

Meperidine depresses respirations by decreasing the tidal volume rather than by depressing the respiratory rate. Hypotension may occur after the IV administration of meperidine, with a compensatory increase in the heart rate.

183 NURSING ORDERS: Patients receiving morphine or meperidine for management of chest pain
1. Watch for hypotension following IV administration.
   —Elevate the patient's legs as indicated.
2. Observe for respiratory depression following administration.
   —Administer with caution in patients known to have limited respiratory reserve, that is, patients with emphysema, asthma, bronchitis, or pneumonia.
3. Administer morphine with caution to the patient with increased vagal tone; have atropine available.
   —IWMI
   —Bradyarrhythmia
4. The following side effects may occur with the administration of morphine or meperidine:
   —Dizziness
   —Sweating
   —Nausea and vomiting

—Weakness
—Syncope
—Palpitations
—Euphoria or dysphoria

Nitrates

184 The nitrates are the only agents equally effective in the management of all forms of angina. They are also well established in clinical use with few reported side-effects. For these reasons, they are currently indicated in the first-line management of effort or mixed angina syndromes. The most commonly used nitrates are nitroglycerin and isosorbide.

LET US REVIEW: Nitrates are *both* to increase coronary _____ and to lower _____. They are therefore effective in the therapy of both _____ and _____ angina. In this way they differ from the beta blockers, which are effective in *(rest/effort)* angina but may aggravate *(rest/effort)* angina by facilitating _____. They also differ from the calcium-channel blockers (calcium antagonists), which are most effective in *(rest/effort)* angina but whose effectiveness in effort angina varies with the specific agent.

supply; demands
effort
rest
effort; rest
spasm

rest

185 The pain of angina is usually rapidly relieved by a rapidly acting nitrate, such as sublingual nitroglycerin or isosorbide. These agents may also be used immediately before anticipated stressful events to *prevent* anginal attacks. The chest pain of unstable angina usually requires the use of intravenous nitrates. Longer-acting nitrates, such as the topical ointment (Nitrol) or oral nitrates (Nitrospan, Nitro-Bid, Iso-Bid, Sorbitrate, and so forth), are used prophylactically on a continuous basis to prevent anginal attacks. Transdermal nitroglycerin patches (Nitrodur, Nitroderm) have more recently been introduced and have become popular in the management of chronic stable angina, since they facilitate patient compliance. However, their absorption rate may be less predictable and/or reliable, making these agents less ideal in the acute setting.

186 The predominant effect of nitrates in chronic stable angina is to *(increase coronary supply/decrease O_2 demands)*. The nitrates act directly on the smooth muscle of the peripheral as well as coronary vascular bed. They act to lower O_2 demands by reducing both preload and afterload (see Frames 139 and 140).

decrease O_2 demands

LET US REVIEW: The nitrates reduce preload by producing *(venous/arterial)* dilation and reduce afterload by producing *(venous/arterial)* dilation. However, the predominant effect is on the *(venous/arterial)* bed.

venous
arterial
venous

187 Reduction of both preload and afterload results in the lowering of myocardial _____ _____ and relief or _____ of anginal chest pain. Reduction of preload and left ventricular filling _____ can also decrease the pulmonary congestion associated with CHF. Cardiac output improves because of the changes in both preload and afterload. For these reasons the nitrates are also commonly used in the acute and chronic management of _____ _____ (see Frames 139 to 142).

    Nitrates also act to increase coronary supply by increasing blood flow in the normal collateral vessels or by relaxing _____. Diseased vessels lose their responsiveness to vasodilators unless spasm is involved. Reductions in LV filling pressure may also facilitate coronary flow by reducing _____ to coronary filling.

    O₂ demands
prevention
pressure

heart failure

spasm

impedance

188 Management of the chest pain of *unstable* angina often requires _____ nitrates. Administration of intravenous nitrates requires more careful monitoring. Intravenous nitroglycerin is administered as a continuous drip. Like other vasodilators, nitroglycerin administration may result in *(hypotension/hypertension)*.

    In this setting hypotension is caused *primarily* by *(arterial/venous)* dilation and is usually preceded by a drop in filling (wedge) pressure or *(preload/afterload)*. Significant hypotension is unusual with continuous IV drip nitroglycerin. Filling pressure is most closely monitored by a(n) *(arterial/Swan-Ganz)* catheter; however, the use of a Swan-Ganz catheter is not critical unless the arterial BP is already low—that is, 100/60. Frequent checking of arterial BP via arterial line *or* cuff is usually adequate with the mean arterial BP as the therapeutic end point.

    intravenous

hypotension
venous

preload

Swan-Ganz

189 Nitrates may also be administered within the first 2 to 4 hours of evolving MI by the intravenous or intracoronary route in an attempt to reverse coronary _____. In this setting intracoronary injection of nitrates precedes the use of thrombolytic agents and/or PTCA (see Frames 267 and 279) but is typically rarely effective.

    Hypotension is also seen with sublingual, oral, or topical administration of nitrates for management of chronic stable angina. The BP endpoint should be established by the physician and communicated to the nurse. Nursing actions in the event of hypotensive episodes should be directed toward supporting *(preload/afterload)* or _____ return. Measures such as lowering the head of the bed and raising the feet may provide rapid symptomatic relief. Patients should also be observed for reflexive tachycardias, especially in the presence of normal or low filling pressures. Orthostatic

    stenosis

preload
venous

hypotension is often reported with sublingual nitroglycerin. Patients should be instructed to sit or lie down before taking sublingual nitroglycerin and remain in this position for at least 15 minutes.

190 NURSING ORDERS: Patients receiving a nitrate (nitroglycerin or isosorbide) for the management of chest pain
1. Check BP before administering a vasodilator for chest pan.
2. Watch for episodes of symptomatic hypotension and tachyarrhythmias after the administration of nitrates.
   —Put the head of the bed down.
   —Elevate the patient's legs.
3. Repeat nitroglycerin as ordered by the physician if chest pain is still not relieved; administer a narcotic as prescribed.
4. Report closely recurrent episodes of chest pain to the physician; administration of nitrates on a continual basis may be necessary.
5. Teaching considerations regarding the administration of nitroglycerin:
   —Caution the patient always to sit or lie down when taking sublingual nitroglycerin.
   —Caution the patient to report chest pain that is unrelieved by taking nitroglycerin three successive times at 5-minute to 10-minute intervals.
   —Caution the patient that nitroglycerin tablets may deteriorate and lose effectiveness in as short a time as 3 months; thus the tablets should be replaced every 3 months with a fresh supply.
   —Inform the patient that potent tablets characteristically produce a transient headache because of meningeal vasodilation, a burning sensation under the tongue, or both. The headaches can be treated with aspirin or a decrease in nitroglycerin dosage but may also disappear over a period of time.
6. Instruct the patient in the proper application of the dermal patch to ensure adhesion and proper absorption. Make the patient aware that any site having access to blood flow is adequate, and encourage the rotation of sites.

Beta blockers

191 Beta blockers are indicated in the therapy of (*effort/rest*) angina. They relieve chest pain by lowering O_2 demands and restoring O_2 _____.

effort

balance

Beta blockers such as propanolol reduce myocardial O_2 consumption or demands by decreasing *heart rate* and *depressing contractility*.

REMEMBER: MVO_2 is a function of _____, rate _____, _____, and preload; afterload _____. Beta blockers may also indirectly increase contractility supply by prolonging diastolic filling time as a result of the decrease in rate.

Drugs that block the beta receptors of the *(sympathetic/para-* sympathetic *sympathetic)* nervous system produce these effects on the heart and lungs:

1. *(Increased/Decreased)* heart rate — Decreased
2. *(Increased/Decreased)* AV conduction — Decreased
3. *(Increased/Decreased)* contractility — Decreased
4. *(Increased/Decreased)* automaticity — Decreased
5. *(Bronchoconstriction/Bronchodilation)* — Bronchoconstriction

192 Although beta blockade is effective in relieving the chest pain of effort angina, it may aggravate chest pain caused by coronary spasm or _____angina. — rest

Coronary vascular tone is thought to be maintained by a balance of alpha-adrenergic and beta-adrenergic (sympathetic) activity. Alpha-adrenergic activity causes coronary vasoconstriciton, and beta-adrenergic activity causes coronary _____. Beta — vasodilation blockade allows alpha-adrenergic activity to predominate, which may result in _____ _____. — coronary spasm

NOTE: Beta blockade may also aggravate peripheral vascular spasm. Therefore beta blockers should be used with caution in patients with vasospastic peripheral vascular disease.

193 The administration of beta blockers in Prinzmetal (variant) angina has potential risk and is best avoided.

REMEMBER: Variant angina is primarily caused by _____ _____. — coronary spasm

But, the use of beta blockers in unstable angina is well established.

REMEMBER: Unstable angina probably represents a _____ of fixed disease and spasm. Concurrent ad- — mixture ministration of nitrates or calcium antagonists may offset any negative vasospastic effects.

194 Nine beta blockers are currently available in the United States. All are equally effective in angina control, although not all are officially approved for this purpose by the FDA. These specific drug agents are propranolol (Inderal), metoprolol (Lopressor), nadolol (Corgard), atenolol (Tenormin), timolol (Blocadren), pindolol (Visken), labetolol (Normodyne/Trandate), acebutolol (Sectral), and esmolol (Brevibloc). Additional agents under investigation include oxprenolol, sotalol, acebutolol, and tolamolol.

195 All beta-blocking agents are also effective in the control of arrhythmias (see Frame 40) and hypertension. Control of hypertension may provide further benefits in angina control because of the reduction in *(preload/afterload)*.

afterload

REMEMBER: Angina occurs caused by a critial imbalance in O_2 supply and demand. Hypertension may precipitate angina because of an increase in O_2 _____.

demand

The primary mechanism of action is thought to be a lowering of cardiac output. Peripheral vascular resistance may actually increase initially in response to the fall in cardiac output. Inhibition of renin secretion from beta cells in the kidney is likely to be a contributing factor. Full antihypertensive effect may take as long as 1 to 4 weeks to develop.

196 The more recently released labetolol (Normodyne/Trandate) has the unique property of alpha blockade in addition to beta blockade.

REMEMBER: Alpha receptors are located in the peripheral and coronary _____ _____. Stimulation of the alpha receptors causes vasoconstriction. Blockade of the alpha receptors, therefore, causes _____.

blood vessels

vasodilation

Labetolol, thus, lowers peripheral vascular _____, is available in IV form, and acts more rapidly on severe hypertension than any other beta blocker administered intravenously. These properties make it a useful alternative to Nipride for the management of hypertensive crisis. Labetolol may also be continued in oral form and combines the effects of beta blockade with vasodilation. However, labetolol is not cardioselective (See Frames 198, 199).

resistance

197 Beta blockers may also be used during or following myocardial infarction to preserve ischemic myocardium, prevent extension, and prevent complication (see Frames 227 to 229). They are also currently used in the management of other cardiovascular disorders such as arrhythmias (see Frames 11, 39, and 89 to 96), mitral valve prolapse, IHSS, (see Unit 12) migraine, and aortic dissection.

198 The nine available beta blockers differ in their specific beta-blocking activity. Metoprolol, atenolol and acebutolol are more "cardioselective," acting predominantly as B_1 blockers. However, this selectivity is dose dependent and is lost at higher doses.

REMEMBER: Beta receptor sites can be further differentiated into B_1 sites in the _____ and B_2 sites on _____ smooth muscle.

heart
bronchial

B_2 blockade produces _____. Selective B_1 blockers, such as _____ and

bronchospasm
metoprolol

_____, have less bronchospastic, vasospastic, and metabolic side effects.

atenolol

199 B_2 receptors also control glucose release from glycogen stores in response to hypoglycemia. Nonselective beta blockers may prolong insulin-induced hypoglycemia in diabetic patients. Therefore cardioselective beta-blocking agents may be preferred.

Cardioselective beta blockers block (B_1/B_2) receptors with minimal or decreased effects on (B_2/B_2) receptors.

B_1
B_2

200 The beta blockers pindolol (Visken) and acebutolol (Sectral) differ from the others in possessing some intrinsic sympathetic activity (ISA). Of these two _____ is cardioselective, while _____ is non-selective. The ISA activity of acebutolol is also milder. This activity is evident primarily when overall sympathetic tone is low, that is at rest rather than at exercise.

acebutolol
pindolol

Reduction in resting heart rate induced by the beta blockade would be balanced by this slight beta stimulation. Therefore administration of this beta blocker would produce *(more/less)* resting bradycardia. Vasodilation occurs as a result of beta 2 stimulation decreasing the risk of coronary and peripheral _____ and more effectively lowering the peripheral vascular resistance in hypertensive disease. This mild inherent sympathetic stimulation may also minimize the typically aggravating effect of beta blockade in CHF but has not yet proven clinically significant. Intrinsic beta 2 activity may produce tremors.

less

spasm

201 The side effects of beta-blocking agents may be categorized as affecting the cardiovascular system, pulmonary system, metabolism, sexual function, and CNS.

The most frequent, significant effects are cardiopulmonary. They include *(bradycardia/tachycardia)*, *(hypotension/hypertension)*, CHF, and *(bronchodilation/bronchospasm)*.

bradycardia; hypotension
bronchospasm

All beta blockers should be avoided in patients with severe COPD or asthma. In less severe lung disease the "cardioselective" beta blockers provide the least risk.

Patients with mild CHF may benefit from the rate-reducing effects of beta blockade. However, beta blockers *(should/should not)* be administered to the patient with severe CHF.

should not

202 CNS effects include insomnia, nightmares, hallucinations, and depression. These effects may be prevented or minimized by the use of beta blockers that do not penetrate the blood/brain barrier, such as nadolol (Corgard) or atenolol (Trenormin).

Fatigue may occur caused by bradycardia, hypotension, CHF, or altered skeletal muscle metabolism.

507

Beta blockers such as propanolol lower free fatty acids, which act as a skeletal muscle energy source. Beta blockers also inhibit the catecholamine-induced breakdown of muscle glycogen stores in response to hypoglycemic or increased energy demands. Switching to another beta blocker may decrease the fatigue.

The combination of beta blockers and insulin therapy may make the patient more prone to *(hypoglycemia/hyperglycemia)*.

hypoglycemia

Impotence caused by impaired ejaculation has also been reported, but this is considered rare, since ejaculation is usually under the control of alpha receptors.

203 NURSING ORDERS: Patients receiving a beta blocker for the management of chest pain
1. Check pulse and BP before administering each dose. Watch for bradycardia and/or hypotension. Establish a target pulse rate and BP with the physician. Hold for a heart rate of less than 40 beats per minute.
2. Ausculate for wheezes or increased rales with each set of vital signs. So not administer to patients with a history of asthma.
3. Administer with caution to patients with
   • CHF
   • Diabetes, who are receiving insulin therapy or oral hypoglycemics
   • Peripheral vascular disease
4. Do not discontinue beta blocker abruptly, to avoid potential withdrawal syndrome.
5. Instruct patient not to stop taking these medicines abruptly, and explain why.
6. Observe patient for (or instruct patient to report):
   • Increased peripheral vascular spasm (claudication, paresthesias, and so forth)
   • Increased angina (especially rest angina)
   • Excessive fatigue
   • Nightmares
7. Watch for interaction with disopyramide.

Calcium antagonists (calcium channel blockers)

204 Calcium antagonists are indicated in the therapy of both rest and effort angina. All three currently available calcium antagonists are equally effective in the management of rest angina or angina caused by _____ _____. However, their effec-

coronary system

tiveness in effort angina varies according to the mechanism and ability of the specific agent in lowering demands in individual patients.

REMEMBER: Effort angina is triggered by increased O_2 _____. It is most effectively treated by rest or drugs that

demands

(raise/lower) O_2 demands.

lower

Rest angina is triggered by coronary spasm or decreased O_2 _____. It is most effectively treated by drugs that relieve the coronary spasm, thus *(increasing/decreasing)* O_2 supply.

supply
increasing

Calcium antagonists can *both* increase coronary (O_2) supply and lower O_2 demands. They are therefore potentially effective in both effort and rest angina or a mixture of the two.

205 The calcium antagonists are either selectively *vasoactive* or both *cardioactive* and *vasoactive*. The vasoactive properties are the most significant when these agents are used in the management of either rest or effort angina.

REMEMBER: The traditional key role of calcium is in the contraction of _____ muscle (mechanical ativity). However, calcium also plays a significant role in the contraction of the *smooth* muscle of the peripheral and coronary arterial bed. It therefore has a *vasoactive* as well as *cardioactive* role. Calcium also plays a significant role in cardiac _____ as well as mechanical activity (see Unit 4).

cardiac

electrical

Calcium antagonists act by blocking the entry of calcium into _____ or _____ cells. Cardiovascular cells especially depend on the movement of extracellular calcium into the cells as a calcium source because of poor _____ stores. These drugs are also referred to as "calcium _____-blocking agents" and *(do/do not)* significantly alter total serum calcium (see Fig. 10-3).

cardiac; vascular

intracellular
channel; do not

206 The physiological consequences of calcium-channel blockade in cardiovascular cells can be classified as either electrical or mechanical. The electrical effects include suppression of slow cell activity, especially in the _____ _____ and _____ _____. The mechanical effects include actions on the cardiac muscle and/or _____ muscle of the arterial vascular bed.

SA node; AV node

smooth

207 Contraction of the arterial smooth muscle maintains normal and abnormal peripheral and _____ artery tone.

coronary

A manifestation of increased (abnormal) coronary artery tone is coronary artery _____.

spasm

A manifestation of increased peripheral artery tone is an *(increased/decreased)* BP or the syndrome of _____. An increased BP may also reflect an increased arterial systemic vascular resistance or *(preload/afterload)*. Calcium-channel blockade results in decreased contraction of both the coronary and peripheral arterial muscles, thus relaxing coronary spasm and lowering arterial systemic vascular resistance, BP, and afterload.

increased
hypertension

afterload

Calcium-channel blockade also results in *(increased/decreased)* myo-

decreased

Ca^{++} CHANNEL BLOCKADE

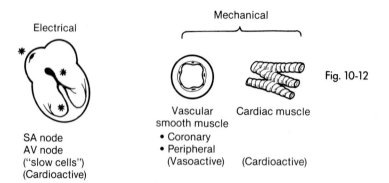

Fig. 10-12

Electrical

SA node
AV node
("slow cells")
(Cardioactive)

Mechanical

Vascular
smooth muscle
• Coronary
• Peripheral
(Vasoactive)

Cardiac muscle

(Cardioactive)

cardial contractility. However, this effect has few specific therapeutic indications at this time. Significant side effects related to this action, such as CHF, are not usually seen in common therapeutic dose ranges.

208 There are four major categories of calcium channel blockers: 1) the cardioactive agents; 2) the dihydropyridine vasoactive a gents; 3) the piperazine vasoactive agents; and 4) the mixed Na$^+$ and Ca^{++} channel blockers. The two currently available calcium channel blockers with cardioactive effects are verapamil (Isoptin/Calan) and diltiazem (Cardizem).

These agents *(do/do not)* act similarly. Agents within this category still under investigation include tiapamil and gallopamil.

do

Nifedipine (Procardia) is the only currently available dihydropyridine. There are many other agents under investigation within this category including nitrendipine (Baypress), nicardipine, nisoldipine, and felodipine. The piperazine vasoactive agents and mixed Na$^+$ and Ca^{++} blockers are all under investigation. These include perhexiline, lidoflazine, and bepridil which produces significant Q-T prolongation.

209 Verapamil is the most balanced of the currently available calcium-channel blockers. It has both electrical and mechanical effects and is both _____ active and _____ active. Therefore it has the widest spectrum of potential clinical usage. Verapamil is currently used in the management of supraventricular tachyarrhythmias, both rest and effort angina, and hypertension. For its use in supraventricular tachyarrhythmias see Frames 69 to 81.

cardio-; vaso-

Diltiazem has both cardioactive and vasoactive properties *(similar to/different from)* verapamil. Therefore, its indications for use are also similar. Its therapeutic effects are weaker, but its side effects are fewer than with either verapamil or nifedipine. It has been rapidly gaining popularity the last few years.

similar to

210 Nifedipine is a selectively *vasoactive* calcium-channel blocker. Therefore it *(does/does not)* have significant clinical effects on cardiac electrical and/or mechanical activity. Nifedipine *(is/is not)* effective in the management of supraventricular tachyarrhythmias. However, it *is* effective in the management of both rest and effort angina and hypertension.

does not

is not

The calcium channel blockers are also effective in many cardiovascular disorders other than arrhythmias, angina, and hypertension.

REMEMBER: These disorders include _____ headaches, _____ spasm, _____ vascular spasm (Raynaud's disease), _____ hypertension, and _____ cardiomyopathy.

migraine

cerebrovascular; cardio

pulmonary

hypertrophic

Effects in inhibiting platelet function may also be beneficial in coronary artery disease. Cardioprotective effects post MI are still under investigation, but the results of preliminary studies are not encouraging.

211 Calcium channel blockers are usually used for hypertension in the patient with coronary artery disease. However, they are more recently gaining popularity as a third line agent after diuretics and beta blockade, in patients without coronary artery disease as well. They may also be used as an equally effective alternative to beta blockade in the elderly patient, the patient at risk for pulmonary, vascular, or metabolic side effects, or where these or other side effects have already occurred.

The major mechanism of action in hypertension is to *(raise/lower)* peripheral vascular resistance, which is a characteristic of *(early/end stage)* hypertensive disease. Most beta blockers act primarily on *(heart/blood vessels)* to lower the _____ _____ and at least initially *(increase/decrease)* peripheral vascular resistance.

lower

end stage

heart; cardiac output

increase

212 There is some recent evidence that the calcium channel blockers may be more effective in patients with low renin levels, while beta blockers are more effective in patients with high serum renin levels. High serum calcium levels appear to interfere with calcium channel antagonism. Patients with low renin levels have also been found to have low serum Ca^{++} levels, so that the effects of calcium channel blockade are enhanced rather than suppressed. Blood pressure in these patients may also be more sensitive to ECF Ca^{++} changes.

Nifedipine produces a rapid drop in blood pressurer due to its more prominent *(cardioactive/vasoactive)* effects. However, the duration of this effect if often limited by reflex sympathetic stimulation, which may also produce *(tachycardias/bradycardias)*. The combination of nifedipine with a beta blocker may decrease these effects while augmenting the effect of beta blockade.

vasoactive

tachycardias

213 The specific effects of the calcium channel-blocking agents in effort angina vary.

REMEMBER: Effort angina is most effectively treated by drugs that *(increase coronary O_2 supply/lower O_2 demands)*.

lower O_2 demands

The determinants of myocardial demands of O_2 consumption (MVO_2) are the following:
1. Heart _____

rate

2. Preload
3. _____

Afterload

4. Contractile state

Calcium-channel blockers can act to lower myocardial O_2 demands (MVO_2) by any of the following mechanisms:
1. Decreased afterload caused by peripheral arterial _____

dilation

2. Decreased heart rate (negative _____ effect)

chronotropic

3. Decreased contractility (negative _____ effect)

inotropic

NOTE: The last two mechanisms occur primarily with cardioactive agents.

214 Although nifedipine has the strongest peripheral dilating action, it has no direct effect on heart rate or contractility. It's major mechanism of action in effort angina is to decrease *(afterload/preload)*. In fact it may increase heart rate in seleected cases as a reflex response to the vasodilation, thus limiting its antianginal action. Nifedipine is thus safer than the cardioactive agents in patients with SA or AV node disease or those receiving other cardiac depressant medications.

afterload

Verapamil probably decreases O_2 demands by a combination of these mechanisms. Thus the mode of action of verapamil in effort angina is to decrease *(afterload/preload)*, decrease heart _____, and decrease _____. For this reason, verapamil may prove effective in cases in which nifedipine has not proved beneficial. It is most ideal for patients requiring a combination of arrhythmia and angina control.

afterload
rate; contractility

Diltiazem also has a potential combined mode of action in angina effort but is *(stronger/weaker)* than verapamil. Its use is ideal for cases in which side effects from either nifedipine or verapamil prevent their use.

weaker

215 Side effects seen with calcium antagonists are related to cardiovascular, CNS, and GI actions. The cardiovascular effects include hypotension, headache, and dizziness. These symptoms are noted most commonly in agents that are peripherally vasoactive. The currently available calcium antagonist with the strongest peripheral vasoactivity is _____. Therefore side effects more likely to be seen with nifedipine administration are _____,

nifedipine
hypotension

_____, and _____. Reflex *(tachy-cardia/bradycardia)* has also been reported with nifedipine.

headache; dizziness; tachycardia

Verapamil is also vasoactive. Therefore _____, _____, and _____ may also occur with verapamil therapy.

headache
hypotension; dizziness

216 Bradycardia can occur with cardioactive agents, especially when used in combination with other cardiac depressants or in the presence of conduction system disease. The currently available calcium antagonist with the strongest cardioactivity is _____. Therefore bradycardia is most likely to be seen with verapamil administration. The administration of verapamil is best avoided in the presence of sick sinus syndrome or AV block greater than first degree.

verapamil

Bradycardia occurs most commonly if this agent is administered intravenously in conjunction with cardiac depressants. The IV route is indicated primarily in arrhythmia control (see Frames 66 to 78).

217 CNS effects include tremors, nervousness, and mood changes. Currently they are less commonly reported than the CNS effects occurring with beta blockers.

Peripheral edema is often reported, especially with nifedipine. However, this edema is not thought to be related to cardiovascular deterioration. The exact mechanism is unclear but may be related to local protein shifts.

The GI side effect of constipation has been primarily reported with oral verapamil therapy. The agent with the lowest incidence of reported side effects is currently diltiazem; this may be because of its selectivity.

REMEMBER: Although diltiazem has been both cardioactive and vasoactive properties, its _____ properties are weaker than those of verapamil, and its _____ properties are more selective than those of nifedipine.

cardioactive
vasoactive

218 Therapy with calcium antagonists offers certain distinct advantages over therapy with beta blockers alone, especially with reference to side effects. None of the calcium antagonists possess any broncho-constricting activity. They are therefore safer in the patient with _____. Even the cardioactive agents produce less myocardial depressant effects than do the beta blockers in dosages used for either arrhythmia or angina control, despite some blockade of myocardial calcium channels. They are therefore safer in the patient with _____.

asthma

CHF

Calcium blockade relaxes coronary and peripheral vascular spasm, wherreas beta blockade may aggravate it. Thus calcium blockade is safer than beta blockade in the patient with *(rest/effort)* angina or _____ vascular disease. Coronary spasm probably complicates unstable angina even in the presence of fixed disease or with a previous history of effort angina. The addition of calcium blockade to beta blockade at this time can minimize any detrimental effects on coronary supply while maximizing lowered demands.

REMEMBER: Calcium antagonists lower O_2 demands primarily by decreasing *(afterload/preload)*. Selected calcium antagonists also decrease heart rate and _____.

219 LET US REVIEW: Other, less serious side effects reported with beta blockade include fatigue, CNS changes such as nightmares and depression, alterations in serum lipoproteins, and sexual dysfunction. The incidence and significance of these side effects is currently being reevaluated in light of the younger and more extensive population now receiving these agents; they have been reported less frequently or not at all with calcium blockade.

Although calcium blockade does not replace beta blockade in the therapy of effort angina, combined therapy can provide distinct advantages. For example, this regimen may allow for the use of reduced dosages of beta-blocking agents, thus minimizing any of the previously mentioned side effects.

220 Calcium blockade does not currently offer advantages over nitrate therapy in the first-line management of effort or mixed angina syndromes.

REMEMBER: Nitrates act primarily to decrease *(afterload/preload)* but can also relax coronary spasm. Therefore they act both to decrease O_2 demands and to increase _____, as the calcium antagonists do. However, fewer significant side effects have been reported with the use of nitrates, despite extensive use of these drugs over many years. The lower incidence of side effects may be caused by the absence of any myocardial depressant activity and the lessening of peripheral arterial activity.

Calcium blockade may complement the action of nitrates in angina. They may be added to the therapeutic regimen in patients unresponsive to nitrate therapy or combined nitrate and beta-blocker therapy.

REMEMBER: Calcium antagonists decrease O_2 demands primarily by decreasing *(afterload/preload)*. Cardioactive calcium antagonists may also act to decrease _____ _____ and _____. Combined nitrate and calcium-blocker therapy may be especially beneficial in the unstable angina syndrome, which is often complicated by _____ _____.

rest

peripheral

afterload

contractility

preload

supply

afterload

heart rate

contractility

coronary spasm

514

221 LET US REVIEW: Calcium antagonists may be used in the therapy of both rest and effort angina. However, these drugs *(are/are not)* first-line agents in the management of effort angina. They *(are/are not)* first-line agents in the management of rest angina. The effectiveness of calcium antagonists in effort angina may vary according to the ability of specific agents to *(increase coronary supply/decrease O_2 demands)*.

Calcium antagonists are also commonly used in the management of arrhythmia and/or hypertension. The effectiveness of these agents in these syndromes and their related side effects depends on their relative cardioactivity, as opposed to their _____. Other cardiovascular disorders in which these agents may be used include migraine headaches, cerebrovascular spasm after aneurysmectomy, and pulmonary hypertension.

are not

are

decrease O_2 demands

vasoactivity

222 NURSING ORDERS: Patients receiving a calcium-channel blocker/antagonist for the management of chest pain:
1. Check BP before administering each dose. Watch for *(hypotension/hypertension)* and establish target BP with the physician.
2. Also check the pulse rate before verapamil administration. Establish a target pulse rate with the physician. Hold for a heart rate of less than 40 beats per minute.
3. Instruct the patient to report dizziness, headache, or constipation.
4. Evaluate the effectiveness in anginal relief and document it.

hypotension

ANTIANGINAL AGENTS (SUMMARY)

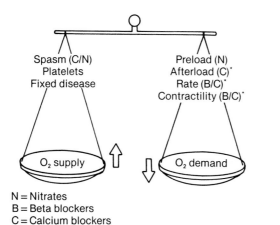

Spasm (C/N)
Platelets
Fixed disease

Preload (N)
Afterload (C)*
Rate (B/C)*
Contractility (B/C)*

Fig. 10-13

O_2 supply

O_2 demand

N = Nitrates
B = Beta blockers
C = Calcium blockers

*REMEMBER: The effects of calcium blockade on O_2 demands vary with the specific agent.

DRUG THERAPY REVERSING STRUCTURAL AND/OR METABOLIC CHANGES
Preservation of ischemic myocardium

223 Drugs used in the management of chest pain may also prevent acute MI, limit infarct size, decrease the rate of reinfarction, and reduce mortality after acute MI. They act by reversing the immediate structural functional, and/or metabolic changes occurring during acute MI, thus preserving ischemic myocardium and minimizing related complications.

REMEMBER: The chest pain of evolving acute MI or angina represents an _____ crisis secondary to coronary artery narrowing. This coronary artery narrowing results in a decreased blood supply or _____ and hypoxia. Hypoxia produces cellular _____ changes that result eventually in the _____ of tissue.

energy

ischemia
metabolic
death

224 The current focus of therapy to prevent or limit myocardial infarction has two dimensions: reversal of coronary stenosis and management of related metabolic changes. This focus represents an evolution from earlier modes of preserving ischemic myocardium and preventing or limiting acute MI. These earlier methods were primarily directed toward control of _____ and mechanical complications and lowering of O_2 _____.

electrical
demands

Therapy to prevent acute MI and/or reduce mortality may be instituted (1) before any acute symptomatology, (2) during stable or unstable angina, (3) once an infarction is in progress, or (4) following acute myocardial infarction (to prevent recurrence, extension, and complications). Although infarction may begin earlier, significant death of tissue occurs within about 2 to 4 hours after acute obstruction. Therefore, once an infarction is in progress, intervention to prevent or limit infarction size should be instituted within this time period to maximize effectiveness.

225 Drugs that can act to reverse coronary stenosis and relieve the obstruction include the nitrates, calcium blockers, antilipemic agents, antithrombotic (platelet) agents, and thrombolytic agents.

LET US REVIEW: Although the exact mechanism of acute coronary obstruction is not conclusively established, the three most common theories are (1) _____ _____ (atherosclerosis), (2) _____ aggregation, and (3) coronary _____. This triad of atherosclerosis, _____ (thrombi), and spasm has been implicated in the related syndromes of angina and acute _____ _____.

lipid infiltration
platelet
spasm
platelets
myocardial infarction

226 Platelet and antilipemic agents are most effective in the long-term prevention of coronary artery disease. Therapy may be begun before any acute symptomatology. Related risk factor control can also support the effectiveness of these agents. Nitrates and calcium blockers are most effective in reversing anginal changes but may lose their effectiveness once an infarction is in progress.

227 When an infarction is in progress, effective reversal of coronary stenosis usually responds more effectively to thrombolytic agents administered by either the intravenous or intracoronary route (see Frames 267 to 279). The effects of these agents may be complemented by percutaneous coronary angioplasty (PTCA) in the presence of an accessible fatty lesion. Reversal of acute obstruction has been shown to coincide with relief of chest pain, reversal of acute ECG changes, and recovery of normal wall motion. Myocardial infarction may be limited or prevented if this mode of therapy is instituted within 2 to 4 hours.

REMEMBER: Significant death of tissue occurs within about _____ to _____ hours after acute, severe _____ obstruction. This time period also corresponds to the rise of _____ isoenzymes (see Unit 6, Frames 18 to 24). Establishment of reperfusion with either pharmacological or mechanical therapy may be associated with transient ventricular arrhythmias.

2; 4
coronary
CPK

228 Mortality immediately after acute MI (that is, hours to days later) is probably related to the metabolic effects of acute ischemia. Long-term complications and/or mortality may relate more to either infarct size or the extent of the underlying coronary disease.

The metabolic consequences of acute MI extend beyond the initial, critical 2 to 4 hours. The initial area of necrosis is usually surrounded by an unclearly defined, critically ischemic zone, which may remain for hours or days. Patchy areas of infarction often develop within this ischemic border zone, thus extending the initial area of infarction. The approach to preserve ischemic myocardium after an MI is multifaceted and is directed toward protecting and preserving this ischemic zone.

Factors contributing to infarction of the ischemic zone include (1) increases in myocardial O_2 demand, (2) decreases in myocardial O_2 supply, and (3) metabolic changes related to hypoxia. Infarction size may be further limited by the use of metabolic intervention or the antianginal agents, which act either to increase _____ _____ or to lower _____.

coronary supply
demands

229 Cardioprotective agents that may minimize the metabolic consequences of ischemia include the beta blockers, the calcium blockers, and steroids. Beta blockers act to lower myocardial free fatty acids (FFA), and to increase glucose uptake.

REMEMBER: Under normal conditions the primary energy source of the myocardium is *(fat/glucose)* in the form of _____. Fatty acids require the presence of _____ to act as an energy source. In hypoxia myocardial FFA utilization is *(stimulated/inhibited)*, causing serum levels to *(rise/fall)*. Increased serum FFA levels have been associated with increased myocardial O_2 _____, chest pain, _____ arrhythmia, and *(increased/decreased)* contractility (see Unit 6, Frames 138 to 145).

fat; FFA

oxygen

inhibited

rise

consumption; ventricular

decreased

230 Hypoxia also depletes intracellular ATP stores that effectively pump out calcium. Accumulation of intracellular calcium within the mitochondria has been associated with myocardial necrosis. These calcium changes may be detected within 12 hours after MI with _____ scanning (see Unit 6, Frames 109 to 112).

technetium-99m-pyrophosphate

The use of calcium antagonists in the period immediately after MI may prevent this intracellular calcium accumulation and protect the machinery of contraction. Benefits of preventing postarrest cerebral necrosis look promising. However, there is no current evidence that these drugs prevent myocardial infarction or decrease mortality.

231 Hypoxia also acts as a local stressor to the myocardial tissues, triggering an inflammatory response (see Unit 4, Frames 69 and 70 and Unit 6, Frame 147). This response, if excessive, may compress and further compromise the normal tissue. Inflammation is also associated with the release of additional chemical toxins, which can irritate or injure nerve or muscle cells.

Steroids can act to decrease local inflammatory responses and stabilize cell membranes, lysosomes, and mitochondria. However, they also *(increase/decrease)* capillary fragility and *(inhibit/promote)* tissue healing and scar formation. They may thus increae the risk of rupture and/or tamponade. Therefore the use of steroids after MI to preserve myocardial tissue remains highly controversial and is best avoided.

increase; inhibit

232 Beta blockers are the major agents with currently documented benefits after MI, primarily beyond the acute phase. The use of intravenous beta blockers in the acute phase (that is, within the first 24 hours) is currently under active clinical investigation.

Three major studies in the United States and abroad have documented the effectiveness of beta blockers in the reduction of mortality after MI. The three beta blockers studied were propanolol, metoprolol, and timolol. Benefits reported were similar, although the specific protocols varied significantly. Onset of therapy (oral) ranged from 24 hours to 4 weeks after MI. Duration of therapy ranged from 3 to 33 months. Oral therapy was preceded by intravenous therapy in the metoprolol study only.

233 The specific mechanism of the reported benefits is not clearly established, currently.

LET US REVIEW: Mortality immediately after acute MI is probably related to the _____ effects of *(acute/chronic)* ischemia—especially within the critical ischemic _____ zone. Long-term complications and mortality may relate more to infarct _____ or to the extent of underlying *(acute/chronic)* coronary disease. The symptoms of chronic ischemic disease respond best to agents that *(increase coronary supply/decrease O₂ demands)*.

metabolic; acute

border

size; chronic

decrease O₂ demands

Therefore agents effective in reducing mortality in the various phases after MI should (1) alter acute _____ changes, (2) reduce or limit infarct _____, and/or (3) lower _____ _____.

metabolic
size
O₂ demand

234 Beta blockers have proved *most* beneficial to a subgroup of patients following acute MI: that is, patients with hypertension or recurring angina, suggestive of further underlying ischemic disease. Benefits in these patients appear related at least in part to a lowering of O₂ demands. Therefore patients sustaining an acute myocardial infarction who continue to have hypertension, angina, or both should probably be placed on long-term beta-blocker therapy for at least 1 year and possibly several years. A broader population may also benefit. The choice of beta blocker does not seem critical and may be

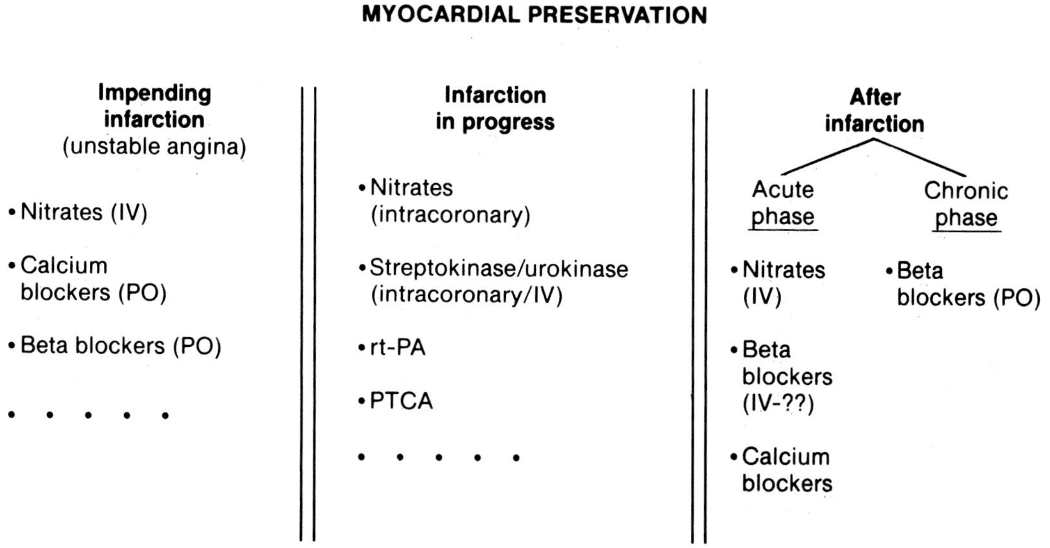

MYOCARDIAL PRESERVATION

Impending infarction (unstable angina)	Infarction in progress	After infarction
		Acute phase / Chronic phase
• Nitrates (IV)	• Nitrates (intracoronary)	
• Calcium blockers (PO)	• Streptokinase/urokinase (intracoronary/IV)	Acute phase: • Nitrates (IV) Chronic phase: • Beta blockers (PO)
• Beta blockers (PO)	• rt-PA	• Beta blockers (IV-??)
• • • • •	• PTCA	• Calcium blockers
	• • • • •	

Fig. 10-14

individually adjusted according to side effects and patient compliance. The benefits of extended (that is, over several years) beta-blocker therapy require further investigation, since there is some evidence from experience in the chronic hypertensive population that long-term beta-blocker therapy may increae serum lipoproteins, thus potentiating atherosclerotic disease.

The use of intravenous beta blockers in the acute phase (especially within the first 2 to 24 hours) remains controversial and is currently under active clinical investigation. In this setting other agents, such as the nitrates, or calcium antagonists, may prove to have equal benefits via different mechanisms. Perhaps it will be a combination of these agents, adapted for the particular phase of the acute process, that will eventually prove the most effective.

Antithrombotic agents

235 Drugs that alter the clotting process may be referred to collectively as antithrombotic agents. These drugs have a potential role in reversing acute coronary stenosis and preventing or minimizing myocardial infarction and its thrombotic complications. The process of sealing potential vascular leaks with a clot is also referred to as *hemostasis*. It is a major body defense mechanism designed to prevent the escape of blood and involves a process of clot formation *balanced* by a process of clot lysis (Fig. 10-15).

Disruption of this balance leads to an abnormal response, resulting in either *thrombosis* or *hemorrhage*. The focus of this discussion will be *thrombosis*, since this is the major disorder affecting the patient with coronary artery disease.

CLOTTING PROCESS:
OVERVIEW

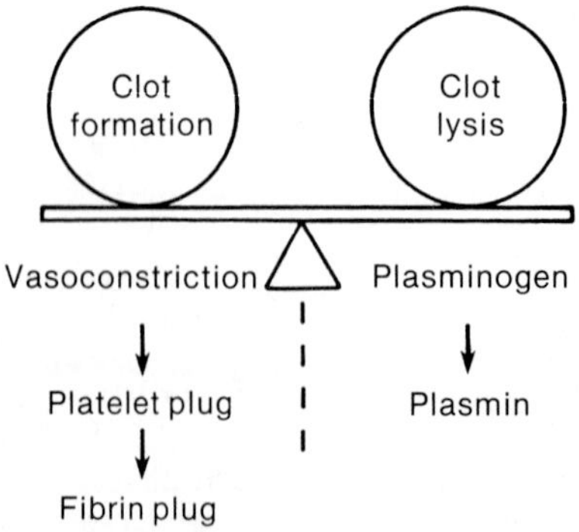

Fig. 10-15

236 The process of clot formation is activated in response to either extravascular or intravascular injury and involves three interrelated steps: a vascular response, platelet activation, and formation of a fibrin clot.

The primary purpose of this clotting, hemostatic mechanism, is to provide a simple seal (plug) in the presence of vessel breaks or disruption. Thrombosis is defined as inappropriate or exaggerated _____. Thrombosis is triggered by an endothelium vascular injury and is no longer limited to the simple sealing off of a vascular break. The normal process of repair is extended or _____ until an abnormal mass develops. This mass obstructs the lumen of the artery or vein, limiting or arresting blood flow.

hemostasis

exaggerated

237 It is an interplay between five major factors that determines whether a significant thrombus will form within the vascular system; they are the following:
1. State of the _____ wall
2. Activity of the blood _____
3. Activity of the _____ factors
4. Rate of blood flow
5. Activity of the fibrinolytic or clot lysis system

vessel
platelets
clotting

Like the normal h emostatic mechanism, thrombus formation involves the initial deposition of a primary _____ plug. This primary plug may or may not be followed by the formation of a fibrin _____ (the secondary plug).

platelet

clot

238 Three types of thrombi may occur in the setting of coronary artery disease: arterial, venous, and mural. Arterial thrombi are triggered by *vessel wall* changes such as those occurring in the proces of atherosclerosis. Venous and mural thrombi are primarily triggered by *stasis* and may or may not be associated with vascular wall injury or change.

LET US REVIEW: The process of clot formation is balanced by a process of _____ _____. The most common disorder of hemostasis in the setting of CAD is *(hemorrhage/thrombosis)*. Thrombus formation may include the depositions of a _____ plug and a(n) _____ (secondary) plug.

clot lysis

thrombosis

platelet; fibrin

Venous and mural thrombi are usually triggered by _____. Arterial thrombi are usually triggered by _____ _____ changes.

stasis
vessel wall

239 The site of origin of an arterial thrombus is usually a roughened intimal lining such as occurs in the setting of _____. This vessel wall abnormality predisposes to _____ activation, and a thrombus slowly forms.

atherosclerosis
platelet

There is usually a minimal deposition of fibrin in an initial arterial thrombus because rapid flow rates in arteries allows for washout of the required clotting factors.

The amount of fibrin deposited in an arterial thrombus thus relates to the degree to which blood flow has been *(slowed/accelerated)* by the atherosclerotic process.

    slowed

REMEMBER: Atherosclerosis narrows the lumen of the coronary _____. Fibrin thrombus formation is often the final event resulting in complete or significant occlusion (see Unit 6, Frame 5).

    artery

The anticoagulants most effective in preventing coronary artery disease are thus those that inhibit *(platelet activation/fibrin formation)*. Drugs that inhibit platelet aggregation include aspirin, clofibrate Atromide-S, dipyridamole (Persantine), sulfinpyrazone (Anturane), and dextran 40 (Rheomacrodex).

    platelet activation

240 Thrombus formation in the venous system is usually slower and involves extensive deposition of fibrin.

The slow-flow venous system promotes stasis, allowing time for the clotting factors to accumulate and react.

Activity restriction in the patient with acute MI promotes venous _____. This predisposes to thrombus formation with potential embolization. Emboli from a venous thrombus can travel rapidly to the pulmonary circulation, resulting in _____ _____ and infarction.

    stasis

    pulmonary embolus

241 When MI occurs, contractility is diminished, resulting in areas of relative stasis within the left ventricular wall. Thrombi formed on these areas of ventricular wall stasis are known as *mural thrombi*. Emboli from a left ventricular mural thrombus can travel rapidly to the _____ circulation, resulting in a _____ embolus and infarction.

    cerebral

    cerebral

REMEMBER: Stasis predisposes to *(more/less)* complete thrombus formation with the deposition of _____. Anticoagulants used to prevent the formation of venous and mural thrombi are those that inhibit *(platelet activation/fibrin formation)*. The two drugs most commonly used in the setting of coronary care for this purpose are _____ and _____.

    more

    fibrin

    fibrin formation

    warfarin; heparin

NOTE: These drugs have no effect on an established thrombus. However, once a thrombus has occurred, anticoagulant treatment aims to prevent further clot formation and minimize embolization.

242 Let us now review in more detail the normal processes of platelet activation and fibrin formation to understand the exact mechanism of action of drugs altering the clotting process.

REMEMBER: Hemostasis is a function of 3 interrelated processes: a

_____ response, _____ activa-tion, and the formation of _____.

vascular; platelet
fibrin

The vascular response to vessel disruption primarily involves contraction of the smooth muscle within the vessel wall and probably does not play a significant role in coronary artery disease.

243 Platelet activation is triggered when the smooth inner lining of the blood vessel (endothelium) is disrupted or roughened. The first re-sponse to the disruption of the endothelial tissue is platelet adhesion. "Adhesion" refers to the process by which platelets are attracted to and stick to something other than platelets. Following adhesion, platelets undergo a change in shape and become activated. With ac-tivation, a complex series of reactions occurs, resulting in the release of compounds that promote platelet aggregation. "Aggregation" re-fers to the process by which platelets are attracted to and stick to other platelets, forming larger clumps. Platelet release factors have also been implicated as contributing to coronary artery spasm and the development of atherosclerosis. Platelets may contribute to the development of atherosclerosis by altering permeability and thus al-lowing for lipid deposition and/or aggravating smooth muscle prolif-eration (medial layer changes).

LET US REVIEW: Platelet activation is initially triggered by a break or roughening within the _____ layer of the blood vessel. The process by which platelets stick to exposed subendothe-lial tissue is known as platelet _____.

Platelet aggregation follows platelet _____ and results in the formation of larger _____. Many substances, such as epinephrine, collagen fibers, immune complexes, serotonin, adenosine phosphate, thrombin, and microorganisms, can induce platelets to aggregate. Risk factors associated with coronary artery disease have also been implicated in promoting platelet aggregation. Included are high serum cholesterol values, Type II hyperlipidemia, cigarette smoking, stress, birth control pils, diabetes, and a high-fat diet.

endothelial

adhesion

adhesion
clumps

244 Let us now consider the process of fibrin clot formation in more de-tail. Fibrin formation occurs in three major stages: thromboplastin activity, conversion of prothrombin to thrombin, and conversion of fibrinogen to fibrin (Fig. 10-16).

Thromboplastin activity may be generated by either the intrinsic or the extrinsic clotting factor pathways. The intrinsic pathway is stimulated by intravascular trauma that results in disruption or roughening of the endothelial layer of the blood vessels.

REMEMBER: _____ activation is also triggered by intravascular damage. Platelets therefore exert a major influence on the (intrinsic/extrinsic) pathway.

Platelet

intrinsic

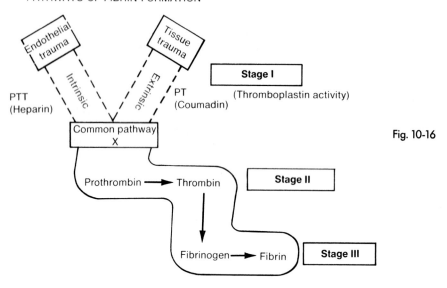

PATHWAYS OF FIBRIN FORMATION

Endothelial trauma

Tissue trauma

Intrinsic

Extrinsic

Stage I
(Thromboplastin activity)

PTT
(Heparin)

PT
(Coumadin)

Fig. 10-16

Common pathway
X

Prothrombin → Thrombin

Stage II

Fibrinogen → Fibrin

Stage III

245 The extrinsic pathway for the generation of thromboplastin activity is stimulated by extravascular trauma (that is, tissue trauma). With tissue trauma a "tissue juice" is released, which activates the extrinsic pathway. Most often fibrin deposition is probably a result of simulataneous activation of both pathways.

There are certain clotting factors unique to each pathway. However, there is a common point or junction at which the two pathways become one. This common pathway begins with factor X (see Fig. 10-4).

Immediately following the activation of factor X, stage II of the fibrin formation process begins, with the conversion of _____ to _____.

prothrombin; thrombin

Thrombin subsequently converts fibrinogen to _____, completing stage III.

fibrin

246 Fibrin formation is accompanied by activation of a *fibrin breakdown* or *fibrinolytic (clot lysis) system.*

A delicate balance normally exists between the fibrin formation and _____.

fibrinolysis

The presence of a *thrombus* in the vascular system indicates that the rate of fibrin formation has exceeded the body's _____ capacity.

fibrinolytic

Let us now consider the fibrinolytic system in more detail. The proteolytic enzyme *plasmin* is the active component of the fibrinolytic system. The action of plasmin is to digest fibrin clots.

Plasminogen is the inactive precursor of plasmin. Conversion of plasminogen to plasmin depends on contact with specific activator substances.

Plasminogen activators have an affinity for fibrin threads, thus allowing for _____ to be generated at the site of thrombus formation.

247 LET US REVIEW: The active component of the body's fibrinolytic system is _____.

Production of plasmin depends on activation of its precursor _____.

The action of plasmin is to break up or digest existing _____ _____. The end products of this process are referred to as *fibrin split* or *fibrin degradation products* (FSP/FDP).

Anticoagulant agents whose mode of action is fibrinolytic are currently under investigation in the acute management of coronary artery disease.

Therapeutically induced fibrinolysis may succeed in dissolving a thrombus in either the venous or arterial system.

REMEMBER: Although platelet deposition is primarily implicated in the genesis of an arterial thrombus, limited _____ deposition may also occur.

Therapeutic implications: overview

248 The major focus of antithrombotic therapy in coronary artery disease is directed toward one or more of the following:
1. Prevention of thrombus formation
2. Prevention of embolic complications
3. Disruption of existing thrombi

Three major categories of drugs may be effective. They include the antiplatelet, antifibrin, and fibrinolytic agents.

The antiplatelet agents are most effective in the prevention of coronary artery thrombosis, since thrombus formation in arteries consists primarily of _____.

Agents that prevent arterial thrombi have a potential role in the _____ of acute MI.

REMEMBER: Although the exact pathogenesis of acute coronary artery occlusion is not conclusively established, the triad of atherosclerosis, _____, and _____ are implicated in the syndromes of angina and myocardial infarction.

Antiplatelet agents have also been shown to prevent closure of vein grafts after bypass surgery.

249 The antifibrin agents _____ and _____ are effective in preventing venous and _____ thrombi. These agents potentially decrease the growth of and embolization from thrombi forming in these areas.

plasmin

plasmin

plasminogen

fibrin clots

fibrin

platelets

prevention

spasm; thrombus

warfarin
heparin
mural

Heparin and warfarin are generally throught to be *ineffective* in preventing arterial thrombi or rersolving a thromboembolic event unless flow is compromised as with stenosis or the presence of mechanical devices, such as the IABP or arterial line catheters.

The thrombolytic drugs streptokinase, urokinase, and tissue plasminogen activator (rt-PA) have been shown to be effective in disrupting or lysing existing thrombi.

All three drugs are currently used to achieve coronary reperfusion in the setting of acute coronary artery occlusion.

250 Successful reperfusion with thrombolytic agents supports the role of
_____ in the pathogensis of **thrombosis**
_____ _____ occlusion (see Frames 219 **coronary artery**
to 221).

The antiplatelet, antifibrin, and fibrinolytic agents may be collectively referred to as antithrombotic agents. Although the drugs discussed within this classification differ pharmacologically, all interfere with clot formation and/or support clot lysis in the cardiovascular system.

Antiplatelet agents

251 Many agents have been demonstrated to inhibit platelet activity and thus have potential as antithrombotic agents. Three antiplatelet agents currently in common use are aspirin, dypyridamole (Persantine) and sulfinpyrazone (Anturane).

REMEMBER: Antilatelet agents may be used to prevent the formation of *(arterial/venous)* thrombi, which consist primarily of **arterial**
_____. **platelets**

Aspirin

252 Aspirin inhibits the formation of arterial thrombi by preventing the release of platelet-activator substances.

REMEMBER: When platelets adhere to a roughened endothelium, they release *platelet-activator substances,* which cause platelets to clump, or _____. Arterial thrombi are primarily **aggregate**
composed of _____ _____. **platelet aggregates**

The use of aspirin in the prophylaxis of angina and/or myocardial infarction remains controversial, although it is extensively used for this purpose. Aspirin is also prescribed to prevent vein graft closure after bypass surgery. Aspirin is commonly prescribed in the setting of cerebrovascular disease for the prevention of transient ischemic attacks (TIAs) or strokes.

The antithrombotic effects of aspirin do not usually cause bleeding unless a history of ulcers or bleeding disorder exists. The use of aspirin is contraindicated in this setting.

253 LET US REVIEW: Aspirin acts as an antithrombotic agent by inhibiting the release of ———————— substances and thus inhibits platelet ————————.

    REMEMBER: Arterial thrombi are primarily composed of ———————— ————————. Aspirin can thus potentially prevent the formation of *(arterial/venous)* thrombi. Although its beneficial effects in coronary artery disease *(are/are not)* clearly established, aspirin *(is/is not)* commonly prescribed in this setting. It is *(common/uncommon)* to bleed with aspirin therapy.

Dipyridamole and sulfinpyrazone

254 Although pharmacologically different, both dipyridamole (Persantine) and sulfinpyrazone (Anturan, Anturane) act as antiplatelet agents. Both are currently under clinical investigation in the prophylaxis of acute MI as well as the prevention of vein graft closure after bypass surgery. Dipyridamole, a coronary vasodilator, was initially used in the treatment of angina pectoris. Side effects associated with its use are primarily related to its peripheral vasodilating ctions; they include headache, dizziness, weakness, hypotension, flushing, and fainting. Sulfinpyrazone is classified as a uricosuric agent because it promotes the excretion of uric acid. Side effects associated with its use primarily relate to its antithrombotic effects; they include epigastric pain, blood loss, and reactivation of peptic ulcers.

Antifibrin agents

255 Agents that inhibit the formation of fibrin can also act as antithrombotic agents. The traditional, more familiar anticoagulants heparin and coumadin fall within this category.

    REMEMBER: Antifibrin agents are most effective in preventing formation of *(arterial/venous)* and ———————— thrombi. They thus prevent pulmonary or ———————— emboli in the patient with an acute MI.

Heparin

256 Heparin sodium is a naturally occurring substance found in many tissues, including the liver, lung, and intestine. Heparin inhibits the formation of fibrin clots primarily by inactivating thrombin.

    REMEMBER: The main role of the enzyme thrombin is to convert ———————— to fibrin. Heparin also exerts a significant inhibitory effect on the clotting factors within the intrinsic pathway.

257 Heparin may be administered intravenously as a bolus or as a continuous infusion. It may also be given subcutaneously. It is generally not given intramuscularly because of the risk of intramuscular or retroperitoneal hematomas. The administration of small amounts of

Margin answers:
platelet-activator
aggregation

platelet aggregates
arterial
are not
is
uncommon

venous; mural
cerebral

fibrinogen

527

heparin at 12-hour intervals is known as "minidose heparin" and is currently preferred for prophylactic use in acute MI. It has been shown that small dosages are all that is required to block the coagulation process at the start of the common pathway (factor X).

258 Therapeutic higher dosages of heparin are required once a coagulation disorder, such as thrombophlebitis or pulmonary emboli, is established in the setting of acute MI; once thrombophlebitis or pulmonary emboli have been established, *(higher/lower)* dosages of heparin are indicated. High-dose heparin may be administered every 4 hours or in the form of a continuous infusion at a rate of approximately 1000 units an hour.

higher

   Heparin may neutralize the effects of many other agents because of its acid pH. It therefore *should not* be administered in conjunction with other drugs by the intravenous route.

259 LET US REVIEW: Heparin exerts its anticoagulant effect by inactivating the enzyme _____. Heparin exerts its predominant effects on the *(intrinsic/extrinsic)* pathway for fibrin deposition. Small doses of heparin administered at 12-hour intervals are known as _____ therapy. It is used to *(prevent/treat)* thrombus formation. Once the clotting process has been established, *(high/low)* dosages of heparin are required.

thrombin
intrinsic

minidose; prevent
high

260 The anticoagulation study most commonly used to control heparin therapy is the partial thromboplastin time (PTT). This study tests for the clotting factors unique to the intrinsic pathways as well as those involed in the common pathway.

   REMEMBER: Heparin exerts a significant effect on the *(intrinsic/extrinsic)* pathway. Maintenance of the PTT between 1.5 and 2.5 times the control values has been shown to ensure anticoagulation in most patients.

intrinsic

   The plasma recalcification time (PRT) may also be used to monitor heparin therapy. This study tests the overall fibrin formation process or clotting time. This normally slow process is accelerated by the addition of the clotting factor Ca^{++} to the patient's blood sample.

261 The most common complication of heparin therapy is bleeding. Monitoring coagulation studies as well as observing for signs and symptoms of bleeding is a primary nursing responsibility (see Frame 268). If rapid reversal of the effects of heparin is required, protamine sulfate is the specific antidote; it is usually administered as a slow IV bolus. Protamine in excessive amounts may itself act as an anticoagulant.

Warfarin

262 The most commonly used anticoagulant of the coumarin group is warfarin sodium (Coumadin). Warfarin drugs compete with vitamin K and thus depress the synthesis of vitamin K–dependent clotting factors in the liver. There are four vitamin K–dependent clotting factors, the most well known of which is prothrombin (factor II).

263 Warfarin is usually given orally. It may take several days to achieve the full anticoagulant effect. Therefore, when a switch from heparin to warfarin is desired, the two drugs must be given concomitantly for 3 to 5 days. The coagulation study most commonly used to control warfarin therapy is the prothrombin time (PT). The PT tests for the factors unique to the extrinsic pathway as well as for those of the common pathway.

Of the five factors tested, three are vitamin K–dependent and thus are depressed by _____. These factors are also influenced by liver function.   *warfarin*

Warfarin thus exerts its main influence on the *(intrinsic/extrinsic)* pathway of fibrin formation. Maintenance of the PT at approximately 1.5 to 2 times the control value ensures anticoagulation in most patients.   *extrinsic*

264 LET US REVIEW: The most commonly used coumarin derivative is _____. Warfarin exerts its anticoagulant effect by   *warfarin*
depressing the synthesis of the _____   *vitamin K*
_____–dependent clotting factors in the _____.   *liver*
The test used to control warfarin therapy is the
_____ _____. This test checks the factors   *prothrombin time*
unique to the *(intrinsic/extrinsic)* pathway. Of the five factors tested in   *extrinsic*
the PT, _____ are vitamin K dependent.   *three*

265 Many commonly used drugs interact withthe coumarin anticoagulants. Some drugs antagonize the action, producing warfarin resistance, and may lead to overdosage when they are withdrawn. Commonly used drugs that antagonize coumarins are the barbiturates and oral contraeptives. Other drugs may potentiate the action of the coumarins. Commonly used drugs that may potentiate the action include aspirin, quinidine, neomycin, chloral hydrate, clofibrate, indomethacin, and allopurinol. A complete list of drugs with which warfarin can interact should be available to the physician as he prescribes. Readjustment of the warfarin dosage will be required as interacting drugs are withdrawn or prescribed.

266 The most common complication of warfarin therapy is bleeding. Patient education regarding covert signs of bleeding as well as the importance of follow-up coagulation studies is crucial for patients receiving warfarin at home.

REMEMBER: Warfarin exerts its anticoagulant effect by competing with _____ _____. Thus the antidote for bleeding resulting from warfarin therapy is _____ _____, or phytonadione (Aquamephyton).

vitamin K
vitamin K

THROMBOLYTIC AGENTS

267 Three agents: streptokinase (Kabbinase, Streptase), urokinase (Abbokinase, Breokinase, Win-Kinase), and recombinant tissue-type plasminogen activator or rt-PA (Activase) are currently approved for use as thrombolytic agents in acute MI.

The goal of thrombolytic therapy in acute MI is to achieve sustained reperfusion of the infarct related vessel theraby maintaining left ventricular function, limiting infarct size and improving immediate and long term survival. Reperfusion is accomplished by reversing the thrombotic component of coronary thrombosis or occlusion.

REMEMBER: It is the triad of _____, _____, and _____ that contributes to the coronary stenosis or occlusion associated with acute myocardial infarction.

lipids
vasospasm; thrombosis

268 Thrombolytic therapy was first attempted in acute MI in the 1950's using streptokinase. However without the benefit of coronary arteriography to confirm pathology and results of therapy, the findings were inconclusive and this mode of intervention was abandoned.

Enthusiasm for the use of thrombolytic drugs was rekindled in the 1970s by the work of Chazov and later Rentrop who dramatically showed the opening of a coronary artery in acute MI with intracoronary streptokinase. The rationale for the use of thrombolytic therapy in acute MI was even more clearly established by the work of DeWood and associates in 1980. They performed coronary arteriograms within six hours of the onset of symptoms of acute MI and demonstrated that a thrombus was present in 87% of those patients evaluated. Their work also confirmed the safety of catheterization in acute MI, which had been controversial until this time.

269 Since 1980, many large scale trials using thrombolytic drugs in acute MI have been conducted, and results support that these goals are being accomplished. It has been repeatedly demonstrated that the time from onset of symptoms till reperfusion of the involved muscle is the critical factor in achieving success. One large study involving over 12,000 patients in Italy (GISSI) demonstrated that beyond six hours there was very little difference in mortality between those treated and those not treated. The lowest mortality at one year was in the group treated the earliest from the onset of symptoms. Other studies have also demonstrated that the earlier thrombolytic therapy is initiated the better the preservation of left ventricular function.

Despite reperfusion in a large percentage of patients with the use of thrombolytic drugs, re-occlusion is encountered in 20% to 40% of patients. The most important determinant for acute re-occlusion appears to be the degree of residual stenosis.

270 The common denominator of all thrombolytic drugs is that they in some way activate the body's own clot lysis or *fibrinolytic* system. For this reason these agents may also be referred to as _____ agents.　　　　　　　　　　　　　　　　fibrinolytic

REMEMBER: The proteolytic enzyme *plasmin* is the active component of the fibrinolytic system. The action of plasmin is to _____ fibrin clots.　　　　　　　　　　　　　　　digest

Plasminogen is the inactive _____ to plasmin.　precursor
Conversion of plasminogen to _____ depends on contact　plasmin
with _____ substances. Plasminogen activators　activator
have an affinity for fibrin threads thus allowing for _____　plasmin
to be generated at the site of thrombus formation.

Plasmin is a non-specific proteolytic enzyme and depletes many circulating proteins, including fibrinogen and other clotting factors. The end products of fibrinogen breakdown are known as fibrin split or _____ products. These exert an anticoagulant　degradation
effect themselves.

Streptokinase

271 Streptokinase is an extract of non-pathogenic hemolytic streptococi. It is the most economical thrombolytic drug and has been studied extensively in the United States and Europe.

Streptokinase had no fibrin selectivity and exerts its action systematically converting plasminogen to _____ in the circu-　plasmin
lating blood pool. This results in very high levels of plasmin, which ultimately depletes the blood pool of fibrinogen and other clotting factors for as long as 24 to 36 hours. High levels of fibrin split and _____ products are also present, which, together　degradation
with depletion of clotting factors, potentially exposes the patient to serious bleeding complications.

Streptokinase is recognized as a foreign protein by the body and is thus antigenic. Therefore resistance or allergic reactions may develop with the use of the drug. Streptokinase may produce serious hypotension with initial administration in some patients requiring vasopressor support.

272 Streptokinase has been administered by both the intracoronary and _____ route in the setting of acute MI. With intra-　intravenous coronary administration the reperfusion success rate is approximately 75%. However because of the lack of catheterization labs in most hospitals the intravenous route has been studied more extensively. Successful reperfusion with intravenous streptokinase is approximately 50%. The GISSI trial with IV streptokinase demonstrated a 50% reduction of in hospital mortality in the group who received IV streptokinase.

REMEMBER: The Italian GISSI study demonstrated very little difference in mortality when treatment was initiated beyond _____ hours (see Frame 267). However, *(positive/negative)* results were obtained with earlier administration.

six; positive

A second generation thrombolytic drug related to streptokinase is known as plasminogen streptokinase activator complex (APSAC) is currently under investigation.

273 The largest USA study on thrombolysis is known as Phase I of the Thrombolysis in Myocardial Infarction (TIMI) study, which compared IV streptokinase and IV recombinant tissue plasminogen activator (rt-PA). This study was terminated prematurely because of the superiority of rt-PA over streptokinase. Tissue plasminogen activator elicited reperfusion in twice as many occluded arteries as compared with streptokinase.

Recombinant tissue plasminogen activator rt-PA

274 Tissue plasminogen activator (rt-PA) is a naturally occurring substance found in the endothelium, circulating blood, and other human tissue, which normally plays a role in the fibrinolytic system.

It was first isolated in the 1940s, but it was not until the 1980s through recombinant DNA genetic engineering techniques that it could be produced in quantities sufficient for commercial use. It still costs approximately fifteen times as much as streptokinase. Tissue plasminogen activator is non-antigenic and, unlike streptokinase, no allergic reactions have been reported as yet.

Unlike both streptokinase and urokinase, the action of rt-PA is clot specific. It activates only the plasminogen that is incorporated into the thrombotic fibrin clot and *(does/does not)* alter circulating plasminogen.

does not

275 Because of its selectivity for the plasminogen within the fibrin clots, it has been referred to as the "magic bullet." Due to its short half life of only four to ten minutes, it is usually infused over a period of three hours and heparin therapy is initiated concomitantly. The heparin infusion is continued after the rt-PA infusion is completed to reduce the incidence of re-occlusion.

Tissue plasminogen activator has been shown to have approximately a 75% success rate when administered intravenously, compared to a _____ success rate with streptokinase. Though there is less serious depletion of fibrinogen and clotting factors than occurs with streptokinase and urokinase, the occurrence of bleeding episodes is comparable (see Frame 277).

50%

Recombinant tissue plasminogen activator is currently being studied extensively in the United States in combination with other thrombolytic drugs, angioplasty, and beta blockers.

Thrombolysis in Myocardial Infarction (TIMI) Phase II looks at the role and optimal timing of angioplasty in combination with rt-PA administration and beta blockers using a larger dose of rt-PA than with TIMI Phase I. The dosage of rt-PA was immediately reduced at the beginning of this study due to the incidence of intracranial bleeds. The protocol for immediate angioplasty was also abandoned due to problems encountered early in the study.

Urokinase

276 Urokinase is a naturally occurring human enzyme derived from kidney cells and is a direct activator of plasminogen. It is about ten times as expensive as streptokinase. Like streptokinase but unlike rt-PA, urokinase *(is/is not)* clot specific and exerts its action systemically on circulating plasminogen. Urokinase is non-antigenic and is generally well tolerated when administered intravenously with no reports of allergic reactions. Fewer bleeding episodes are reported with the use of intracoronary urokinse than with streptokinase. Comparable reperfusion success rates are reported. Limited experience with IV urokinase shows a success rate of 60%. A single recent German trial using urokinase in larger than usual dosages has shown a nearly identical patency rate as with tissue plasminogen activator, providing a challenge to the superiority of this agent. A clot specific derivative of urokinase, prourokinase, is currently being investigated.

The use of urokinase in combination with rt-PA is currently being investigated in the Thrombolysis and Angioplasty in Myocardial Infarction (TAMI) Study.

is not

Complications of thrombolytic therapy:

277 The major complication associated with the use of thrombolytic drugs is _____. Periaccess bleeding or bleeding at puncture sites may be serious and can occur with all of the thrombolytic drugs in use including rt-PA. This bleeding occurs most commonly at femoral access sites used for catheterization or arterial or venous sheaths. Limiting venous and arterial punctures is recommended. Anticoagulants administered to maintain patency, such as _____, may also be implicated in the bleeding episodes. Intracranial hemorrhages have been reported with all the thrombolytic drugs in use with high risk patients. Risk factors for

bleeding

Heparin

bleeding include female sex, advanced age, and longstanding or acute hypertension. The incidence is approximately one out of every 200 patients.

278 Indications of effective reperfusion include abrupt cessation of chest pain, a rapid fall in the ST segments and rapid peaking of the CPK enzymes 3 to 4 hours after treatment. The major complications associated with any form of reperfusion is arrhythmias. These include AIVR, VT, VF, and bradycardia primarily with IWMI. *(Hypotension/ hypertension)* may also occur.

hypotension

279 NURSING ORDERS: Patients receiving antithrombotic therapy for coronary artery disease
   1. Check for a history of bleeding disorders, GI ulcers, gastritis, and liver disease before initiating therapy.

NOTE: Antiplatelet and antifibrin agents may be used within a specified time frame after surgery in selected cases (for example, after bypas surgery or valve replacement).

   2. Check other medications for possible interactions with anticoagulants—especially with warfarin and heparin.

REMEMBER: Intravenous _____ should not be infused with other drugs.

heparin

   3. Regularly inspect the patient for signs of bleeding with hemostat of urine, stools, and emesis; check the gums and nose and watch for bruising, ecchymotic areas, and so forth.
   4. Report any new pericardial friction rub to the physician; withdrawal of anticoagulant therapy may be required.
   5. Follow coagulation studies closely: PTT with _____ therapy should be _____ to _____ times normal; PT with _____ therapy should be _____ to _____ times normal.

heparin
1.5; 2.5
warfarin
1.5; 2

   6. During thrombolytic therapy:
      • Support the patient and family and provide them with information as required regarding the therapy.
      • Watch for markers of reperfusion during intravenous administration of thrombolytic drugs, arrhythmia, sudden end to chest pain, hypotension and bradycardia with IWMI, early peaking of the CPK enzyme; note CPK higher than normal and falls faster than normal.
      • Monitor on a lead where ST elevation can be monitored carefully. Note any increases or decreases with therapy.
      • Be alert for the development of life-threatening reperfusion arrhythmias—V.T., V.F., AIVR
      • Monitor clinical signs of ischemia closely i.e. chest discomfort, ST segment shifts, arrhythmias,

- Report continued chest discomfort post thrombolytic therapy or any ECG changes suggestive of further ischemia that could signal re-occlusion. Alert the physician immediately if these occur.
- Monitor carefully at catheter insertion sites for signs of bleeding, hematoma formation, unusual bruising. Monitor lab values that may indicate covert bleeding.
- Limit IV puncture by use of large gauge intracaths for blood sampling and IV therapy.
- Maintain heparin infusion and follow PTT's carefully.
- Monitor neurological status carefully for subtle signs of possible bleed.

7. After thrombolytic therapy:
- Maintain pressure at the catheter-introducer site as prescribed to avoid excessive bleeding.
- Handle the patient gently to avoid bruising.
- Administer no intramuscular medications until the effects of therapy have been resolved.

REMEMBER: There is no exact antidote for thrombolytic drugs.

8. Administer subcutanoues heparin between the iliac crests in the lower abdomen. Rotate the injeciton sites and do not massage. Use of a standardized card is desirable for this purpose. Obtain PTT approximately 30 minutes before the next dose of heparin. The antidote for bleeding from heparin therapy is _____ _____. **protamine sulfate**

9. Give warfarin at the same time daily. The elderly and those patients with renal and liver disease are particularly susceptible if given warfarin; they should wear a bracelet. The antidote for bleeding from warfarin therapy is _____ _____. **vitamin K**

10. Patient teaching considerations:
- A Medic Alert bracelet should be worn by patients receiving anticoagulants at home.
- A "vial of life" with medical information and a list of all cardiac medications should be kept in the refrigerator of cardiac patients.
- Teach patients the subtle signs and symptoms of bleeding.
- Avoid over-the-counter medications that may potentiate anticoagulant effects.
- Instruct patients to take warfarin at the same time daily.
- Instruct patients to use an electric razor and a soft tooth brush.
- Instruct patients to report any changes in menses.
- Stress to patients the importance of a pressure dressing or bag.
- Maintain poststreptokinase therapy.

Table 15. Antithrombotic drugs

	Antiplatelet	Antifibrin	Thrombolytic
Name	Acetylacetic acid (aspirin)	Warfarin sodium (Coumadin)	Streptokinase (Streptase, Kabikinase)
	Dipyridamole (Persantine)	Heparin	Urokinase
	Sulfinpyrazone (Anturane)		rt-PA (Activase)
Major use in CAD	Prevent arterial thrombus/vein graft closure before and after MI and after bypass surgery	Prevent venous/mural thrombus after MI; prevent LA thrombus in chronic atrial fibrillation	Disrupt coronary arterial thrombus with acute obstruction
Severity of associated side effects	Mild	Moderate	Potentially severe
Antidote(s) for treatment of complications	Withdraw medication; no specific therapy usually required	Administer medication: for warfarin, Vitamin K; for heparin, protamine sulfate; for extreme cases, fresh frozen plasma (FFP)	Stop drug Administer blood products
Related coagulation test(s)	Platelet count	PT: warfarin; PTT: heparin	PTT: concomitant heparin administration

*Potential use—not approved.

Table 16. Pharmacological management of cardiac arrest

Arrhythmias	CHF/Shock	Chest pain	Metabolic complications
Antiarrhythmics —Lidocaine* (Xylocaine) —Procainamide* (Pronestyl) —Bretylium tosylate* (Bretylol) Sympathetic (beta) stimulators —Isoproterenol (Isuprel) —Epinephrine (Adrenalin) Sympathetic (beta) blocker —Propranolol (Inderal) Parasympathetic stimulator —Digitalis (Digoxin, Lanoxin) Parasympathetic blocker —Atropine sulfate* Calcium blocker —Verapamil* (Isoptin, Calan)	Diuretic agents —Furosemide (Lasix) —Ethacrynic acid (Edecrin) Vasodilators —Nitroglycerin —Na$^+$ nitroprusside (Nipride) Tinotropic agents —Digitalis (Digoxin, Lanoxin) —Amrinone (Inocor) Sympathetic (beta) stimulators (inotropic agents) —Dopamine (Intropin) —Dobutamine (Dobutrex) Sympathetic (alpha) stimulators —Norepinephrine (Levophed) —Metaraminol (Aramine)	Narcotic —Morphine sulfate* Nitrates —Nitroglycerin	Oxygen* Na$^+$ bicarbonate* Corticosteroids Nitrates (MI) —Nitroglycerin Calcium blockers†
		Electromechanical dissociation	
		—Epinephrine* (Adrenalin) —Na$^+$ bicarbonate*	

*Currently designated as emergency drugs by the American Heart Association.
†Potential use—not approved.

536

280 In Summary:

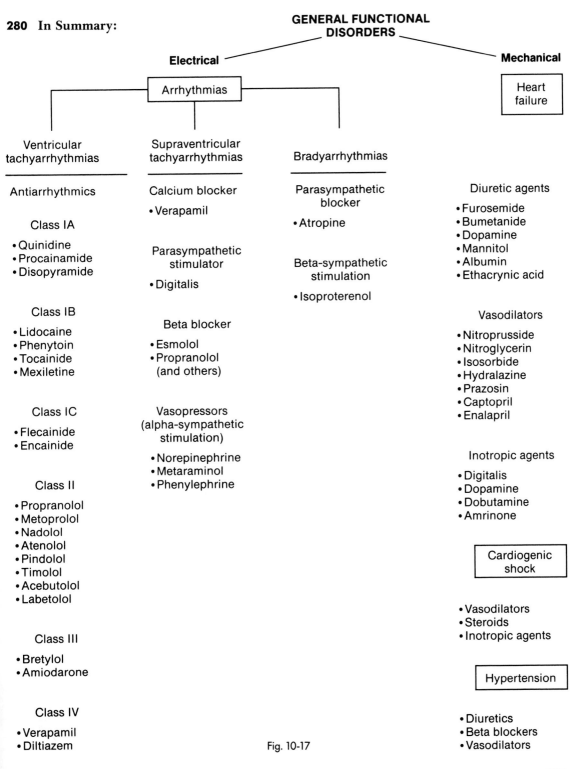

GENERAL FUNCTIONAL
DISORDERS

Electrical   **Mechanical**

Arrhythmias   Heart
                                                                 failure

Ventricular   Supraventricular
tachyarrhythmias   tachyarrhythmias   Bradyarrhythmias

Antiarrhythmics   Calcium blocker   Parasympathetic   Diuretic agents
                        • Verapamil   blocker
                                                • Atropine   • Furosemide
  Class IA   • Bumetanide
• Quinidine   Parasympathetic   • Dopamine
• Procainamide   stimulator   • Mannitol
• Disopyramide   • Digitalis   Beta-sympathetic   • Albumin
                                                stimulation   • Ethacrynic acid
                                                • Isoproterenol
  Class IB   Beta blocker
• Lidocaine   • Esmolol   Vasodilators
• Phenytoin   • Propranolol
• Tocainide   (and others)   • Nitroprusside
• Mexiletine   • Nitroglycerin
                                                                       • Isosorbide
                        Vasopressors   • Hydralazine
  Class IC   (alpha-sympathetic   • Prazosin
• Flecainide   stimulation)   • Captopril
• Encainide   • Norepinephrine   • Enalapril
                        • Metaraminol
                        • Phenylephrine
  Class II   Inotropic agents
• Propranolol   • Digitalis
• Metoprolol   • Dopamine
• Nadolol   • Dobutamine
• Atenolol   • Amrinone
• Pindolol
• Timolol
• Acebutolol   Cardiogenic
• Labetolol   shock

  Class III   • Vasodilators
• Bretylol   • Steroids
• Amiodarone   • Inotropic agents

  Class IV   Hypertension
• Verapamil
• Diltiazem   Fig. 10-17   • Diuretics
                                                                    • Beta blockers
                                                                    • Vasodilators

537

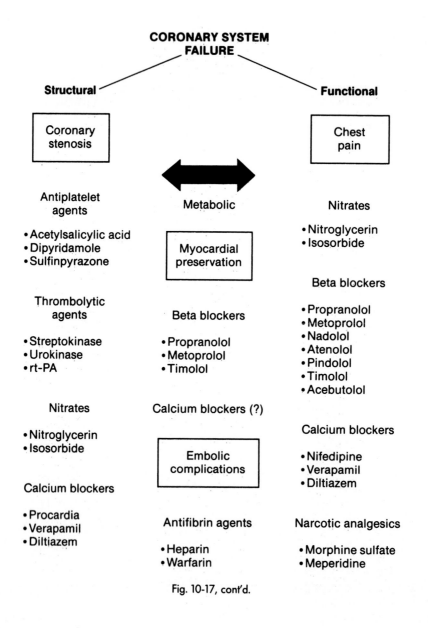

CORONARY SYSTEM FAILURE

Structural   **Functional**

| Coronary stenosis | | Chest pain |

⟷

Metabolic

| Myocardial preservation |

Antiplatelet agents

- Acetylsalicylic acid
- Dipyridamole
- Sulfinpyrazone

Nitrates

- Nitroglycerin
- Isosorbide

Beta blockers

Thrombolytic agents

- Streptokinase
- Urokinase
- rt-PA

Beta blockers

- Propranolol
- Metoprolol
- Timolol

- Propranolol
- Metoprolol
- Nadolol
- Atenolol
- Pindolol
- Timolol
- Acebutolol

Nitrates

- Nitroglycerin
- Isosorbide

Calcium blockers (?)

Calcium blockers

| Embolic complications |

- Nifedipine
- Verapamil
- Diltiazem

Calcium blockers

- Procardia
- Verapamil
- Diltiazem

Antifibrin agents

- Heparin
- Warfarin

Narcotic analgesics

- Morphine sulfate
- Meperidine

Fig. 10-17, cont'd.

SUGGESTED READINGS
General

Alpert J: The pharmacologic management of coronary artery disease in 1986, Heart Lung 15(6):558, 1986.

Braunwald E, editor: Heart disease: a textbook of cardiovascular medicine ed. 3, Philadelphia, 1988, WB Saunders Co.

Cardiac therapy: digitalis glycosides, diuretics, antianginals, and anti-arrhythmics, Nursing 16(11):92, 1986.

Eberts MA: Advances in the pharmacologic management of angina pectoris, J Cardiovasc Nurs 1(1):15, 1986.

Klamerus KJ: Current concepts in clinical therapeutics: congestive heart failure, Clin Pharm 5(6):481, 1986.

Labin I and others: New approaches to the treatment of angina pectoris, Compr Ther 12(6):14, 1986.

Opie LH and others: Drugs for the heart ed. 2, Philadelphia, 1987, WB Saunders Co.

Riegel B: The role of the nurse in limiting myocardial infarct size, Heart Lung 14(3):247, 1985.

Smith S: How drugs act: drugs in angina and myocardial infarction, Nurs Times 83(22):52, 1987.

Standards and guidelines for cardiopulmonary resuscitation (SPR) and emergency cardiac care (ECC), JAMA 255:2905, 1986.

Textbook of advanced cardiac life support, 1987, American Heart Association.

Antiarrhythmic drugs

Campbell RWF: Clinical pharmacology of new antiarrhythmic drugs: I. encainide, flecainide, propafenone, mexiletene, Symposium proceedings of Ventricular Arrhythmias Update, Washington D.C., 1987, Boehringer Ingelheim Pharmaceuticals.

Dicarlo LA Jr and others: Cardiac arrest and sudden death in patients treated with amiodarone for sustained ventricular tachycardia or ventricular fibrillation: risk stratification based on clinical variables, Am J Cardiol 55(2):372, 1985.

Greenspan AM: Combination antiarrhythmic drug therapy for ventricular tachyarrhythmias, PACE 9(4):565, 1986.

Kelliher GJ, and others: Clinical pharmacology of antiarrhythmic agents, Cardiovasc Clin 16(1):287, 1985.

Kienzle MG and others: Antiarrhythmic drug therapy for sustained ventricular tachycardia, Heart Lung 13(6):614, 1984.

Mason JW: Clinical pharmacology of new antiarrhythmic drugs: II. Amiodarone, Sotalol, Symposium proceedings of Ventricular Arrhythmias Update, Washington D.C., 1987, Boehinger Ingelheim Pharmaceuticals.

Morganoth J and others: A review of the uses and limitations of tocainide—a class IB antiarrhythmic agent, Am Heart J 110(4):856, 1985.

Moser SA and Flaker G: Get ready: the new antiarrhythmics are coming, Nursing 15(9):56, 1985.

Muhiddin KA and Turner P: Is there an ideal antiarrhythmic drug? A review—with particular reference to class I antiarrhythmic agents, Postgraduate Med J 61:665-678, 1985.

Nestico PF: Cardiac arrhythmias in the elderly: antiarrhythmic drug treatment, Cardiol Clin 4(2):285, 1986.

Pepper GA: New antiarrhythmic agents, Nurse Pract 11(7):62, 1986.

Podrid PJ: Antiarrhythmic drug therapy: benefits and hazards, Part I, Chest, 88(3):453, 1985.

Podrid PJ: Antiarrhythmic drug therapy: benefits and hazards, Part II, Chest 88(4):618, 1985.

Pohl JE: Flecainide: a positive advance in antiarrhythmic therapy, Intensive Care Nurs 1(2):111, 1985.

Rosen MR: Subclassificationof antiarrhythmic drugs, Symposium proceedings of ventricular arrhythmias update, 1987, Boehringer Ingelheim Pharmaceuticals Inc.

Roden DM: Antiarrhythmic drugs: clinical pharmacology of the old and the new agents, Postgrad Med J 78(4):28, 1985.

Siddoway LA and others: Clinical pharmacology of old and new antiarrhythmic drugs, Cardiovasc Clin 15(3):199, 1985.

Somberg JC and others: The treatment of ventricular rhythm disturbances, Am Heart J 111(6):1162, 1986.

Somberg JC: Antiarrhythmic drugs: making sense of the deluge, Am Heart J 113(2):408, 1987.

Smith A: Amiodarone: clinical considerations, Focus 11(5):30, 1984.

Thielbar S: Antiarrhythmic drug therapy: an overview, CCQ 7(2):21, 1984.

Vaughan WEM: A classification of antiarrhythmic actions reassessed after a decade of new drugs, J Clin Pharmacol 24:129-47, 1984.

Weng JT and others: Antiarrhythmic drugs: electrophysiological basis of their clinical usage, Ann Thorac Surg 41(1):106, 1986.

Wettrell G and others: Cardiovascular drugs I: Antidysrhythmic drugs, Ther Drug Monit 8(1):59, 1986.

Zipes D: Proarrhythmic effects of antiarrhythmic drugs, Am J Card 59(11):26E, 1987.

Sympathetic and parasympathetic nervous system/inotopic agents

Antman EM: Digitalis toxicity, Mod Concepts Cardiovasc Dis 55(6):26, 1986.

Applefeld MM and Roffman DS: Digitalis and other positive catecholamine-like inotropic agents in the management of congestive heart failure, Am J Med (suppl)80:28, 1986.

Benotti J and others: Comparative vasoactive therapy for heart failure, Am J Cardiol 56:19B, 1985.

Braunwald E: A symposium: amrinone—introduction, Am J Cardiol 56(3):1B, 1985.

Butler V: Immunologic treatment of digitalis toxicity: a tale of two prophesies, Annals of Int Med 105(4):613, 1986.

Catalano JT: Antiarrhythmic medications classified by their autonomic properties, Crit Care Nurse 6(3):44, 1986.

Chellingsworth M: Digitalis in the elderly, J Clin Hosp Pharm 11(1):15, 1986.

Cole PL and others: Use of digoxin-specific Fab fragments in the treatment of digitalis intoxication, Drug Intell Clin Pharm 20(4):267, 1986.

Colucci WS and others: New positive inotropic agents in the treatment of congestive heart failure, Part 1, N Engl J Med 314(5):290, 1986.

Colucci WS and others: New positive inotropic agents in the treatment of congestive heart failure, Part 2, N Engl J Med 314(6):349, 1986.

Doherty JE: Clinical use of digitalis glycosides: an update, Cardiology 72(5-6):225, 1985.

Gever LN: Treatment with dopamine, Nursing 16(3):93, 1986.

Guimond JG and others: Augmentation of cardiac function in end-stage heart failure by combined use of dobutamine and amrinone, Chest 90(2):302, 1986.

Krell MJ: Intermittent, ambulatory dobutamine infusions in patients with severe congestive heart failure, Am Heart J 112:787, 1986.

Maekawa K and others: Comparison of dobutamine and dopamine in acute myocardial infarction: effects of systemic hemodynamics, plasma catecholamines, blood flows, and infarct size, Circulation 67:750, 1983.

Mancini DM: Inotropic drugs for the treatment of heart failure, J Clin Pharmacol 25(7):540, 1985.

Marcus F: Pharmokinetics between digoxin and other drugs, JACC 5(5):82A, 1985.

Monrad ES: Milrinone, dobutamine, and nitroprusside: comparative effects on hemodynamics and myocardial energetics in patients with severe congestive heart failure, Part 2, Circulation 73(3):III168, 1986.

Muller JE and others: Digoxin therapy and mortality after myocardial infarction: experience in the MILIS Study, N Eng J Med 314(5):265, 1986.

Norsen LH and others: Understanding cardiac output and the drugs that affect it, Nursing 15(4):31, 1985.

Rackow EC: Hemodynamic effects of digoxin during acute cardiac failure: a comparison in patients with or without acute myocardial infarction, Crit Care Med 15(11):1001, 1987.

Roberts R: Inotropic therapy for cardiac failure associated with acute myocardial infarction, Chest (Suppl)93(1):22S, 1988.

Selzer A: Role of serum digoxin assay in patient management, JACC 5(5):106A, 1985.

Smith T and others: Digitalis glycosides: mechanisms and manifestations of toxicity, Part I, Prog Cardiovasc Dis 26(5):413, 1984.

Smith T and others: Digitalis glycosides: mechanisms and manifestations of toxicity, Part III, Prog Cardiovasc 27(1):21, 1984.

Sonnenblick E and others: New positive inotropic drugs for the treatment of congestive heart failure, Am J Cardiol 55:41A, 1985.

Sundqvist K and others: Effect of digoxin on the electrocardiogram at rest and during exercise in healthy subjects, Am J Cardiol 57:661, 1986.

Surawicz B: Factors affecting tolerance to digitalis, JACC 5(5):69A, 1985.

The failing heart: role of inotropic agents in its

management, 1986, Eli Lilly and Co.

Tommaso CL: Non-glycoside, non-catecholamine inotropic agents in the treatment of congestive heart failure, Am J Med (Suppl) 80:36, 1986.

Treadway G: Clinical safety of intravenous amrinone—a review, Am J Cardiol 56:39B, 1985.

Wade OL: Digoxin 1785-1985, Part I. Two hundred years of digitalis, J Clin Hosp Pharm 11(1):3, 1986.

Diuretics

Brater DC and Chennavasin P: Diuretics: comparing the effect of bumetanide and furosemide, Clin Pharmacol Ther 34:207, 1983.

Carvalho F: Diuretic therapy in congestive heart failure for the elderly patient, Drugs (Suppl) 31(4):165, 1986.

Hill MN: Diuretics for mild hypertension: still the best choice? Nursing 17(9):62, 1987.

Jacobson HR: Diuretics: mechanisms of action and uses, Hosp Pract (Off) 22(12):129, 1987.

Lant A: Diuretic drugs: progress in clinical pharmacology, Drugs (Suppl) 31(4):40, 1986.

Kuchar DL and ohters: High dose furosemide in refractory cardiac failure, Eur Heart J 6(11): 954, 1985.

Melby JC: Selected mechanism of diuretic-induced electrolyte changes, Am J Cardiol 58:1A, 1986.

Ramires JA and others: Diuretics in cardiac edema, Drugs (Suppl) 31(4):68, 1986.

Smith S: How drugs act—diuretic agents, Nurs Times 83(23):53, 1987.

Whelton A: An overview of national patterns and preferences in diuretic selection, Am J Cardiol 57:2A, 1986.

Whelton P and Watson A: Diuretic-induced hypokalemia and cardiac arrhythmias, Am J Cardiol 58:5A, 1986.

Whelton PK: Systemic hypertension, diuretic drugs, arrhythmias, and death, Am J Cardiol 55:221, 1985.

Vasodilators

Abrams J: Vasodilator therapy for chronic congestive heart failure, JAMA 254(21):3070, 1985.

Abrams J: A reappraisal of nitrate therapy, JAMA 259(3):396, 1988.

Andrien P and Lemberg L: An unusual complication of intravenous nitroglycerin, Heart Lung 15(5):534, 1986.

ACE inhibitors: enalapril and captopril compared, Drug Ther Bull 23(23):89, 1985.

Charase B and Scheidt S: The controversy over transdermal nitroglycerin: an update, Am Heart J 112(1):207, 1986.

Cohn J: Nitrates for congestive heart failure, Am J Cardiol 56:19A, 1985.

Cohn PF: Total ischemic burden: effect of vasoactive agents, Part 1, Am Heart J 115(1):215, 1988.

Deans KW and others: Nitrates in the treatment of coronary artery disease, J Cardiovasc Nurs 1(1):81, 1986.

DiBianco R: Angiotensin converting enzyme inhibition: unique and effective therapy for hypertension and congestive heart failure, Postgrad Med J 78(5):231, 1985.

Flaherty J: Clinical revelance of nitrate hemodynamic attenuation, Am Heart J 112(1):216, 1986.

Fogarty A and others: Finding the facts on glycerin trinitrate tablets, Nursing Times 82(3):37, 1986.

Frishman WH: Pharmacology of the nitrates in angina pectoris, Am J Cardiol 56(17):8I, 1985.

Gever LN: Sodium nitroprusside: fast-acting antihypertensive, Nursing 12(2):114, 1982.

Gever LN: ACE inhibitors improve compliance, Nursing 17(10):143, 1987.

Lee WH and Packer M: Prognostic importance of serum sodium concentration and its modification by converting-enzyme inhibition in patients with severe chronic heart failure, Circulation 73(2):257, 1986.

Levine TB: Role of vasodilators in the treatment of congestive heart failure, Am J Cardiol 55:32A, 1985.

Matthewson MA: Current vasodilator therapy, Focus on Crit Care 10(1):49, 1983.

Purcell JA: Intravenous nitroglycerin, Am J Nurs 82(2):254, 1982.

Sanders JB and others: A comparison of plasma renin activity levels in patients with and without congestive heart failure after myocardial infarction, Heart Lung 14(1):1, 1985.

Sutton F: Vasodilator therapy, Am J Med (Suppl)80:2B:54, 1986.

Thadani U: Current status of nitrates in angina pectoric, Mod Concepts Cardiovasc Dis 56(9):49, 1987.

Valladares BK and Lemberg L: Intravenous nitroglycerin in acute infarction, Part I, Heart Lung 11(4):383, 1982.

Valladares BK and Lemberg L: Intravenous nitroglycerin in acute infarction, Part II, Heart Lung 11(5):490, 1982.

Morphine and merperidine

Brown S: Morphine: the benefits are worth the risks, RN 50(3):20, 1987.

Coyle N: Analgesics and pain: current concepts, Nurs Clin N Am 22(3):727, 1987.

Gorman ES: The use of opiods in the management of pain, Hosp Pract (Off) 21(6):48A, 1986.

Goldfrank L and others: Clinical aspects of drug intoxication: opiods and opiates, Heart Lung 12:114, 1983.

Harrison M and others: Pain: advances and issues in critical care, Nurs Clin N Am 22(3):691, 1987.

Lee G and others: Comparative effects of morphine, meperidine, and pentazocine on cardiocirculatory dynamics in patients with acute myocardial infarction, Am J Med 60:949, 1976.

Talbert R: Pharmacotherapeutic modification of the stress response: analgesics, CCQ 7(4):27, 1985.

Semenkovich CF and Jaffe AS: Adverse effects due to morphine sulfate—challenge to previous clinical doctrine, Am J Med 79:325, 1985.

Beta blockers

Abrams J and others: Efficacy and safety of esmolol vs. propanolol in the treatment of supraventricular tachyarrhythmias: a multicenter double-bind clinical trial, Am Heart J 110(5):913, 1985.

Bigger JT and Coromilas J: How do beta-blockers protect after myocardial infarction? Annals Int Med 101(2):256, 1984.

Cohn JN: Clinical implications of the hemodynamic effects of beta blockade, Am J Cardiol 55:125D, 1985.

Dalgas P: Understanding drugs that affect the autonomic nervous system, Nursing 15(10):58, 1985.

DiBianco R: Role of cardioselectivity and intrinsic sympathomimetic activity in beta-blocking drugs in chronic coronary artery disease, Am J Cardiol 59:38F, 1987.

Frishaman WH and others: Beta-adrenergic blockade: an update, Cardiology 72(5):280, 1985.

Frishman WH and others: Beta-adrenergic blockers in the prevention of sudden death, Cardiovasc Clin 15(3):249, 1985.

Frishman WH and others: Use of beta-blocking agents after myocardial infarciton, Postgrad Med J 78(8):40, 1985.

Frishman WH: Beta-adrenergic blocker withdrawal, Am J Cardiol 59:26F, 1987.

Gerber JG and others: Beta-adrenergic blocking drugs, Ann Rev Med 36:145, 1985.

Johnson G and Johanson B: B blockers, Am J Nur 83(7):1034, 1983.

Kendall MJ: Impact of beta1 selectivity and intrinsic sympathomimetic activity on potential unwanted noncardiovascular effects of beta blockers, Am J Cardiol 59:44F, 1987.

Lauler DP: Symposium: potassium, catecholamines, and beta blockade, Am J Cardiol 56(6):1D, 1985.

Lowenthal DT: Mechanisms of action and the clinical pharmacology of beta-adrenergic blocking drugs, Am J Med 77(4A):119, 1984.

Man In'T Veld AJ: Effect of beta blockers on vascular resistance in systemic hypertension, Am J Cardiol 59:21F, 1987.

Mauro VF and Zeller F: Early use of beta-adrenergic blocking agents in acute myocardial infarction, Drug Intell Clin Pharm 20(1):14, 1986.

Mann HJ and others: Cost analysis of substituting labetolol for nitroprusside, Am J Hosp Pharm 43(6):1501, 1986.

Michelson E: A comparison of esmolol and verapamil in the treatment of atrial fibrillation/flutter, (Abstracts), JACC 7(2):157A, 1986.

Michelson L: Labetolol: an alpha- and beta-adrenoceptor blocking drug, Annals Int Med 99(4):553, 1983.

Moore LC: An on-the-spot guide to antihypertensive drugs, Nursing 16(1):54, 1986.

Norris RM: B eta-adrenoreceptor blockers—an update on their role in acute myocardial infarction, Drugs 29(2):97, 1985.

Opie L: Effect of beta-adrenergic blockade on biochemical and metabolic response to exercise, Am J Cardiol 55:95D, 1985.

Pas DA and others: Beta-blocker agents: an update, JEN 12(1):18, 1986.

Pearle DL: Beta blockers and calcium channel blocking agents in acute myocardial infarction, Cardiovasc Clin 16(3):29, 1986.

Singh B and others: Beta-adrenergic blockade in unstable angina pectoris, Am J Cardiol 57:992, 1986.

Taylor SH: Late intervention studies with beta-blocking drugs in myocardial infarction: a critical appraisal, Eur Heart J (Suppl) 7:41, 1986.

The Esmolol Research Group: Intravenous esmolol for the treatment of suprventricular tachyarrhythmia: results of a multicenter, baseline-controlled safety and efficacy study in 160 patients, Am Heart J 112:498, 1986.

Valladares B and Lemberg L: Catecholamines, potassium, and beta-blockade, Heart Lung 15(1):105, 1986.

Vliestra R and McGoon M: Beta-adrenergic blockers: choosing among them, Postgraduate Med J 76(31):71, 1984.

Calcium-blocking drugs

Bonow R: Effects of calcium-channel blocking agents on left ventricular diastolic function in hypertrophic cardiomyopathy and coronary artery disease, Am J Cardiol 55:172B, 1985.

Doyle A: Comparison of calcium antagonist with other antihypertensive agents, Am J Cardiol 57:90D, 1986.

Fleckenstein A and otheres: Antihypertensive and arterial anticalcinotic effects of calcium antagonists, Am J Cardiol 57:1D, 1986.

Frishman W and others: Comparison of diltiazem and nifedipine for both angina pectoris and systemic hypertension, Am J Cardiol 56:41H, 1985.

Gelmers HJ: Calcium-channel blockers: effects on cerebral blood flow and potential uses for acute stroke, Am J Cardiol 55:144B, 1985.

Katz A: Basic cellular mechanisms of action of the calcium-channel blockers, Am J Cardiol 55:2B, 1985.

Katz A: Mechanisms of action and differences in calcium channel blockers, Am J Cardiol 58:20D, 1986.

Kennedy GT: Slow channel calcium blockers in the treatment of chronic stable angina, CV Nursing 20(1):1, 1984.

Kendall MJ: Calcium antagonism—with special reference to diltiazem, J Clin Hosp Pharm 11:159, 1986.

Lute E: Calcium blockers: the important differences, RN, pp. 36-39, 1984.

Massie B: Antihypertensive therapy with calcium-channel blockers: comparison with beta blockers, Am J Cardiol 56:97H, 1985.

Mehta J: Influence of calcium-channel blockers on platelet function and arachnidonic acid metabolism, Am J Cardiol 55:158B, 1985.

McAllister RG and others: Pharmacokinetics of calcium-entry blockers, Am J Cardiol 55:30B, 1985.

Orekhov A and others: Evidence of antiatherosclerotic action of verapamil from direct effects on arterial cells, Am J Cardiol 59(5):495, 1987.

Resnick L and Laragh J: Renin, calcium metaboism and the pathophysiologic basis of antihypertensive therapy, Am J Cardiol 56:68H, 1985.

Schamroth L: The clinical use of intravenous verapamil, Am Heart Journal 100:1070, 1980.

Singh B and others: Second-generation calcium antagonists: search for greater selectivity and versatility, Am J Cardiol 55:214B, 1985.

Singh BN: The mechanism of action of calcium antagonists relative to their clinical applications, Br J Clin Pharmacol (Suppl) 21(2):109S, 1986.

Soward AL: The hemodynamic effects of nifedipine, verapamil, and diltiazem in patients with coronary artery disease, Drugs 32(1):66, 1986.

Stone K and Cordo K: Understanding the calcium channel blockers, Heart Lung 13(5):563, 1984.

Stowe HO: Review of calcium-channel blockers, Nurse Pract 11(4):57, 1986.

Touloukian JE: Calcium channel blocking agents: physiologic basis of nursing intervention, Heart Lung 14(4):342, 1985.

Urthaler R: Role of calcium channel blockers in clinical medicine, Am J Med Sci 292(4):217, 1986.

Winniford MD and others: Calcium antagonists for acute ischemic heart disease, Am J Cardiol 55:116B, 1985.

Antithrombotic drugs

Becker L and Ambrosio G: Myocardial consequences of reperfusion, Prog Cardiovasc Dis 30(1):23, 1987.

Bhatnagar S and Al Yusuf A: Left ventricular thrombi after acute myocardial infarction, Postgrad Med J 59:495-499, 1983.

Brewer CC and Markis JE: Streptokinase and tissue plasminogen activator in acute myocardial infarction, Heart Lung 15(6):552, 1986.

Chesebro JH and others: Thrombolysis in myocardial infarction (TIMI) trial, phase I: a comparison between intravenous tissue plasminogen activator and intravenous streptokinase, Circulation 76(1):142, 1987.

Chierchia S and Patrono C: Role of platelets and vascular eicosanoids in the pathophysiology of ischemic heart disease, Fed Proceedings 46(1):81, 1987.

Collen D and others: Coronary thrombolysis with recombinant human tissue-type plasminogen activator: a prospective, randomized, placebo-controlled trial, Circulation 70(6):1012, 1984.

Collen D and others: Human tissue-type plasminogen activator: from the laboratory to the bedside, Circulation 72:1, 1985.

Draccup K and Bryan-Brown C, editors: Symposium proceedings of Critical Care Nursing Update 1988. Thrombolytic therapy for acute myocardial infarction, Heart Lung 17(2):6, 1988.

De Gaetano G and others: Current issues in thrombosis prevention with antiplatelet drugs, Drugs 31(6):517, 1986.

Fitzgerald DJ: Platelet activation in unstable coronary artery disease, New Eng J Med 315(16):983, 1986.

Gallino A and others: Fibrin formation and platelet aggregation in patients with acute myocardial infarction: effects of intravenous and subcutaneous low-dose heparin, Am Heart J 112(2):285, 1986.

Garabedian HD and others: Comparative properties of two clinical preparations of recombinant human tissue-type plasminogen activator in patients with acute myocardial infarction, JACC 9(3):599, 1987.

Gersch B: Role of thrombolytic therapy in evolving myocardial infarction, Mod Concepts Cardiovasc Dis 54(3):13, 1985.

Gold HK and others: Acute coronary reocclusion after thrombolysis with recombinant human tissue-type plasminogen activator: prevention by maintenance infusion, Circulation 73(2):347, 1986.

Goldberg RJ and others: Long-term anticoagulant therapy after acute myocardial infarction, Am Heart J 109:616, 1985.

Gruppo Italiano Per ho Studio Della Streptochinasi Nell Infarcto Miocardiaco (GISSI): Effectiveness of intravenous thrombolytic treatment in acute myocardial infarction, Lancet I:397, 1986.

Huerta BJ and Lemberg L: Anticoagulation in atrial fibrillation, Heart Lung 14(5):521, 1985.

Jaffee AS and Sobel BE: Thrombolysis with tissue-type plasminogen activator in acute myocardial infarction, potentials, and pitfalls, JAMA 255(2):237, 1986.

Kaplan K and others: Role of heparin after intravenous thrombolytic therapy for myocardial infarction, Am J Cardiol 59(4):241, 1987.

Levine MN and others: Hemorrhagic complications of long-term anticoagulant therapy, Chest (Suppl) 89(2):16S, 1986.

Miller HI and others: Early intervention in acute myocardial infarction: significance for myocardial salvage of immediate intravenous streptokinase therapy followed by coronary angioplasty, JACC 9(3):608, 1987.

Milligan KS: Tissue-type plasminogen activator: A new fibrinolytic agent, Heart Lung 16(1):69, 1987.

Molyneaux R and others: Coagulation studies and the indwelling heparinized catheter, Heart Lung 16(1):20, 1987.

Nursing interventions in limiting infarct size in the acute myocardial infarction patient: nursing implications, Symposium proceedings of the Pre-National Teaching Institute Conference, Part 2, Heart Lung (Suppl) 16:6, 1987.

Ong YSC and Wescott BL: Intravenous fibrinolytic therapy in a community hospital, Focus Crit Care 13(1):33, 1986.

Patel B and Kloner R: Analysis of reported randomized trials of streptokinase therapy for acute myocardial infarction in the 1980's, Am J Cardiol 59(6):501, 1987.

Reskenov L and others: Antithrombotic agents in coronary artery disease, Chest (Suppl) 89(2):54S, 1986.

Schroder R: A prospective placebo-controlled double blind multicenter trial of intravenous streptokinase in acute myocardial infarction (ISAM) long term mortality and morbidity, JACC 9(1):97, 1987.

Sheehan FH: Determinants of improved left ventricular function after thrombolytic therapy in acute myocardial infarction, JACC 9(4):937, 1987.

Sherry S: Recombinant tissue plasminogen activator (rt-PA): is it the thrombolytic agent of choice for an evolving acute myocardial infarction ?, Am J Cardiol 59(9):984, 1987.

Sobel BE: Coronary thrombolysis with tissue-type plasminogen activator t-PA: emerging strategies, JACC 8(5):1220, 1986.

Swither CM: Tools for teaching about anticoagulants, RN 51:157, 1988.

Topol EJ: Thrombolytic therapy for myocardial infarction, Practical Card 14:53, 1988.

The thrombolysis in myocardial infarction (TIMI) trial, phase I findings, New Eng J Med 312(14):932, 1985.

Verstraete M and others: Double blind randomized trial of intravenous tissue-type plasminogen activator versus placebo in acute myocardial infarction, Lancet 2:965, 1985.

Weinreich DJ and others: Left ventricular mural thrombi complicating acute myocardial infarction: long-term follow-up with serial echocardiography, Ann Intern Med 100:789, 1984.

Willerson JT and Winniford M: Speculation regarding mechanisms responsible for acute ischemic heart disease syndromes, J Am Coll Card 8(1):245, 1986.

Williams DO: Intravenous recombinant tissue-type plasminogen activatory in patients with acute myocardial infarction: a report from the NHLBI thrombolysis in myocardial infarction trial, Circulation 73(2):338, 1986.

Electrical Intervention in Coronary Artery Disease

Electrical intervention is used primarily in the management of cardiac arrhythmias and consists of either *countershock* or *pacemakers*.

COUNTERSHOCK

1 Let us first consider *countershock*. Countershock is the delivery of a high-intensity charge to the heart that results in complete depolarization of the myocardium. This charge has the potential for interrupting certain arrhythmias and thus allows the normal pacemaker, the SA node, to resume control of the rhythm.

NOTE: If the SA node is depressed, it may not resume control of the rhythm. If this occurs, lower centers having the property of automaticity may assume control of the rhythm, or total electrical failure may occur.

There are two types of countershock: cardioversion and defibrillation.

Definitions

2 *Cardioversion* refers to the delivery of a *synchronized* charge to the myocardium. *Synchronization* means that the countershock machine is programmed to deliver its charge *only* after "sensing" the patient's major QRS deflection.

3 The term *synchronization* therefore implies that there is a(n) _____ mechanism.

A synchronized charge will be released *only* after the machine senses the major _____ deflection.

The charge is then released *during* the QRS phase of the cardiac cycle. A synchronized charge *(will/will not)* be delivered during the T wave. A synchronized charge *(will/will not)* cause VF.

4 *Cardioversion* is used in the management of fast arrhythmias when a QRS complex is present. Therefore cardioversion *(may/may not)* be

sensing

QRS

will not
will not

may

used in the management of atrial fibrillation with a rapid ventricular response. Cardioversion *(may/may not)* be used in the management of VT. Cardioversion *(may/may not)* be used in the management of VF.

may

may not

5 The other form of countershock is *defibrillation. Defibrillation* refers to the delivery of a *nonsynchronized* charge to the myocardium. The term *nonsynchronized* implies that there *(is/is not)* a sensing mechanism.

is not

6 A *nonsynchronized* charge is indicated *only* for fast arrhythmias where there is no QRS complex present. The only fast arrhythmia in which there is *no* QRS complex present is _____.

VF

   Therefore defibrillation is used only in the treatment of _____. Defibrillation *(may/may not)* be used in the management of atrial fibrillation with a rapid ventricular response. In VF there *(is/is not)* a QRS complex present.

VF; may not

is not

   A *synchronized* charge, then, *(would/would not)* fire during VF.

would not

   An unsynchronized charge, however, *(will/will not)* fire during VF.

will

7 NOTE: Another form of unsynchronized shock may be delivered by a blow to the precordium. This mechanical shock, although of low intensity, can also result in complete depolarization of the myocardium and can terminate certain arrhythmias.

8 The amount of electrical voltage required for the delivery of countershock is dependent on the characteristics of the arrhythmia.
   NOTE: The countershock charge is registered in watt-seconds.

9 Abolishing *supraventricular arrhythmias generally* require smaller amounts of charge, such as 10 to 100 watt-seconds.
   VT may be abolished with the same voltage. However, because of its rapid disintegration into VF, larger amounts of voltage may be required.
   VF represents the most deteriorated electrical activity. Therefore abolishing it usually requires the highest voltage—200 to 400 watt-seconds (joules).

10 REMEMBER: Cardioversion and defibrillation differ in these ways:
   1. Synchronized as opposed to nonsynchronized charge
   2. Degree of voltage required
   3. Indications (absence or presence of a QRS complex)

11 LET US REVIEW: Cardioversion is used in the management of *(fast/slow)* arrhythmias when there is still a _____ complex present. Cardioversion is the delivery of a(n) *(synchronized/nonsynchronized)* charge to the myocardium.

fast

QRS

synchronized

The term *synchronized* implies that there *(is/is not)* a *sensing* mechanism. A synchronized charge will always be delivered during the _____ _____. Synchronization may be used in all fast arrhythmias, except _____.

Defibrillation is the delivery of a(n) *(synchronized/unsynchronized)* charge.

Another form of unsynchronized shock is the _____ _____. An electrical charge will abolish arrhythmias by causing complete myocardial _____.

is

QRS complex
VF
unsynchronized

precordial blow

depolarization

12 The mechanical equipment necessary for cardioversion and defibrillation is:
1. A power generator, which builds up the charge
2. A set of paddles to deliver the charge
3. A monitor scope or ECG write-off to document the ECG patterns

Preparation for countershock

13 There are common principles that must be considered before the delivery of countershock. Following the delivery of a countershock charge to the myocardium, there is always a period of *electrical instability,* which may result in arrhythmias. Therefore any factors that enhance electrical instability should be managed before the delivery of the charge, if possible. The following have been identified as factors that enhance electrical instabiliy:
1. Hypokalemia
2. Hypoxia
3. Digitalization
4. Acidosis or alkalosis

14 Following countershock, there is a period of _____ _____.

Electrical instability is enhanced in the presence of _____, _____, _____, and _____ or _____. Countershock in the presence of these abnormalities may result in _____.

electrical
  instability
hypokalemia
hypoxia; digitalis; acidosis
alkalosis
arrhythmias

15 NURSING ORDERS:
1. Check serum K^+ levels before cardioversion.
2. Assess the patient's respiratory status by an ABG analysis (P_{O_2} levels), auscultation of the lungs, and observation of the rate and character of respirations.
3. If the patient is digitalized:
   —Know when the last dose was given.
   —Know the cumulative total of digitalis administered.

4. Check the acid-base balance by ABG analysis (pH, P_{CO_2}, HCO_3^- levels).
5. Anticipate ventricular arrhythmias after cardioversion; have lidocaine at the bedside.

NOTE: These orders are especially indicated in the setting of elective cardioversion.

16 Another factor to be considered is *premedication,* which is required if countershock is an elective procedure. Two drugs commonly used in this setting are (1) diazepam (Valium) and (2) sodium methohexital (Brevital). Other short-acting barbiturates have also been used. The more recently introduced (Versed), a member of the valium family may also be used, but causes greater respiratory depression.

NOTE: These drugs are primarily used for their transient amnesic effect rather than for general anesthesia.

17 Respiratory depression and hypoventilation can occur following the administration of either of these drugs. Hypoventilation can then lead to hypoxia and respiratory acidosis.

REMEMBER: Hypoxia and acidosis can *(increase/decrease)* electrical instability.

increase

The major side effect associated with the IV administration of diazepam and methohexital is _____ _____.

respiratory depression

Respiratory depression results in _____, which can lead to the development of _____ and _____.

hypoventilation

hypoxia

acidosis

18 NURSING ORDERS:
1. The patient must have a patent and stable IV line.
2. Watch for hypoventilation.
3. Have an Ambu bag, airway, and supplementary oxygen at the bedside.
4. Stimulate the patient and encourage him or her to breathe deeply and cough following the cardioversion.
5. Provide for physical safety until the patient has recovered from the effects of the drugs.
6. Be aware that paradoxical reactions may be seen following IV administration of diazepam (irritability, hyperactive behavior, confusion).

19 Other factors to be considered are related to the *preparation* of the *patient,* preparation of the *equipment,* and *monitoring* and *safety* aspects.

NURSING ORDERS:

1. Explain the procedure to the patient; avoid the use of frightening terms such as *electric* and *shock* when describing the procedure.
    —The patient should be aware that the procedure will make his or her heart slower and more regular and will relieve his or her symptoms.
    —Some patients may benefit by observing precardioversion and postcardioversion strips of their rhythm.
    —The cardioversion procedure may be described as being analogous to a "message" delivered to the heart.
2. Place the patient in a supine position, if possible.
3. Remove dentures.
4. Securely attach electrodes, and obtain clear ECG trace with no artifact.

21
5. Check for synchronization, if required.
6. Charge the machine to the desired voltage.
7. Apply conductive paste to paddles.
8. Position the paddles correctly.
    NOTE: In the setting of elective cardioversion, *anteroposterior* paddles are usually preferred because a discharge directly through the heart is usually more effective. Paddles are also designed to be placed on the precordium in a *transverse* position. In emergency settings, *transverse* paddles are usually preferred because one person can apply them rapidly. The correct positioning for both types of paddles is presented in Fig. 11-1.
9. Apply the paddles firmly to the patient's chest wall.

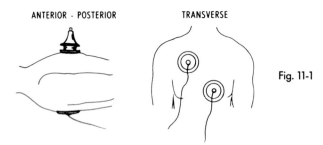

ANTERIOR - POSTERIOR   TRANSVERSE

Fig. 11-1

22
10. Before delivering the charge, make certain that no one is in contact with the bed or patient; avoid contact with wet areas, which may conduct the current.
11. After delivery of the charge, immediately evaluate the rhythm and corresponding mechanical activity by checking for pulses; subsequent shocks may be necessary if the arrhythmia is not abolished.

NOTE: Failure of a properly delivered high-intensity charge to convert the arrhythmia may indicate the presence of a secondary problem, such as *hypoxia, acidosis,* or *alkalosis,* or *drug toxicity.*

12. Following the delivery of the charge, continue monitoring to observe for the development or recurrence of arrhythmias.

13. In patients who have had long-standing atrial fibrillation, observe for signs of embolism to brain, lung, or extremities after cardioversion.

Automatic implantable cardioverter defibrillator (AICD)

23 The automatic implantable cardioverter derbrillator was developed as a life saving device for use in those patients at risk for sudden death from ventricular arrhythmias. It was approved for use in the United States in 1985. Earlier models of this device were only capable of defibrillation, but newer models are able to deliver a synchronized charge and are thus also known as _____.   cardioverters

All patients elected to receive the AICD have survived one or more episodes of sudden cardiac death resulting from ventricular tachycardia or ventricular fibrillation not associated with an acute MI (see Unit 12, Frames 11 and 12, Malignant ventricular arrhythmias). Most have undergone extensive electrophysiologic testing and failed multiple trials or antiarrhythmic drugs before the AICD is implanted. Despite extensive therapy, they still have recurrent life-threatening ventricular arrhythmias. The AICD has dramatically decreased the death rate in this group of high risk patients.

Patients who have multiple daily episodes of ventricular tachycardia or fibrillation are not considered candidates for the AICD because the lithium powered battery pack only lasts for approximately 100 shocks.

24 Unlike the traditional manual cardioverter/defibrillatory systems, the AICD *selectively detects* ventricular tachyarrhythmias as well as *terminates* these arrhythmias. It *(is/is not)* used for the control of supraven-   is not tricular tachyarhythmias.

Detection of arrhythmias by the AICD is dependent upon the sensing of the electrical activity of these impulses from their intracardiac ECG patterns or *electrograms.*

The *electrograms* are analyzed for both QRS morphology and heart rate by the sensing circuitry in the AICD. Most AICDs require that both *heart rate* and *QRS morphology* criteria be fulfilled before a shock is generated and released. Some older units, however, only require that a heart rate criteria be met before defibrillation is initiated.

25 The major components of an AICD system are a *pulse generator* and *four electrodes.* These components are similar to those of artificial pacing systems (see Frames 52, 53, and 56 to 85). For this reason, the AICD units have been incorporated into the latest proposed revision of the International Pacing Code (see Frames 83-91, 168).

Automatic Implantable Cardioverter Defibrillator

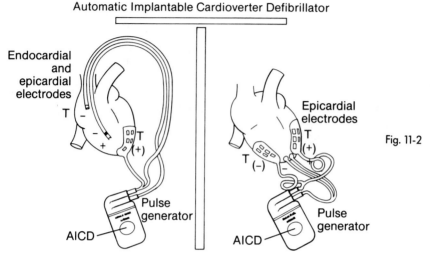

Fig. 11-2

T = "Transcardiac electrodes"

The *pulse generator* produces, stores, and releases the charge and contains the sensing circuitry for detection of heart rate and QRS morphology. It weighs approximately ½ pound and is surgically implanted within a subcutaneous pocket in the left paraumbilical area.

Two electrodes (one negative and one positive) are used as a bipolar system to detect and transmit the *heart rate* to the pulse generator. These electrodes may be contained within a single catheter or lead, which is threaded transvenously into the heart and positioned against the inner (endocardial) surface of the right ventricle. These electrodes may also be separately attached to the outer or _____ surface of the heart.

epicardial

26 The *other two electrodes* also act as a bipolar system and are used to detect transmit *QRS morphology* to the pulse generator and deliver the _____ current to the heart. These electrodes are usually contained within separate catheters or "leads." They are positioned so that the current will transverse the heart and are known as "transcardiac leads."

defibrillation

A *spring lead* may serve as the *negative* electrode. It is placed at the junction of the superior vena cava and right atrium. It is inserted transvenously through the left subclavian vein. The defibrillation current actually *exits* from this lead.

NOTE: In some settings the spring electrode is replaced by a second epicardial patch electrode sewn to the epicardium of the right ventricle (see Fig. 11-2).

The lower ventricular *patch lead* acts as a *positive* electrode and is sutured to the epicardium at the apex of the elft ventricle. This lead is place via a thoracotomy and completes the defibrillation circuit.

27 LET US REVIEW: The AICD is a complex electronic device capable of detecting _____ tachyarrhythmias and delivering a _____ to terminate these arrhythmias.
    It should only be implanted in patients with refractory _____ arrhythmias who have failed extensive trials of _____ drugs.
    Detection of ventricular tachyarrhythmias by the AICD is accomplished by sensing of _____, which are analyzed for heart _____ and _____ _____ by the sensing mechanism of the AICD.
    The AICD is composed of a _____ generator and _____ electrodes. Two electrodes detect and transmit the _____ _____ while the other two detect and transmit the _____ _____ and deliver the _____ current to the heart.

> ventricular
> shock
>
> ventricular
> antiarrhythmic
>
> electrograms
> rate; QRS
>   morphology
> pulse
> four
> heart rate
> QRS morphology
> defibrillation

28 *QRS morphology detection* by the transcardiac leads allows the AICD to differentiate between "sinus like" supraventricular rhythms and ventricular tachycardia and fibrillation.
    NOTE: Sinus rhythms with *wide* QRSs may be mistakenly recognized as ventricular in origin by the QRS morphology detector of the AICD but are not likely to meet the heart rate criteria. Conversely, some ventricular tachycardias with "narrow QRSs" may be mistakenly recognized as supraventricular in origin causing the AICD not to fire.
    If the rhythm detected is ventricular tachycardia, this sensing enables the "shock" to be synchronized to the QRS.
    REMEMBER: When a shock is synchronized, it is known as _____.

> cardioversion

29 The *rate sensing channel* of the AICD provides protection against inappropriate firing for sinus rhythm with a wide QRS and allows for earlier detection of a life-threatening arrhythmia. Intracardiac signals are averaged for heart rate. If the rate is above a preset value (usually 155) for a long enough period of time when the rhythm is sensed.
    REMEMBER: The upper rate limit for sinus rhythms is usually about _____ BPM. Most AICDs are programmed with preset cutoff rates of approximately 155 or higher so that sinus rhythms will not meet this criteria. The cutoff rate is set by the manufacturer and cannot be reprogrammed after insertion. However, newer mod-

> 155

els under investigation allow for reprogramming by the physician and will be the type inserted in the future.

30 If the rate of the arrhythmia is *lower* than the cutoff rate the arrhythmia *will not* be sensed. If the arrhythmia is *faster* than the cutoff rate and the QRS morphology is abnormal the rhythm *will* be sensed and the AICD will charge and defibrillate/cardiovert.

31 LET US REVIEW: The two criteria that must be met before a shock is delivered by the AICD are *QRS morphology* suggesting ventricular ectopy and/or _____ _____ greater than the _____ rate.

The *cutoff rate* for the AICD is usually around _____ BPM. This means rhythms with heart rates below 155, this cutoff will not be _____.

A potential hazard of AICDs that are activated *only* by heart rate detection is that a _____ tachycardia could activate the defibrillator.

heart rate

cutoff

155

sensed

supraventricular

32 It takes the AICD approximately *5-20* seconds to diagnose the rhythm and another *5-15* seconds to build up a charge. If the rhythm is not terminated with the initial shock, then the device can recharge and deliver three more subsequent shocks for a total of four shocks. This is known as *recycling*. After that time the AICD will be dormant until at least *35 seconds* of a rhythm other than VT or VF is sensed.

Therefore if the patient is having a life-threatening arrhythmia and the fourth shock delivered by the AICD is ineffective, external countershock should be applied immediately.

33 The usual voltage required to terminate a ventricular rhythm with an AICD is much less than with an external defibrillator because the charge is delivered directly to the myocardium. Testing of defibrillation threshold is done at the time of the surgical procedure with an external cardioverter/defibrillator.

The standard AICD is only capable of delivering approximately *25 to 35 joules*. If a VT or VF cannot be consistently terminated with 10 joules less than the mid-range of this voltage at the time of implantation, then the transcardiac leads are repositioned or replaced with *two large* epicardial patches.

The defibrillation threshold is then retested with the new leads. If the arrhythmias still cannot be consistently terminated with *10 joules less* than the maximum energy, then the leads are left in place but the pulse generator is not implanted at that time. The patient will be retested at a later time after changes in antiarrhythmic regimen.

34 LET US REVIEW:

It takes the AICD approximately _____ to 5
_____ seconds to diagnose a rhythm and another 20
_____ to _____ seconds to charge. 5; 15

The AICD can potentially deliver up to _____ consecu- 4
tive shocks. If the arrhythmia is still not terminated the AICD requires _____ seconds of a rhythm other than VT or VF 35
before it will be activated again.

The AICD can potentially deliver _____ to 25
_____ joules with cardioversion/defibrillation. If the pa- 35
tient's arrhythmias cannot be consistently terminated with approximately _____ joules less than the mid range of this voltage 10
then implantation of the pulse generator is delayed.

35 Placement of an AICD at this time requires a thoracotomy because
of placement of the _____ electrode(s) on the surface of patch
the heart and tunneling of the electrode wires to the pulse generator. A chest tube is left in place postoperatively.

The surgical approach will depend on whether other procedures,
such as bypass or aneursymectomy, will be done or if the AICD is a single procedure. The subxyphoid, left lateral thoracotomy, and median
sternotomy approaches have all been utilized. The pulse generator is
placed in the left paraumbilical area of the left upper quadrant of the
abdomen and the three wires are tunneled down to this area.

A single percutaneous system is currently under investigation and will probably be all that is necessary to implant the AICD
and a _____ may not be required. Later models thoracotomy
will also serve as demand pacemakers and antitachycardia pacemakers.

36 The AICD has an *audiofunction* that signals when it is in the active
and inactive mode with the application of a ring magnet. Placing the
ring magnet over the upper part of the pulse generator for a minimum of thirty seconds will activate or deactivate the device.

When the AICD is in the *active mode,* it will beep with each QRS,
showing that it is sensing the QRS. When the AICD is in the *inactive
mode* there is a continuous electronic tone.

37 Nursing staff taking care of patients with an AICD should be familiar with how to inactivate the device in case an emergency arises
where it is inappropriately firing.

To deactivate the AICD a magnet is held over the device for a
minimum of _____ seconds. A continuous electronic tone 30
would indicate that the device is _____. inactivated

The AICD is usually left in the inactive mode in the immediate
post-operative period. This is because it is not unusual to have su-

praventricular tachyarrhythmias and/or short burst of ventricular tachycardia due to manipulation of the heart and pericardium during the surgery.

38 LET US REVIEW:

To activate the AICD a _____ _____ is placed over the upper part of the pulse generator for a minimum of _____ seconds. Activation of the AICD is denoted by an audiosignal, which beeps in synchrony with the patient's _____ complex.

To deactivate the AICD a _____ is placed over the pulse generator for a minimum of 30 seconds. There will be a _____ electronic tone when the unit is inactivated.

The AICD is usually left in the *(active/inactive)* mode in the immediate post-operative period.

ring magnet

30

QRS

magnet

continuous

inactive

39 If external cardioversion or defibrillation is required during this time, there may be difficulty in transmission of the charge due to the placement of the patch electrodes. If there is a difficulty then a switch to anterior posterior paddle position is recommended. However, no damage to the AICD will occur.

Pacemakers utilizing *unipolar catheters* should not be implanted in patients with the AICD because they emit larger signals, which may interfere with interpretation of intracardiac signals. These large signals may result in double sensing by the AICD and thus meet the *(heart rate/QRS morphology)* activation criteria. Because ventricular paced beats usually have *(narrow/wide)* QRSs the QRS morphology criteria could also be met resulting in inappropriate firing of the AICD.

During ventricular fibrillation, the AICD could interpret the pacing signals as normal impulses and be inhibited.

heart rate

wide

40 Many factors could potentially interfere with appropriate sensing and firing of the AICD. Factors related to the "hardware" of the unit include: component failure, battery failure, fracture of the battery unit or any of the leads, and thrombus formation on the leads.

Antiarrhythmics can also potentially alter the functioning of the device. A drug induced rise in the defibrillation threshold could prevent the arrhythmias from being terminated. Antiarrhythmic drugs may also alter QRS morphology and/or heart rate of the ventricular arrhythmia making recognition more difficult and resulting in malfunctioning of the device.

41 Shocks from the AICD are unpleasant and the patient needs to be prepared for what they will feel like. A test shock is usually administered in the EPS laboratory so the patient can experience the feeling in a controlled environment. The shocks are usually described as feeling like "being hit in the chest" but are psychologically well tolerated by the patient.

Following surgical recovery a final electrophysiologic study is performed to further evaluate functioning of the AICD. The patient may also be given an exercise tolerance test to determine the average rate achieved during peak exercise. This is to ensure that sinus tachycardia will not be improperly _____. If the patient   sensed
is having supraventricular arrhythmias that exceed the cutoff rate they should be treated pharmacologically.

42 NURSING ORDERS:

The patient with an AICD

1. Explain purpose of the AICD, surgical procedure and basic mode of operation of the AICD. The patient needs to know he will have a bulge in the paraumbilical area from the pulse generator. Show model of the AICD pulse generator if possible.

2. Explain reason for chest tube post-operatively and importance of breathing exercises and coughing postoperatively. Some patients may require ventilator support for short periods depending on prior state of health.

3. Provide patient with order blank for Medic Alert bracelet and explain importance of wearing it at all times. Also provide patient with manufacturers information card to carry in his wallet.

4. Instruct patient to report first shock that is felt to physician. It depends on the circumstances of the shock whether physician will require the patient to be seen.

5. Inform family of risks of driving—consult with physician on specific restrictions. NOTE: Some states may have laws prohibiting driving with such devices.

6. Tell patients to avoid lifting, isometric type movement, and driving for first six weeks after the operation to allow for healing. Tight clothing should be avoided in the waist area to prevent fracture of the lead wires. Tell patient to expect early mobilization in the post-operative period and stress importance of compliance to prevent respiratory and other complications of immobility.

7. Tell patients to avoid things in the environment that may generate electromagnetic fields and interfere with functioning of the AICD: arc welders, electrocautery, electric smelting furnaces, large outboard motors, timer lights, airport metal detectors and radio frequency transmitters, including radar and power plants.

8. With physician approval, instruct patient and/or family member on technique for deactivating the device with a ring magnet. Instruct patient to never carry the magnet on his body or near the pulse generator. Storing the magnet on the refrigerator is suggested. Describe to patient how a shock may feel and allow him to ventilate his feelings about dependence on this device.

9. Instruct patient to report and observe for signs of infection—i.e., fever, redness, excessive tenderness or drainage from incisions.

10. Inform patient of importance of checking about antibiotic coverage for any dental work, sore throat, "flu like" or febrile illness—i.e., SBE prophylaxis advised.

11. Instruct patient/family member on what to do if the device is firing repeatedly, or if it fails to terminate an arrhythmia—i.e., when to call the emergency rescue personnel, physician, etc.

The patient with an AICD—cont'd

12. Tell patients that if they hear the device beeping they are near a electromagnetic field and should walk away in the opposite direction. The device could accidentally be deactivated in the presence of an electromagnetic field.

13. Inform family members that they may "feel" the shock through the chest wall if they are doing CPR when the device discharges. The feel has been described as a startle type reaction and is not dangerous. Inform patient that sexual activity can usually be resumed when he or she is comfortable.

14. Instruct patient on importance of avoiding contact sports after device is implanted because of potential disruption of the lead wires.

PACEMAKERS

43 REMEMBER: Electrical intervention in the management of cardiac arrhythmias consists of either countershock or _____.

    pacemakers

    The function of a cardiac pacemaker is to provide an artificial electrical stimulus when the heart's own electrical system is failing.

44 REMEMBER: The heart has an intrinsic electrical system that allows for the origination and conduction of electrical energy. When the heart's electrical system is failing, there will be disturbances in these electrical properties. The most significant manifestations of this failure are bradyarrhythmias, or *(slow/fast)* rates. Therefore pacemakers are used primarily in the management of _____ _____.

    slow
    slow
      rates

45 LET US REVIEW: Electrical failure may result from disturbances in the ability of the heart to _____ and _____ electrical impulses. The most significant manifestation of this electrical failure is _____, or _____ rates.

    originate
    conduct
    bradyarrhythmias
    slow

    The device that is used in the management of slow rates secondary to electrical failure is known as a _____.

    pacemaker

INDICATIONS FOR PACING

46 The current indications for pacing may be grouped into 4 major categories:

1. Symptomatic bradyarrhythmias
2. Tachyarrhythmias
3. Prophylaxis
4. Diagnosis

    The presence of *symptomatic bradyarrhythmias* is the oldest and still most important indication for both temporary and permanent pacing. These arrhythmias involve either the SA node or AV conduction system (see Unit 7, Frames 148 to 177). They can occur in both acute MI and chronic conduction system disease, or may be drug induced.

47 When the SA node fails, *atrial* activation is impaired. When the AV conduction system fails, _____ activation is impaired. In the presence of SA node disease, *(atrial/ventricular)* pacing is indicated. In the presence of AV conduction system disease, *(atrial/ventricular)* pacing is indicated. SA and AV conduction disease often coexist. In this setting, support of _____ activation is the most critical in maintaining cardiac output.

> REMEMBER: The function of a cardiac pacemaker is to provide an artificial electrical stimulus when the heart's own electrical system _____. The most critical factor in the maintenance of cardiac output is *(atrial/ventricular)* activation.

ventricular
atrial

ventricular
ventricular

fails
ventricular

48 The pacemaker provides a *substitute* electrical signal to the heart. It may provide this substitute signal or stimulus to a single chamber—the _____ or _____ or *both* chambers. Pacing of single chamber is referred to as _____ chamber pacing. Pacing of *both* chambers is referred to as _____ chamber pacing.

atria; ventricles
single-
dual-

Dual-chamber stimulation is most often indicated in AV conduction disease when both the atrial and ventricular contributions to cardiac output are critical or when single-chamber pacing induces pacemaker syndrome (see Frame 109). Atrial contribution is most easily maintained by bifocal, sequential, dual-chamber pacing.

49 An artificial pacemaker may also be inserted *prophylactically* in anticipation of a significant bradyarrhythmia or loss of AV synchony.

The potential for significant bradyarrhythmia typically exists after acute MI in the presence of a warning _____ _____ or _____ _____ blocks. It may exist following cardiac surgery because of edema or the inability of the electrical system to compensate for postoperative changes in stroke volume and cardiac output.

AV
node; bundle branch

Prophylactic pacing may also be indicated when there is the risk of electrical suppression caused by the effects of drug therapy.

Pacemakers may be used in patients requiring intraaortic balloon pumping who have irregular rhythms such as atrial fibrillation. They can provide a substitute regular rhythm to help the ECG trigger balloon deflation.

50 The *diagnostic* uses of pacemakers include (1) assessment of SA and AV conduction in electrophysiological labs, (2) hemodynamic evaluation at varying rates, and (3) identification of mechanisms of onset and termination of tachyarrhythmias, including the role of accessory pathways and effectiveness of drug therapy.

Pacemakers with *antitachycardia* functions are becoming more easily available. However, these pacemakers are still in their infancy.

51 LET US REVIEW: Pacemakers are currently used in the management of bradyarrhythmias and _____, in the _____ of bradyarrhythmias, and in _____ labs.

tachyarrhythmias
anticipation
electrophysiological

Pacemakers provide an electrical stimulus that can either interrupt a tachyarrhythmia or provide a substitute signal to either the _____ or _____ in bradyarrhythmias.

atria; ventricles

Pacemakers can also offer sequential or synchronous _____ chamber support to maximize the _____ contribution to cardiac output.

dual-; atrial

BASIC COMPONENTS/FUNCTION

52 An artificial pacemaker consists of two essential components: a pulse generator, which acts as an energy source for the stimulus, and a minimum of two electrodes, which are often but not always contained within a catheter. The electrodes deliver and return the electrical stimulus. Some temporary pacing units also utilize a bridging cable as an extension between pulse generator and the catheter.

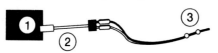

Fig. 11-3

1. Pulse generator
2. Bridging cable
3. Electrodes

The placement and specific characteristics of the pulse generator and electrode systems vary depending upon the type of pacemaker (see Frames 58-82).

53 Pacemakers provide a(n) _____ electrical signal, which, like the heart's natural pacemakers, allows for _____ and _____ of this electrical energy.

substitute

origination; conduction

Normal basic pacemaker function involves:
1. Release of a stimulus
2. Response to the stimulus (atrial, ventricular, or both)
3. Sensing (of natural impulses)

This function is reflected in the specific characteristics of the pulse generator and the ECG assessment of pacemaker patterns (see Frames 68 to 73, 81, 82, and 136 to 162).

TYPES OF PACEMAKERS

54 Pacemakers are generally categorized as: 1) *single-*or *dual*-chamber; and 2) *temporary* (external) or *permanent* (internal). Pacemakers may be utilized on a temporary or permanent basis, depending upon the clinical setting.

The pulse generators of permanent pacemakers are implanted subcutaneously—i.e., *(internally/externally)*. The electrodes are contained within a catheter(s), which may also be referred to as lead wires. The catheter is positioned in contact with the endocardium or epicardium. Endocardial positioning, similar to that of temporary pacemakers, is by far the most common positioning.

internally

In contrast with permanent pacemakers, temporary pacemakers use an *(internal/external)* energy source. Depending upon the setting, the electrodes may or may not be contained within a _____. The transvenous route is preferred when pacing for extended periods of time in settings other than postoperative thoracic surgery. When using this route, the physician threads a catheter transvenously into the right side of the heart, so that contact is established with the *(endocardium/epicardium)*. The ideal, most stable position for the catheter tip in ventricular endocardial pacing is in the RV apex (see Frame 59).

external

catheter

endocardium

55 Pacemaker catheters may be either unipolar or bipolar. Bipolar catheters are more common in temporary pacing, whereas unipolar catheters are common in permanent pacing (although bipolar catheters are usually preferred).

Bipolar catheters contain two electrode sites (positive and negative) on the catheter. When the catheter is in the proper position, both electrode sites lie within the heart.

The electrical signal stimulating the myocardium exits from the negative terminal of the pulse generator and returns through the positive terminal (see Frame 61). With bipolar catheters, it is recommended that initially the distal electrode be connected to the negative terminal. However, this method of connection is not essential for pacer function. In the event of inadequate stimulation or sensing, the poles may be reversed, allowing the impulse to exit from the proximal electrode. If the proximal tip is in better contact with the endocardial wall, better functioning will be achieved.

56 Unipolar catheters contain one electrode site on the catheter itself, which functions as the negative electrode when attached to the *(negative/positive)* terminal of the pulse generator. The electrical signal *(exits from/returns through)* this negative electrode. An external site on the pulse generator or outer skin surface serves as the positive electrode in this system. When the catheter is in the proper position, *(one/both)* electrode site(s) lie within the heart.

negative

exits from

one

The major advantage of the unipolar system is a greater sensitivity to intracardiac signals. However, a major corresponding disadvantage is a greater sensitivity to outside interference. This outside interference may take the form of either oversensing or electrical competition (see Frames 180, 152 to 168). Muscle stimulation may also occur due to the larger signal emitted.

57 The principles of pacing are similar for both _____ and _____ pacemakers. Both are currently used in patients with acute MI or chronic conduction system disease and are therefore commonly seen in coronary care and progressive care areas.

temporary; permanent

SINGLE-CHAMBER PACING SYSTEMS

58 Single-chamber pacing refers to systems designed to stimulate *(one/ both)* chamber(s)—i.e., either the _____ or _____. These systems may be either temporary or permanent and deliver their signals to either the endocardium or epicardium utilizing transvenous, transthoracic, or direct access routes. The most common single chamber paced is the *(atrium/ventricle)*.

one
atria
ventricles

ventricle

Endocardial

59 The most commonly used form of single chamber pacing is ventricular endocardial pacing using a transvenous route.

REMEMBER: In endocardial pacing, the _____ is in contact with the endocardium. In single chamber ventricular pacing, it is threaded _____ into the _____ side of the heart with the tip ideally positioned in the RV _____. Transvenous endocardial pacing is commonly used in both temporary and _____ pacing systems.

catheter

transvenously; right

apex
permanent

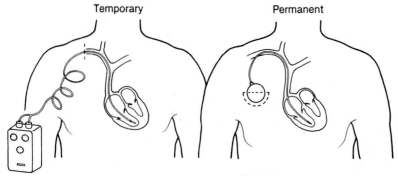

SINGLE-CHAMBER PACING

Temporary   Permanent

Fig. 11-4

Effective endocardial atrial pacing for extended periods of time requires specialized catheters adapted to maintain contact with the smoother atrial wall. These adaptations include a "J" shaped tip and spikes referred to as tines. Short term atrial pacing for tachycardia control or diagnostic purposes can be accomplished with catheters similar the those used with ventricular pacing. Atrial catheters are also threaded transvenously with the catheter tip ideally positioned in the right atrial appendage, which contains some trabeculae (see Fig. 11-11).

60 Temporary versus permanent single-chamber pacing systems differ primarily with regard to the pulse generator.

REMEMBER: Temporary pacemakers use an *(internal/external)* energy source, or _____ _____ (see Fig. 11-4). The pulse generator contains only the essential control dials, which are easily visible and accessible. Although the opposite was true in earlier years, these units are currently simpler to set initially and evaluate or adjust later than were the internal units.

external
pulse generator

Internal (permanent units) are adjusted and evaluated extensively in the outpatient setting. However, the focus of this discussion is inpatient nursing assessment and intervention.

61 Two terminals are provided to connect the pulse generator to the more commonly used *(unipolar/bipolar)* catheter. One terminal is marked *positive* and the other *negative*. Extension cables are also provided with these markings.

bipolar

REMEMBER: With bipolar catheters, it is recommended that initially the *distal* electrode be connected to the *(positive/negative)* terminal. However, this method *(is/is not)* essential for pacemaker function. The distal electrode is usually designated on the catheter ending. This mode of connection allows the impulse to exit from the electrode on the distal end or tip of the catheter, which is more likely to be in close contact with the myocardium (Fig. 11-5).

negative
is not

BIPOLAR CATHETER SYSTEM

Fig. 11-5

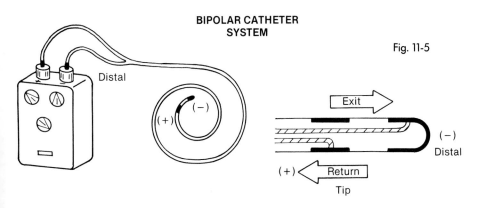

REMEMBER: The electrical signal stimulating the myocardium exits from the _____ terminal and returns via the _____ terminal.

negative
positive

62 A temporary bipolar pacing system can be converted to a unipolar system to maximize sensing. A bipolar system is converted to a unipolar system by disconnecting one catheter end from the pulse generator, so that only one functional electrode remains inside the heart. The catheter end attached to the positive terminal is disconnected and capped, and the negative terminal remains connected to the endocardial pacing catheter. The positive terminal is then connected by means of a needle adapter and an alligator clamp to the metal portion of a monitoring electrode applied to the outer skin surface (see Fig. 11-6).

CONVERTING BIPOLAR SYSTEMS TO UNIPOLAR

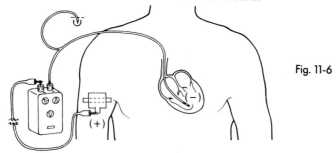

Fig. 11-6

REMEMBER: The electrical signal _____ from the negative terminal. Therefore in a unipolar system it is essential that the negative terminal remain connected to an electrode in contact with the cardiac wall. An external site on the pulse generator or outer _____ _____ serves as the positive electrode.

exits

skin surface

63 NURSING ORDERS:
During temporary (endocardial) pacemaker insertion

1. Explain the procedure to the patient.
2. Position the patient.
3. Assist the physician with obtaining venous access (usually brachial, subclavian, or femoral).
4. Connect the catheter to the pulse generator.
5. Monitor for RV PVCs caused by mechanical stimulation.
6. Adjust the pulse generator dials.
7. Assess the ECG rhythm for confirmation of proper stimulus release, capture, and sensing.
8. Request an X-ray film.
9. Validate the catheter position on the monitoring leads and 12-lead ECG.
10. Monitor for unusual complications, such as perforation.

After temporary pacemaker insertion
1. Provide immediate and follow-up care.
2. Inspect the insertion site for signs of infection.
3. Maintain catheter and system stability without restricting patient mobility.
4. Assess the ECG patterns, especially during patient position changes.
5. Adjust the pulse generator dials if necessary.
6. Insulate the exposed metal catheter ending to minimize external electrical interference.
7. Instruct the patient about activity limitations, and discuss with the patient questions and concerns related to the purpose and risks of the pacing system.

Epicardial

64 Epicardial pacing is currently being used more with temporary rather than permanent pacing systems. Both the transthoracic and direct access routes are utilized.

Noninvasive epicardial pacing using a transthoracic route has re-emerged recently and is rapidly gaining popularity for short term emergency management of bradyarrhythmia. Direct access to the heart is available during thoracic surgery allowing for the use of specialized pacing systems in that setting.

Although temporary and permanent pacemakers differ primarily with regard to the _____ _____, endocardial and epicardial pacing systems differ primarily with regard to the electrode system. In these forms of epicardial pacing, the electrodes remain separate rather than within a catheter. Therefore, a catheter *(is/is not)* utilized.

pulse generator

is not

65 Noninvasive epicardial pacing utilizes two large electrode pads similar to monitoring system electrodes, which are attached to the pulse generator by cables or "lead wires". The pads are positioned on the outer chest wall in a transverse (anterior-anterior) or anterior-posterior fashion (see Fig. 11-7). Although neither electrode is actually in the heart, these pads function as a *(unipolar/bipolar)* pacing system.

REMEMBER: The electrical signal exits from the *(positive/negative)* terminal and adjoining electrode. To allow the signal to directly activate the heart, this electrode is best placed over the apex. The signal is delivered through the chest wall to both the ventricles and atria simultaneously. However, the ventricular response dominates giving the ECG appearance of single chamber ventricular pacing (see Frame 104).

bipolar

negative

The pulse generators of non-invasive transthoracic pacemakers may attach to monitor-cardioverter-defibrillator units as in Fig. 11-7 or may remain separate. An attached cardiac monitor is also optional depending on the specific modes utilized. Since the signal is delivered across the skin surface of the chest wall, this form of transthoracic pacing is also referred to as *transcutaneous* pacing. This form of transthoracic pacing has for all practical purposes replaced the former invasive mode of transthoracic pacing.

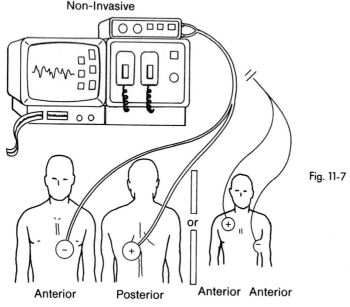

Non-Invasive

Fig. 11-7

Anterior   Posterior   Anterior   Anterior

Single-chamber pacing (ventricular)

Epicardial

66 Direct access to the heart is available during thoracic
_____.

surgery

    Thoracic surgical wires may be used for either single-chamber or dual-chamber pacing. These pacing wires are specialized, coated suture wires that are positioned against the *(endocardial/epicardial)* wall during thoracic surgery, including but not limited to coronary artery surgery. A minimum of two wires and a maximum of four wires are usually left in position and should be labeled as either atrial or ventricular. They are usually sutured to the outer thoracic wall but are not sutured to the epicardial walls and are thus easily removed after the operation. Instead, they may be threaded through the epicardial (pericardial) lining or through the sutures used to redirect the blood flow during the bypass (see Fig. 11-8).

endocardial

67 Surgical pacing wires may be used for either bipolar or unipolar, single-chamber or _____ chamber pacing. Bipolar pacing requires connecting *(one/two)* epicardial pacing wire(s) to the terminals on the pulse generator. Unipolar pacing also requires connecting two pacing wires to the pulse generator terminals. However, only

dual

two

566

one of these wires is an epicardial wire. The other is a wire sutured to the outer skin surface, often labeled as the "ground" wire. At least one epicardial wire from the chamber to be paced is connected to the *(negative/positive)* terminal.

negative

THORACIC SURGICAL PACING WIRES

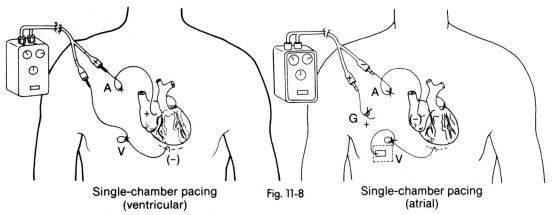

Single-chamber pacing
(ventricular)

Fig. 11-8

Single-chamber pacing
(atrial)

NOTE: 2 ventricular wires may also be used.

NOTE: 2 atrial wires may also be used for bipolar pacing.

REMEMBER: The electrical signal *(exits from/returns through)* the negative terminal. The negative terminal thus controls stimulus _____. The positive terminal may be connected to a second epicardial wire from any chamber for bipolar pacing or may be connected to the suture (or "ground") wire on the _____ _____ for *unipolar* pacing (see Frame 66). An adapter cable is often used to facilitate connecting the suture wires to the pulse generator terminals.

exits from

release

skin
surface

Atrial pacing in this setting is typically done using a unipolar system since it facilitates sensing (see Fig. 11-8).

NURSING ORDERS: In cases involving thoracic epicardial wires
1. Provide site care, including inspection for signs of infection.
2. Correct the labeling of suture wires as either atrial or ventricular (initially as well as after each dressing change) or designate them by marking the chest wall.
3. Insulate exposed suture endings. When disconnected, the wires can be coiled and capped within an empty needle cap.
4. Maintain an adapter cable for connection to the pulse generator at the bedside.

Pulse generator control dials

68 The typical control dials of a single-chamber temporary unit are illustrated in Fig. 11-9. They represent and ensure minimal basic pacemaker function.

REMEMBER: Normal basic pacemaking involves (1) stimulus
_____, (2) stimulus response or   release
_____, and (3) _____ (see Frame   capture; sensing
53). There is a key dial for each of these on the pulse *generator*.

69 Stimulus release is controlled primarily by the *rate* dial. This dial also
determines the automatic (pulse) interval on the ECG trace.

The automatic (pulse) interval corresponds to the
_____ at which the pacemaker is _____   rate; releasing
stimuli (see Frame 93). Initial adjustment of an on/off switch may be
required, depending on the manufacturer. It is also important to
verify that there is a battery pack in the proper position within the
pulse generator, since they are currently removable.

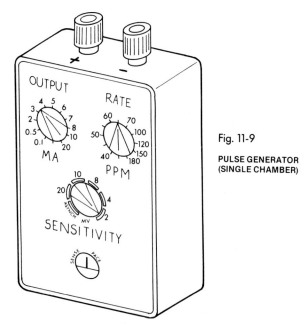

Fig. 11-9

**PULSE GENERATOR
(SINGLE CHAMBER)**

REMEMBER: It is the battery pack within the pulse generator that
_____ and _____ the electricity.   creates; releases
The initial rate at which to set the pacemaker is determined by the
physician and is usually just above that at which symptoms are anticipated to disappear.

70 Adequate stimulus response or capture is ensured by proper catheter position and adjustment of the *output* dial. The output dial controls the strength or intensity of the electrical signal, which is determined by its mulliamperage. The initial milliamperage at which the
pacemaker is set is also determined by the physician but is usually at

0.2 to 0.4 mamp. The output may be gradually increased until capture is confirmed by the ECG. The minimal milliamperage producing capture is referred to as *threshold*. A lower threshold usually indicates a more stable catheter position and is preferred. Higher thresholds, although sometimes necessary, may result in chest wall twitching and patient discomfort.

71 Sensing is controlled by the third key dial, which may or may not be labeled "*sensitivity*."

The property of sensing may be added, depending on the specific _____ of pacing selected. In the inhibited or _____ mode, sensing *(is/is not)* required (see Frame 68). Since ventricular demand pacing is currently the most common mode of temporary pacing, adjustment of the sensing dial, or _____, is usually required. Sensitivity is increased by turning the dial *away* from the asynchronous or fixed rate (F) position.

mode
demand; is

sensitivity

Sensitivity is determined by the strength of the myocardial signals usually in millivolts mV, detectable by the pacemaker. If the pacemaker is able to detect weaker signals (less than 2 mV) as well as strong ones, it is *(more/less)* sensitive. Therefore, if numbers are provided on the sensing dial, the *(higher/lower)* numbers will indicate greater sensitivity and will correspond to positions *(closer/farther)* from the asynchronous position.

more
lower
farther

72 Pace/sense indicators are also provided on external pacing units. The pace indicator will move or light as each stimulus is released. This stimulus release is also easily visible and best confirmed on the ECG. The sense indicator will move or light as each stimulus is being inhibited *as the result of proper sensing*. Proper sensing is often assumed in the prsence of adequate rates but is difficult to confirm on the ECG if paced beats are not also seen. Monitoring the sense indicator adds reassurance, but accuracy is best obtained from the ECG trace.

73 The control dials of a non-invasive transthoracic pulse generator differ slightly from those of other *(single-/dual-)* chamber units. There is a rate and output dial.

single-

However, the output required to pace through the chest wall is much greater—i.e., usually 50-75 mamps, initially. This greater amplitude produces discomfort in the alert patient.

There is no sensing dial since the sensing signal is obtained from the voltage of the monitored ECG complex. Therefore, for sensing to occur a monitor *(does/does not)* have to be attached to the system. Newer, less expensive units are available without the ability to sense. In these units monitors *(are/are not)* attached. However, their use is limited to the immediate cardiac arrest setting.

does

are not

74 Temporary pacing systems differ from permanent systems primarily with regard to the _____ _____. Permanently implanted pulse generators are currently *(more/less)* difficult to evaluate and adjust than temporary units. These units are initially set in the operating room by the physician. They are evaluated in the CCU or progressive care area by assessment of the ECG pattern, application of a pacemaker magnet (see Frames 138, 139, and 144), or *interrogation* (see Frame 75) of the pacemaker. They are adjusted by external *reprogramming.* An extensive variety of modes and specific functional parameters may be readjusted or reprogrammed, depending on the manufacturer's exact specifications. Many of these parameters are unfamiliar to the average coronary care nurse, who works to a much greater extent with external units that have only *(two/three)* adjustable dials. Frequently used manufactuerer's specifications should be kept on file as a resource. Common programmable parameters include "pulse width" (see Frame 126) and refractory periods.

pulse generator
more

three

NOTE: This is an example of one manufacturer's system. The systems of other manufacturers utilize the same principles but are often more compact.

**REPROGRAMMING/INTERROGATING
THE PACEMAKER**

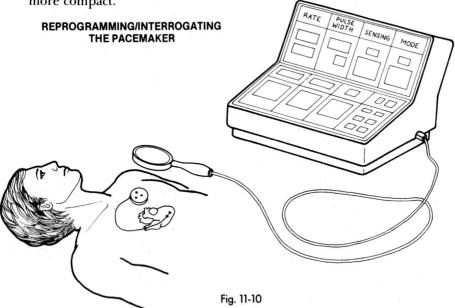

Fig. 11-10

75 Although the bedside nurse should be familiar with the general purpose and function of an external programming unit, reprogramming should be reserved for the physician, manufacturer, or pacemaker nurse specialist trained and experienced in the use of each specific unit. Unlike the magnet, programming units are manufacturer specific and sometimes model specific. A bedside recorder is preferred during the procedure. The programmer is applied over the area of the implanted pulse generator. The desired adjustment is then selected on the computerized programming module and is verified by the ECG pattern or *interrogation*. Interrogation is a feature whereby a computer printout of the currently set parameters is obtained—usually from the same programmer unit. This procedure is illustrated in Fig. 11-10. Refer to Frame 163 for additional nursing considerations in caring for the patient with a recently implanted pacemaker.

DUAL-CHAMBER PACING SYSTEMS

76 Dual-chamber pacing refers to systems designed to stimulate *(one/ both)* chamber(s) of the heart. These systems may be either temporary or _____ and deliver their signals to either the endocardium or the _____ utilizing transvenous or direct access routes.

both

permanent
epicardium

Endocardial

77 As in single-chamber pacing, the most commonly used form of dual-chamber pacing is endocardial pacing using a _____ route.

Two sets of electrodes are used. One set is positioned in atria and the other set in the _____. These electrodes may be contained within a single catheter or within two separate catheters.

transvenous

ventricles

78 External (temporary) units are used in conjunction with either a single catheter used for both PA monitoring and pacing (see Unit 9, Fig. 9-5) or with two catheters contained within the same sheath.

With the PA pacing catheter, three atrial electrodes are provided any two of which can be connected for *(unipolar/bipolar)* pacing. The two ventricular electrodes are located at a distance from the distal tip to allow their positioning in the RV apex while the distal balloon tip is positioned for hemodynamic monitoring in the _____ _____ (see Fig. 9-5).

With the two catheter system the atrial catheter is J-shaped, facilitating its more stable position in the right atrial appendage.

bipolar

pulmonary artery

79 Two separate catheters are used for permanent pacing.

The atrial catheter is most often a tined, or pronged, catheter positioned in the right atrial appendage. The ventricular catheter tip is ideally positioned, as usual, in the _____ of the _____ ventricle.

To allow for smaller catheter diameters, with permanent pacing only unipolar catheters are currently being used; because of this, oversensing is a commonly seen problem (see Frame 140).

apex
right

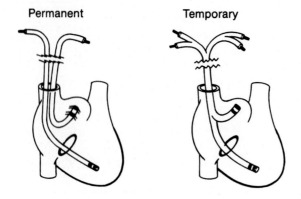

Permanent   Temporary

Transvenous catheter placement,
dual-chamber pacing

Fig. 11-11

REMEMBER: Small-diameter bipolar catheters are in the process of development and should decrease the incidence of this problem.

Epicardial

80 Dual-chamber epicardial pacing utilizes the direct access to the heart available during _____ surgery. Dual-chamber external (temporary) pacing units are used frequently in conjunction with surgical pacing wires. Four wires are used—two in the _____ and two in the _____, mimicking *(unipolar/bipolar)* pacing. The principles are similar to single-chamber epicardial pacing (see Fig. 11-8 and Frames 66 and 67).

thoracic

atria; ventricles

bipolar

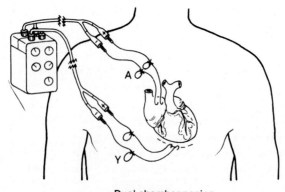

Dual-chamber pacing
(bifocal)

Fig. 11-12

Pulse generator control dials

81 Dual-chamber external pacing units (pulse generators) are characterized by four terminals for catheter connection (Fig. 11-13). Two terminals are provided to connect to a bipolar atrial catheter or its equivalent. The other two terminals are provided to connect to a bipolar _____ catheter or its equivalent. The dials of dual-chamber pacing units are similar to those of single-chamber units and are illustrated in Fig. 11-13.

    The key to this pacing system is the *(atrial/ventricular)* component. The three key dials controlling minimal ventricular functions are identical to those on a single-chamber unit. Thus stimulus release is

ventricular

ventricular

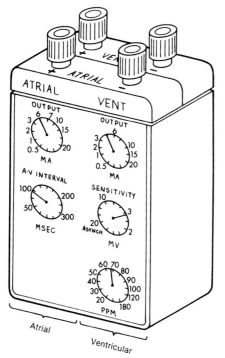

Fig. 11-13

**PULSE GENERATOR
(DUAL CHAMBER)**

controlled by a(n) _____ dial, stimulus response is controlled by a(n) _____ dial, and sensing is controlled by a(n) _____ dial.

rate
output
sensitivity

82 Two dials control minimal atrial function: stimulus release and stimulus response. An atrial sensing dial is not provided with these units.

    Stimulus release is controlled by the AV *interval* dials. This dial allows for the release of the atrial spike at a prescribed time before each ventricular spike establishing an artificial PR interval.

    REMEMBER: The PR intervals represent the delay between _____ and _____ activation. The normal PR interval is _____ to _____ seconds. Therefore

atrial; ventricular

0.12; 0.20

this dial is usually set between _____ and _____   120; 200
*milli*seconds (msec).

The AV interval dial reflects the dependency on and close relationship with the ventricular component. Thus the atrial rate should equal the ventricular rate, and the atrial automatic (pulse) interval should equal the _____ automatic (pulse) interval.   ventricular

Stimulus response in the atria is controlled by an _____ dial similar to its ventricular parallel.   output
This dial controls the _____ and   strength
_____ of the electrical signal in   intensity
_____.   milliamperage

CLASSIFICATION OF PACEMAKERS

83 Pacemakers were formerly classified according to their stimulating *location* (chamber paced) and *sensing function* (chamber sensed and mode of response).

A three-letter international coding system was established in 1974 to reflect these parameters. In 1981 an international group expanded this to the current five-letter code and classification system to reflect recent advancements in pacemaker technology (see Suggested readings). However, most pacemakers are commonly referred to by only the first three letters.

In 1987 a revised code was proposed jointly by the North American Society of Pacing and Electrophysiology (NASPE) and British Pacing and Electrophysiology Group (BPEG) (see Table 17).

84 The complete five-letter code addresses the following parameters:
1. Chamber sensed
2. Chamber paced
3. Mode of response (sensing function)
4. Programmable function/Rate modulation
5. Special tachyarrhythmia (Antitachyarrhythmia) functions

85 LET US REVIEW: Normal basic pacemaker function involves:
1. Stimulus _____   release
2. Stimulus _____ (capture)   response
3. _____, which is dependent on the pacing   sensing
_____   mode
     The pulse generator acts as the _____   energy
_____ for the pacing stimulus.   source

86 The stimuli are delivered to the heart from _____,   electrodes
which are located on the cathter tip. These electrodes are referred to as the *stimulating*, or *pacing*, *electrodes*. When the stimulating electrodes are located in the ventricles, they become the chambers paced, and the

pacemaker is classified as a(n) _____ pacemaker.   ventricular
When the stimulating electrodes are located in the atria, the atria become the chambers paced, and the pacemaker is classified as
_____.   atrial

Table 17. Pacemaker identification codes

Chamber(s) paced	Chamber(s) sensed	Mode of responses (sensing function)	Programmable functions	Special tachyar-rhythmia functions
1974				

V = Ventricle
A = Atrium
D = Double (dual)
	V = Ventricle
	A = Atrium
	D = Double (dual)
	O = None
		T = Triggered
		I = Inhibited
		  (demand)
		O = None
		  (continuous)		

1981				

V = Ventricle
A = Atrium
D = Double
  (dual)
	V = Ventricle
	A = Atrium
	D = Double
	  (dual)
	O = None
		T = Triggered
		I = Inhibited
		  (demand)
		D = Double (dual
		  function:
		  T and I)
		O = None
		  (continuous)
		R = Reverse
			P = Programmable
			M = Multipro-
			  grammable
			O = None (Perma-
			  nent pacemakers
			  only)
				B = Bursts
				N = Normal rate
				  competition
				  (dual demand)
				S = Scanning
				E = External

Table 18. The NASPE/BPEG Generic (NBG) Pacemaker Code (1987)

Position	I	II	III	IV	V
Category	Chamber(s) paced	Chamber(s) sensed	Response to sensing	Programmability, rate modulation	Antitachyarrhythmia function(s)

	O = None
	A = Atrium
		O = None
		A = Atrium
			O = None
			T = Triggered
				O = None
				P = Simple Pro-
				  grammable
					O = None
					P = Pacing
					  (antitachy-
					  arrhythmia)

	V = Ventricle	V = Ventricle	I = Inhibited	M = Multipro- grammable	S = Shock

	D = Dual
	  (A + V)
		D = Dual
		  (A + V)
			D = Dual
			  (T + I)
				C = Communi-
				  cating
				R = Rate
				  modulation
					D = Dual (P + S)

Manufacturers designation only	S = single
	  (A or V)
		S = single
		  (A or V)			

Note: Positions I through III are used exclusively for antibradyarrhythmia function.

87 The three oldest modes of pacing are:
1. Continuous (asynchronous, fixed rate)
2. Inhibited (demand)
3. Triggered (synchronous)

The *modes* of pacing are differentiated by the presence and function of a(n) _____ mechanism.

sensing

88 The *continuous* pacemaker fires continuously without regard for the patient's own rhythm. It therefore *(is/is not)* sensitive to the patient's own rhythm and *(does/does not)* have a sensing mechanism. Continuous pacing is also referred to as asynchronous or fixed rate. The two other modes of pacing all have sensing mechanisms, but their sensing *functions* differ.

is not
does not

REMEMBER: The continuous pacing mode is also referred to as the _____ rate or _____ mode and *(does/does not)* require sensing. Therefore, when in this mode of sensing the dial is *(on/off)*.

fixed; asynchronous; does not
off

In the *inhibited* mode the sensing mechanism allows the pacing spike to be _____ in the presence of the patient's own rhythm. Therefore the pacemaker fires only when needed, or on *demand*. For this reason, the inhibited mode of pacing is referred to as *true* _____ *pacing*.

inhibited

demand

In the *triggered* mode the sensing mechanism controls the timing of the next stimulus release. Therefore this stimulus is actually *synchronized to* or *triggered by* the sensing mechanism.

89 The two newest modes of pacing are *dual* and *reverse*. Dual function *combines two* traditional modes of pacing: inhibited and triggered. It refers to the ability of the sensing mechanism in one chamber (the ventricle) to inhibit a stimulus while the sensing mechanism in the other chamber (the atrium) triggers a stimulus. It is best illustrated in the presence of ventricular ectopy with universal dual-chamber (DDD) pacing (see Frames 108 and 110).

"Reverse function" refers to a pacemaker that fires opposite to what is normally expected.

REMEMBER: Pacemakers were first designed to fire during *(tachycardia/bradycardia)* and remain dormant during *(tachycardia/bradycardia)*. However, this pacemaker fires during tachycardia and *does not fire* during bradycardia. It is an antitachycardia mode, closely related to the traditional triggered mode, and may be more logically classified under the fifth category of the five-letter code. However, it has minimal clinical applicability at this time and is not widely available. The other antitachycardia modes are discussed in Frames 164 to 168.

bradycardia
tachycardia

The fourth position of the pacing code addresses characteristic of permanent pacemakers only. The addition of the letter "R" to this fourth position, representing "rate modulation" has been proposed to encompass the new implantable physiologically responsive pacemakers (see Frame 83). The fifth position of the pacing code addresses antitachycardia modalities. The revised code in this section has been proposed to include the AICD as an electrical antitachycardia device.

90 LET US REVIEW: Pacemakers are classified according to _____ and specific _____ of _____.

    location; mode action

    Classification according to location (chamber paced) depends on the site of the _____, or pacing, electrodes.

    stimulating

    Classification according to specific mode of action depends on the presence and function of the _____ mechanism. Sensing is separately coded as _____ *sensed* and *mode of* _____.

    sensing
    chamber
    response

91 The most common modes of either temporary or permanent pacing are the following:
    1. QRS-inhibited (demand)—ventricular pacing (VVI)
    2. Atrial continuous pacing (AOO)
    3. Dual-chamber pacing
       —Noncommitted (DVI)
       —Committed (DVI)
       —Universal (DDD)

Normal function of each of these pacemakers is discussed in the following sections in this order. Familiarity with atrial pacing patterns facilitates the recognition and solving of problems in these patterns when incorporated into dual-chamber pacing.

    NOTE: Atrial inhibited (AAI) pacing is also used with varying frequency for temporary or permanent pacing depending upon the clinical setting and/or institutional preference. Atrial demand pacing patterns are contrasted with AOO patterns (see Frames 112 and 113).

    Triggered atrial pacing will be discussed in the context of the DDD pacer.

    REMEMBER: The code letter *D*, when used to indicate mode of response, refers to one of the newest, available modes _____ function. Dual function refers to the ability of the *(sensing/pacing)* mechanism in the *ventricles* to _____ a stimulus while the sensing mechanism in the atria _____ a stimulus.

    dual
    sensing
    inhibit
    triggers

ECG ASSESSMENT: NORMAL FUNCTION
Overview

92 Normal basic pacemaker function involves:
    1. Release of a _____

    stimulus

2. _____ to the stimulus

3. _____ (depending upon the sensing mode)

Systematic ECG assessment should evaluate at least these parameters.

Response
Sensing

93 When the pacemaker signal or stimulus is released, a sharp, narrow deflection is seen on the ECG. This is known as the *stimulus artifact* or *pacing spike*.

The pacemaker stimulus is seen on the ECG as a pacing _____.

spike

The interval between the spikes of two consecutively paced beats is the *automatic,* or *pulse, interval.* This interval should approximately correspond to the rate at which the pacemaker is set to fire on the pulse generator. This interval should be measured to confirm that stimuli are being released at the prescribed automatic rate.

The rate at which the pacemaker releases stimuli is known as the _____ interval.

automatic (pulse)

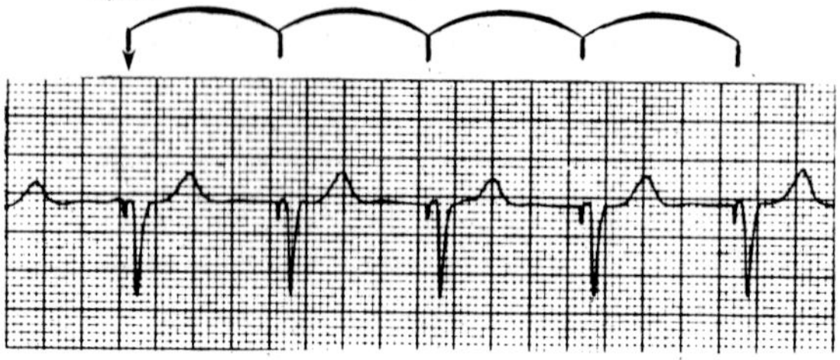

Fig. 11-14

According to this trace, the pacemaker stimulus *(is/is not)* released. The automatic pacing interval is measured from _____ to _____. It corresponds to the _____ at which the pacemaker is set. Therefore the rate of the pacemaker is _____.

is

spike; spike
rate
72

94 Although the battery pack within the pulse generator creates and releases the electricity, the stimulus is delivered to the heart from *electrodes,* which are usually located in the *catheter.*

When the pacing catheter is in the ventricle, each pacing spike should be expected to produce a(n) _____ electrical response. Therefore each spike should be followed by a(n) _____ complex.

ventricular

QRS

This response is referred to as *capturing* the ventricles. The impulse is delivered ectopically by the _____ to the ventricular muscle wall. Therefore it can be expected that the QRS complex will be *(wide/narrow)* and *(the same as/different from)* the patient's own natural QRS pattern.

catheter (electrodes)

wide; different from

Ventricular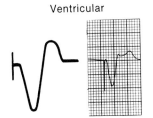

Fig. 11-15

Atrial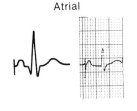

Fig. 11-16

In the trace in Fig. 11-15, stimulus response *(is/is not)* normal. Therefore this pacemaker *(is/is not)* "in capture."

is
is

95 When the pacing catheter is in the atria, each pacing spike should be expected to produce a(n) _____ electrical response. Therefore each spike should be followed by a(n) _____ wave (Fig. 11-16).

This response is referred to as _____ the atria.

atrial

p

capturing

96 With dual-chamber pacing *(one/two)* pacing spike(s) should be visible in the ECG trace. The first spike should be followed by a(n) _____ _____. The second spike should be followed by a(n) _____ _____, which is *(narrow/wide)* and *(the same as/different from)* the patient's natural QRS pattern.

two

p wave
QRS complex; wide
different from

Dual

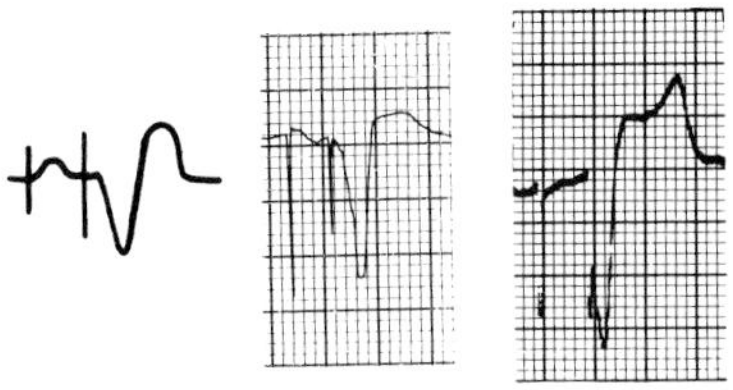

Fig. 11-17

(Bifocal/sequential)

NOTE: The p wave following the atrial spike is usually difficult to see.

This ECG pattern reflects the capture of *(one/both)* chambers. It represents the basic ECG pattern of normal _____ chamber (sequential) pacing.

both
dual-

97 The property of *sensing* may be added, depending upon the specific mode of the pacing selected.

The sensing mechanism allows the pacemaker to be sensitive to the patient's own natural impulses. In this way the pacemaker *receives* signals from these impulses. These signals can then be interpreted by the pulse generator and used to alter subsequent stimulus release.

98 If the sensing electrodes are located in the ventricles, the pacemaker senses the patient's _____ _____. If the

QRS complex

sensing electrodes are located in the atria, the pacemaker senses the patient's _____ _____. The same set of electrodes (catheter) may be used to transmit both sensing as well as stimulating signals.

p wave

In QRS-inhibited (demand) pacing, as well as the commonly used dual-chamber pacing, when a patient's natural QRS complex is sensed, the next stimulus release is _____. Therefore the pacemaker fires only when needed, or on _____.

inhibited

demand

99 The automatic pacing interval is also *reset* by the sensed beats. Therefore there will be a pause or interval between a sensed beat and the next automatically paced beat. This interval is referred to as the *escape interval* and should approximately equal the automatic (pulse) interval (see Fig. 11-18 for an ECG example and Frame 102 for an exception).

If a second natural impulse occurs before the lapsed time, it may again inhibit and _____ the pacemaker interval. However, if another impulse does *not* occur, the pacemaker will escape and automatically fire at an interval corresponding to the minimally set rate. Thus the escape interval ensures that the patient's heart rate will never fall below a certain _____ _____.

reset

minimal rate

100

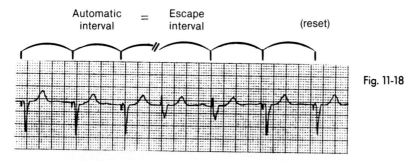

Fig. 11-18

In this trace (same patient as in Fig. 11-6) natural ventricular impulses are evident. Therefore on this tracing there is an opportunity to evaluate sensing.

When the patient's natural QRS complex occurs, the next automatic stimulus release *(occurs/is inhibited)*. The automatic pacing interval is also _____.

is inhibited

reset

Therefore the pacemaker *(is/is not)* sensing and is firing only on _____.

is

demand

The interval between the sensed beat and the next automatically paced beat is known as the _____ _____. This interval should correspond to this pacemaker's minimal automatic rate of _____ (see Frame 93).

escape

interval

72

This patient's pacemaker is best described as a *QRS-inhibited ventricular demand pacemaker*. It is the most common form of pacing currently utilized in both temporary and permanent pacing (see Frames 101 to 109 and 136 to 158 for more detail including an ECG assessment of malfunction).

ECG ASSESSMENT: SINGLE-CHAMBER PACING
QRS-inhibited (demand) ventricular pacemaker

Identification code (1981)

Chamber paced	Chamber sensed	Mode of response	Programmable functions	Special tachyarrhythmia functions
V	V	I	Varies with manufacturer	

A

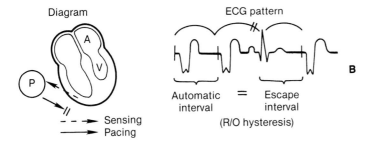

Diagram

ECG pattern

- - - → Sensing
———→ Pacing

Automatic interval = Escape interval
(R/O hysteresis)

B

ECG TRACE: NORMAL FUNCTION

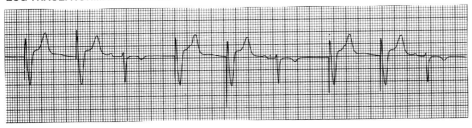

C

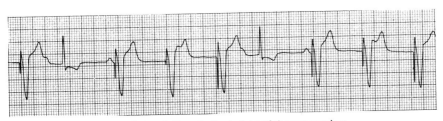

NOTE: The variations in the height of the pacemaker spikes are commonly seen and are probably caused by respiratory artifact

101 The mode of pacing currently being used most frequently in the setting of coronary care is the *QRS-inhibited ventricular pacemaker*. This pacemaker has both *stimulating* and *sensing* mechanisms and is coded VVI. Both stimulating and sensing are accomplished by means of electrodes located in the _____.

ventricles

   Therefore the *chamber paced* should be the _____, and each pacing spike (stimulus *release*) should be followed by a _____ _____ (stimulus *response*).

ventricles
QRS complex

   This pacemaker should be sensitive to the patient's natural *(atrial/ ventricular)* impulses *(chamber sensed)*. The pacing stimulus is _____ by the patient's own QRS complex *(mode of response* to sensing), and the automatic pacing interval is _____.

ventricular

inhibited

reset

   REMEMBER: With temporary pacing, stimulus release is controlled by the _____ dial on the pulse generator. Stimulus response is controlled by the _____ dial. Sensing is set by turning the _____ dial *(towards/away from)* the asynchronous or fixed rate (F) position. With permanent pacing, these features are _____. Stimulus response is adjusted by pulse _____ (duration) as well as amplitude (output).

rate
output
sensitivity; away from

programmable
width

102 The interval between the sensed beat and the next automatically paced beat is known as the _____ _____. The escape interval should be approximately _____ to the automatic interval—unless the pacemaker has a special feature known as *hysteresis*.

escape
interval
equal

   Hysteresis is an optional programmable feature available in permanent pacemakers in which escape interval is extended slightly beyond the automatic interval. The word hysteresis means "a lagging behind." A longer escape interval allows for natural beats to have an extra second chance to inhibit the pacemaker; however, undesiruable ectopic beats are also given the chance. Therefore the appropriate use of hysteresis must be carefully evaluated.

103 Physiologic rate responsive/rate adaptive ventricular demand pacing is now available in permanent pacing systems and has been rapidly gaining popularity. This pacemaker can adjust or *modulate* its stimulus release or pacing rate in response to an increase in the patient's physical activity. Thus, this property is also referred to as rate _____, and has been recently singled out with its own pacing code. Physical activity is sensed as muscle vibrations, increased respiratory rate, or other factors. When the patient's activity exceeds a selected threshold (low, medium, or high), the pacemaker rate will progressively increase within a selected programmed range.

modulation

Although stimulus release can vary with this form of ventricular pacing, stimulus response and sensing of cardiac electrical activity occur in the same way as other VVI pacemakers. Therefore, ECG assessment is, for the most part, *(the same/different)*.

the same

104 With at least one popular transthoracic pacing unit, a sensing marker is provided on the ECG trace to confirm sensing. This marker appears like another pacing spike (see Fig. 11-20), and may be initially mistaken for dual-chamber pacing. Arrows correspond with the actual stimulus release.

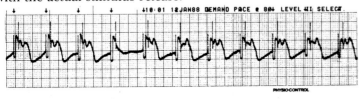
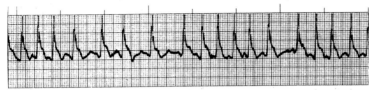

Fig. 11-20

REMEMBER: Although both chambers are paced simultaneously with transthoracic pacing, the _____ response dominates thus acting as a *(single/dual)*-pacing system.

ventricular
single

This maker appears with each natural (sensed) QRS complex mimicking the ECG pattern of ventricular-triggered pacing or pacer malfunction associated with an irregular stimulus release. The large stimulus released may also at times make it difficult to evaluate the ventricular response and confirm *(capture/sensing)*.

capture

Fusion beats

105 When the rate of the underlying rhythm (natural beats) is about the same as that of the pacemaker, *fusion beats* can occur. These beats are *normal* but can distort the QRS *response* following the pacing spike, giving the appearance of malfunction (Fig. 11-21).

LET US REVIEW: Fusion beats result when two foci simultaneously depolarize part of the _____ chamber. The resulting complex is a _____ of the contributing impulses in _____ and _____.

same
blend
contour; duration

Fusion beats typically represent simultaneous depolarization of the same chamber of the heart (ventricles) by both _____ and _____ impulses. They are best demonstrated on the ECG in the presence of *(ventricular/atrial)* pacing (see Unit 7, Frames 90 to 98).

supraventricular; ventricular
ventricular

583

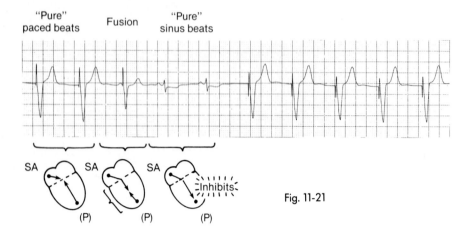

"Pure" paced beats   Fusion   "Pure" sinus beats

SA   SA   SA

Inhibits

(P)   (P)   (P)

Fig. 11-21

106 In ventricular endocardial pacing the catheter and sensing electrodes are ideally positioned in the apex of the right ventricle. Therefore natural ventricular impulses cannot be sensed until they have completely activated the ventricles and reached the apex. Complete ventricular activation *(is/is not)* thus required to inhibit and reset the pacing spike.

    When the rate of the underlying natural rhythm is about the same as that of the automatic pacer rhythm, both impulses will attempt to control the ventricles at the same time. If the natural impulse has begun to activate the ventricles at the time of stimulus release, a "shared," or _____, beat occurs.

is

fusion

107 This mutual or shared activation results in a distortion of the QRS complex *(preceding/following)* the spike. The resulting QRS morphology resembles either the paced or sinus beats or both.

    Any change in QRS morphology following pacemaker spikes should be assumed to be normal and to represent fusion even when complete confirmation is not present.

    REMEMBER: Confirmation of fusion require identification and comparison of the morphology of the separate contributing foci.

    True loss of sensing (abnormal function) will always appear as a spike or spikes *after* a fully formed QRS complex (see Frames 152 and 153).

following

Evaluating catheter position

108 When the catheter is properly positioned in the _____ of the right ventricle, pacing should produce a positive complex in lead I and a negative complex in leads II and aV_F (ALAD; see Unit 8). The QRS complex in lead V_1 should also be negative.

apex

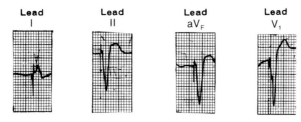

Lead I   Lead II   Lead aV_F   Lead V_1

Fig. 11-22

Pacemaker syndrome

109 Although ventricular pacing is used to eliminate symptomatic hypotension and sometimes improve symptoms of CHF, it can ironically also induce these very symptoms. This phenomenon has been referred to as "pacemaker syndrome," and occurs at adequate ventricular rates. It is becoming progressively better recognized. It's incidence has been reported to be from 7% to 30% depending upon the existence of SA as well as AV disease. Symptoms include fatigue, uncomfortable neck pulsations, shortness of breath, and pedal edema. These symptoms, if minor may not be reported masking the true incidence. Slight drops in cardiac output probably occur more commonly but are tolerated asymptomatically. However, they can be observed in critically ill patients with arterial lines in place. Loss of AV synchrony and the presence of ventriculoatrial conduction have both been implicated. Both of these factors result in loss of _____ contribution to cardiac output and increases in left atrial pressure with _____ congestion. Patients with valvular incompetence or decreased compliance due to acute MI, LV hypertrophy, or cardiomyopathy are particularly sensitive to this loss.

atrial

pulmonary

When this syndrome occurs, VVI pacing should be replaced with either AAI or dual-chamber pacing depending upon the status of the AV conduction system. The pacemaker rate can also be reduced to allow for more normally conducted beats to occur.

Atrial continuous (fixed rate, asynchronous) pacemaker

110 The mode of atrial pacing most commonly used in external (temporary) pacing system is the *continuous atrial pacemaker*. This pacemaker is referred to as an _____ pacemaker according to the American Heart Association pacemaker code. It has a stimulating mechanism accomplished by means of electrodes located in the _____.

AOO

atria

Therefore the _____ should be *chamber paced*, and each pacing spike (stimulus *release*) should be followed by a _____ _____ (stimulus *response*).

atria

p wave

A

Chamber paced	Chamber sensed	Mode of response	Programmable functions	Special tachyarrhythmia functions
A	O	O	Varies with manufacturer	

Fig. 11-23

B

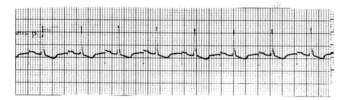

Diagram   ECG pattern

Automatic interval

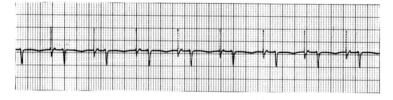

ECG TRACE: NORMAL FUNCTION

Fig. 11-24

Lack of visible p waves

111 The p waves of atrial pacemakers are commonly not easily visible following the spike (see Fig. 11-25). However, their presence may be implied and assumed when "related" QRS complexes have supraventricular characteristics.

    REMEMBER: Supraventricular impulses usually produced a *(narrow/ wide)* and *(changing/unchanging)* QRS complex (Fig. 11-25).

narrow

unchanging

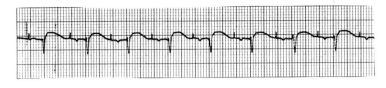

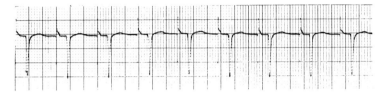

Fig. 11-25

The fixed spike—QRS interval confirms that the narrow, unchanging QRS complexes are related to the pacing spikes although separate from them. Actual validation of atrial activity may require multilead assessment, esophageal leads, atrial electrogram, or echocardiographic visualization of atrial contraction.

Lack of atrial sensing

112 In AOO pacing sensing *(does/does not)* occur. Lack of sensing appears as a spike following a natural, _____ _____ complex or wave. Therefore lack of atrial sensing (competition) should appear as a spike *following* each of a series of _____ waves. These p waves may be shaped differently than the p waves preceded by spikes, since they usually represent the sinus or natural nonpaced atrial impulse (Fig. 11-23).

does not
fully formed

p

    In AAI pacing sensing *(does/does not)* occur. Thus this pattern *(should/should not)* be seen with normal AAI pacing. Atrial demand (AAI) pacing occurs most commonly with thoracic pacing or with permanent pacing systems.

does
should not

113 Sensing is turned off on the pulse generator by turning the _____ dial *(towards/away from)* asynchronous/fixed rate.

sensitivity; towards

    Failure to sense a *series* of beats is referred to as competition (see Frames 153). In continuous pacing loss of sensing and competition is *(normal/abnormal)*. The danger of the disregard for the patient's own rhythm is that a pacing spike may fall in the _____ period of the cardiac cycle, causing repetitive firing, or _____. Therefore, a normal risk of continuous atrial pacing is atrial _____ caused by firing in the vulnerable period of the _____.

normal

vulnerable
fibrillation
fibrillation
atria

NOTE: For an actual trace, see DVI, Figs. 11-27 and 11-28.

    Since p waves are often not this clearly seen with atrial pacing, atrial competition may be difficult to confirm. However, any unexplained sudden onset of atrial fibrillation occurring in the presence of continuous atrial pacing should initially be assumed to be secondary to atrial competition, whether or not earlier unsensed waves can be documented.

DUAL-CHAMBER PACING
Overview

114 Dual-chamber stimluation is most often indicated in AV conduction system disease in which the _____ contribution to cardiac output is critical. When the AV conduction system fails, *(atrial/ventricular)* activation is primarily impaired. Atrial activation can remain normal but is no longer always related to or synchronized with ventricular activation.

    AV conduction system disease is usually managed by single-chamber ventricular (VVI) pacing. Ventricular pacing restores ventricular activation, thus maintaining the critical component of cardiac output, but *(does/does not)* restore AV synchrony. Ventricular pacing can also induce ventriculo-atrial conduction. Either or both of these can result in the symptoms of _____ syndrome (see Frame 109).

atrial
ventricular

does not

pacemaker

115 REMEMBER: Atrial contraction occurs during ventricular *(systole/diastole)*, allowing for a(n) _____ boost to cardiac output. Atrial contribution normally sustains about 25% of the cardiac output. However, this proportion can increase to as much as 80% in the presence of cardiac disease. Patients with mitral regurgitation (insufficiency) and/or decreased _____ are particularly sensitive to loss of atrial contribution.

    After cardiac surgery AV synchrony is often desirable to maximize compensation for changes in stroke volume and to maintain optimal _____ _____.

diastole
extra

compliance

cardiac output

116 SA and AV conduction disease can also coexist. Lack of atrial stimulation can result in atrial stasis and the development of mural thrombi, which can later embolize. Artificial dual-chamber stimulation may help minimize this complication.

    LET US REVIEW: Sequential dual-chamber pacing can restore AV _____ and maintain atrial stimulation in the presence of coexisting _____ conduction system disease. These pacemakers, when implanted, are also the most versatile pacing units, since they can be reprogrammed to *either* single-chamber or dual-chamber function as needed. However, they are significantly more costly due both to more sophisticated circuitry as well as the extra catheter required.

synchrony
AV

117 The two most common forms of dual-chamber pacing are 1) DVI and 2) DDD pacing. Only DVI pacing is currently available in both temporary (external) as well as permanent (internal, implanted) pulse generators. DVI pacing is more completely described as QRS-inhibited (demand), AV sequential bifocal pacing, but is more commonly referred to by its more compact 3-letter code. DDD pacing is more completely described as dual-sensing, dual-function (demand), AV sequential bifocal pacing but is also more commonly referred to by its 3-letter code.

DVI pacing is used more in *(temporary/permanent)* pacing, while DDD pacing is used more in *(temporary/permanent)* pacing although temporary units are now being clinically tested. However, DVI pacing patterns may be seen in permanent pacing as well since DDD units are at times reprogrammed to this mode.

temporary
permanent

118 Dual-chamber pacers have common as well as differentiating ECG patterns. In the absence of any natural impulses, all dual chamber pacemakers release two stimuli firing in sequence. For this reason, these pacemakers are all referred to as AV _____.

sequential

The distance between the atrial spike and the ventricular spike is referred to as the AV interval. It refers to the time from beginning of _____ activation to beginning of _____ activation, acting as an artificial _____ interval. This interval should also be noted at the time that stimulus release is evaluated. It is set by the _____ dial on temporary pulse generators and is usually a programmable parameter with permanent pacers (see Frame 74).

atrial; ventricular
P-R

A-V interval

119 Two corresponding pacing spikes are seen on the ECG. The first spike is the *(atrial/ventricular)* impulse and the second spike is the *(atrial/ventricular)* impulse. When stimulus response is adequate, a QRS complex should follow the *(first/second)* spike and a p wave should follow the *(first/second)* spike (see Fig. 11-25). However, as with single-chamber atrial pacemakers, the p waves are commonly not easily visible following the atrial spike. Multilead assessment is usually not helpful in this setting.

atrial
ventricular
second
first

REMEMBER: The p waves of single-chamber atrial pacemakers are commonly not visible following the spike but can be assumed to be present because of _____ QRS complexes with _____ characteristics. However, in dual-chamber pacing this QRS clue is lost because of the combined _____ pacing.

related
supraventricular

ventricular

Validation of atrial activity may require _____ leads, _____ electrograms, or _____ visualization of atrial contraction. If these measures are inaccessible,

esophageal
atrial; echocardiographic

atrial capture is assumed to be normal, and the focus of ECG assessment is on the second (ventricular) spike response.

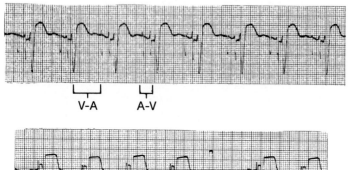

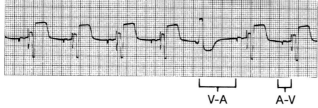

Fig. 11-26

120 All dual-chamber pacers are also QRS-inhibited. Naturally occurring QRS complexes can completely inhibit both pacing spikes. (See Fig. 11-27). The interval from a paced or natural QRS complex to the atrial spike is referred to as the *V-A* interval and is used by many pacemaker manufacturers and clinicians to evaluate pacer function. The V-A interval is a calculated perameter. It is determined in most pacemakers by subtracting the AV interval from the pacer R-R (automatic, pulse) interval. The authors prefer to focus on the AV interval since it is a directly set parameter. This approach appears to also work effectively in problem-solving.

The major distinguishing characteristics between dual-chamber pacemakers are the ability to sense the atria and the ability to sense within the AV interval (see Frames 122 to 127).

QRS-inhibited (demand), AV sequential bifocal pacemaker

Identification code (1981)

Chamber paced	Chamber sensed	Mode of response	Programmable functions	Special tachyarrhythmia functions	
D	V	I	Varies with manufacturer		**A**

Fig. 11-27

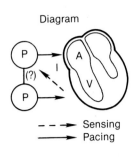

Diagram

ECG pattern

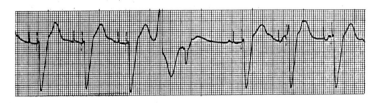

Automatic release: both spikes

QRS inhibition: both spikes

B

Fig. 11-27, cont'd.

*Lack of atrial sensing

- - - → Sensing
——→ Pacing

ECG: normal function

Fig. 11-28

121 The earliest available mode of dual-chamber pacing was the DVI pace-maker, referred to more completely as the QRS-*inhibited AV sequential bifocal pacemaker.* These pacemakers have *stimulating* mechanisms in *both* the atria and ventricles, but they have a *sensing* mechanism only in the *ventricles* and are, therefore, *(able/unable)* to sense in the atria. **unable** Thus, an atrial spike *(may/may not)* normally appear after a natural p **may** wave (see Fig. 11-27). In a sense, these pacemakers combine VVI and AOO pacing.

REMEMBER: Lack of atrial sensing results in atrial _____, which can trigger atrial **competition** _____. Therefore unexplained sudden-onset atrial **fibrillation** fibrillation is a potential complication of this form of dual-chamber pacing. Further episodes can be prevented by reprogramming the pacemaker to the VVI (single-chamber) mode or by disconnecting and capping the atrial wires in temporary units.

Committed versus noncommitted versus modified ("semi") committed DVI pacing

122 DVI pacemakers are further divided into committed, non-committed, and modified ("semi") committed. These forms of DVI pacing are differentiated by their ability or inability to sense within the AV interval.

Committed pacing was introduced because of complications with the earlier (non-committed) pacemakers, which sensed freely within the AV interval. Large atrial spikes were occasionally interpreted as ventricular impulses with subsequent inhibition of the second most critical ventricular spike. This phenomenon is referred to as "cross-talk" and occurs more frequently with unipolar pacing since larger stimuli are emitted. Unfortunately, this is the only currently available form of catheter for permanent dual-chamber pacing.

To avoid this complication, pacemakers were developed without the ability to sense within the AV interval. The sensing ability was literally "blanked out" for the entire duration of the _____ interval. Thus once an atrial stimulus was released, the ventricular stimulus was *committed* to fire also regardless of the presence of a natural QRS complex during this period. Since the spikes are either inhibited together or _____ together, mode of pacing became nicknamed as the "double or nothing" pacemaker.

AV

released

123 Although the inadventent inhibition of the ventricular spike was avoided, this mode of pacing introduced new, confusing normal ECG patterns.

Since QRS complexes occuring after the atrial spike (i.e., within the AV interval) cannot inhibit the second spike, this second (ventricular) spike may *normally* appear after a fully formed QRS complex—unlike what occurs in any other form of QRS-inhibited pacing.

ECG trace: DVI-C

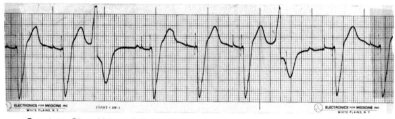

Fig. 11-29

Courtesy Chea Haran, A.P.S. Inc., Miami.

REMEMBER: In QRS-inhibited (demand) ventricular pacing the ventricular spikes are inhibited and reset by _____ formed QRS complexes to prevent the spikes from falling within the _____ period. This vulnerable period is typically designated by the _____ wave.

fully

vulnerable

T wave

124 Because of a carefully predetermined, fixed PR (AV spike) interval duration, the ventricular spike of the committed pacemaker should not extend into the critical vulnerable period.

The atrial spike may be difficult to locate at times. When both spikes are released, the first spike may become buried and hidden within the QRS complex, leaving the appearance of a single spike (see Fig. 11-29). This phenomenon is referred to as pseudofusion, since it represents two chambers separately activated instead of one. The electrical activity is superimposed instead of blended.

125 To decrease the incidence of these disturbing ECG patterns, modified ("semi") committed pacing was introduced. This is currently the most common form of DVI permanent pacing and is the one most frequently built into DDD systems as well. It is rapidly replacing committed pacing, but has not totally replaced it as yet, especially in patients with older pulse generators.

A shorter, programmable "blanking period" occurs with this type of DVI pacing. Thus only those QRS complexes that occur *early* within the AV interval are not sensed.

LET US REVIEW: Committed pacers *(do/do not)* have a blanking period. However, this period *(is/is not)* programmable and extends over the *(initial part of/entire)* AV interval.

do
is not
entire

Committed patterns still occur with this modification, but with less frequency.

126 With both noncommitted and modified committed pacing, QRS complexes occuring within the AV interval (i.e., after the release of the atrial spike) may still inhibit the second, ventricular spike. This gives the appearance on the ECG of single chamber atrial pacing. The simpler non-committed pacing is the only form available in temporary dual chamber pacing units since the bipolar pacing utilized with these systems is not associated with "cross-talk." Atrial pacing patterns *(are/are not)* seen with these pacemakers. The nurse working with temporary dual-chamber pacing units should be particularly familiar with this pattern.

are

For a summary of the major possible variations in ECG patterns with DVI pacing, see Fig. 11-30.

NOTE: The addition of the letters *C, MC and NC* to the standard codes is our personal method of differentiation.

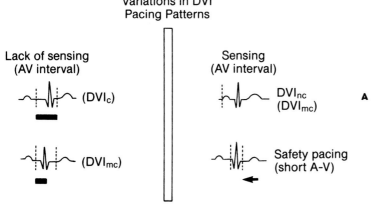

Fig. 11-30

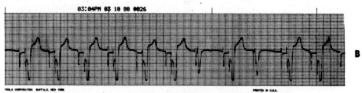

B

DVI mc pacing (blanking period = .038 seconds)

Fig. 11-30, cont'd

127 The most recently introduced variation in DVI pacing is *safety pacing*. This feature was introduced when the short blanking periods of modified committed pacing failed to totally prevent crosstalk and/or similar phenomena.

REMEMBER: Crosstalk refers to the inadvertent _____ of the atrial spike with subsequent _____ of the more critical ventricular spike.

sensing
inhibition

The blanking process itself may increase the sensitivity of the pacer to electrical interference in the period immediately following it. With safety pacing, impulses sensed immediately after the blanking period but still within the early part of the AV interval trigger rather than inhibit the second ventricular spike. This second spike is released at a shorter AV interval to minimize the risk of an "r on t" phenomenon and ventricular _____. This type of pacing is provided by two major pacemaker manufacturers. The diagnostic hallmark on the ECG is this variation of the AV interval. Another helpful diagnostic clue is that the shorter AV interval in safety pacing is always 110 ms. or .11 sec.

fibrillation

Dual-sensing, dual function (demand) AV sequential bifocal pacemaker (universal pacing) = DDD

Identification code (1981)

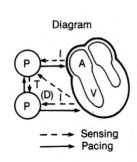

Diagram

P ⇢ A
T
(D)
P

- - -→ Sensing
——→ Pacing

Chamber paced	Chamber sensed	Mode of response
D	D	D
Programmable functions	Special tachyarrhythmia functions	
M	O	

Fig. 11-31

128 The universal pacemakers are the newest and most versatile of the dual-chamber pacemakers. They are classified and more commonly referred to by their code letters DDD. Implantable (permanent) units are currently available. External (temporary) units are in clinical trial.

The two key innovations in this pacing system are the addition of *atrial sensing* and *dual function*. Atrial sensing prevents the atrial competition and fibrillation seen with DVI pacing and provides a necessary ingredient for dual function.

LET US REVIEW: Dual function combines two traditional modes of pacing, inhibited and _____, in separate chambers (see Frame 53); that is, it refers to atrial (p wave) triggered ventricular pacing capabilities plus ventricular (QRS) inhibition.

triggered

129 Atrial triggered pacing is also referred to as atrial synchronized pacing or "p wave tracking." The atrial triggered pacing mode allows this pacemaker to increase its pacemaker rate in response to increased sinus rates, thus further maximizing cardiac output. It mimics the body's normal physiological response to increased demands for cardiac output. This mode of pacing was formerly available as a single-chamber pacing mode and used primarily in children. It was referred to by the code letters VAT. (Fig. 11-30). Although VAT pacemakers paced the _____, as designated by the first code letter, they sensed only the _____, as designated by the second code letter. Thus only one chamber was paced, with the other one sensed. Two separate catheters were necessary.

ventricles
atria

A thoracotomy was usually required to secure the atrial wire by suturing it to the epicardial wall. In this way the close, sustained contact necessary for atrial *(capture/sensing)* was maintained.

sensing

Identification code (1981)

Diagram

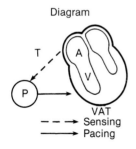

VAT
- - - → Sensing
——— → Pacing

Chamber paced	Chamber sensed	Mode of response
V	A	T

Fig. 11-32

ECG pattern:

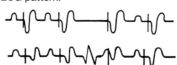

130 The VAT pacemakers *(did/did not)* sense natural ventricular impulses. Because of the lack of ventricular sensing, ventricular _____ could occur, predisposing to ventricular _____.

did not

competition
fibrillation

Because of the need for a thoracotomy and this risk of ventricular competition, the former use of this mode of pacing was very limited.

However, newer developments in atrial catheters have eliminated the need for a thoracotomy. The addition of ventricular sensing (QRS inhibition) in the _____ sensing mode has eliminated the risk of ventricular competition.

    NOTE: Lack of ventricular sensing with VAT pacing is best illustrated in the presence of PVCs (Fig. 11-32, *B*)

131 The code DDD implies that the *chamber(s) paced* are _____; that is, *both* the _____ and _____ are paced. Therefore during automatic pacing there should be *(one/two)* visible pacing spikes, as with DVI pacing. Each pacing spike (stimulus *release*) should be followed by an electrical response (stimulus *response*) corresponding to the activated chamber. Therefore the first spike should be followed by a _____ _____ and the second spike followed by a _____ _____ (see Fig. 11-31, *B*).

As designated by the second code letter, the *chamber(s) sensed* are also _____: *both* the _____ and _____. Unlike DVI pacing, this pacemaker should be sensitive to both _____ and _____ impulses. As in VVI or DVI pacing the ventricular pacing spike should be inhibited by fully formed _____ _____. However, unlike any mode of DVI pacing, the atrial pacing spike should also be inhibited by fully formed _____ _____.

    REMEMBER: The pacing spikes of dual-chamber DVI pacing may be inhibited by _____ _____ only. The process of atrial inhibition occurring in DDD pacing is not clearly designated in the code letters. The chambers sensed and the corresponding mode of sensing denoted by the second code letter are best described as a combination of AAI and DVI (noncommitted) pacing (see Figs. 11-31 and 11-32).

132 Following inhibition of an atrial spike, the pacemaker immediately converts to *dual function,* as designated by the _____ code letter.

    LET US REVIEW: Dual function combines two traditional modes of pacing—_____ and _____. It refers to the ability of the sensing mechanism in one chamber (the ventricles to inhibit a stimulus (or stimuli) while the sensing mechanism in the other chambers (the _____) triggers a stimulus. Thus dual function combines atrial (p wave)-triggered ventricular pacing capabilities with ventricular (QRS) _____. The ventricular inhibition is best illustrated in the presence of ventricular ectopy (see Fig. 11-33, *B*).

Right margin answers:

dual

dual
atria; ventricles
two

p wave
QRS complex

dual; atria
ventricles
atrial; ventricular

QRS complexes

p waves

QRS complexes

third

inhibited; triggered

atria

inhibition

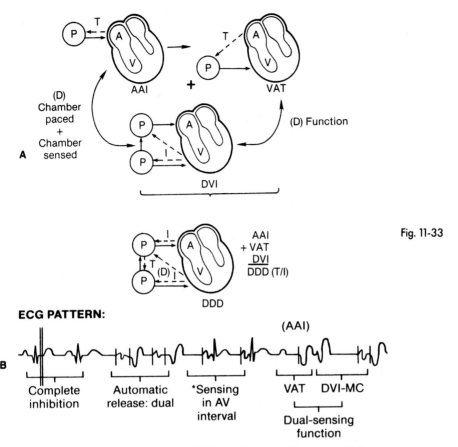

Fig. 11-33

ECG PATTERN:

Complete inhibition | Automatic release: dual | *Sensing in AV interval | VAT   DVI-MC

Dual-sensing function

(AAI)

*This pattern is seen only when DDD pacing is built upon a DVInc or DVImc system. However, the majority are built upon DVImc systems.

133 In the presence of sinus p waves the atrial spikes are *(inhibited/triggered),* and the DDD pacemaker immediately converts to the _____ mode. In the initial (VAT) phase of the dual-sensing mode, the sensed p waves *(inhibit/trigger)* the ventricular spike. Thus the rate of the ventricular spike will *normally* vary according to the rate of naturally occurring p waves. This phenomenon is also commonly referred to as *p wave tracking* and will usually result in irregular ventricular spike intervals (Fig. 11-32).

REMEMBER: The atrial triggered pacing mode allows the pacemaker to increase its pacemaker rate in response to increased _____ rates, thus maximizing _____ _____ and facilitating a normal _____ response.

inhibited

dual

trigger

sinus; cardiac output

physiological

134 The universal, or DDD, pacemaker is the most versatile of the currently available modern pacemakers. This pacemaker provides a variety of pacing modes, either instantaneous or programmable. It is essential to differentiate between the instantaneous or programmable modes before analyzing the ECG pattern. The "instantaneous" modes of DDD pacing refer to those that should be available when the pacemaker is programmed to full ("fully automatic") DDD function. These include AAI, VAT, and DVI (usually committed or "semi" committed), as illustrated in Fig. 11-33, A. The corresponding normal variations in ECG pattern are illustrated in Fig. 11-30, A.

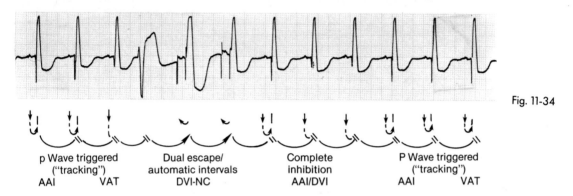

Fig. 11-34

p Wave triggered ("tracking")	Dual escape/ automatic intervals	Complete inhibition	P Wave triggered ("tracking")
AAI VAT	DVI-NC	AAI/DVI	AAI VAT

The DDD pacemakers may also be selectively reprogrammed to many other programmable modes, such as DVI (committed, "semi" committed), VDD, VVI, DOO, and VOO. The exact programmable modes available vary according to the specific manufacturer. If the pacemaker is programmed to the VVI mode, *(one/two)* pacing spike(s) would be expected. If the pacemaker is programmed to the DVI mode, only *(atrial/ventricular)* sensing would be expected. Thus the ECG pattern in a programmable mode *(would/would not)* appear significantly different from fully automatic DDD pacing. If the patient has a DDD pacemaker implanted, check to confirm that it is programmed to full DDD function before assuming malfunction.

one

ventricular

would

Many other programmable parameters may also be available. These include rate, sensitivity, pulse width and amplitude, AV delay, atrial and ventricular refractory periods, and maximal rate limit (during triggered function). These programmable parameters also vary widely according to the specific manufacturer and may influence potential intervention for complications and/or malfunction. Information on frequently used manufacturer' models should be filed for easy access.

135 Because of its dual *function* the DDD pacemaker is often misleadingly referred to as and confused with dual-demand pacing an antitachycardia mode (see Frame 166). The true dual-demand pacemaker automatically escapes at *either* fast or slow rates, as needed. It utilizes the antitachycardia function known as normal rate competition, designated by the code letter *N*. Although the DDD pacemaker may be legitimately considered a demand pacemaker because of its properties of QRS or p inhibition, it is merely a highly versatile bradycardia control pacemaker. True dual-demand function is currently a *programmable* mode of only one manufacturer's DDD pacemaker.

ECG ASSESSMENT: PROBLEM/SOLVING (SINGLE/DUAL CHAMBER)

136 Systematic ECG assessment of both normal and abnormal pacemaker function should evaluate the following:

1. Stimulus _____   release
2. Stimulus _____ or _____   response; capture
3. _____   Sensing

     The major ECG problems that occur as a result of pacemaker malfunction may be classified as follows:

1. Related to stimulus *release*
2. Related to stimulus response, or _____   capture
3. Related to *sensing*

     All three are commonly seen with ventricular inhibited (demand) pacing, whether temporary or permanent.

     Tachyarrhythmias may also be inadvertently produced by pacemakers. Assessment of these arrhythmias should be the fourth step in problem solving for abnormal function. Single chamber ventricular pacemakers typically generate ventricular arrhythmias. Single chamber atrial and dual chamber pacemakers typically generate atrial arrhythmias.

Problems related to stimulus release

137   LET US REVIEW: The power source, or pulse generator, contains the electrical energy that generates the electrical _____. The rate of stimulus release is adjusted to   stimulus the individual need and is selected by means of an external programmer or dial on an external (temporary) pulse generator.

     The release of the stimulus appears on the ECG as a(n) _____ _____. The interval between the   pacing spike spikes of two consecutively paced beats is known as the _____ _____. This interval   automatic (pulse) interval should approximately correspond to the rate at which the pacemaker is set or programmed to fire on the _____   pulse generator _____. The automatic (pulse) interval is therefore measured to confirm that stimuli are being released as prescribed. Some variation inthe automatic (pulse)interval can be expected with normal pacemaker function. Marked variation in the automatic interval indicates malfunction.

138 A high-powered magnet, provided by most pacemaker companies, may be used to elicit the pacing spike at normal heart rates with implanted demand pacemakers.

LET US REVIEW: In ventricular inhibited (demand) pacing, when a patient's natural QRS complex is *sensed*, the next stimulus release is _____. Therefore this pacemaker normally *(fires/remains dormant)* at adequate heart rates.

inhibited; remains dormant

In the presence of adequate sensing, therefore, stimulus release *(can/cannot)* be effectively evaluated.

cannot

139 Application of this magnet over the implanted pulse generator site creates a magnetic field that adjusts the pacemaker reed switch, temporarily eliminating sensing. In the absence of sensing, the pacemaker should escape and automatically fire, thus allowing evaluation of stimulus release. The "magnetic rate" is usually slightly faster than the basic automatic rate. The exact magnetic rate is manufacturer dependent. Most current implanted pacemakers are responsive to external magentic influence. This property may also be used in tachyarrhythmia control (see Frame 165) or to inhibit a runaway pacemaker (see Frame 143).

140 Problems with stimulus release may be manifested by the intermittent or complete absence of a pacing spike.

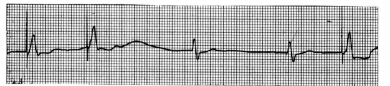

Fig. 11-35

This problem may be the result of battery failure, loose connections, disconnections, or oversensing.

Loose connections or disconnections may occur within or between the _____ and pulse generator or extension cables.

catheter

Oversensing may occur with unipolar pacing systems or in early battery or pulse generator failure. External chest wall twitching or local myocardial electrical changes are interpreted as impulses, thus inhibiting the pacemaker stimuli and resulting in pauses. Application of a pacer magnet over the pulse generator should eliminate this problem and can be used as a test for oversensing in permanent pacing systems without reprogramming. Eventual reprogramming is required.

NOTE: It is our opinion that reprogramming should not be a skill expected of the average coronary care nurse, although he or she should be aware of the potential programmability of the different units. Reprogramming should be performed only by manufacturer representatives, physicians, or nurse specialists trained and experienced in the use of each specific unit.

141 True malfunction of implanted dual chamber pacemakers is uncommon because of their sophisticated circuitry and shielding. More often, unexplained complex ECG patterns represent variations in normal function. However, intermittent inhibition of *stimulus release* has been reported with enough frequency to warrant careful monitoring. This phenomenon is usually associated with oversensing secondary to the *(unipolar/bipolar)* pacing system currently used (see Frame 55) and results most commonly in inhibition of the ventricular spike due to *crosstalk* (see Frame 127).

unipolar

REMEMBER: Only unipolar catheters are currently used with permanent dual-chamber systems to allow for smaller catheter _____.

diameter

142 Another manifestation of improper stimulus release is gross variation in the automatic interval. This phenomenon does not require emergency intervention but should be reported as a possible sign of battery and/or pulse generator failure, especially with internal units.

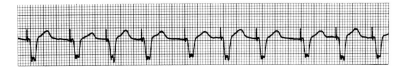

Fig. 11-36

143 When marked acceleration of the stimulus rate occurs, the pacing unit is referred to as a *runaway pacemaker*. Appropriate intervention in the management of this problem is to disconnect the pacing unit to terminate the arrhythmia if the pulse generator is external (temporary). However, this phenomenon occurs most commonly with battery failure in implanted (permanent) pacemakers. In this setting, application of a pacemaker magnet over the pulse generator site may inhibit the rapid stimuli until the unit can be replaced. The exact mechanism of this action is unclear, since external application of a magnet usually allows for rather than inhibits stimulus release.

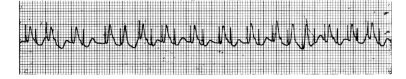

Fig. 11-37

144 NURSING ORDERS: Problems with stimulus release

    1. With external (temporary) units, verify that the battery pack is inside the pulse generator, since such packs are currently removable. This should be considered as a possible solution when no spikes are released.

    2. Check the integrity of the catheter and connections between the catheter and pulse generator, especially the negative terminal.

    3. Evaluate the adequacy of the patient's own rhythm: is the patient symptomatic? Have an isoproterenol drip on standby and/or have atropine available.

    4. To test for oversensing:

       —*With external (temporary) units* turn down the sensitivity by adjusting the sensitivity dial, and note the effect on the pauses (see Fig. 11-39, Frames 68 and 71).

       —*With internal (implanted) units* apply the pacemaker magnet over the pulse generator site as a test and note the effect on pauses. Remove it if competition occurs (see Frame 79) and report to physician. Reapply only if patient is symptomatic from pauses.

    5. *To correct oversensing:*

       —*With external (temporary) units* turn down the sensitivity dial and replace the battery pack and/or pulse generator. If the system is unipolar and convertible to bipolar, convert it.

       —*With internal (implanted) units* reprogram sensitivity down if trained to do so, or contact the physician and/or discuss possible replacement of the pulse generator if the system not unipolar.

Problems related to stimulus response (capture)

145 When a pacemaker is stimulating adequately, each pacing spike should produce a(n) _____ response. When each   myocardial
pacing spike produces a myocardial response, the pacemaker is said to be *in capture.* If the stimulating electrode are in the atria, each spike should produce a(n) _____ _____. If the   p wave
stimulating electrodes are in the ventricles, each spike should produce a(n) _____ _____.   QRS complex

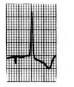 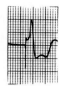

Fig. 11-38

When a pacing spike fails to produce a myocardial response, the pacemaker is said to be *out of* _____.

capture

146 When a ventricular pacemaker is *out of capture,* the pacing spike will fail to produce a(n) _____ _____. This phenomenon indicates improper stimulus _____.

QRS complex

response

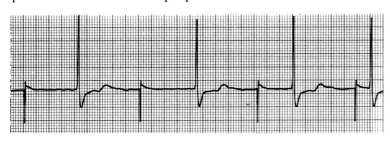

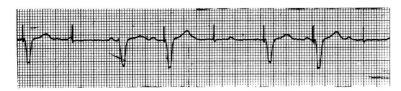

Fig. 11-39

147 Failure to capture may be the result of battery or pulse generator failure, increased voltage (amplitude) requirements, or poor catheter contact with the chamber wall. Perforation of the ventricles is a less commonly seen cause of loss of capture and is often accompanied by unexplained hiccups corresponding to the pacemaker rate. These hiccups are caused by subsequent pacing of the diaphragm. Perforation occurs most commonly during the actual insertion or in the first week after insertion.

Effective capture requires close catheter contact with the chamber wall. This is especially difficult to maintain with transvenous endocardial catheter systems, particularly when they are inserted for short-term, or temporary, rate control. In these cases the ideal, most stable position for the catheter tip is in the RV apex.

A frequent cause of failure to capture with temporary pacing systems is a floating catheter, since there is an inability to place the catheter tip in the ideal, most stable position, that is, in the RV _____. Catheters that are not positioned in the RV _____ are more susceptible to losing contact with the chamber wall with simple patient position changes and/or movements.

apex

apex

148 Although catheter position may remain stable, voltage or amplitude requirements often increase over time because of changes in the electrode tissue interface. These changes include edema and fibrosis around the electrode tip, local ischemia, and drug and/or electrolyte changes. With internal (implanted) systems, the increase in voltage requirements is highest in the first 2 weeks after implantation and then declines slightly and stabilizes. The reverse energy output of the pulse generator is usually able to compensate for this phenomena. However, in external (temporary) units loss of capture occurs more commonly, requiring manual adjustment of the output dial to increase the voltage or milliamperage (ma). In permanent pacemakers the pulse width (or duration) can also be adjusted.

149 The major ECG manifestation of single-chamber atrial pacemaker malfunction is loss of stimulus response or _____.
A pacemaker is said to be out of capture when the pacing spike *(does/does not)* produce a myocardial response. When an *atrial* pacer is *out of capture,* the pacing spike will fail to produce a _____ _____. (Fig. 11-40). Loss of ventricular capture is reported rarely with dual-chamber systems, except for external (_____) ones. Intervention is identical to that for VVI pacing.

capture
does not

p wave

temporary

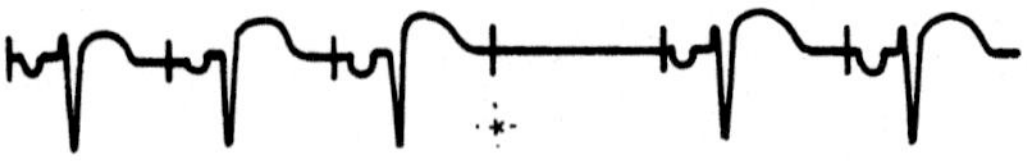

Fig. 11-40

150 LET US REVIEW: Effective capture requires close catheter contact with the _____ _____. The ideal, most stable position for the catheter tip is in the _____ _____.

chamber wall
RV apex

Failure to capture may be the result of battery or _____ _____ failure, increased _____ or _____ requirements or poor _____ contact with the chamber wall.

pulse
generator; voltage
milliamperage
catheter

Corrective intervention includes increasing the _____ or voltage, repositioning the _____, and/or changing the _____ or pulse generator.

milliamperage
patient
battery

A less commonly seen cause of failure to capture is _____ of the chamber wall. This phenomenon is characteristically accompanied by _____ caused by pacing of the _____.

perforation
hiccups
diaphragm

151 NURSING ORDERS: Problems with stimulus response (capture)
1. With external (temporary) units:
   —Increase the voltage or milliamperage by adjusting the output dial (see Fig. 11-9, Frames 68 and 70).
   —Reposition the patient.
   —Change the battery pack and/or pulse generator.

—Call the physician to reposition the catheter.

2. With internal (implanted units):
   —Reprogram the output if trained to do so or notify the physician and/or discuss possible replacement of the pulse generator.
3. Evaluate the adequacy of the underlying rhythm: is the patient asymptomatic?
   —Obtain an order for standby atropine or isoproterenol.
   —If the patient loses consciousness, start supportive cardiopulmonary resuscitation.
4. With bipolar pacing, try switching polarity.

Problems related to undersensing

152 The purpose of a sensing mechanism is to interpret information about the patient's own rhythm. In ventricular inhibited (demand) pacing when the patient's natural QRS complex is sensed, the next stimulus release is _____, and the automatic pacing interval is _____. Therefore, when sensing adequately, this pacemaker should *(fire/remain dormant)* in the presence of natural beats and/or adequate heart rates.

    REMEMBER: Complete ventricular activation by the natural beat *(is/ is not)* usually required to inhibit and reset the pacing spike. Therefore failure to sense or loss of sensing will always appear as a spike or spikes released *(before/after)* a fully formed QRS complex (see Frames 106 and 107).

    inhibited

    reset
    remain dormant

    is

    after

153 When the sensing mechanism fails, the pacemaker will fire *(with/without)* regard for the patient's own beats or rhythm. the danger of the disregard for the patient's own rhythm is that a pacing spike may fall during the vulnerable period of the cardiac cycle or _____ wave, causing _____ _____ or _____.

    without

    T
    repetitive firing
    fibrillation (VF)

    Failure of the sensing mechanism may be manifested by failure to sense *occasional* impulses (Fig. 11-41, *B*) or failure to sense an entire *series* of beats or rhythm. The pacemaker then *competes* with the patient for control of the rhythm. This manifestation of failure to sense is known as competition (Fig. 11-41, *A*).

154 Most problems with sensing occur because of failure of the sensing mechanism within the pulse generator or even light changes in catheter position. Since the underlying rhythm is usually adequate in true competition, the pulse generator may be gradually turned off while the unit and/or battery pack is replaced. The sensitivity may also be increased by adjusting the sensitivity dial or reprogramming the pacemaker (see Frame 151 for additional nursing action).

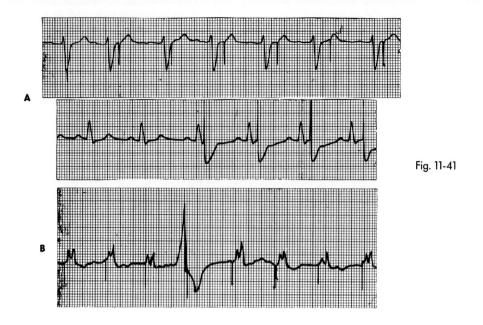

A

B

Fig. 11-41

155 Loss of sensing is most hazardous in acute, unstable patients or when allowed to continue uncorrected for long periods of time. Short-term loss of sensing and/or competition is not usually associated with serious hazard, especially in patients with chronic heart disease.

    REMEMBER: Application of a magnet over the implanted pulse generator site creates a magnetic field that temporarily _____ sensing, thus creating short-term _____. The magnetic response is used to elicit the pacing spike with demand pacers at normal rates, confirming normal stimulus _____. This magnetic property is safely used on an outpatient basis in offices or clinics or as part of patient telephone follow-up systems. It is also a component of most reprogramming systems.

eliminates

competition

release

156 Pacemakers may be intentionally set on continuous, or fixed, rate for short periods of time to interrupt or overdrive tachyarrhythmias.

    REMEMBER: When the pacemaker is set on the continuous mode, sensing is turned *(on/off)*. In this case loss of sensing would be *(normal/abnormal)*. Continuous pacing is also referred to as _____, or _____, rate. If the sensitivity dial of a pulse generator is adjusted to read fixed rate or asynchronous, sensitivity has been turned *(on/off)*, and the pacemaker *(is/is not)* set on demand.

off; normal

fixed; asynchronous

off; is not

157 With dual-chamber pacemakers true loss of sensing will appear two spikes after a fully formed _____ _____.

    LET US REVIEW: It is normal for one spike to follow a fully formed QRS complex in DVI *(committed/noncommitted)* pacing only. However,

QRS complex

committed

both spikes should never normally appear following a QRS complex while _____ is intact.

sensing

Loss of sensing: dual-chamber pacemaker

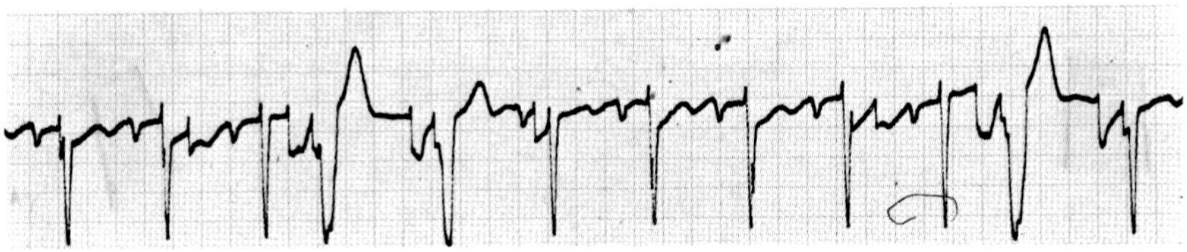

Fig. 11-42

158 NURSING ORDERS: Failure to sense
1. Make sure that the pacemaker is not set on the continuous mode.
2. Increase sensitivity by adjusting the sensitivity dial or by reprogramming.
3. Reposition the patient.
4. With failure to sense occasional beats:
   — Turn up the pacemaker rate to override.
   — Lidocaine can be given if the beat is ventricular
   — Change the pulse generator or battery.
5. If the system is bipolar it can be converted to unipolar (see Frame 62).
   NOTE: A bipolar system can be transformed into a unipolar system by connecting the positive terminal of the pacemaker to an electrode on the body surface instead of to the proximal catheter electrode.

Pacemaker tachyarrhythmias

159 Although pacemakers prevent bradycardias, they may generate as well as prevent or correct _____.

tachycardias

LET US REVIEW: Single-chamber *ventricular* pacemakers are most typically associated with *(atrial/ventricular)* arrhythmias. Pacemaker induced ventricular arrhythmias are usually right ventricular, producing an *(upright/negative)* complex on V_1 similar to that of the paced beat. They are corrected with lidocaine and/or repositioning of the catheter or are left untreated unless sustained VT occurs. Ventricular arrhythmias occuring immediately after pacemaker insertion often subside without therapy.

ventricular

negative

Single-chamber *atrial* pacemakers are most typically associated with *(atrial/ventricular)* arrhythmias. The most common atrial arrhythmia induced by these pacemakers is _____ _____ due to the lack of atrial sensing.

atrial
atrial
fibrillation

Dual-chamber pacemakers are most typically associated with *(atrial/ventricular)* arrhythmias. The most common atrial arrhythmia

atrial

associated with DVI pacing is atrial *(tachycardia/fibrillation)* due to the lack of atrial _____. When this occurs, the pacemaker is best converted to a VVI mode.

fibrillation

sensing

Problem solving: atrial tachycardia

160 Although the DDD pacemaker does not trigger atrial fibrillation, two forms of atrial tachycardia are typically associated with this mode of pacing. Appropriate corrective intervention is facilitated by their recognition. These two forms are (1) atrial tachycardia with antegrade p wave tracking and (2) atrial tachycardia caused by retrograde p wave tracking (pacemaker-mediated tachycardia). The first is the result of a normal p wave-triggered response to a spontaneous atrial tachycardia (Fig. 11-33).

ATRIAL TACHYCARDIA
WITH p-WAVE TRACKING

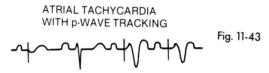

Fig. 11-43

The second is caused by the unintended tracking of retrogradely conducted p waves, usually associated with PVCs. In this case, the arrhythmia is sustained as well as induced by the pacemaker.

PACEMAKER-MEDIATED TACHYCARDIA: "PMT"

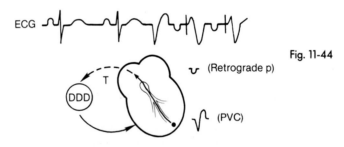

ECG

(Retrograde p)

Fig. 11-44

T

DDD

(PVC)

161 These two pacemaker rhythms may be difficult to distinguish without documentation of their onset. The rapid ventricular rate may be corrected similarly in both cases by eliminating atrial sensing (i.e., converting to the DVI or VVI mode). Atrial tachycardia with p-wave tracking may be more simply corrected by lowering the maximum (upper) rate limit. Pacemaker-mediated atrial tachycardia is more simply corrected by reprogramming the post ventricular atrial refractory period (PVARP) if this is a programmable feature. Further episodes may also be prevented by these adjustments.

LET US REVIEW: Normal dual-chamber pacing may be complicated by selected *(atrial/ventricular)* arrhythmias. DDD pacing is typically associated with *(atrial fibrillation/atrial tachycardia)*. This tachycardia is

atrial

atrial tachycardia

the result of either antegrade or retrograde _____   tracking
of p waves. Further episodes may be prevented by adjusting the
atrial _____ period or rate limit or by eliminating   refractory
atrial _____.   sensing

SUMMARY: SYSTEMATIC APPROACH—ECG ASSESSMENT AND CLASSIFICATION OF PACEMAKERS

162
    I. Evaluate *stimulus release* ("automatic interval).
       A. Is there ever too long a pause without a stimulus being released?
       B. Identify pacing spikes and automatic pacing interval, including discharge rate and regularity and A-V interval with dual chamber pacemakers.
       C. *Problems identified*
          1. Absence of stimulus (intermittent/sustained)
          2. Changes in stimulus rate and/or regularity
   II. Evaluate *stimulus response* ("capture").
       A. Does each pacemaker stimulus away from a potential refractory period produce a myocardial response ("capture")?
       B. Is the response atrial, ventricular, or both (dual)?: *Classification Criteria 1* (chamber paced)
       C. With variations in QRS response R/O fusion.
       D. *Problem identified:* loss of capture
  III. Evaluate adequate *sensing*.
       A. Is the pacemaker given the opportunity to sense (presence of natural beats from same chamber or chambers)?: *Classification Criteria 2* (chamber sensed)
       B. Evaluate *ventricular* sensing
          1. Is/are the spike(s) ever completely inhibited by natural QRS complexes?: *Classification Criteria 3* (mode of sensing)
          2. Is the automatic interval reset by these natural QRS complexes?
          3. Identify escape interval and correlate it with automatic interval. (with dual-chamber pacing correlate with A-V or V-A interval)
          4. Is there ever a spike(s) after a fully formed natural QRS complex?
          5. With dual chamber pacing, evaluate sensing within the A-V interval to detect normal committed, non-committed vs. modified committed pattern variations
       C. Evaluate *atrial* sensing
          1. Can natural p waves be clearly seen? On any other lead?
          2. Do atrial spikes appear after these natural p waves?
          3. Do the p waves appear to be "tracking" single chamber ventricular spikes? *Classification Criteria 3* (mode of sensing)

D. *Problem identified:* Loss of sensing/competition
IV. Evaluate any *arrhythmias* present (independent or pacemaker-induced).
V. Determine if the pacemaker is implanted.
  A. Are programmable options available?
  B. Does it have antitachycardia capabilities?
    1. Primary: major pacemaker function
    2. Secondary: programmable functions

SINGLE-CHAMBER PACING:

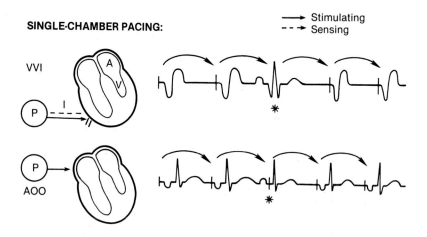

DUAL-CHAMBER PACING:

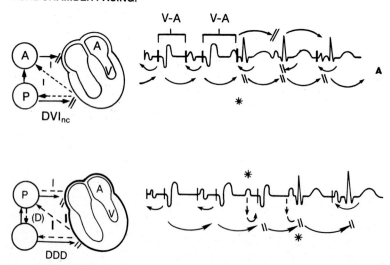

Fig. 11-45

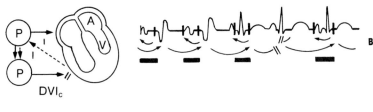

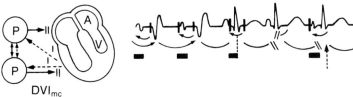

Fig. 11-45, cont'd

ADDITIONAL ASSESSMENT PARAMETERS

163 Additional problem areas to consider when caring for the patient with an external (temporary) or internal (permanent) pacemaker include:

1. Evaluation of any arrhythmias present:
   —Is it independent or pacemaker induced?
   —Is it correct by pacemaker adjustment?
2. If the pacemaker is implanted, consider the following:
   —What are the programmable options?
   —What are the antitachycardia capabilities?
3. Potential electrical interference, especially with temporary units
4. Potential infection of insertion and/or incision site
5. Restriction of movement depending on catheter position
6. Patient instruction and follow-up:
   —Provide the patient with Medic Alert card; write down the pacing mode as well as manufacturer/model number and explain their significance to the patient.
   —Identify the follow-up system.
   —Discuss local and national patient/family support groups with the physician.
   —Specify how to care of site and any activity limitation before the first follow-up visit.

ANTITACHYCARDIA FUNCTIONS

164 Antitachycardia functions are currently available only in selected, highly specialized temporary or permanent pacing units and are currently used only minimally. They are reflected by the fifth category of the International Pacing Code and Classification System (see Frames 83 to 91).

LET US REVIEW: The major antitachycardia functions are referred to by the following letter codes in the 1981 pacing code:
E (_____), N (_____ _____), S (_____ _____), and B (_____).

external; normal rate
competitive scanning
bursting

165 *External* is the earliest antitachycardia function available and refers to *external control*. The fixed rate mode is activated by external application of a magnet or radiofrequency unit over the pulse generator during attacks by the patient or physician. The pacemaker signals fall at different times during the tachycardia, eventually interrupting the tachycardia circuit.

REMEMBER: A high-powered magnet, provided by most pacemaker companies, may be used to elicit the pacing spike at normal (or rapid) rates with implanted demand pacemakers. Application of this magnet over the implanted pulse generator site creates a magnetic field that temporarily eliminates _____, thus converting the system to the continuous, or _____, mode and allowing for stimulus release.

sensing
fixed-rate

Since all demand pacemakers (single-chamber or dual-chamber) are magnetically responsive, the only easily available method for interruption of a tachycardia is by external control. Although awkward for sustained use, this method may be very practical and effective in an emergency.

166 Normal rate competition is true *dual-demand* pacing. It is available as a programmable mode in one manufacturer's implanted DDD unit.

LET US REVIEW: Because of its dual function, the DDD pacemaker is often misleadingly referred to and confused with _____ pacing—an antitachycardia mode. The true dual-demand pacemaker *automatically* escapes at *either* _____ or _____ rates as needed. It utilizes an antitachycardia function known as _____ competition, designated by the code letter _____.

dual-demand

fast; slow
normal rate

N

Fast rates automatically activate the pacemaker's magnetic fixed-rate mode without the need for external influence or control. The pacemaker stimuli—*firing at a normal rate range*—fall at different times during the tachycardia, eventually interrupting the tachycardia circuit.

167 *Scanning* refers to the delivery of carefully timed pacemaker extrasystoles during the tachycardia. The pacemaker automatically recognizes the rapid rate and emits timed stimuli (1 to 16, as programmed) at progressively longer coupling intervals until the tachycardia is interrupted.

Bursting refers to *short, rapid* overdrive fixed-rate pacing with progressive hysteresis, that is, progressively longer automatic intervals. Tachycardia control, similar to bursting, may now be obtained in at least one manufacturer's temporary (external) unit by pressing a "×5" button on the pulse generator. This increases the rate of stimulus release to 5 times the rate indicated on the rate dial for a short period of time.

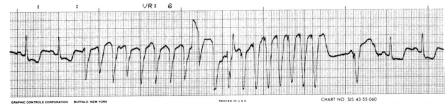

Fig. 11-46

NOTE: Implanted Antitachycardia pacemaker which recognizes the ventricular tachycardia and then delivers a "burst" of stimuli at a fixed interval that interrupts the tachycardia. This pacemaker is also a VVI Antibradycardia pacer, which escapes at a rate of approximately 60 following the termination of VT.

168 These antitachycardia functions have been grouped together in the proposed 1987 revision of the pacing code under the one letter "p" for "pacing" control of tachyarrhythmias. The use of "S" in this category has changed from "scanning" to "shock" to refer to automatic implantable cardioverter/defibrillator (AICD) units, which control tachyarrhythmias by the purposeful delivery of a higher voltage electrical discharge or _____. Currently available AICD   shock
units may now be classified in this system by the code OOOPS.

The letter "D" has been proposed to refer to the availability in the near future of antitachycardia systems, which can *both* pace and/or shock separately as needed.

SUGGESTED READINGS
Cardioversion and defibrillation/AICD

Alexander S: Landmark perspective: The new era of cardioversion, JAMA 256(5):628, 1986.

Clyde C and others: Defibrillators in general practice, Br Med J (Clin Res) 289(6455):1351, 1984.

Crocetti SS: AICD: some lifesaving advice, AJN 86(9):1006, 1986.

Cooper DK and others: Care of the patient with the automatic implantable cardioverter defibrillator: a guide for nurses, Part 6, Heart Lung 16(1):640, 1987.

Chapman PD and others: The automatic implantable cardioverter-defibrillator: evaluating suspected inappropriate shocks, J Am Coll Cardiol 7(5):1075, 1986.

Dalzell GW: Ventricular defibrillation: the Belfast experience, Br Heart J 58(5):441, 1987.

Echt DS and others: Clinical experience, complications, and survival in 70 patients with the automatic implantable cardioverter defibrillator, Circulation 71:287, 1985.

Eysmann SB and others: Electrocardiographic changes after cardioversion of ventricular arrhythmias, Circulation 73(1):73, 1986.

Flores B and Hildebrandt M: the automatic implantable defibrillator, Heart Lung 13(6):608, 1984.

Fye WB: Ventricular fibrillation and defibrillation: historical perspectives with emphasis on the contributions of John MacWilliam, Carl Wiggers, and William Kouwenhoven, Circulation 71(5):858, 1985.

Grogan EW and others: Management of supraventricular tachycardias, Cardiovasc Clin 16(1):261, 1985.

Greco A: An expert's guide to using a defibrillator, Nursing 17(8):60, 1987.

Karch SB: Morphologic effects of defibrillation: a preliminary report, Crit Care Med 12(10):920, 1984.

Leclerq JR and others: Clinical use of automatic implantable defibrillators, Eur Heart J (SupplD)8:143, 1987.

Lake CL and others: Low-energy defibrillation: safe and effective, Am J Emerg Med 3(2):104, 1985.

Marchlinski FE and others: The automatic implantable cardioverter-defibrillator: efficacy, complications, and device failures, Arch Intern Med 104(4):481, 1986.

Mirowski M: The automatic implantable cardioverter/defibrillator: an overview, J Am Coll Cardiol 6:461, 1985.

Mirowski M and others: Recent clinical experience with the automatic implantable cardioverter-defibrillator, Cardiol Clin 3(4):623, 1985.

Moss PM and others: An implantable defibrillator: help for ventricular arrhythmias, AORN J 40(4):551, 1984.

Mower MM and others: Automatice implantable cardioverter-defibrillator structural characteristics, Part 2, PACE 7(6):1331, 1984.

Noel D: Challenging concerns for patients with automatic implantable cardioverter defibrillators, Focus Crit Care 13(6):50, 1986.

Pancoast P and others: Electrical interventions in cardiopulmonary resuscitation: cardioversion, Emerg Med Clin North Am 1(3):535, 1983.

Paros RJ and Goren CC: The precordial thump: an adjunct to emergency medicine, Heart Lung 12:61, 1983.

Reid PR: Implantable cardioverter-defibrillator: patient selection and implantation protocol, Part 2, PACE 7(6):1338, 1984.

Saksena S and others: Developments for future implantable cardioverters and defibrillators, PACE 10(6):1342, 1987.

Seger JJ and others: Electrical therapy of arrhythmias, Cardiol Clin 3(4):617, 1985.

Valladares B and Lemberg L: A new device for the prevention of sudden death, Heart Lung 14(6):632, 1985.

Valladares B and Lemberg L: Problem solving for complications with the AICD, Heart Lung 16(1):105, 1987.

Ventriglia WJ and others: Electrical interventions in cardiopulmonary resuscitation: defibrillation, Emerg Med Clin North Am 1(3):515, 1983.

Vlay SC: The automatic internal cardioverter-defibrillator comprehensive clinical follow-up, economic and social impact (Stony Brook experience), Am Heart J 112(1):189, 1986.

Waldecker B and others: Disrhythmias after direct-current cardioversion, Am J Cardiol 57(1):120, 1986.

Winkle RA and others: Practical aspects of automatic cardioverter/defibrillator implantation, Am Heart J 108:1335, 1984.

Yee BH and others: Elective cardioversion: a standard for patient care, Crit Care Nurse 5(3):11, 1985.

Pacemakers

Akiyama T: Ventricular safety pacing in DDD and DVI pacemakers, Medtronic News, pp. 9-13, March 1984.

Activitrax becomes world's most prescribed pacemaker, Medtronic News 26(2):16, 1986/87.

Ausubel K and others: Pacemaker syndrome: definition and evaluation, Cardiol Clin 3(4):587, 1985.

Barold SS and others: Oversensing by single-chamber pacemakers: mechanisms, diagnosis, and treatment, Cardiol Clin 3(4):565, 1985.

Bass LS and others: Temporary epicardial electrodes, Dimens Crit Care Nurs 5(2):80, 1986.

Beyersdorf F and others: Increase in cardiac output with rate-responsive pacemakers, Ann Thorac Surg 42(2):201, 1986.

Berman N: antiarrhythmic therapy in the elderly: pacemakers and drugs, Geriatrics 41(2):61, 1986.

Bernstein A and others: The NASPE/BPEG generic pacemaker code for antibradyarrhythmia and adaptive-rate pacing and antitachycardia devices, PACE 10:794, 1987.

Birdsall C: How do you manage epicardial wires?, AJN 86(3):252, 1986.

Clarke D and Popp S: Activitrax—how does it work?, Medtronic News 25(4):12, 1986.

Clinton JE: Emergency non-invasive external cardiac pacing, J Emerg Med 2(3):155, 1985.

Conover MB: Understanding electrocardiography: physiologic and interpretive concepts, ed. 5, St. Louis, 1984, The CV Mosby Co.

den Dulk K and others: Is there a universal anti-tachycardia pacing mode? Am J Cardiol 57(11):950, 1986.

Duncan J and others: Initial experience with universal pacemakers, PACE 6:806, 1983.

Falk R and Ngai STA: External cardiac pacing: influence of electrode placement on pacing threshold, Crit Care Med 14(11):931, 1986.

Griffin JC: Pacemaker follow-up: its role in the detection and correction of pacemaker system malfunction, PACE 9(3):387, 1986.

Gupta AK and others: Variety of pacemakers and monitoring systems, part I, PACE 9(1):143, 1986.

Hauser RG: Programmability: a clinical approach, Cardiol Clin 3(4):539, 1985.

Haffajee CI: Temporary cardiac pacing: modes, evaluation of function, equipment, and trouble shooting, Cardiol Clin 3(4):515, 1985.

Hedges J and others: Developments in transcutaneous and transthoracic pacing during brady-asystolic arrest, Ann Emerg Med 13(9):822, 1984.

Hammond C: Pacemakers: seeing to it they work right. . . and keep on doing it, RN 45(12):33, 1982.

Hayes D and Fetter J: Pacemaker syndrome: recognition and management, Medtronic News 1984.

Isicoff C: Understanding upper rate responses of DDD pacers, Heart Lung 14(4):327, 1985.

Keung E and Sudduth B: Arrhythmias in single-chamber pacemakers, Cardiol Clin 3(4):551, 1985.

Levine PA and Seltzer JP: Fusion, pseudo-fusion, pseudo-pseudo fusion and confusions: normal rhythms associated with atrioventricular sequential "DVI" pacing, Clin Prog Pacing Electrophysiology 1(1):70, 1983.

Levine PA: Normal and abnormal rhythms associated with dual-chamber pacemakers, Cardiol Clin 3(4):595, 1985.

Mickus D and others: Exciting external pacemakers, AJN 86(4):403, 1986.

Murdock DK and others: Pacemaker malfunction: fact or artifact, Heart Lung 15(2):1504, 1986.

Niemann J and others: External non-invasive cardiac pacing: a comparative hemodynamic study of two techniques with conventional endocardial pacing, PACE 7:230, 1984.

Owen P: Defibrillating pacemaker patients: how to safeguard the fail-safe device, AJN 84(9):1129, 1984.

Parker MM and Lember L: Pacemaker update 1984, Part I, Introduction to electrocardiographic analysis of pacing function and site, Heart Lung 13(3):315, 1984.

Parker MM and Lemberg L: Pacemaker Update 1984, Part III, Pacemaker arrhythmias in normally functioning pacemakers, Heart Lung 13(5):589, 1984.

Parker MM and Lember L: Pacemaker Update 1984, Part IV, DDD pacemaker—electrocardiographic assessment and problem solving, Heart Lung 13(6):687, 1984.

Parsonnet V and Bernstein AD: Cardiac pacing in the 1980's: treatment and techniques in transition, J Am Coll Cardiol 1:339, 1983.

Parsonnet V: Wanted—a pacemaker lexicon, PACE 10:1385, 1987.

Patros RJ: Temporary ventricular pacemakers demonstrating bipolar and unipolar modes, Heart Lung 12(3):277, 1983.

Phibbs B and others: Indications for pacing in the treatment of bradyarrhythmias, JAMA 252(10):1307, 1984.

Rosenquist M and others: Atrial vs. ventricular pacing in sinus node disease: a treatment comparison study, Am Heart J 111(2):292-7, 1986.

Seger J and Griffin J: Electrical therapy of arrhythmias, Cardiol Clin 3(4):617, 1985.

Shilling E: The external pacemaker: what the nurse needs to know, Medtronic News June 1982.

Shively B and Goldschlager N: Progress in cardiac pacing, Part I, Arch Intern Med 145(11):2103, 1985.

Shively B and Goldschlager N: Progress in cardiac pacing, Part II, Arch Intern Med 145(12):2238, 1985.

Spielman S and Segal B: Pacemakers in the elderly: new knowledge, new choices, Geriatrics 41(2):13, 1986.

Spielman S: Pacemakers: abnormal function, Geriatrics 40(10):99, 1985.

Sukhum P: Pacemakers of the 1980's, Postgrad Med 79(4):173, 1986.

Sutton R and others: Physiologic benefits of atrial synchrony in paced patients, PACE 6:327, 1983.

Syverud SA and others: Hemodynamics of transcutaneous cardiac pacing, Am J Emerg Med 4(1):17, 1986.

Van De Water J and others: Physiologically responsive cardiac pacemakers: a role for electrical impedence? Chest 9(2):194, 1987.

Videen JS and others: Emodynamic comparison of ventricular pacing, atrioventricular sequential pacing, and atrial synchronous ventricular pacing using radionuclide ventriculography, Am J Cardiol 57(15):1305, 1986.

Wingate S: Levels of pacemaker acceptance by patients, Heart Lung 15(1):93, 1986.

Wulff KS: Use of temporary epicardial electrodes for atrial pacing and monitoring, Cardiovasc Nurs 18(1):1, 1982.

Zipes DP: Cardiac pacemakers. In Braunwald E, editor: Heart disease: a textbook of cardiovascular medicine, ed. 3, Philadelphia, 1988, WB Saunders Co.

The Patient Without Coronary Artery Disease in the Coronary Care Unit

1 Chronic electrical or mechanical cardiac disorders often occur in the absence of acute coronary artery disease. Patients with these disorders can present with potentially life-threatening complications. They may thus require the acute monitoring and intervention or diagnostic expertise provided in the coronary care unit. Malignant ventricular tachyarrhythmias, including torsades de pointes and the supraventricular tachyarrhythmias of pre-excitation syndrome, are frequently seen electrical disorders. Two frequently seen mechanical disorders with both electrical and mechanical complications are mitral prolapse, and cardiomyopathy. Although the complications of mitral prolapse are usually benign, they can be disturbing enough to warrant evaluation in a coronary care unit.

REMEMBER: Arrhythmias are manifestations of abnormal _____ activity of the heart.   electrical

Abnormal mechanical activity may also trigger electrical complications or can present as either congestive _____ failure or   heart
_____ shock.   cardiogenic

ELECTRICAL DISORDERS
Malignant ventricular arrhythmias

2 Chronic ventricular arrhythmias may be classified as either benign, potentially malignant, or malignant according to severity, accompanying symptoms/heart disease, and ultimately prognosis.

Ventricular arrhythmias are considered *benign* when they occur singly rather than in couplets or VT, in the absence of any identifiable form of structural heart disease. They are typically tolerated asymptomatically except for complaints of palpitations. Prognosis is good without therapy. Couplets or unsustained VT (i.e., short bursts), which usually occur in the setting of some form of structural heart disease (i.e., coronary artery disease, valvular disease, ventricular hypertrophy, or myopathy), are considered *potentially malignant* arrhyth-

617

mias. Although also typically tolerated asymptomatically, they are associated with a moderate risk of sudden death in spite of effective suppression with therapy.

Both benign and potentially malignant ventricular arrhythmias are typically tolerated (*symptomatically/asymptomatically*). Treatment (*does/does not*) have a significant effect on prognosis. Structural heart disease, but not necessarily coronary artery disease, is usually present in the setting of (*benign/potentially malignant*) ventricular arrhythmias.

asymptomatically
does not

potentially malignant

3 Uniform (monomorphic) or multiform (polymorphic), sustained VT and ventricular fibrillation (VF), which usually occur in the setting of structural heart disease and/or the prolonged Q-T syndrome, are considered the *malignant* ventricular arrhythmias. They are typically associated with symptoms of dizziness and/or syncope and with a high risk of sudden death.

Forms of structural heart disease where these may occur include coronary artery disease, _____ heart disease, hypertrophy, and _____. Patients with the prolonged Q-T syndrome are at high risk even with normal LV function (see torsades de pointes, Frames 13 to 21). Therapy (*does/does not*) have a significant effect on prognosis.

valvular
myopathy

does

Role of EPS/antiarrhythmic therapy

4 Antiarrhythmic drug therapy is the initial treatment of choice for patients with chronic malignant ventricular arrhythmias. Due to the variety of individual responses, the effectiveness of the therapy should be evaluated by either Holter monitoring or serial electrophysiologic studies (EPS). Exercise testing may also be used.

LET US REVIEW: The most significant chronic ventricular arrhythmias are _____ and _____. They have been associated with symptoms of _____ and _____, especially in patients (*with/without*) heart disease. The treatment of choice is _____ therapy, which is monitored by _____ monitoring and _____.

VT; VF
dizziness
syncope; with
arrhythmias
Holter
EPS

5 Holter monitoring can evaluate the effect of the drug(s) in suppressing the number of episodes of spontaneous VT or frequent PVCs. It is best used in patients who have frequent episodes of VT.

Electrophysiologic studies (EPS) evaluate the effectiveness of the drug in suppressing electrically induced VT. It is best used in patients whose episodes of VT are more sporadic.

6 Electrophysiologic studies (EPS) include both invasive and non-invasive methods. Intracardiac electrophysiologic studies evaluate the electrical characteristics of the conduction system and selected brady-

and tachyarrhythmias from multiple recording sites on specialized catheters threaded transvenously into the heart. The patterns obtained (including atrial and His bundle electrograms) are correlated with the surface ECG.

Arrhythmias are induced in this controlled situation using specialized artificial pacing systems, which deliver single and/or multiple electrical stimuli to different sites within the heart. This technique is referred to as *programmed* _____ _____. Hemodynamic responses may be evaluated by monitoring level of consciousness, BP, skin temperature and moisture, and by obtaining simultaneous arterial blood gases.

electrical stimulation

7 These studies may be indicated in patients with symptomatic ventricular or _____ tachyarrhythmias, which are difficult to diagnose and/or control, or difficult to diagnose bradyarrhythmias associated with SA or AV block. Potential candidates for specialized antitachycardia pacemakers, AICD implantation, and/or transcatheter ablation may require prior EPS studies to predict the effectiveness of these measures.

supraventricular

Non-invasive or less invasive electrophysiologic techniques include Holter monitoring, exercise testing, body surface mapping, and esophageal atrial electrograms or AEG's (see Unit 7).

8 Pharmacologic therapy for malignant ventricular arrhythmias is most typically initiated with Class IA agents. A Class IB or IC agent may then be tried alone or in combination. The Class III agent amiodarone is considered when none of these have been effective.

REMEMBER: The Class I antiarrhythmic agents act by decreasing the rate at which _____ enters the cell. The Class IA agents include: quinidine, _____, and _____. The Class IB agents include Xylocaine, _____, and _____. Class IB agents differ from Class IA agents in that they shorten repolarization and *(do/do not)* depress normal ventricular conduction.

Na$^+$
Pronestyl
Norpace
Tonocard; Mexitil

do not

The two currently approved Class IC agents are _____ and _____. Class IC agents differ from IA agents in that they do not delay repolarization, and they differ from IB agents in that they prolong normal ventricular conduction resulting in widening of the _____ complex.

Tambocor; Enkaid

QRS

9 Class IB agents are not usually as effective alone. Disopyramide and flecainide are not good choices in the patient with CHF due to their more significant negative _____ effects.

Amiodarone is not an ideal initial choice due to its diffuse action on the heart, duration of action, and side effects.

inotropic

REMEMBER: The onset and duration of action of amiodarone is *(short/long)*. Side effects include: _____ toxicity, GI symptoms, skin photosensitivity, corneal microdeposits, pseudocyanosis, hyper and hypothyroidism, pneumonitis, and _____ fibrosis.

long; neurologic

pulmonary

Concept of proarrhythmia

10 Ironically the very drugs designed to suppress or correct arrhythmias have the potential to generate them. This ability of a drug to *produce* arrhythmias is referred to, logically, as a _____ effect. Drugs such as digitalis, while controlling the ventricular rate of supraventricular tachycardia, may produce heart blocks, ventricular and even other new supraventricular arrhythmias.

proarrhythmic

   Antiarrhythmic agents are particularly notorious for producing malignant ventricular arrhythmias—the very type of arrhythmia they are supposed to effectively treat. The concept of proarrhythmia is used most commonly when referring to the toxic effects of these agents. One of the most common proarrhythmic effects is the production of torsades de pointes (see Frames 13 to 23). Proarrhythmic effects are more likely to occur in the presence of severe LV function. These effects must be taken into consideration when evaluating the mechanisms and therapy of malignant ventricular arrhythmias.

Nonpharmacologic therapy

11 Current nonpharmacologic therapy for malignant ventricular arrhythmias includes surgical isolation, excision, and/or cryoablation of the ectopic site, transcatheter ablation, or the insertion of an automatic implantable cardioverter/defibrillator (AICD). Transcatheter ablation of the ectopic site and/or critical pathway is effective in selected patients but is still investigational. Serious complications, as well as a recurrence rate of arrhythmia up to 40%, have been reported. The use of the AICD is extensively discusses in Unit 11, Frames 23 to 42.

12 **In Summary:** Malignant ventricular arrhythmias include sustained, symptomatic _____ and/or _____, occurring in the context of structural heart disease or the prolonged _____ syndrome.

VT; VF

Q-T

   Available modes of therapy include Class _____ or _____ antiarrhythmic agents administered alone or in combination, surgery, transcatheter _____ (investigational), and _____ implantation.

I

III

ablation

AICD

   The indications for and/or effectiveness of these modes of therapy are best evaluated by intracardiac _____ studies and/or _____ monitoring.

EPS

Holter

Torsades de pointes

13 Torsades de pointes (TDP) is a malignant ventricular tachyarrhythmia—intermediary between VT and VF—associated with a prolonged QT(U) interval. It is named for its ECG appearance, which most typically gives the appearance of cyclically *twisting* from negative to upright or vice versa (see Fig. 12-1). The typical pattern may appear only on selected leads, so obtaining a 12-lead ECG or multi-lead trace may be helpful.

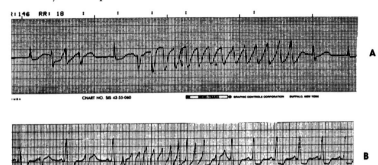

Fig. 12-1

Regretfully, torsades is also used to describe the spindle-like pattern seen in true ventricular fibrillation as well (see Fig. 12-2). The spindle pattern is thought to be produced by a more gradual shift in the polarity of the deflections.

Since the syndrome can appear to mimic both ventricular tachycardia and ventricular fibrillation, it has been referred to as: multiform (polymorphous) VT, atypical VT, ventricular fibrilloflutter, and paroxysmal or transient ventricular fibrillation. It has also been referred to as cardiac ballet and/or delayed repolarization syndrome.

14 LET US REVIEW: Torsades de pointes can mimic both ventricular tachycardia and ventricular _____. It is associated with a prolonged _____ interval. The complexes in torsades appear to twist back and forth from _____ to _____.

fibrillation
QT
upright
negative

The normal QT interval is less than 0.40 sec. for men and less than 0.44 for women at a heart rate of 60 beats per minute. It prolongs with slower heart rates and shortens with faster heart rates. QT(U) intervals greater than 0.50 are diagnostic for this syndrome at any heart rate. Borderline QT intervals should be corrected for heart rate by calculating the "QTc" or QT interval *corrected* for heart rate, or using available conversion charts. QTc intervals greater than 0.44 sec. are also considered diagnostic for this syndrome (see Fig. 12-1B).

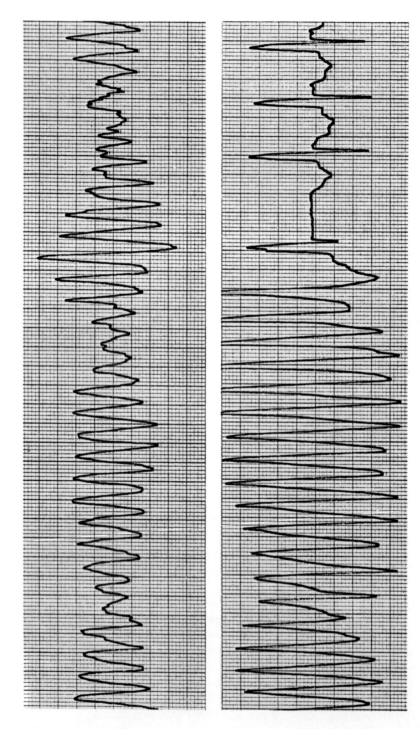

Fig. 12-2 (From Conover MB: Understanding Electrocardiography, ed. 5, St. Louis, 1988, The CV Mosby Co.)

622

The appearance of broad T waves is a clue to the presence of a prolonged QT.

An "R on T" phenomenon is usually the triggering factor. However, in the presence of a prolonged QT, PVCs do not have to be significantly early to create this phenomenon. A typical characteristic of TDP is the initiation of the arrhythmia by a PVC late in diastole.

15 Factors that can significantly prolong the QT intervals include: Class IA or Class III antiarrhythmics, electrolyte imbalance, selected psychotropic agents, bradycardia, CNS disorders, high protein diets, coronary spasm, and occasionally mitral valve prolapse. Electrolyte imbalances associated with prolonged QT or QU intervals include _____, hypocalcemia, and _____   *hypokalemia; hypomagnesemia* (see Unit 5). Normal serum K levels below 3.9 may also contribute to this syndrome. Psychotropic agents producing this effect include the phenothiazines, such as Thorazine, Compazine, Trilafon, and Mellaril and tricyclic antidepressants, such as Elavil, Tofranil, and Nardil. Congenital QT prolongation has also been recognized and associated with torsades. Changes in sympathetic tone, bradycardia secondary to elevated systolic BP, or both are implicated in CNS disorders. Prolonged QT intervals in patients with coronary artery disease have also been associated with an increased risk of sudden death.

16 The most popularly theorized mechanism of torsades is thought to be re-entry. The triggering of torsades by an "R on T" phenomenon is supportive of the reentry theory.

REMEMBER: If a reentrant impulse exits early in repolarization when the _____ in recovery is still pronounced, the im-   *disparity* pulse may recycle within the circuit producing a _____   *chain reaction* _____ response. Reentrant tachycardia is also typically triggered by _____ electrical impulses (see Unit 7,   *single* Frames 39-50).

Prolonged repolarization is associated with increased disparity of refractory periods, which is thought to contribute further to this phenomenon. The QT interval reflects ventricular (*repolarization/depolar-*   *repolarization* *ization*). Bradycardia and/or long R-R cycles are also associated with a prolonged refractory period and potentially increased disparity. Thus, bradycardia may enhance the effects of a prolonged QT interval and torsades is typically triggered by PVCs preceded by (*short/long*)   *long* R-R cycles (see Fig. 12-1).

17 Other possible mechanism of torsades include sympathetic induced after depolarizations in susceptible individuals, bifocal and/or multifocal ventricular activity in competition, and biventricular tachycardia. The concept of bifocal or biventricular ectopy may explain the directional changes in the ECG pattern.

REMEMBER: RV PVCs produce a(n) *(negative/upright)* deflection on lead V_1 and a(n) *(negative/upright)* deflection on lead V_6, while LV PVCs produce a(n) *(negative/upright)* on lead V_1 and a(n) *(negative/upright)* on lead V_6.

negative
upright
upright; negative

18 Torsades often terminates spontaneously. However, it has been associated with episodes of syncope, seizures, and sudden death if not terminated spontaneously. It is usually not responsive to conventional antiarrhythmic therapy and may actually be caused or aggravated by it. Countershock remains an effective mode of therapy.

The antiarrhythmic drugs most commonly producing torsades are the Class _____ agents. Examples of these agents include _____, Pronestyl, and _____. These drugs act to prolong ventricular repolarization/refractory periods as evidenced by the effect on the _____ interval.

IA
Quinidine; Norpace

QT

This effect has been referred to as _____ effect and *(is/is not)* thought to be associated with toxic levels of these drugs. It represents a sensitivity to the drug instead, which may occur with even the first usual dose. If the QT interval is exceedingly prolonged (i.e., greater than _____ sec., or greater than _____ for QTc) an episode of TDP may be triggered.

Quinidine
is not

.50
.44

19 When any of these drugs are initiated, the individuals should be carefully monitored in a CCU or telemetry unit. If an episode of torsades occurs or the QT interval exceeds .50 sec, the drug is best discontinued. Episodes of torsades after prolonged therapy are unusual unless another complicating factor, such as electrolyte imbalance or bradycardia, occurs. Patients taking Class IA antiarrhythmics should be regularly monitored for these factors as well.

Class III antiarrhythmic agents also act to prolong ventricular _____ periods. QT prolongation with TDP has been associated with amiodarone therapy. The additional side effects of AV block and bradycardia further increase susceptibility. The long half-life of this drug necessitates that therapy for torsades be continued up to 5-10 days. Ironically, the other major Class III agent bretylium does not cause TDP and has actually been effective in its therapy. This may be explained by its differential effect on normal versus ischemic or abnormal cardiac tissue, which, unlike amiodarone, may promote uniformity of refractoriness.

refractory

20 Therapy is initially directed at shortening the QT interval by increasing the heart rate. The heart rate may be increased with overdrive pacing, Isuprel, or atropine. Although overdrive atrial pacing is preferred, cautious ventricular overdrive pacing at the lowest effective VR (@90-150) may be more practical in this emergency setting. The

use of the newer external transcutaneous pacing systems can further facilitate this (see Unit 11, Frame 65). After the normal rhythm is restored, transvenous pacing may be used to prevent any further bradycardia that may trigger TDP or until the QT (QTc) interval has returned to normal.

Class IB agents may also be effective in the therapy of TDP since they act to *(shorten/prolong)* repolarization. Examples of Class IB agents include: _____, _____, and _____. Reports are currently available primarily on the use of Xylocaine although the use of Tonocard and Mexitil has also been mentioned. Xylocaine is often unsuccessful due to its different effect on normal vs. ischemic or abnormal cardiac tissue. Xylocaine shortens refractory periods primarily in *(normal/abnormal)* tissues. Due to this differential effect also Xylocaine occasionally has been reported actually cause TDP (see Unit 10, Frame 28). Further studies are needed in this area, particularly with regard to the effects of the other Class IB agents.

shorten
Xylocaine; Tonocard
Mexitil

normal

21 Magnesium sulfate has been used more recently, proving effective in abolishing TDP. This effect can occur without any alteration in the QT intervals or Mg blood levels. Reactivation of the Na^+/K^+ pump with restoration of intracellular K^+ may be the mechanism.

REMEMBER: Magnesium is important in the breakdown of _____ for energy and is thus necessary for the normal functioning of the _____ pump.

ATP
Na^+/K^+

Patients with congenitally prolonged QT, mitral valve prolapse, and CNS disorders exhibit an increased sensitivity to autonomic stimulation. Physical or emotional stress, loud noises, and/or pregnancy can trigger episodes of torsades. Therefore, in this setting Isuprel *(is/ is not)* indicated. In contrast, they respond best to sympathetic blocking agents, such as the _____ blockers. Surgical removal of the left stellate ganglion can be performed as a last resort if there is no response to beta blockade.

is not

beta

22 Polymorphous VT has also been documented in the presence of a normal QT interval. This pattern has been reported in the setting of coronary artery disease and cardiomyopathy. However, the treatment and clinical significance in these settings is very different from settings in which the QT intervals are prolonged. In this setting, the arrhythmia is responsive to conventional antiarrhythmic therapy, but the prognosis is very poor. Therapy with sympathetic agents, such as Isuprel, is often harmful. This rhythm behaves clinically as true VT or VT and is best treated as such. For this reason, some authorities have suggested that the term polymorphous VT be used to describe this pattern and the term torsades be reserved for the pattern occurring in the presence of a prolonged QT (QTc) interval.

REMEMBER: Classic torsades *(is/is not)* responsive to conventional antiarrhythmic therapy. However, the prognosis is often *(poor/good)* if the contributing factor can be corrected or eliminated. Therapy with sympathetic agents, such as Isuprel, is often *(harmful/beneficial)*.

is not
good

beneficial

23 Since the significance and management of this arrhythmia can vary depending upon the corresponding QT interval, and since true VF and TDP mimic each other so closely (see Fig. 12-3 and Fig. 12-2, Frame 13), a conservative approach is best. If the QT is unknown, or normal, or there is any doubt, the rhythm is best diagnosed as _____ VT or VF *resembling* TDP and it is initially treated as classic VT or _____.

polymorphous
VF

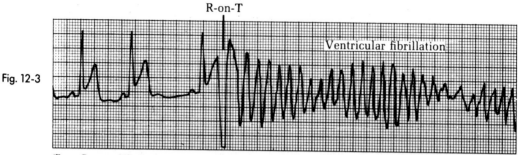

R-on-T

Ventricular fibrillation

Fig. 12-3

(From Conover MB: Understanding Electrocardiography, ed. 5, St. Louis, 1988, The CV Mosby Co.)

The use of Isuprel is best avoided since negative effects may occur in the presence of a normal QT, congenitally prolonged QT or CNS disease. Alternate approaches, such as overdrive pacing or the administration of Class IB agents, bretylium, or magnesium sulfate, appear to be associated with far less risk.

PRE-EXCITATION SYNDROME (WPW, ETC.)

24 Pre-excitation syndrome refers to the presence of a congenital bypass of part or all of the normal AV conduction system, since the normal AV delay is avoided, atrial impulses can reach the ventricles through this extra pathway earlier than through the normal conduction pathways. The ventricles may thus be _____-excited by atrial impulses using this pathway, predisposing the patient to *(supraventricular/ventricular)* tachyarrhythmias.

pre
supraventricular

Because these congenital pathways bypass part or all of the normal conduction system, they are referred to as extra or *accessory* pathways or _____ tracts.

bypass

25 There are three major forms of pre-excitation syndrome: Wolff-Parkinson-White (WPW), Lown-Ganong-Levine (LGL), and Mahaim. They are differentiated by the characteristics of their _____ pathways or bypass _____.

accessory; tracts

626

REMEMBER: These congenital tracts bypass _____ or _____ of the normal AV conduction system.

part
all

A second major characteristic of the pathway is the insertion into either the free ventricular wall or the normal conduction system. The term *tract* is more strictly reserved for pathways with one end attached to normal conductive tissue.

26 The congenital pathway in Wolff-Parkinson-White (WPW) syndrome is referred to as the Kent Bundle. It completely bypasses the normal AV conduction system, inserting into the ventricular wall, and thus connecting the atria directly into the ventricles (see Fig. 12-4).

ECG Characteristics

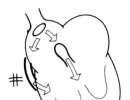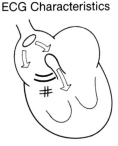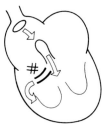

Fig. 12-4

Kent (W-P-W)
short P-R with
Δ wave

James (L-G-L)
short P-R without
Δ wave

Mahaim
normal P-R with
Δ wave

The congenital pathway in Lown-Ganong-Levine (LGL) syndrome is referred to as the James Bundle. It partially bypasses the AV node, inserting into the normal AV conduction system below the node, and thus connecting the atria directly to the lower portion of the AV node. This pathway may also be referred to in the strictest sense as a bypass _____ since one end remains attached to the normal _____ tissue (see Fig. 12-4).

tract
conductive

Mahaim fibers originate below the AV node, bypass part or all of the ventricular conduction system, and insert into the ventricular wall. They thus connect the lower AV node or Bundle of His directly to the ventricular muscle (see Fig. 12-4).

27 Accessory pathways, which bypass the AV node, eliminate the major part of the AV delay, resulting in a *(short/long)* P-R interval.

short

Accessory pathways, which insert directly into ventricular muscle, produce a *delta* (δ) wave pattern in sinus rhythm or sinus tachycardia.

28 The Kent Bundle of the WPW syndrome *(does/does not)* bypass the AV node. Therefore, the P-R interval is *(short/normal)*. The Kent Bundle also inserts directly into the _____ _____. Therefore, a delta wave pattern *(should/should not)* be expected in sinus rhythm or sinus tachycardia.

does
short
ventricular muscle
should

The James Bundle of the LGL syndrome *(does/does not)* bypass the AV node. Therefore, the P-R interval is *(short/normal)*. The James Bundle also inserts into the lower portion of the _____.

does
short

AV node

Therefore, a delta wave pattern *(should/should not)* be expected in sinus rhythm or sinus tachycardia.

should not

Mahaim fibers *(do/do not)* bypass the AV node. Therefore, the P-R interval is *(short/normal)*. Mahaim fibers insert directly into the ventricular wall. Therefore, a delta wave pattern *(should/should not)* be expected in sinus rhythm.

do not
normal
should

29 Delta waves are seen with both _____ and _____ pathways. The delta wave is the result of a *fusion complex*.

Kent; Mahaim

REMEMBER: Fusion beats occur when _____ or more impulses are attempting to control the ventricles at the _____ time.

two
same

Fusion complexes

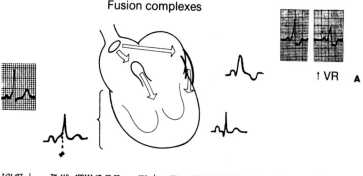

↑VR **A**

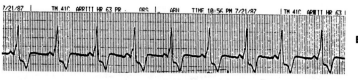

B

Fig. 12-5

During sinus rhythm in WPW the atrial impulse travels down both the normal conduction and Kent pathways simultaneously (see Fig. 12-5). However, the ventricles are activated by the accessory pathway first since there is no AV delay.

The Kent pathway inserts into _____ _____, which conducts slowly. Thus the initial part of the QRS complex is wide. The remainder of the QRS complex is produced by activation through the normal conduction pathways and is, therefore, *(narrow/wide)*.

ventricular muscle

narrow

The completed QRS complex reflects a blending or _____ of the two potential complexes. The initial slurring of this fusion complex mimics the Greek triangular symbol—delta (δ)

fusion

and is thus referred to as a _____ wave. This initial part of the QRS complex reflects activation through the *(Kent pathway/AV node)*.

delta
Kent pathway

30 The delta wave becomes more pronounced either during very slow or rapid atrial rates due to increased refractoriness and delay within the normal AV conduction system. When conduction through the normal AV pathway is delayed, conduction through the accessory pathway is unopposed or a longer period of time.

Slight increases in heart rate may cause a delta wave to disappear. In fact, the delta wave may be totally dormant during normal sinus rates, when the AV node conduction time is *(normal/increased)*. Rapid atrial pacing or vagal stimulation can be used to elicit the delta wave in a patient with a suspect history during normal sinus rates.

normal

Complete activation by the accessory pathway can occur at rapid atrial rates producing a totally *(narrow/wide)* QRS complex (Fig. 12-5).

wide

31 WPW syndrome is the most common form of pre-excitation. The most common tachyarrhythmias occurring in patients with WPW syndrome are paroxysmal atrial tachycardia (PAT), presenting most typically with a narrow QRS, and atrial fibrillation, presenting most typically with a wide QRS (see Fig. 12-6).

The atrial tachycardia seen in WPW is an AV re-entrant supraventricular tachycardia. Patients with a James pathway (_____ syndrome) may also present with this form of supraventricular tachycardia.

LGL

REMEMBER: Re-entry is one of the major mechanism of arrhythmia formation. Re-entry is defined as the ability of an impulse to _____ a region of the heart through which it has _____ _____ (see Unit 7, Frames 39-43).

re-excite
already passed

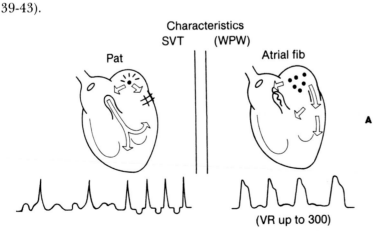

Characteristics
SVT   (WPW)

Pat   Atrial fib

A

(VR up to 300)

Fig. 12-6

Continued.

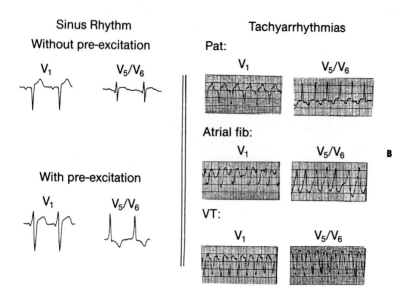

Sinus Rhythm

Without pre-excitation

V_1 V_5/V_6

With pre-excitation

V_1 V_5/V_6

Tachyarrhythmias

Pat:

V_1 V_5/V_6

Atrial fib:

V_1 V_5/V_6 B

VT:

V_1 V_5/V_6

Fig. 12-6, cont'd

AV re-entry utilizes macro circuits connecting the atria and ventricles to re-excite either the atria or ventricles after already leaving the chamber. Thus the exciting impulse may originate in either the atria or the ventricles.

In WPW, the macrocircuit is formed by the AV node, bundle branches, and the accessory (Kent) pathway (see Fig. 12-6).

32 During sinus rhythm, the impulse travels simultaneously through both the _____ conduction system and the _____ pathway, colliding with itself in the ventricles. However, ectopic impulses do not always travel simultaneously down both pathways. PACs are often selectively unable to conduct through the accessory pathway due to its longer refractory period.

normal; Kent

NOTE: Kent pathways typically conduct faster but recover more slowly than the AV node.

Thus *block* occurs within this part of the *circuit*. The PAC is, instead, transmitted exclusively through the AV node and bundle branch system to the ventricles. At the same time, it is conducted in a retrograde fashion back to the atria via the accessory pathway. Since the AV node has a natural *delay*, the atria are given the time to recover and be able to again accept this impulse. They are thus re-excited by the original impulse, limited only by the refractory period of the accessory pathway and atria. This impulse can easily recycle again and again, resulting in a *(tachycardia/bradycardia)*.

tachycardia

REMEMBER: The three conditions necessary for a re-entry to occur are 1) a potential _____, 2) _____ within part of

circuit; block

630

the circuit, and 3) _____ conduction within the remainder of the circuit.

delayed

33 The ECG characteristics of an AV reentrant tachycardia are 1) a p wave that changes direction at the onset, 2) a long p-r interval at the onset and 3) a short r-p interval during the tachycardia.

The p wave changes direction since the atria are activated initially in an antegrade direction and subsequently in a _____ direction. This change may be seen an any lead with clear p waves, such as V_1 (MCL1), lead II, or sometimes lead I, depending on the exact location of the accessory pathway.

retrograde

The *r-p interval* is the distance from the beginning of the QRS of one impulse to the p wave of the next impulse. It reflects retrograde conduction from the ventricles through the Kent pathway in contrast with the p-r interval, which reflects _____ conduction _____ the ventricles through the _____ _____ and bundle branches. There *(is/is not)* a natural delay at the AV node. This is reflected in the normal p-r interval delay of up to _____ seconds. There *(is/is not)* a natural delay within the Kent pathway. Therefore, the r-p is *(shorter/longer)* than the p-r.

antegrade
to; AV node
is

.20; is not
shorter

34 Since the ectopic impulses are usually conducted to the ventricles using only the normal AV conduction pathway, the delta wave *(is/is not)* present. Thus the QRS complex during the tachycardia is typically *(narrower/wider)* than in sinus rhythm.

is not

narrower
atrial fibrillation

Totally wide QRS complexes are usually associated with the *(PAT/ atrial fibrillation)* of WPW. However, AV reentrant PAT may result in a wide QRS less commonly when rate-dependent bundle branch block occurs. This further delay in the AV macrocircuit may trigger a reentrant tachycardia, which could not be triggered in the presence of AV node delay alone. Rate-dependent bundle branch block can also uncover the presence of an accessory pathway, which is concealed in sinus rhythm due to sustained antegrade block in the accessory pathway. This phenomenon is appropriately referred to as _____ WPW. AV reentrant tachycardias may also result in wide QRS complexes, even less commonly if the ectopic impulse is conducted antegrade via the accessory pathway and retrograde via the AV node.

concealed

In the setting of a wide QRS tachycardia the 12 lead ECG may be useful in confirming the presence of a bundle branch block vs. ectopic pattern (see Unit 7 and Unit 8).

35 Since the original impulse *returns back* to the atria via the accessory pathway, AV re-entrant PAT is also referred to as a *reciprocating tachy-*

cardias. A single reciprocal beat or the first beat of a potential reciprocating tachycardia is called an "echo" beat, since like a true echo, the same message that is sent out is returned to its source. This beat has also been referred to as a "sandwiched" beat since the QRS appears to be sandwiched between the two related p waves.

An AV reciprocating tachycardia may also be initiated, less commonly, by a PVC. The PVC conducts selectively through the accessory pathway in a retrograde fashion, then antegrade back into the ventricle through the normal AV conduction system. In the first beat of this tachycardia the P wave appears sandwiched between two related _____ _____.

QRS complexes

36 Atrial fibrillation also occurs commonly in the WPW syndrome. The multiple, rapid impulses of atrial fibrillation bombard the AV node, prolonging its refractory period to a greater extent than that of the accessory pathway. These impulses are, therefore, preferentially conducted exclusively through the accessory pathway. The ventricular rate is *(slow/rapid)*, limited only by the _____ period of the accessory pathway.

slow; refractory

REMEMBER: The Kent pathway typically recovers slowly but _____ more rapidly than the AV node.

conducts

In this rhythm, the accessory pathway does not act as part of a circuit. It is merely a point of entry to the ventricles, controlling the ventricular response. Therefore this rhythm *(does/does not)* represent an AV reentrant tachycardia. The QRS complex remains *(regular/irregular)*.

does not

irregular

37 Since ventricular conduction occurs totally via the _____ pathway, the resulting QRS complex is *(narrow/wide)*. This wide QRS tachycardia mimics VT, especially with very rapid rates where the irregularity is not so easily seen. The 12 lead ECG patterns may again be helpful.

accessory/Kent; wide

The rapid ventricular response in atrial fibrillation may deteriorate into ventricular fibrillation in time and, is therefore, a particularly significant though only potentially life-threatening rhythm. When a VR of 300 or more is sustained in a wide QRS tachycardia without immediate deterioration into VF, WPW should be highly suspected.

38 The supraventricular tachycardias of WPW (pre-excitation) syndrome may be treated pharmacologically, electrically, or surgically. Pharmacologic therapy is the initial treatment of choice. The AV re-entrant PAT is prevented and/or interrupted by drugs, which prolong the refractory period of the AV node (see Fig. 12-7). Prolongation of the retrograde refractory period of the accessory pathway is also helpful but less consistently effective.

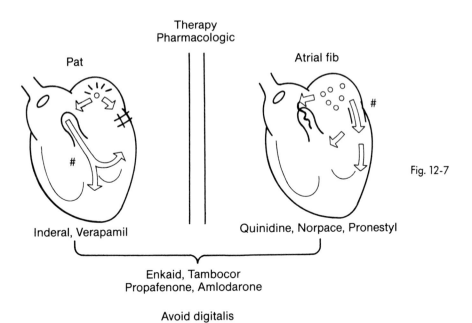

Therapy
Pharmacologic

Pat

Atrial fib

#

#

Fig. 12-7

Inderal, Verapamil

Quinidine, Norpace, Pronestyl

Enkaid, Tambocor
Propafenone, Amlodarone

Avoid digitalis

REMEMBER: Atrio-ventricular conduction in PAT typically occurs over the AV node, but ventriculo-atrial conduction occurs via the _____ _____.

accessory pathway

The ventricular response of atrial fibrillation in WPW is decreased by agents that prolong the antegrade refractory period of the accessory pathway or totally block antegrade conduction via this pathway. Agents prolonging the refractory period of the AV node can facilitate conduction via the accessory pathway, thus further increasing the ventricular response. These rapid ventricular responses can deteriorate into _____ _____. Therefore, agents acting primarily at the AV node *(are/are not)* indicated in the therapy of atrial fibrillation. The therapy of atrial fibrillation in WPW is *(the same/different from)* the therapy of PAT.

ventricular fibrillation
are not

different from

39 This drug-induced acceleration of the ventricular response in atrial fibrillation occurs primarily in patients with short antegrade accessory pathway refractory periods (i.e., less than 250 ms). The length of this refractory period can be estimated non-invasively by observing the length of the shortest r-r cycle in spontaneous or induced atrial fibrillation. Blocking of the accessory pathway conduction during exercise testing or with Pronestyl administration indicates a long refractory period and *(low/high)* risk of sudden death (see Frame 25-26). This effect may be confirmed by the disappearance of the _____ wave in sinus rhythm or sinus tachycardia.

low
delta

Agents that block both the AV node and the accessory pathway may be preferred in the management of PAT since there is less risk of an accelerated VR in the event of unexpected atrial fibrillation.

40 Examples of drugs that prolong the refractory period of the AV node include digitalis, verapamil, and the beta blockers. These drugs are most effective in the management of the *(PAT/atrial fibrillation)* of WPW. They are potentially contraindicated in the presence of atrial fibrillation due to the risk of _____ conduction through the accessory pathway and an *(increased/decreased)* ventricular rate. This risk is greatest with digitalis, which also has a direct effect on the accessory pathway, shortening its refractory period. These drugs may be used in this setting only in the presence of a documented long accessory pathway refractory period.

PAT

accelerated

increased

Examples of drugs that prolong the antegrade refractory period of the accessory pathway include quinidine, Pronestyl, and Norpace. These drugs are all classified Class *(IA/IB)* antiarrhythmic and are most effective in the management of the *(PAT/atrial fibrillation)* of WPW. Of these drugs, only _____ may be administered IV to quickly control the rapid, life-threatening wide QRS tachycardias seen in this type of SVT. These tachycardias can mimic ventricular tachycardia and/or flutter, which *(are/are not)* also controlled by this drug.

IA

atrial fibrillation

Pronestyl

are

41 Class IB antiarrhythmics, such as lidocaine, have variable effects on the accessory pathway. Lidocaine acts to prolong the refractory period and/or block conduction in the accessory pathway primarily in the presence of long initial refractory periods (i.e., greater than 380 ms). However, lidocaine has also been reported to shorten the refractory period of the accessory pathway in individuals with short initial refractory periods, resulting in an increased ventricular response and deterioration into ventricular fibrillation. It is best avoided in patients with WPW.

Class IA agents appear more consistently effective in individuals with both short and long accessory pathway refractory periods, offering a safer alternative. Thus the drug of choice in the management of wide QRS tachycardia is the IV Class IA agent _____.

Pronestyl

42 Examples of drugs that prolong the refractory period of both the AV node and the accessory pathway include amiodarone, flecainide, encainide, and propafenone. These agents are effective in *both* the _____ _____ and PAT of WPW. They may be preferred when the properties of the accessory pathway are unknown. Among these agents encainide seems to have the fewest side effects since there are minimal negative inotropic and fewer

atrial fibrillation

proarrhythmic effects. The diffuse effect of amiodarone on the conduction system as well as its delayed onset of action, long half-life, and side effects, limits its use in this setting where less toxic agents are now available.

43 Surgical intervention in WPW consists of division of the accessory pathway or pathways during precise electrophysiologic mapping to determine this location. Cryoablation has also been used. Although this procedure is no longer experimental and its success rate is high, it is reserved for individuals refractory to drug therapy, or, more recently young otherwise healthy individuals facing a lifetime of antiarrhythmic therapy. Ironically, the procedure is less well tolerated in physically conditioned individuals, such as athletes. A period of preoperative deconditioning has been suggested.

Electrical intervention consists of specially designed pacemakers including burst atrial pacing and dual chamber pacemakers with short AV delays.

44 The 12 lead ECG may also be helpful in identifying the presence and approximate location of the accessory pathway. The direction of the delta wave on V_1 and V_6 can suggest an RV versus LV location.

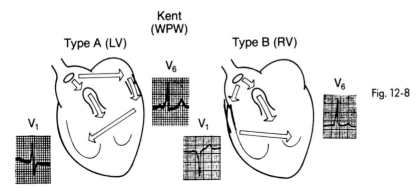

Fig. 12-8

REMEMBER: The positive electrode on lead V_1 is on the *(right/left)* side of the chest. The positive electrode on lead V_6 is on the *(right/left)* side of the chest.

With an RV pathway, the impulse travels away from this electrode producing a *(negative/positive)* deflection on V_1. A positively deflected wave is recorded on lead V_6. Conversely, with an LV pathway, the impulse travels toward lead V_1, producing a *(negative/positive)* deflection and away from lead V_6, producing a *(negative/positive)* deflection. Posterior pathways produce a positively deflected delta wave on both V_1 and V_6 (see Fig. 12-8).

When the presence of an LV pathway is identified, the syndrome is designated as Type A WPW. When an RV pathway is identified, the

right
left

negative

positive
negative

syndrome is designated as Type B WPW. Type B WPW was formerly considered more surgically accessible. The direction or axis of the delta wave on the limb leads can suggest and inferior or lateral location. However, this finding has little added clinical significance.

Multiple pathways may also be present in a single individual. The location of these is best made in the electrophysiologic laboratory.

CARDIOMYOPATHIES

45 The cardiomyopathies are primary diseases of the heart muscle, occurring independently of any other cardiovascular pathology. Myocardial changes secondary to coronary artery disease, hypertension, other congenital, or valvular disease are excluded from this classification.

Myocardial infarction *(is/is not)* considered a form of cardiomyopathy.

is not

46 There are three forms of cardiomyopathy: dilated (congestive), hypertrophic, and restrictive. All three are associated with stiff (noncompliant) left ventricular walls, resulting in difficulty filling and a rise in left ventricular *(systolic/diastolic)* pressure.

diastolic

Changes in LV cavity size, systole, specific myocardial changes, signs and symptoms, and therapy vary. Either genetic or immunologic mechanisms are implicated in all three forms.

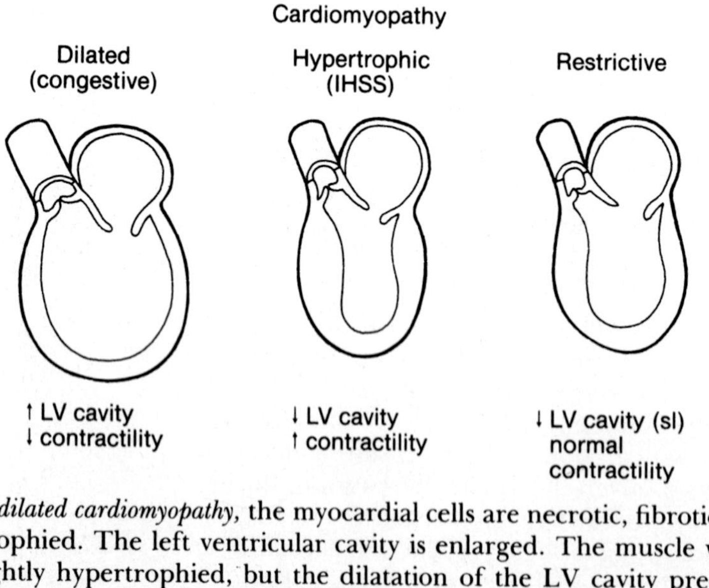

Cardiomyopathy

Dilated (congestive)	Hypertrophic (IHSS)	Restrictive

Fig. 12-9

↑ LV cavity ↓ contractility	↓ LV cavity ↑ contractility	↓ LV cavity (sl) normal contractility

47 In *dilated cardiomyopathy,* the myocardial cells are necrotic, fibrotic, and atrophied. The left ventricular cavity is enlarged. The muscle wall is slightly hypertrophied, but the dilatation of the LV cavity predominates. Dilated cardiomyopathy is associated with decreased contractility and ineffective emptying in systole. Cardiac output and ejection fractions are decreased.

REMEMBER: As a result of ineffective emptying, blood becomes dammed up within the left ventricle. This produces _____ in the heart, and results in symptoms of _____ _____ _____.

For this reason, dilated cardiomyopathy is also referred to as _____ cardiomyopathy.

congestion
congestive heart failure

congestive

48 Specific causes of congestive cardiomyopathy include viral diseases, alcoholism, chemotherapy, and toxicity of pregnancy. The diagnosis can be made by cardiac biopsy.

Typical signs and symptoms include dypsnea, crackles (rales), fatigue, and an S_3 gallop.

REMEMBER: An S_3 gallop is indicative of _____. Distended neck veins, peripheral edema, and hepatomegaly are also seen.

CHF

REMEMBER: These are signs of *(RV/LV)* failure.

RV

Murmurs of mitral and tricuspid regurgitation may be heard.

REMEMBER: These murmurs are *(systolic/diastolic)*. They occur because of incomplete closure associated with ventricular dilatation.

systolic

49 In *hypertrophic cardiomyopathy*, the myocardial cells are typically in disarray with fibrosis and hypertrophy of the individual muscle fibers present. The muscle wall is thickened at the expense of left ventricular cavity.

The hypertrophy is often asymmetrical, occurring predominantly in the septal area and resulting in a narrowed left ventricular outlet. Narrowing is also referred to as _____. Since the narrowed outlet is below the aortic valve, this form of hypertrophic cardiomyopathy is referred to as idiopathic hypertrophic subaortic stenosis (IHSS).

stenosis

50 Hypertrophic cardiomyopathy is congenital and is thought to be related to a disturbance in the autonomic (sympathetic) nervous system, resulting in ineffective regression of fetal hypertrophy. It is associated with increased contractility resulting in systolic obstruction and/or "oversqueezing" of the left ventricle. Although the presence of true obstruction is currently being questioned due to a normal ejection fraction, the signs and symptoms of this syndrome correlate with this hypercontractility.

The cardiac output is decreased due to the difficulty filling and small ventricular cavity size. However, since ventricular emptying is effective, signs and symptoms of CHF *(are/are not)* present. Typical signs and symptoms include chest pain, dyspnea, fatigue, and syncope. These symptoms are more pronounced during physical exertion or times of increased *(sympathetic/parasympathetic)* activity.

An S_4 gallop may also be heard.

are not

sympathetic

REMEMBER: This gallop correlates with decreased ventricular _____. A systolic murmur may also be present due to the increased turbulence. The murmur becomes louder with maneuvers that increase contractility and/or decrease preload or afterload.

compliance

51 In *restrictive cardiomyopathy,* there is an inflammatory response in the endocardial and myocardial cells. It is associated with an increased wall thickness and small cavity size similar to but not as small as the LV cavity size associated with hypertrophic cardiomyopathy. Ejection fractions are normal, and cardiac output is decreased secondary to *(systolic/diastolic)* changes. However, contractility is normal and the diastolic stiffness is more pronounced.

diastolic

Since ejection fractions are normal, congestion *(is/is not)* present. However, signs and symptoms of heart failure are present secondary to the severe compliance changes and increases in the left ventricular and left atrial pressure. These signs and symptoms include dypsnea, fatigue, hepatomegaly, and peripheral edema.

is not

Equilibration of diastolic pressures within the cardiac chambers may occur similar to constrictive pericarditis. However, x-ray and echocardiographic findings differ.

Restrictive cardiomyopathy is the rarest form. Specific causes include endomyocardial fibrosis, Loeffler disease (eosinophilic endomyocardial disease), and amyloidosis. Both ventricles may be involved.

52 Treatment of dilated cardiomyopathy is directed toward controlling the CHF. Medical therapy includes diuretics, vasodilators, inotropic agents, and salt restriction. However, long-term prognosis is poor. End stage CHF may be reached within 2 years of the initial diagnosis. At this time, the only effective mode of therapy is cardiac transplantation.

In peripheral cardiomyopathy, the heart may return to normal within 6 months. When it does not, the prognosis is poor especially with another pregnancy.

53 Heart failure is also present in *(hypertrophic/restrictive)* cardiomyopathy. However, it is more difficult to treat since many of the agents commonly used for heart failure cannot be used.

restrictive

Inotropic agents are not indicated since contractility is *(high/ normal).* Venous vasodilators cannot be used since they may further decrease ventricular filling and cardiac output by a decrease in *(pre-load/afterload).* Symptomatic hypotension can result.

normal

preload

The use of calcium channel blockers may assist in improving myocardial relaxation but needs to be further investigated. Immunosuppressive therapy (steroids, etc.) has not proven successful.

638

Surgical resection of the fibrotic tissue carries a high mortality rate. Cardiac transplantation is an alternative.

54 Hypertrophic cardiomyopathy *(is/is not)* associated with significant signs of CHF. Signs and symptoms are associated with *(hypo/hyper)* contractility and increased *(sympathetic/parasympathetic)* activity. Therefore inotropic agents *(are/are not)* indicated.

is not
hyper
sympathetic
are not

Beta blockers are used to block the sympathetic activity and *(increase/decrease)* the rate and force of ventricular contraction. Ventricular filling time is increased and ventricular stiffness may be decreased.

decrease

Ca^{++} channel blockers may also be used to decrease the hypercontractility and promote ventricular relaxation. However, these agents must be used with caution since the vasodilating effect may result in reflex stimulation of contraction. Conduction defects may also be enhanced especially if the patient is also on beta blockade.

Surgical treatment consists of myotomy (incision of the septum) or myectomy (removal of part of the tissue). Cardiac transplantation *(is/is not)* indicated.

is not

55 Arrhythmias and ECG changes may occur in any of the three forms of cardiomyopathy. Malignant ventricular arrhythmias are associated with sudden death. Rapid supraventricular arrhythmias, such as atrial fibrillation with a rapid ventricular response, may further compromise diastole resulting in hemodynamic compromise. These arrhythmias must be rapidly corrected. Their control represents a therapeutic challenge.

Amiodarone (Cardorone) has proven effective when these patients have significant ventricular arrhythmias.

Abnormal Q waves may be present on the ECG in patients with either congestive or hypertrophic cardiomyopathy.

REMEMBER: Abnormal Q waves correlate with areas of _____. Abnormal Q waves in patients with hypertrophic myopathy correlates with abnormal septal depolarization rather than necrosis.

necrosis

56 Anticoagulant therapy is used in patients with dilated cardiomyopathy to prevent mural thrombi and embolization. Formation of mural thrombi also occurs in patients with restrictive myopathy.

MITRAL VALVE PROLAPSE

57 Mitral valve prolapse is the most common valvular disorder and may be defined functionally, clinically, or anatomically. It is defined *functionally* as a disorder in which there is a pronounced displacement of one or both of the mitral leaflets back up into the left atrium during systole. The posterior leaflet is most often affected.

Unlike the cardiomyopathies, mitral prolapse is considered a primary *(systolic/diastolic)* disorder. The heart muscle may not be directly affected.

systolic

Mitral Prolapse

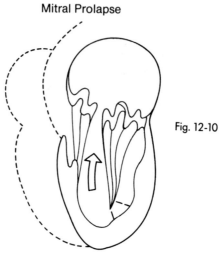

Fig. 12-10

58 Mitral valve prolapse is defined *clinically* by its ausculatory findings (see Frames 61-63). It is defined *anatomically* as degeneration of the myxomatous and collagen tissue layers of the valve producing weakened leaflets with a larger than necessary (i.e., redundant) surface area, similar to a furled sail (see Fig. 12- 10). Degenerative changes also occur within the chordae tendonae. They are thin and long, and are further weakened by the strain of the prolapsing valve.

These changes are considered primary valvular changes. The most commonly proposed mechanism is genetically transmitted connective tissue disease. Skeletal deformities are common in these individuals, confirming the presence of systemic _____ tissue disease.

connective

Mitral valve prolapse may also occur secondary to papillary muscle changes as in acute MI or myocardial changes, such as myocarditis, endocarditis, or cardiomyopathy, where the left ventricular diameter is disproportionately smaller than the valve ring.

59 This syndrome has also been referred to as Barlow's syndrome, floppy mitral valve syndrome, billowing mitral leaflet syndrome, flailed mitral valve, or the mitral click-murmur syndrome.

LET US REVIEW: Mitral prolapse is associated with _____ valve leaflets, which are displaced back up into the _____ _____. It is thought to be due to _____ tissue disease and is transmitted _____. It is defined clinically by its _____ findings.

weakened
left atrium
connective
genetically
auscultatory

60 The *functional* diagnosis of mitral valve prolapse is confirmed by visualization of valve movements on M-mode or two-dimensional (2D) echocardiogram. Because of the availability of both forms of echocardiography, mitral prolapse is now diagnosed more frequently and is recognized as highly prevalent in many otherwise normal individuals.

It is generally considered a benign disorder, but may be complicated by the disturbing symptoms of chest pain, palpitations, and syncope. The incidence of these complications may be no greater than that of the general population. They have been explained in some individuals by the coexistence of a congenital hyperadrenergic state. Asymptomatic prolapse is more common, and requires no therapy except occasional antibiotic prophylaxis (see Frame 72).

61 Although some arching back into the left atrium is normal during systole, pronounced displacement can prevent the valve leaflets from approximating and closing tightly, thus predisposing to mitral regurgitation.

Mitral regurgitation is diagnosed by the presence of a *(systolic/diastolic)* murmur. In mitral prolapse the murmur is accompanied by a characteristic mid to late systolic "click." It is best heard over the apex and lower left sternal border. This click-murmur combination can be the first diagnostic clue in asymptomatic patients, and confirms the _____ diagnosis of mitral prolapse.

systolic

clinical

62 The click is produced by a sudden tightening of the chordea tendonae with ventricular contraction. It has been said to be similar to a "parachute snapping open."

Changes in ventricular volume affect the pressure, timing, and intensity of the click and murmur. Both the click and murmur are usually louder in intensity and occur earlier—i.e., in mid rather than late systole—with maneuvers that decrease venous return and/or left ventricular volume. This is thought to occur because the chordae are in a more ventricle position earlier than the time of contraction, and may allow the click/murmur to be more clearly heard. Examples of such manuevers include standing, performing a Valsalva maneuver, tachycardia, and inspiration, which increases RV filling but decreases LV filling. Hemodynamically these measures can be said to decrease LV *(preload/afterload)*.

The degree/extent of prolapse also occurs earlier and is accentuated by measures that increase the force of contraction, such as sympathetic stimulation related to stress. Unlike these other measures, vasodilators, such as the nitrates or amyl nitrite, decrease the intensity of the murmur because of a simultaneous decrease in afterload, which *(impedes/facilitates)* systole.

preload

facilitates

63 Conversely manuevers that increase ventricular volume by impeding ejection or increasing *(afterload/preload)* delay the click and murmur until *(mid/late)* in systole. The intensity is louder due to increased turbulence. These measures include lying down, squatting, isometric hand grip, and the use of vasopressors. Variation in the intensity and timing at different times and/or different conditions in the same individual is a hallmark of mitral prolapse.

afterload
late

A "whoop" or "honk" may also be present in late systole, but is not as common a finding. These are murmurs due to thin jets of regurgitant blood striking the non-prolapsed leaflet.

64 LET US REVIEW: Auscultatory findings confirm _____ diagnosis of mitral prolapse. The typical auscultatory findings are a systolic _____ and _____. These are heard in midsystole with manuevers that *(increase/decrease)* venous return or preload. They are heard in late systole with manuevers that *(increase/decrease)* afterload. Measures that decrease venous return *(increase/decrease)* the extent of prolapse. Both decreased preload and increased afterload *(increase/decrease)* the intensity of the murmur for different reasons. But combined decrease in both preload and afterload, such as with nitrates, *(does/does not)* decrease the intensity.

clinical

click; murmur
decrease
increase
increase
increase

does not

Both the functional and clinical definitions of mitral prolapse can be confirmed diagnostically. Neither are considered more accurate. The presence of both has the highest accuracy and may be considered major criteria in the diagnosis of significant mitral valve prolapse.

65 Mitral regurgitation produces an increased *(pressure/volume)* on the heart. When the heart is presented with an increased volume load that it is unable to pump, _____ _____ can occur. Significant mitral regurgitation and CHF is unusual unless the chordae tendonae have ruptured. Symptoms of fatigue and shortness of breath are common but do not necessarily correlate with the presence of CHF. Treatment for severe mitral regurgitation is mitral valve replacement. The term "floppy mitral valve" is often reserved for this variant of the syndrome.

volume

heart failure

Patients with mitral regurgitation with or without congestive heart failure are at higher risk for bacterial endocarditis, TIAs, progressive mitral regurgitation, and/or chordae rupture. Both symptomatic and asymptomatic patients should receive antibiotic prophylaxis. Mitral valve prolapse is a major cause of TIAs in patients under the age of 45. Thrombotic lesions collect on the angle of the leaflet and their attachment to the atrial wall. These patients should receive antiplatelet therapy to prevent stroke. Examples of antiplatelet agents are _____ and _____. Patients with progressing mitral regurgitation or chordae rupture should be monitored for signs of _____.

ASA; Persantin

CHF

642

66 Chest pain is the most common symptom in symptomatic mitral valve prolapse. This pain can be precordial, either sharp or dull, is often localized, can occur during rest or exertion, and may be relieved by lying down. It most typically occurs during times of combined physical and emotional stress, lending support to an autonomic component. It can last for seconds, hours, or days. Chest pain is considered a non-specific, though highly suspect finding. Auscultatory and echocardiographic findings must also be present to make the diagnosis.

The pain is thought to be due to the stretching of the chordae tendonae and papillary muscles with increased rate and force of contractions, and/or blood pressure.

REMEMBER: Stress is associated with stimulation of the _____ nervous system, which in turn increases heart _____, _____, and _____. Adrenergic sensitivity in these individuals may generate or further magnify this response. Esophageal spasm related to esophageal motility disorders has also been implicated.

> sympathetic
> rate; contractility; BP

67 Patients with adrenergic sensitivity can also exhibit other forms of autonomic dysfunction, parasympathetic as well as sympathetic, such as prolonged bradycardia in response to a Valsalva maneuver, resting bradycardia, irregular pupil size, and orthostatic hypotension. These responses are thought to be due to an impaired central response to baroreceptor reflexes.

REMEMBER: Stimulation of the pressoreceptors (baroreceptors) results in both hormonal and nervous responses. The nervous system affected is the _____ nervous system via the _____ nerve (see Unit 4, Frame 34). Orthostatic hypotension or arrhythmias may be responsible for the symptoms of dizziness or syncope. Psychological factors and arrhythmias have also been implicated. Vagal sensitivity may respond to small doses of phenobarbital, which has a central effect on the vagal system.

> parasympathetic
> vagus

Other symptoms indicating adrenergic hypersensitivity include hypersensitivity to noise or body language, coldness and paresthesias of the extremities, and tachyarrhythmias (see Frame 71). Urinary and plasma catecholamines are often elevated, correlating with an increased activity of the _____ nervous system (see Unit 10, Frame 52).

> sympathetic

68 Psychological neuroses have long been attributed to the mitral valve prolapse syndrome. Anxiety and panic disorders, including sensations of choking, smothering, dypsnea, diaphoresis, and dizziness, have been commonly reported. These have been also explained by the presence of autonomic dysfunction. These patients may be merely more "psychologically vulnerable" to the natural fear that accompanies palpitations and chest pain. Blood lactate levels have also been implicated. Findings from actual studies as to the correlation with mitral prolapse with anxiety disorders are contradictory. A sense of sustained fatigue seemingly unrelieved by rest may be accompanied by unexplained depression. Antidepressants, such as amitriptyline HCl (Elavil) or imipramine HCl (Tofranil), may be helpful.

69 Both ventricular and supraventricular arrhythmias complicate mitral valve prolapse in selected individuals. The most common arrhythmias are PVCs. Malignant ventricular arrhythmias, although rare, have been associated with sudden death. These arrhythmias, like the chest pain, are thought to be generated from _____ of   stretching
the papillary muscles or _____ dysfunction or both.   autonomic

Since there is a strong association with WPW syndrome, the presence of this disorder as well should be ruled out in the presence of supraventricular tachyarrhythmias. Evidence of delta wave indicating a left-sided bypass tract may be present on the ECG.

REMEMBER: WPW syndrome is typically associated with rapid *(ven-*   supraventricular
tricular/supraventricular) arrhythmias. Determination of the presence of a left versus right-sided bypass tract is best made on lead
_____. In this lead, the delta wave of an LV tract would be V_1
(upright/negative) (see Frame 44).   upright

70 T wave inversion in leads II, III, and AVF is seen on the ECG and is thought to correlate with stretching and ischemia to the inferoposterior papillary muscle.

REMEMBER: The valve leaflet most typically involved in mitral prolapse is the _____ leaflet. This leaflet is supported   posterior
by the posterior papillary muscle, which is attached to inferior wall of the LV. Leads II, III, and AVF reflect the _____   inferior
wall of the LV. These changes are augmented when standing.

Prolonged QT intervals have also been reported mitral prolapse, especially in symptomatic patients. This may contribute to the presence of ventricular arrhythmias and/or sudden death, but more studies need to be done since current findings are contradictory. Prolonged QT intervals are associated with _____ syn-   torsades de pointes
drome (see Frames 13 to 23). Specific QT patterns have also been associated with increased catecholamines and need to be more closely examined.

71 Beta blockers are the treatment of choice for the chest pain and arrhythmias of mitral prolapse. Both of these symptoms are thought to be associated at least in part with increased _____   sympathetic
activity. Beta blockers act to block *(sympathetic/parasympathetic)* effects   sympathetic
on the heart, resulting in decreased autonomic tone, heart rate, and contractility. The decreased heart rate and contractility decrease LV

volume, causing less prolapse and stretch of the chordae and papillary muscles. The most commonly used beta blocker is _____. Recent evidence shows that the alpha receptors as well as beta receptors may play a role in these arrhythmias. In these patients, a beta blocker with combined alpha and beta blockade may be more effective. The only currently available beta blocker is _____. Additional antiarrhythmic therapy is often required with malignant arrhythmias.

Propanolol (Inderal)

Labetolol (Normodyne/Trandate)

Manuevers that increase venous return and/or afterload may also be helpful in relieving the chest pain of mitral prolapse, since an increase in LV volume alters the position of the chordae. Examples of these manuevers are raising the legs, _____, _____, and *(isometric/isotonic)* exercises. Stress management should be a goal of therapy in the management of all symptomatic mitral prolapse.

lying
squatting; isometric

72 Asymptomatic prolapse without auscultatory findings *(does/does not)* require therapy. Asymptomatic prolapse with auscultatory findings only intermittent _____ prophylaxis and follow-up for possible _____ or progressive mitral _____. Hypertension should be kept under control since it can aggravate the disorder and may result in ruptured chordae. Hypertension produces and increased *(afterload/preload)* on the heart, which increases the _____ during systole as evidenced by an increased _____ of the systolic murmur.

does not

antibiotic
TIAs
regurgitation

afterload
turbulence
intensity

SUGGESTED READINGS
Malignant ventricular arrhythmias/sudden death/EPS

Adler DC: Current management of ventricular tachycardia. Symposium overview from the University of Pennsylvania Hospital, Heart Lung 13(6):595, 1984.

Braunwald E, editor: Heart diseases: a textbook of cardiovascular medicine, ed. 3, Philadelphia, 1988, WB Saunders Co.

Bigger JT: Definition of benign versus malignant ventricular arrhythmias: targets for treatment, Am J Cardiol 52:47C-54C, 1983.

Bigger JT: Indications for antiarrhythmic drug therapy. Proceedings of Ventricular Arrhythmias Update, 1987, Boehringer Ingelheim Pharmaceuticals.

Buxten AC: Sudden cardiac death—1986, Ann Intern Med 104(5):716, 1986.

Cassidy D and others: The use of programmed electrical stimulation in patients with docu-

mented or suspected ventricular arrhythmia, Heart Lung 13(6):692, 1984.

Clay S: Catecholamine-sensitive ventricular tachycardia, Am Heart J 114(2):455, 1987.

Cox J: The status of surgery for cardiac arrhythmias, Circulation 71(3):413, 1985.

DeBasio N and Rodenhausen N: The group experience: meeting the psychological needs of patients with ventricular tachycardia, Heart Lung 13(6):597, 1984.

Finkelmeier and others: Psychologic ramifications of survival from sudden cardiac death, CCQ 7(2):71, 1984.

Fought SG: Holter monitoring and electrophysiologic study, Crit Care Nurs 7(1):8, 1987.

Funk M and others: A compact electrophysiology-studies record, Am J Nurs 86(5):575, 1986.

Horowitz L: Proarrhythmic responses during

electrophysiologic testing, Am J Cardiol 59(11):45E, 1987.

Horowitz L and others: Proarrhythmia, arrhythmogenesis or aggravation of arrhythmia—a status report 1987, Am J Cardiol 59(11):54E, 1987.

Kienzle M and others: Antiarrhythmic drug therapy for sustained ventricular tachycardia, Heart Lung 13(6):614, 1984.

Krol B and others: Electrophysiologic testing in patients with unexplained syncope: clinical and noninvasive predictors of outcome, JACC 10(2):358, 1987.

Markmann PJ: Surgical management of ventricular tachycardia, Heart Lung 13(6):622, 1984.

McGovern B and Ruskin J: Ventricular tachycardia: initial assessment and approach to treatment, Mod Concepts of Cardiovasc Dis 56(3):13, 1987.

Mercer ME: The electrophysiology study: a nursing concern, Crit Care Nurse 7(2):58, 1987.

Morganroth J: Arrhythmiogenicity of antiarrhythmic drugs, Proceedings of Ventricular Arrhythmias Update, 1987, Boehringer Ingelheim Pharmaceuticals.

Moran J: Surgical management of malignant ventricular arrhythmia, CCQ 7(2):49, 1984.

O'Mara SR and Summers C: Care of the sudden death survivor, CCQ 7(2):81, 1984.

Prystowsky EL: Selection of antiarrhythmic drugs based on electrophysiologic studies, Cardiovasc Clinics 16(1):239, 1985.

Rahimtoola SH and others: Consensus statement of the conference on the state of the art of electrophysiologic testing in the diagnosis and treatment of patients with cardiac arrhythmias, Part 1, Mod Concepts of Cardiovasc Dis 56(10):55, 1987.

Rahimtoola SH and others: Consensus statement of the conference on the state of the art of electrophysiologic testing in the diagnosis and treatment of patients with cardiac arrhythmias, Part 2, Mod Concepts Cardiovasc Dis 56(11):61, 1987.

Rogers RR: Your patient is scheduled for electrophysiology studies, Am J Nurs 86(5):573, 1986.

Ruskin J: New approaches to antiarrhythmic therapy. Proceedings of Ventricular Arrhythmias Update, 1987, Boehringer Ingelheim Pharmaceuticals.

Scheinman MM and Davis JC: Catheter ablation for treatment of tachyarrhythmias: present role and potential promise, Circulation 73:10, 1986.

Schmitt C and others: Amiodarone in patients with recurrent sustained ventricular tachyarrhythmias: results of programmed electrical stimulation and long-term clinical outcome in chronic treatment, Am Heart J 114(2):279, 1987.

Surawicz B: Prognosis of ventricular arrhythmias in relation to sudden cardiac death: therapeutic implications, JACC 10(2):435, 1987.

Summers C: Sudden cardiac death, CCQ 7(2):1, 1984.

Valladares BK: Ventricular arrhythmias: A perspective on management, Heart Lung 14(4):417, 1985.

Zheutlin TA and others: Therapy of patients with malignant ventricular arrhythmias, CCQ 7(2):35, 1984.

Zipes D: Proarrhythmic effects of antiarrhythmic drugs, Am J Cardiol 59(11):27E, 1987.

Torsades de pointes

Fontaine G and others: Torsades de pointes: definition and management, Mod Concepts Cardiovasc Dis 51(6):103, 1982.

Fung AY and others: QT prolonged and torsades de pointes: the sole management of CAD, Int J Cardiol 7(1):63-6, 1987.

Griffin J and Most A: Torsades de pointes complicating acute myocardial infarction, Am Heart J 106:169, 1984.

Jackman WM and others: Ventricular tachyarrhythmias in the long QT syndrome, Med Clin North Am 68:1079-1109, 1984.

Johnson CT and Cowan M: Relationship between the prolonged QTc interval and ventricular fibrillation, Heart Lung 15(2):141, 1986.

Kim HS and Chung EK: Torsade de pointes: polymorphous ventricular tachycardia, Heart Lung 12(3):269, 1983.

Lasater MG: Torsades des pointes—etiology and treatment, Focus Crit Care 13(5):17, 1986.

Lynch L: Torsades de pointes—malignant ventricular arrhythmia, AJN 86(7):826-7, 1986.

Martinez R: Torsades de pointes: atypical rhythm, atypical treatment, Ann of Emergency Med 16(8):871, 1987.

Moss A and Schwartz P: Delayed repolarization (QT or QTU prolongation) and malignant ventricular arrhythmias, Mod Concepts Cardiovasc Dis 51(3):85, 1982.

Ngyen P and others: Polymorphous ventricular tachycardia: clinical characterization, therapy, and the QT interval, Circulation 74(2):340, 1986.

Raehl CL and others: Drug-induced torsades de pointes, Clin Pharm 4(6):675-90, 1985.

Roden DM and others: Incidence and clinical features of the quinidine associated long Q-T syndrome: implications for patient care, Am Heart J 111(6):1088-93, 1986.

Scott JL: Torsades de pointes, J Emerg Med 3(4):289-94, 1985.

Steger KE and others: Drug-induced torsade des pointes: case report and implications for the critical care staff, Heart Lung 15(2):200, 1986.

Tzivoni D and others: Torsades de pointes versus polymorphous ventricular tachycardia, Am J Cardiol 52:639, 1983.

Towanen LK and others: Limited effect of magnesium sulfate on torsades de pointes ventricular tachycardia, Int J Cardiol 12(2):260-2, 1986.

Zipes D: Proarrhythmic effects of antiarrhythmic drugs, Am J Cardiol 59(11):26E, 1987.

Pre-excitation (W-P-W syndrome)

Akhtar M and others: Effect of lidocaine on atrioventricular response via the accessory pathway in patients with Wolff-Parkinson-White syndrome, Circulation 63(2):435, 1981.

Cinca J and others: Daily variability of electrically induced reciprocating tachycardia in patients with AV accessory pathways, Am Heart J 114(2):327, 1987.

Colovita PG and others: Frequency, diagnosis and clinical characteristics of patients with multiple accessory atrioventricular pathways, Am J Cardiol 59(6):601, 1987.

Conover MB: Understanding electrocardiography, ed. 4, St. Louis, 1984, The CV Mosby Co.

Conover M: Electrocardiography update: Wolff-Parkinson-White syndrome, Crit Care Update, pp. 19-20, July 1982.

Cox JL and others: Experience with 118 consecutive patients undergoing operation for the WPW syndrome, J Thorac CV Surg 90(4):490, 1985.

Cox JL: The status of surgery for cardiac arrhythmias, Circulation 71(3):413, 1985.

Critelli G and others: Evaluation of noninvasive tests for identifying patients with pre-excitation syndrome at risk of rapid ventricular response, Part 1, Am Heart J 108(4):905, 1984.

Guiraraudon GM: Surgery for WPW syndrome—further experience with an epicardial approach, Circulation 74(3):525, 1986.

Hancock EW: Irregular tachycardia with wide complexes, Hospital Practice 20(2):49, 1985.

Markel ML and others: Encainide for treatment of supraventricular tachycardia associated with WPW syndrome, Am J Cardiol 58(5):41C, 1986.

Marriott HJL and Conover MHB: Advanced concepts in arrhythmias St. Louis, 1983, The CV Mosby Co.

McGovern B: Precipitation of cardiac arrest by Verapamil in patients with WPW syndrome, Ann Intern Med 104(6):791, 1986.

Morady F and Scheinman M: Paroxysmal supraventricular tachycardia, Part I: Diagnosis, Mod Concepts Cardiovasc Dis 51(8):107, 1982.

Morady F and Scheinman M: Paroxysmal supraventricular tachycardia, Part II: Treatment, Mod Concepts Cardiovasc Dis 51(9):113, 1982.

Prystowsky EN and others: Pre-excitation syndromes—mechanisms and management, Med Clinics North Am 68(4):831, 1984.

Ruffy R and others: WPW syndrome, Arch Intern Med 145(3):533, 1985.

Sharma A and others: Sensitivity and specificity of invasive and noninvasive testing for risk of sudden death in Wolff-Parkinson-White syndrome, JACC 10(2):373, 1987.

Shenasa M and others: Efficacy and safety of intravenous and oral diltiazem for Wolff-Parkinson-White syndrome, Am J Cardiol 59(4):301, 1987.

Skorga P: Lown-Ganong-Levine (LGL) syndrome: recognition and nursing care, Crit Care Update, pp. 38-43, June 1983.

Skorga P and Nunnery C: Lown-Ganong-Levine syndrome, Nursing, pp. 37-42, March 1981.

Sweetwood M: Clinical electrocardiography for nurses, Rockville, Md, 1983, Aspen Publishing Co.

Ward D: Ventricular pre-excitation, Eur Heart J (Suppl)5:119, 1984.

Ward DE and others: Use of flecainide acetate for refractory tachycardia in WPW, Am J Cardiol 57(10):787, 1986.

Wellens HJJ: Wolff-Parkinson-White syndrome. Part I: Diagnosis, arrhythmias, and identification of the high risk patient Mod Concepts Cardiovasc Dis 52(11):53, 1983.

Wellens HJJ: Wolff-Parkinson-White syndrome. Part II: Treatment Mod Concepts Cardiovasc Dis 52(12):57, 1983.

Witt AL and Rosen MR: Cellular electrophysiology of cardiac arrhythmias, Mod Concepts Cardiovasc Dis 50:1, 1981.

Cardiomyopathies

Altman GB: Alcoholic cardiomyopathy, Cardiovasc Nur 17(5):25, 1981.

Hess OM and others: Does verapamil improve left ventricular relaxation in patients with myocardial hypertrophy? Circulation 74(3):531, 1986.

Hirota Y and others: Hypertrophic nonobstructive cardiomyopathy: a precise assessment of hemodynamic characteristics, Am J Cardiol 50:989, 1982.

Hurst JW and Logue RB, editors: The heart, arteries, and veins, ed. 6, 1986, WB Saunders Co.

Jarzemsky P: Nursing care of the patient with dilated cardiomyopathy, Crit Care Nurse 6(2):10, 1986.

Likoff MJ and others: Clinical determinants of mortality in chronic congestive heart failure secondary to idiopathic dilated or to ischemic cardiomyopathy, Am J Cardiol 59(6):634, 1987.

Nikolic G: Left bundle branch block with right axis deviation: a marker of congestive cardiomyopathy, J Electrocard 18(4):395, 1985.

Nissen M: The 'holiday heart' syndrome, Heart Lung 13(1):89, 1984.

Orie J and Liedtke AJ: Cardiomyopathy—1. Dilated (congestive) type, Postgrad Med 79(5):83, 1986.

Orie J and Liedtke AJ: Cardiomyopathy—2. Hypertrophic and restrictive/obliterative types, Postgrad Med 79(5):95, 1986.

Porth C: Pathophysiology, concepts of altered health, ed. 2, Philadelphia, 1986, JB Lippincott Co.

Sanzobrino B and Lemberg L: The cardiomyopathies, Heart Lung 15(4):416, 1986.

Stern TN: Dilated cardiomyopathy: current concepts, Compr Ther 12(6):57, 1986.

Wigle ED: Hypertrophic cardiomyopathy 1988, Mod Concepts Cardiovasc Dis 57(1):1, 1988.

Wingate S: Dilated cardiomyopathy, Part I, Focus on Crit Care 11(4):49, 1984.

Wingate S: Dilated cardiomyopathy, Part II, Focus on Crit Care 11(5):59, 1984.

Mitral valve prolapse

Butrous GS and others: Management of ventricular arrhythmias associated with mitral valve prolapse by combined alpha and beta blockade, Postgrad Med J 62(726):259, 1986.

Cash JT and Grissett G: Not life threatening—mitral valve prolapse, Focus on Crit Care 12(6):54, 1985.

Chambers MA and others: The QT and QS2 intervals in patients with mitral leaflet prolapse, Am Heart J 114(2):355, 1987.

Davidson L and Weaver D: Mitral valve prolapse: its recognition and nursing implications, CV Nursing 15(3):7, 1981.

DeCaprio L and others: QT/QS ratio as an index of autonomic tone changes, Am J Cardiol 53:818, 1984.

Grass S and Utz S: Mitral valve prolapse: a review of the scientific and medical literature, Heart Lung 15(5):507, 1986.

Joyner CR: The mitral valve prolapse syndrome: clinical features and management, Cardiovasc Clin 16(2):233, 1986.

Liebson PR: Mitral valve prolapse: recent advances in diagnosis and therapy, Compr Ther 12(6):21, 1986.

Mason D and others: Arrhythmias in patients with mitral valve prolapse, Med Clin North Am 68:1039, 1984.

Mazza DL and others: Prevalence of anxiety disorders in patients with mitral valve prolapse, Am J Psychol 143(3):349, 1986.

Perloff J and others: New guidelines for the clinical diagnosis of mitral valve prolapse, Am J Cardiol 57(13):1124, 1986.

Savage DD and others: Mitral valve prolapse in the general population, Part 2, Clinical Features: the Framingham Study, Am Heart J 106:577, 1983.

Spears P and others: Chest pain associated with mitral valve prolapse—evidence for esophageal origin, Arch Intern Med 146:4, 1986.

Ultz SW and Grass S: Mitral valve prolapse: self-care needs, nursing diagnosis, and interventions, Heart Lung 16(1):77, 1987.

Abbreviations

A-aDo$_2$	alveolar-arterial oxygen difference
ABG	arterial blood gas
ACTH	adrenocorticotropin hormone
ADH	antidiuretic hormone
AIVR	accelerated idioventricular rhythms
ALAD	abnormal left axis deviation
ALMI	anterior-lateral myocardial infarction
ASA	acetylsalicylic acid
ATP	adenosine triphosphate
AV	atrioventricular; arteriovenous
A-VDo$_2$	arterial-venous oxygen difference
aV$_F$	augmented voltage foot lead (of ECG)
aV$_L$	augmented voltage left lead (of ECG)
aV$_R$	augmented voltage right lead (of ECG)
AWMI	anterior wall myocardial infarction
BP	blood pressure
BSA	body surface area
CAD	coronary artery disease
CCU	cardiac care unit
CHB	complete heart block
CHF	congestive heart failure
CI	cardiac index
CK	creatine kinase
CLBB	complete left bundle branch block
CNS	central nervous system
CO	cardiac output
COPD	chronic obstructive pulmonary disease
CPAP	continuous positive airway pressure
CPK	creatinine phosphokinase
CPR	cardiopulmonary resuscitation
CVP	central venous pressure
2,3-DPG	diphosphoglycerate
ECF	extracellular fluid
ECG	electrocardiogram
EMD	electromechanical dissociation
FFA	free fatty acids
FI$_{O2}$	fraction of inspired oxygen
GAS	general adaptation syndrome
GI	gastrointestinal
GIK	glucose-insulin-potassium
GU	genitourinary
Hb	hemoglobin

HCl	hydrochloride
H$_2$CO$_3$	carbonic acid
HCO$_3$	bicarbonate
HLD	high-density lipoproteins
HPO$_4$	phosphate
IAD	indeterminant axis deviation
ICF	intracellular fluid
IHSS	idiopathic hypertrophic subaortic stenosis
IPPB	intermittent positive pressure breathing
ISF	interstitial fluid
IV	intravenous
IVC	inferior vena cava
IVF	intravascular fluid
IWMI	inferior wall myocardial infarction
JG	juxtaglomerular apparatus (of kidney)
LA	left arm
LAD	left axis deviation
LAEDP	left atrial end-diastolic pressure
LAH	left anterior hemiblock
LAS	local adaptation syndrome
LBB	left bundle branch
LBBB	left bundle branch block
LDH	lactic dehydrogenase
LDL	low-density lipoproteins
LL	left leg
LMD	low molecular-weight dextran
LPH	left posterior hemiblock
LV	left ventricle
LVEDP	left ventricular end-diastolic pressure
MAP	mean arterial pressure
MCL$_1$-MCL$_6$	modified chest lead, 1 through 6 (bipolar)
MDP	maximal diastolic potential
MET	metabolic equivalent
Mg	magnesium
MI	myocardial infarction
MLAP	mean left atrial pressure
MPAP	mean pulmonary artery pressure
MVo$_2$	myocardial oxygen consumption
MVP	mean venous pressure

NA	normal axis	**RBBB**	right bundle branch block
PA	pulmonary artery	**RBC**	red blood cells
PAC	premature atrial contraction	**RMP**	resting membrane potential
PAEDP	pulmonary artery end-diastolic pressure	**RPP**	rate pressure product
Pao$_2$	arterial oxygen pressure	**RL**	right leg
PAOP	pulmonary artery occlusion pressure	**RV**	right ventricle
PAT	paroxysmal atrial tachycardia	**S$_1$, S$_2$** etc.	heart sounds
Pco$_2$	carbon dioxide pressure (tension)	**SA**	sinoatrial
PCWP	pulmonary capillary wedge pressure	**SDD**	spontaneous diastolic depolarization
PEEP	positive end expiratory pressure	**SGOT**	serum glutamic oxaloacetic transaminase
PJC	premature junctional contraction	**SL**	sublingual
PO	postoperative	**SV**	stroke volume
Po$_2$	oxygen pressure (tension)	**SVC**	superior vena cava
PRO	protein	**SVR**	systemic vascular resistance
PT	prothrombin time	**SVT**	supraventricular tachycardia
PTCA	percutaneous transluminal coronary angioplasty	**VF**	ventricular fibrillation
PTT	partial thromboplastin time	**VLDL**	very low-density lipoproteins
PVC	premature ventricular contraction	**V/Q**	ventilation-perfusion
PVR	pulmonary vascular resistance	**VR**	ventricular rate
RA	right arm	**VSD**	ventricular septal defect
RAD	right axis deviation	**VT**	ventricular tachycardia
RBB	right bundle branch	**WBC**	white blood cells
		WPW	Wolff-Parkinson-White syndrome

Index

A

a wave
  of atrial electrograms, 345, 346, 347, 348
  in atrial pulse pattern, 404
A-a gradient, 67
  widened, 68
AAI pacemakers, 577, 587
Abbokinase; *see* Urokinase
Aberration, 315-327
  differential diagnosis of, 322-326
  nursing orders for patient with, 326-327
  versus ventricular ectopic beats, 322-326
ABG values
  to assess metabolic imbalances, 161
  to assess respiratory imbalances, 160
  in metabolic acidosis, 168
  in metabolic alkalosis, 169
  and oxygenation, correlation of, 172-176
  in respiratory acidosis, 165
  in respiratory alkalosis, 166
Absolute refractory period, 34
Accelerated idioventricular rhythm, 295, 298-300
  summary of, 351
Accelerated junctional rhythm, 314
Acebutolol, 505
  for chest pain, 505-508
Acetazolamide, 484
  and bicarbonate formation, 168
  and metabolic acidosis, 172
  for metabolic alkalosis, 170
Acetylcholine as mediator of parasympathetic
    nervous system, 459
Acid, 156
  carbonic, 157, 158
  fixed, 157
  noncarbonic, 157
  nonvolatile, 157

Acid—cont'd
  production of, 157
  volatile, 157
Acid-base balance, 156-160
  normal, mechanisms of, 157-159
  potassium in, 138
  role of buffers in control of, 159-160
Acid-base imbalances
  metabolic, 160-161
  respiratory, 160
Acidosis, 139, 157, 162
  lactic, and anion gap, 171
  metabolic; *see* Metabolic acidosis
  respiratory
    clinical signs of, 164
    treatment of, 165
ACTH; *see* Adrenocorticotropin
Actin in muscle cells, 133, 134
Action current, 275
Action potential, 128-131
  phases of, 129-130
  threshold for, 277
Activase; *see* Recombinant tissue plasminogen
    activator
Activation, ventricular, normal, 356-357
Active transport, 122-123
Activity, electrical, "fast-channel," 125
Adaptation syndrome
  general, 236
  local, 236
Adenosine triphosphate and contraction,
    136
Adrenocorticotropin and aldosterone, 111
Adult respiratory distress syndrome, 78
Adventitious sounds, 81-82
AEG; *see* Atrial electrogram
Aerobic exercise, 260-261
Afterload, 379

Airway pressure, continuous positive, for pulmonary edema, 383
Airway resistance, 76
Airways
  compression of, 164
  conducting, 72, 77
  obstruction of, 163
  respiratory, 72-73
Alarm reaction, 237-239
Albumin
  and edema formation, 120
  25%, for heart failure, 482-483, 484
Alcohol consumption and HDL, 244
Aldactone; see Spironolactone
Aldosterone
  adrenocorticotropin and, 111
  and congestive heart failure, 117
  effect of pressoreceptors on, 111
  and hypokalemia, 139
  renin-angiotensin mechanism and, 111
  secretion of, 111-112, 113
  and stress response, 239
Alkalosis, 139, 157, 162
  and hypocalcemia, 148
  metabolic, 160-161, 169-170
  respiratory, 160, 165-167
Alpha-adrenergic agents, 460-461, 462
Alpha lipoproteins, 243
Alpha receptors, 460
Alveolar-arterial oxygen difference, 67
Alveolar-capillary membrane, diffusion and, 73-74
Alveolar oxygen tension, 67
Alveolar sounds, 81
Alveoli, 73
Aminophylline for pulmonary edema, 384
Amiodarone hydrochloride
  as antiarrhythmic, 443, 455-456
    nursing orders for patient taking, 456-457
    side effects of, 456-457
  for cardiomyopathies, 639
  for malignant ventricular arrhythmias, 619, 620
  and torsades de pointes, 624
  for WPW syndrome, 634-635
Amrinone lactate for heart failure, 494-495
Anaerobic metabolism, 422
Anatomy and physiology, 5-27
Anemia, 85
Aneurysms, radionuclide angiography to detect, 220

Angina, 178-179, 497-499
  causes of, 179-180
  characteristic symptoms of, 180
  crescendo, 499
  differential diagnosis of, 182
  drugs for, 496-515
  effort or exertional, 178, 499
  mixed, 178
  rest, 178
  and stress testing, 257
  structural, coronary artery changes in, 208
  therapy for, 498
  unstable, 179, 499
Angiography, 204, 206-207, 219
  radionuclide, 218-222
    exercise, 221
    first-pass, 222-223
    nursing orders for, 223
Angioplasty, coronary, percutaneous transluminal, 209-212
Angiotensin I, 111
Angiotensin II, 111
Angiotensin converting enzyme inhibitors, 490
Anion, 103
  in extracellular fluid, 103
  in intracellular fluid, 103
  major roles of, 104
Anion gap, 105, 170-172
Anterior descending branch of left coronary artery, 22, 23
Anterior hemiblock, left, 356, 363-366
Anterior portion of left ventricle, 18
Anterior wall injury, 19
Anterior wall myocardial infarction, 45, 227
  and bundle branch blocks and hemiblocks, 371-372
  extensive, 192
Anteroseptal wall myocardial infarction, 193
Anterosuperior division of left bundle branch, 16
Anterosuperior fascicular ectopy, 375-376
Antiarrhythmic drugs, 442-458
  arrhythmias caused by, 620
  Class I, 442-443, 444-454
  Class IA, 444-449
    for malignant ventricular arrhythmias, 618-619
  Class IB, 449-453
    for malignant ventricular arrhythmias, 618-619

Fascicular blocks, 356, 371-372
Fascicular ectopy, 375-377
  anterosuperior, 375-376
  posterior, 376-377
"Fast cells," 125, 278-279
Fast-channel depolarization, 125
"Fast-channel electrical activity," 125
Fatty acids, free, 233
  metabolism of, 234
Femoral artery catheter, insertion of, 206
Fenoximone, 495
Felodipine, 510
$F_{I_{O_2}}$; see Fraction of inspired oxygen
Fiberoptics, 91-92
Fibers
  atrial conduction, 13
  Mahaim, 627, 628
  Purkinje, 16
Fibrillation
  atrial; see Atrial fibrillation
  ventricular; see Ventricular fibrillation
Fibrin degradation products, 524
Fibrin formation, 523-525
Fibrin split, 524
Fibrous pericardium, 6, 7
Filling phase, 394
Fine ventricular fibrillation, 296
Firing, repetitive, 34-35
First-degree AV block, 330-331
  summary of, 350
First-pass radionuclide angiography, 222-223
Fixed acids, 157
Fixed ratio second-degree AV block, 335-337
  summary of, 351
Flailed mitral valve; see Mitral valve, prolapse of
Flecainide acetate
  as antiarrhythmic, 443, 453-454
    nursing orders for patient taking, 454
  for malignant ventricular arrhythmias, 619
  for WPW syndrome, 634
Flipped LDH pattern, 187
Floppy mitral valve syndrome; see Mitral valve, prolapse of
Flow/pressure/resistance relationships, 392-393
Fluid
  capillary, movement of, 119-120
  extracellular, 102
  interstitial, 102
  intracellular, 102

Fluid—cont'd
  intravascular, 102
  and particles, definitions and distribution of, 102-103
  "third space," 102
Fluid and chemical balance, maintaining, 102-136
Fluid imbalances, 114-118
Fluid overload causing heart failure, 380
Flutter
  atrial; see Atrial flutter
  ventricular, 296
Forces, electrical, of heart
  normal, magnitude and direction of, 39-42
  recording, 35-46
Fraction of inspired oxygen, 66-67
Free fatty acids, 233
  metabolism of, 234
Frontal plane, 16-17
Functional disorders, general, 439
  pharmacological management of, 537
Furosemide for heart failure, 479-480, 484
Fusion beats, 300-303, 322, 323
  nursing orders for patient with, 303
  and pacemaker function, 583-584
  ventricular, 300-302
Fusion complexes, 628

G

Gain dial of oscilloscope, 51
Gallopamil, 510
Gallops, 410-413
  atrial, 411
  S_3, 411, 412
  S_4, 411-412
  ventricular, 411
Gated blood pool scans, 218-222
Gating, 219
General adaptation syndrome, 236
General functional disorders, 439
  pharmacological management of, 537
Glucose, 484
  as energy source, 234
Glucose-insulin-potassium (GIK) solution, 126-127
  for myocardial infarction, 235
Glycolysis, 238
Gravity and V/Q mismatch, 79

H

Heart
  auscultation of, 409-418
  cells of
    electrical properties of, 28-30
    polarized, 29
    properties of, 12
  damage to, 6
  electrical activity of, 11-12
    relationship of, to mechanical activity, 12
  electrical forces of, normal magnitude and
      direction of, 39-42
  electrical properties of, 267
  electrical structures of, 12-16
  mechanical activity of, 9-11
    relationship of electrical activity to, 12
  mechanical structures of, 6-9, 392
  monitoring of; see Cardiac monitoring
  pacemaker of, 12, 13, 14, 15
  planes of, 16-18
  position of, in chest, 18-19
  primary function of, 5
  sides of, function of, 8
  valves of; see Valves of heart
  wall of, 6, 7
Heart block; see Block
Heart failure, 6, 378-391, 395
  congestive; see Congestive heart failure
  drug therapy for, 477-495
  left ventricular, edema formation and,
      120-121
  management of, 390
  from myocardial infarction, 378-379
    management of, 388-389
  nursing orders for patient with, 390-391
Heart rate, 5
  increases in, 6
  maximal, 249-250
  and stress testing, 256-257
Heart sounds, 10, 409-410
  normal variations in, 414-416
Hematocrit, 85
Hemiblocks, 356, 360-370
  clinical significance of, for nurses, 370-373
  ECG diagnosis of, 363
  left anterior, 356, 363-367
  left posterior, 356, 366-370
Hemodynamic changes in acute myocardial
    infarction, 393-397

Hemodynamic monitoring, 391-409
  nursing orders for patient during,
      407-409
Hemodynamics, 391
Hemoglobin level and oxygen saturation, 85
Hemoglobin-oxygen binding, factors altering, 87,
    95
Heparin sodium
  as antifibrin agent, 527-528
  as antithrombotic agent, 525
  and cardiac catheterization, 211
Hering-Breuer reflex, 75
High-density lipoproteins, 243, 244
  ratio of, to low-density lipoproteins, 243
His, bundle of, 14
His-Purkinje network, 15-16
His-Purkinje system and automaticity, 28, 29
History and diagnosis of myocardial infarction,
    181, 183-184
Holter monitoring, 46, 225-226
  to evaluate antiarrhythmic therapy, 618
Homeostasis, 105
Homeostatic mechanisms
  at cellular level, 105-109
  at systemic level, 109-114
Horizontal plane, 17
Hormonal regulation of calcium, 147
Hormone, antidiuretic; see Antidiuretic hormone
Human response patterns of unitary person, 7
Hydralazine for heart failure, 490-491
Hydrochlorothiazide, 484
Hydrocortisone for shock, 496
Hydrogen ion concentration, changes in,
    156-157
HydroDiuril; see Hydrochlorothiazide
Hygroton; see Chlorthalidone
Hyperacute T wave changes, 189
Hypercalcemia, 151-153
  ECG evidence of, 152
  signs and symptoms of, 151, 152
  summary of, 153
  therapy for, 153
Hyperglycemia from GIK solution, 235
Hyperkalemia, 143-146
  causes of, 143
  ECG evidence of, 144, 145
  from GIK solution, 235
  summary of, 146
  therapy for, 144
Hyperlipidemia, 242, 245-246

Inotropic agents for heart failure, 491-495
  nursing orders for patients taking, 495
Inspection in lung examination, 80
Inspiration, 74-75
Inspired oxygen, fraction of, 66-67
Insulin in FFA metabolism, 234
Interatrial tract, 14
Interference artifact, 60-cycle, 51-52
Intermittent positive pressure ventilation for
      pulmonary edema, 383
Internal respiration, 72
Internodal tracts, 13-14
Interpolated PVC, 293
Interstitial fluid, 102
  excess of, 119
Interstitial fluid colloid osmotic pressure and
      edema, 120
Interstitial fluid pressure, negative, 120
Interstitial fluid spaces, 73-74
Interstitial pulmonary edema, 381
Intraaortic balloon, nursing orders for patient
      with, 433-434
Intraaortic balloon catheter, 426
Intraaortic balloon pump, 426-428
Intraaortic balloon pumping, 426-434
  patient assessment/problem solving in, 431-432
  timing in, 429-431
Intracavitary lead, 46
Intracellular fluid, 102
  anions in, 103
  cations in, 103
Intravascular fluid, 102
Intraventricular conduction disturbances,
      355-377
Intropin; see Dopamine hydrochloride
Intubation, oxygen administration to patient
      without, 70-71
Ionized calcium, 147
Ions, 102-103
Ischemia
  coronary, effects of, 233-236
  in myocardial infarction, 189-190, 191
  radionuclide angiography to detect, 220
Ischemic myocardium, preservation of, 515-519
Isoenzymes, 185-188
Isoproterenol
  for bifascicular block, 372
  for bradyarrhythmias, 476-477
  and cardiogenic shock, 423
  to increase heart rate, 624

Isoptin; see Verapamil
Isordil; see Isosorbide dinitrate
Isorhythmic AV dissociation, 340
Isosorbide dinitrate
    for chest pain, 501-504
        nursing orders for patient with, 504
    for heart failure, 489, 491
Isotonic solutions, 106, 108-109
Isotopes, 213

J

J joint, 33-34
James bundle of Lown-Ganong-Levine
        syndrome, 627, 628, 629
Judkins technique of cardiac catheterization, 206
Junctional arrhythmias, 312-315
    nursing orders for patient with, 314-315
Junctional contractions, premature, 313
    summary of, 350
Junctional rhythm, 313
    accelerated, 314
    summary of, 351
Junctional tachycardia, 313
    summary of, 350
Junctional tissue, AV, 14-15
    and automaticity, 28

K

Kabbinase; see Streptokinase
Kaochlor Preps, 142
Kaon-Cl, 142
Kay Ciel, 142
Kent bundle of WPW syndrome, 627, 628, 629,
        630, 632, 635
Kerley's B lines, 121
Ketoacidosis, 167
Killip classification of heart failure, 389-390
K-Lyte/Cl, 142
Kussmaul's respirations, 168

L

L tubules, 133-134
Labetalol for chest pain, 505-508
Lactated Ringer's solution, 109
Lactic acidosis and anion gap, 171
Lactic dehydrogenase, 184, 185
    isoenzymes of, 185-186, 187
Lactic dehydrogenase pattern, flipped, 187
Lanoxin; see Digitalis
Lasix; see Furosemide

Magnesium sulfate for torsades de pointes, 625
Mahaim fibers, 627, 628
Mahaim syndrome, 626, 627
Malignant ventricular arrhythmias, 617-626
    treatment of, 618-620
Mannitol
    for heart failure, 481-482, 484
    for shock, 496
Manual resuscitators for oxygen administration,
        71
Maslow's framework and patient responses to
        illness, 1
Maximal heart rate, 249-250
MCL leads, 48-49
Mechanical activity of heart, 9-11
    relationship of electrical activity to, 12
Mechanical complications in coronary artery
        disease, 378-435
Mechanical resuscitation, 71
Mechanical structures of heart, 6-9
Membrane, alveolar-capillary, diffusion and,
        73-74
Membrane potential, resting, 276, 277, 278, 279
Meperidine for chest pain, 501
MET, 259
Metabolic acid-base imbalances, 160-161
Metabolic acidosis, 160-161, 167-168
    causes of, 167, 171, 172
    clinical signs of, 168
    role of anion gap in assessing, 170-172
    and shock, 422
    therapy for, 168
Metabolic alkalosis, 160-161, 169-170
    causes of, 169
    clinical signs of, 169
    therapy for, 170
Metabolic assessment, 233-236
Metabolic changes, drug therapy to reverse,
        515-529
Metabolism, 233
    anaerobic, 422
Metaraminol bitartrate for supraventricular
        tachyarrhythmias, 474-475
Metoprolol for chest pain, 505-508
Mexiletine hydrochloride
    as antiarrhythmic, 443, 449-451
        nursing orders for patient taking, 451-452
        side effects of, 450-451
    for malignant ventricular arrhythmias, 619
    for torsades de pointes, 625

Mexitil; see Mexiletine hydrochloride
Microcircuits for reentry, 280-281
Milrinone, 495
Minipress; see Prazosin hydrochloride
Minute ventilation, 76
Mitral click-murmur syndrome; see Mitral valve,
        prolapse of
Mitral regurgitation, 642
Mitral valve, 8, 9
    prolapse of, 639-645
Mixed angina, 178
M-mode echocardiography, 225
Mobitz I block, 331-333, 336
    summary of, 351
Mobitz II block, 333-335, 336, 370, 371
    summary of, 351
Modified committed pacing, 591-594
Monitor in fiberoptics, 93, 94
Monitoring
    cardiac
        components of, 46
        lead concepts applied to, 46-51
    of cardiac output, 405-406
    hemodynamic, 391-409
        nursing orders for patient with,
            407-409
    Holter, 46, 225-226
        to evaluate antiarrhythmic therapy, 618
    of pressure pulse patterns, 402-405
    of pressures, 397-402
    of pulmonary vascular resistance, 406-407
    of systemic vascular resistance, 406-407
    of venous oxygen saturation at bedside,
        continuous, 91-98
Monitoring systems
    three-electrode, 47-49
    two-electrode, 47
Monofascicular block, 334, 335, 336, 370
Monophasic QRS patterns, 321
Morphine
    for chest pain, 500-501
    and venous return, 383
Motion mode echocardiography, 225
Movement and muscle activity artifact, 52
Multifocal PVCs, 290
Multilead assessment of arrhythmias,
        342-345
Multistage exercise stress tests, 253
Mural thrombi, 521, 522
Murmurs, 413-414

Pulmonary oxygen transport, factors interfering
with, 95
Pulmonary valve, 8, 9
Pulmonary vascular resistance, monitoring of,
406-407
Pulse generator
of AICD system, 551-552
for dual chamber pacing, 573-574
for single chamber pacing, 567-571
Pulse interval, problems with, 599-600, 601
Pump, intraaortic balloon, 426-428
Purkinje fibers, 16

Q

Q wave, 31
abnormal, in myocardial infarction, 189,
190
QRS complex, 31, 32, 39
in aberrant conduction, 320
completely negative, 31
and hyperkalemia, 144, 145
in lead aV_R, 41
in sinus rhythm, 55-56
and ventricular impulses, 284
QRS-inhibited AV sequential bifocal pacemaker,
590-591
QRS-inhibited ventricular pacemaker, 581-583
QRS patterns, monophasic or biphasic, 321
QS complex, 31
QT interval, 33
and hypocalcemia, 151
and torsades de pointes, 621-622
Questran; *see* Cholestyramine
"Quinidine effect," 446, 624
Quinidine sulfate
for arrhythmias, 349-351, 442, 444-447
for atrial fibrillation, 633, 634
for malignant ventricular arrhythmias, 619
nursing orders for patient receiving, 448-449
side effects of, 447-448
for supraventricular tachyarrhythmias, 464
for torsades de pointes, 624
Quinidine syncope, 447

R

"R on T" phenomenon, 622
R wave, 31
in myocardial infarction, 189
"Rabbit ear" phenomenon, 317, 325
Radioactive cell tracers, 214

Radionuclide angiography, 218-222
exercise, 221
first-pass, 222-223
nursing orders for patient undergoing, 223
Radionuclide studies
to diagnose myocardial infarction, 213-223
to diagnose right ventricular infarction, 387
Radionuclides, 213, 219
Rales, 81, 82, 382
Rapid filling phase, 394
Rate meter of oscilloscope, 51
Rate pressure product, 248-249
RBC phosphate and hemoglobin-oxygen
binding, 87-88
Reaction, alarm, 237-239
Rebreathing mask, partial, for oxygen
administration, 70
Receptors, 109
Reciprocating tachycardia, 631-632
Recombinant tissue plasminogen activator as
antithrombotic agent, 529, 532
Recording
of electrical forces, 35-46
of surface information, 44-46
Recycling in AICD, 554
Reentry, 280
and arrhythmias, 280-283, 629-631
conditions required for, 280
Reentry circuit, 281
Reflection spectrophotometry, 92-93
Reflex
Bainbridge, 288
Hering-Breuer, 75
Refractory period of ECG, 34-35
absolute, 34
Regurgitation, mitral, 642
Renal failure
chronic, and hypocalcemia, 148
and hyperkalemia, 143
metabolic acidosis in, 167
Renin, 111
Renin-angiotensin mechanism and aldosterone,
111
Repetitive firing, 34-35
Repolarization, 125
atrial, 31
and hypokalemia, 141
role of electrolytes in, summary of, 126
ventricular, 31
Repolarization syndrome, delayed, 621

Resistance, 392-393
   airway, 76
   and pressure and flow relationships, 392-393
   vascular; *see* Vascular resistance
Respiration
   control centers for, 74-75
   external, 71-72
   internal, 72
   Kussmaul's, 168
   stimulus for, 74-75
Respiratory acid-base imbalances, 160
Respiratory acidosis, 160, 162-165
   clinical signs of, 164
   treatment of, 165
Respiratory airways, 72-73
Respiratory artifact, 54
Respiratory alkalosis, 160, 165-167
   clinical signs of, 166
   treatment of, 167
Respiratory centers, suppression of, 162-163
Respiratory distress syndrome, adult, 78
Respiratory failure, 80
Respiratory response to hypoxia, 64
Response
   chain reaction, 34-35
      and reentry, 282
   to critical illness, patient, 1
Rest angina, 178
Resting membrane potential, 276, 277, 278, 279
Resting potential, 128
Restrictive cardiomyopathy, 636, 638
   treatment of, 638-639
Resuscitators
   manual, for oxygen administration, 71
   mechanical, 71
Retrograde atrial depolarization, 312
Reverse function pacemakers, 576-577
Rheomacrodex; *see* Dextran 40
Rhonchus, 82
Rhythm
   idiojunctional, 313, 337
   idioventricular; *see* Idioventricular rhythm
   junctional, 313
      accelerated, 314
      summary of, 351
   sinus, 54
      diagnosis of, 54-60
Right to left shunting, 78
Ringer's solution, lactated, 109
r-p interval, 631

Rule, second-in-a-group, 318-319
Runaway pacemaker, 601
Rytmonorm; *see* Propafenone

S

S wave, 31
S_1, 10, 341-342, 409
   variations in, 415
S_2, 10, 410
   splitting of, 416
S_3 gallop, 411
S_4 gallop, 411-412
SA node; *see* Sinoatrial node
Safety pacing, 594
Sagittal plane, 17
Saline, normal, 109
Saturation, oxygen; *see* Oxygen saturation
Scan, 214
   gated blood pool, 218-222
   thallium-201, 215
Scanning by pacemaker, 613
Scintigraphic image, 213
Scintillations, 213
Sclerosis causing LBBB, 357
Second-degree AV block, 331-335
   fixed ratio, 335-337
   summary of, 350-351
Second-in-a-group rule, 318-319
Secretion, aldosterone, 111-112
Sectral; *see* Acebutolol
Semilunar valves, 8-9
Sensing, problems related to, and ECG
      assessment, 605-607
Sensorium changes
   from hypoxia, 63
   from metabolic acidosis, 168
   from shock, 421
Sepsis, 95
Septal branches of right coronary artery, 21
Septal depolarization, 43-44
Septum, 7
Serum; *see also* Plasma
Serum colloid osmotic pressure and edema, 120
Serum electrolyte tests, routine, 104-105
Serum enzymes to diagnose myocardial
      infarction, 181, 184-188
Serum glutamic oxaloacetic transaminase, 184-185
Serum pH, 156-157
SGOT; *see* Serum glutamic oxaloacetic
      transaminase

Shock, 64, 396, 418, 420
  cardiogenic, 419-420, 423-425
    therapy for, 424
  drug therapy for, 495-496
  hypovolemic, 419
  intervention in, 435
  nursing orders for patient in, 425-426
  stages of, 421-422
  therapy for, 422-423
  vasogenic, 419
Shock syndrome, 418-426
Shunt
  capillary, 78
  incomplete, 78-79
Shunt effect, 78-79
Shunting of blood, 78
  right to left, 78
Single chamber pacing, 559, 562-571
  pulse generator for, 567-571
  nursing orders for patient during, 564-565
Single chamber pacemaker
  arrhythmias caused by, 607
  ECG assessment using, 581-584, 599-609, 610
Sinoatrial block, 328-329
  summary of, 351
Sinoatrial node, 12-14
  and automaticity, 28, 29
  function of, disturbances in, 285-289
Sinus
  coronary, 24, 25
  of Valsalva, 20
Sinus arrest, 328-329
Sinus arrhythmias, 288
Sinus bradycardia, 13, 55, 286-287, 328
  nursing orders for patient with, 287
Sinus rhythm, 54
  diagnosis of, 54-60
Sinus tachycardia, 13, 55, 285-286
  nursing orders for patient with, 286
Six-lead electrocardiogram, 41-42
Skeletal muscle depression, signs of, 151-152
"Slow cell," 278-279
Slow-channel depolarization, 125
Slow-K, 142
Smoking and coronary artery disease, 241-242
Smooth muscle depression, signs of, 151-152
Sodium (Na^+), 103
  and congestive heart failure, 117
  conservation of, 115-116

Sodium (Na^+)—cont'd
  role of
    in conduction disturbances, 278-279
    in disturbances in automaticity, 274-278
  routine tests to measure, 104-105
Sodium bicarbonate for metabolic acidosis, 168
Sodium methohexital before countershock, 549
Sodium nitroprusside
  cyanide poisoning from, 96
  for heart failure, 486-488, 491
Solu-Cortef; see Hydrocortisone
Solution
  glucose-insulin-potassium (GIK), 126-127
  hypertonic, 106-107, 108
  hypotonic, 106-107, 108, 109
  isotonic, 106, 108-109
  polarizing, 126-127, 235
  Ringer's, lactated, 109
Sones technique of cardiac catheterization, 206
Sotacor; see Sotalol
Sotalol, 455, 505
Sounds
  adventitious, 81-82
  alveolar, 81
  breath, 81-83
    abnormal, 382
    decreased, 81, 82-83
    increased, 83
  bronchial, 81, 83
  heart, 10, 409-410
  vesicular, 81
Spectrophotometry, reflection, 92-93
Spironolactone, 484
Splitting of S_2, 416
Spontaneous diastolic depolarization, 275-277
ST segment, 33-34
  depression of, and cardiovascular decompensation, 254-255
  elevation of, in transmural myocardial infarction, 189, 191
  and hypocalcemia, 150-151
Starling's law, 401
Stimulation of antidiuretic hormone, 113
Stimulus artifact and pacemaker function, 578-579
Stimulus release, problems related to, and ECG assessment, 599-602
Stimulus response (capture), problems related to, and ECG assessment, 602-605

Torsades de pointes, 447, 621-626
Total cholesterol level, 243
Total oxygen content of blood, 84-85
Toxicity, digitalis, 469-471
Tracheotomy, oxygen administration to patient
    without, 70-71
Tract
  interatrial, 14
  internodal, 13-14
Trandate; *see* Labetolol
Transducer, 224
Transmural myocardial infarction, 7, 188,
    189
Transport, active, 122-123
Transverse tubules, 134, 135
Treadmill exercise stress testing, 246-247,
    251-259
Triamterene, 484
Tricuspid valve, 8, 9
Tricyclic antidepressants and exercise stress
    testing, 252
Trifascicular block, 334, 356, 371, 372
Trigeminy, atrial, 306
Triggered pacemaker, 576
Triglycerides, 233
  and coronary artery disease, 243, 244, 245
Trousseau sign, positive, 149
TU wave fusion in hypokalemia, 141, 142
Tubules
  longitudinal, 133-134
  transverse, 134, 135
Twelve-lead electrocardiogram, 49
Two-dimensional echocardiography, 225

U

U wave and hypokalemia, 141, 142
Undersensing, problems related to, and ECG
    assessment, 605-607
Unidirectional block, 282
Unifocal PVCs, 289
Unipolar atrial electrogram, 346-347
Unipolar catheters for pacemakers, 561-562
Unipolar leads, 37-38
  for surface recording, 48-49
Universal pacing, 594-599
Unstable angina, 179, 499
Urine osmolality test, 116
Urokinase as antithrombotic agent, 525, 529,
    533

V

V leads, 42
V wave
  on atrial electrograms, 345, 346, 347, 348
  in PA and wedge tracing, 405
Vagomimetic drugs, 463-464
Valium; *see* Diazepam
Valsalva, sinuses of, 20
Valves of heart, 8-9, 25
  aortic, 9
  atrioventricular, 8
  mitral, 8, 9
    prolapse of, 639-645
  pulmonary, 8, 9
  semilunar, 8-9
  tricuspid, 8, 9
Vascular resistance
  pulmonary, monitoring of, 406-407
  systemic
    monitoring of, 406-407
    rise in, 395
Vasoactive role of calcium, 131-136
Vasoconstrictor, 111
Vasodilators
  for cardiogenic shock, 424
  for heart failure, 484-491
    nursing orders for patient receiving, 489
  for pulmonary edema, 383
Vasogenic shock, 419
Vasopressors for supraventricular
    tachyarrhythmias, 474-475
Vasotec; *see* Enalapril
VAT pacemakers, 594-599
Vector(s), 39
  summation, 39
Veins, coronary, 24, 25
Venous oxygen content, 91
Venous oxygen saturation, 89
  continuous monitoring of, at bedside, 91-98
  fall in, factors causing, 94-95
  monitoring of, nursing orders for patient
    during, 97-98
  normal, 86
  and oxygen extraction, 90-91
  rise in, factors causing, 95-96
Venous thrombi, 521
Ventilation
  impaired, causes of, 162-163

ALSO AVAILABLE!

TECHNIQUES IN BEDSIDE HEMODYNAMIC MONITORING, 4th Edition
by Elaine Kiess Daily, R.N., B.S., R.C.V.T.; John Speer Schroeder, M.D.

This new edition includes new and expanded content, new chapters, and new waveforms and exercises to provide the most current and accurate information available. Its step-by-step approach is useful for both students and practitioners.

- Includes new chapters: Clinical Management Based on Hemodynamic Parameters; Vascular Access; Continuous Monitoring of Oxygenation.
- Provides expanded coverage of cardiac output measurements.
- Gives principles and techniques for continuously monitoring Sv_{O2}.
- Gives clear, concise troubleshooting tables in an easily accessible format.

POCKET GUIDE TO CRITICAL CARE ASSESSMENT
by Laura A. Talbot, R.N., C., M.S.; Mary Meyers Marquardt, R.N., B.S.N., CCRN.

This portable, practical assessment tool is designed for quick access to pertinent information at the bedside. Organized by body systems and using an outline format, this guide presents detailed information on critical care assessment, including history taking, physical examination, and diagnostic studies.

- Presents detailed assessment guidelines related to specific diagnostic procedures and disease entities.
- Provides information on bedside monitoring, including quick-reference tables on respirator settings, blood gas determination, ECG interpretation, assessing patient monitoring systems, and diagnostic studies.
- Includes special considerations for the older adult.

UNDERSTANDING ELECTROCARDIOGRAPHY: Arrhythmias and the 12-Lead ECG, 5th Edition
by Mary Boudreau Conover, R.N., B.S.

One of the best known and highly respected texts available on electrocardiography, UNDERSTANDING ELECTROCARDIOGRAPHY: Arrhythmias and the 12-Lead ECG, 5th Edition, completely surveys the heart, heart electrophysiology, arrhythmia genesis, types and classifications of arrhythmias, interpretation of ECG tracings, electrical safety, pacemakers, and arrhythmic drugs.

MANUAL OF CRITICAL CARE: Applying Nursing Diagnoses to Adult Critical Illness
by Pamela L. Swearingen, R.N.; Marilyn Sawyer Sommers, R.N., M.A., CCRN; Kenneth Miller, R.N., Ph.D., CCRN.

MANUAL OF CRITICAL CARE: Applying Nursing Diagnoses to Adult Critical Illness is a unique care planning guide that applies nursing diagnoses to specific critical care disorders.

- Applies NANDA-approved nursing diagnoses to more than 70 specific critical care dysfunctions.
- Includes for each dysfunction: pathophysiology, assessment, diagnostic tests/medical management, nursing diagnoses, desired outcomes, nursing interventions, rehabilitation, and patient-family teaching.
- Includes a detailed index and 60 original tables related to drug administration, assessment, dietary guidelines, pathophysiology, metric conversions for Canadian nurses, and hemodynamic guidelines.

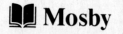 **Mosby**

Experience Mosby's tradition of excellence in critical and cardiac care.
To order, ask your bookstore manager or call toll-free 800-221-7700, ext. 15A.
We hope to hear from you soon!